Symptom Oriented Pain Management

Symptom Oriented Pain Management

Second Edition

Editors

Dwarkadas K Baheti MD
Consultant Anesthesiologist and Pain Physician
Bombay, Lilavati, Shushrusha, and Raheja Hospitals
Mumbai, Maharashtra, India

Sanjay Bakshi MD
President
Manhattan Spine and Pain Medicine
New York, New York, United States

Sanjeeva Gupta MBBS MD DNB FRCA FIPP FFPMRCA
Consultant in Pain Medicine
Bradford Teaching Hospitals NHS Foundation Trust
Spire Leeds Hospital
Nuffield Hospital Leeds
United Kingdom

Raghbir Singh P Gehdoo MD DA
Professor
Department of Anesthesia
Tata Memorial Hospital
Mumbai, Maharashtra, India

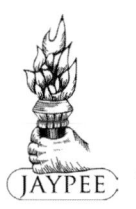

JAYPEE *The Health Sciences Publishers*

New Delhi | London | Panama

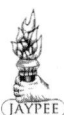 **Jaypee Brothers Medical Publishers (P) Ltd**

Headquarters

Jaypee Brothers Medical Publishers (P) Ltd
4838/24, Ansari Road, Daryaganj
New Delhi 110 002, India
Phone: +91-11-43574357
Fax: +91-11-43574314
Email: jaypee@jaypeebrothers.com

Overseas Offices

J.P. Medical Ltd
83 Victoria Street, London
SW1H 0HW (UK)
Phone: +44 20 3170 8910
Fax: +44 (0)20 3008 6180
Email: info@jpmedpub.com

Jaypee-Highlights Medical Publishers Inc
City of Knowledge, Bld. 237, Clayton
Panama City, Panama
Phone: +1 507-301-0496
Fax: +1 507-301-0499
Email: cservice@jphmedical.com

Jaypee Brothers Medical Publishers (P) Ltd
17/1-B Babar Road, Block-B, Shaymali
Mohammadpur, Dhaka-1207
Bangladesh
Mobile: +08801912003485
Email: jaypeedhaka@gmail.com

Jaypee Brothers Medical Publishers (P) Ltd
Bhotahity, Kathmandu, Nepal
Phone: +977-9741283608
Email: kathmandu@jaypeebrothers.com

Website: www.jaypeebrothers.com
Website: www.jaypeedigital.com

© 2017, Jaypee Brothers Medical Publishers

The views and opinions expressed in this book are solely those of the original contributor(s)/author(s) and do not necessarily represent those of editor(s) of the book.

All rights reserved. No part of this publication may be reproduced, stored or transmitted in any form or by any means, electronic, mechanical, photocopying, recording or otherwise, without the prior permission in writing of the publishers.

All brand names and product names used in this book are trade names, service marks, trademarks or registered trademarks of their respective owners. The publisher is not associated with any product or vendor mentioned in this book.

Medical knowledge and practice change constantly. This book is designed to provide accurate, authoritative information about the subject matter in question. However, readers are advised to check the most current information available on procedures included and check information from the manufacturer of each product to be administered, to verify the recommended dose, formula, method and duration of administration, adverse effects and contraindications. It is the responsibility of the practitioner to take all appropriate safety precautions. Neither the publisher nor the author(s)/editor(s) assume any liability for any injury and/or damage to persons or property arising from or related to use of material in this book.

This book is sold on the understanding that the publisher is not engaged in providing professional medical services. If such advice or services are required, the services of a competent medical professional should be sought.

Every effort has been made where necessary to contact holders of copyright to obtain permission to reproduce copyright material. If any have been inadvertently overlooked, the publisher will be pleased to make the necessary arrangements at the first opportunity.

Inquiries for bulk sales may be solicited at: jaypee@jaypeebrothers.com

Symptom Oriented Pain Management / Dwarkadas K Baheti, Sanjay Bakshi, Sanjeeva Gupta, Raghbir Singh P Gehdoo

First Edition: 2012

Second Edition: **2017**

ISBN: 978-93-86322-48-7

Printed at Sanat Printers

Dedicated to

Chronic Pain Patients

CONTRIBUTORS

EDITORS

Dwarkadas K Baheti MD
Consultant Anesthesiologist and Pain Physician
Bombay, Lilavati, Shushrusha, and
Raheja Hospitals
Mumbai, Maharashtra, India

Sanjay Bakshi MD
President
Manhattan Spine and Pain Medicine
New York, New York, United States

Sanjeeva Gupta MBBS MD DNB FRCA FIPP FFPMRCA
Consultant in Pain Medicine
Bradford Teaching Hospitals NHS Foundation Trust
Spire Leeds Hospital, Nuffield Hospital Leeds
United Kingdom

Raghbir Singh P Gehdoo MD DA
Professor
Department of Anesthesia
Tata Memorial Hospital
Mumbai, Maharashtra, India

CONTRIBUTING AUTHORS

Steve M Aydin DO
Clinical Assistant Professor
Department of Physical Medicine and
Rehabilitation
Hofstra Northwell School of Medicine
Manhattan Spine and Pain Medicine
Manhasset, New York, United States
Email id: steve.aydin@gmail.com

Neeraj D Baheti PT DPT OCS SCS CSCS
Senior Physical Therapist
Department of Sports Medicine Center for
Young Athletes, UCSF Benioff Children's Hospitals
Walnut Creek, California, United States
Email id: Nbaheti76@yahoo.com

Ashish V Bakshi MD DM
Consultant, Department of Medical Oncology
Dr LH Hiranandani Hospital
Mumbai, Maharashtra, India
Email id: baashish@yahoo.com

Krishna A Balkundi DRM MNAMS
Director
Department of Nuclear Medicine
Lilavati Hospital
Mumbai, Maharashtra, India
Email id: drkrish_hinduja@rediffmail.com

Ganesan Baranidharan FRCA FFPMRCA
PG Dip Anesth.
Consultant and Clinical Associate Professor
Leeds Teaching Hospitals NHS Trust
University of Leeds
Leeds, United Kingdom
Email id: g.baranidharan@nhs.net

Sherdil Nath DRCOG FRCA
Chief of Service (Retd)
The Pain Clinic
Umeå, Sweden
Email id: sherdil@hotmail.com

Arun K Bhaskar MSc FRCA FFPMRCA FFICM FIPP
Consultant
Pain Management Centre
Charing Cross Hospital Imperial College Healthcare NHS Trust
London, United Kingdom
Email id: akbhaskar@btopenworld.com

Deepak Chabbra MS DNB MRCSEd
Consultant
Department of Surgical Oncology
Lilavati Hospital and Research Centre
Dr LH Hiranandani Hospital
Mumbai, Maharashtra, India
Email id: drdeepakchhabra@gmail.com

Muthusamy Chandramohan DMRD FRCR
Consultant
Department of Radiology
Bradford Teaching Hospitals NHS Foundation Trust
Bradford, West Yorkshire, United Kingdom
Email id: chandramohanm@hotmail.com

Anjali M Chhabria MD DPM
Director
Department of Psychiatry
Mindtemple
Mumbai, Maharashtra, India
Email id: anjali.chhabria@gmail.com

Joshua D Chrystal NMD DC
Compresive Spine and Sports Centre
San Jose, California, United States

Timothy Connolly MD
Resident
Department of Anesthesiology, Pain Medicine
Weill Cornell Medicine-New York Presbyterian Hospital
New York, New York, United States
Email id: tmc9010@nyp.org

Andrew R Cooper FFARCSI MD FIPP
Consultant
Pain Relief Clinic
Causeway Hospital
Coleraine, Northern Ireland, United Kingdom
Email id: arcooper@btinternet.com

Charles Daknis MD DABPM FABIIP
Spine and Pain Centers
New Jersey, United States
Email id: cdaknis@gmail.com

Samyadev Datta MD FRCA
Director
Center for Pain Management
Hackensack, New Jersey, United States
Email id: sdatta@centerforpain.net

Gerard DeGregoris III MD
Clinical Assistant Professor
Department of Anesthesiology
Hofstra Northwell School of Medicine
Attending Physician
Lenox Hill Hospital
New York, New York, United States
Email id: gdegregoris@manhattanspinepain.com

Nahush P Dilip MD
Chief Resident
Department of Neurology
Bombay Hospital Institute of Medical Sciences
Mumbai, Maharashtra, India
Email id: nahushpatil999@gmail.com

Vasumathi M Divekar BSc DA MD MNAS
Emeritus Professor
Department of Anesthesiology
Dr DY Patil Medical College
Mumbai, Maharashtra, India
Email id: divekarvas@yahoo.co.in

Sudhir Diwan MD
Attending Pain Medicine
Department of Anesthesiology
Lennox Hill Hospital
New York, New York, United States
Email id: Sdiwan63@gmail.com

Kritika M Doshi MD DA FIPP ISSP
In Charge-Pain Clinic
Department of Pain Clinic
Jupiter and Bethany Hospitals
Thane, Maharashtra, India
Email id: drkritikadoshi@gmail.com

Contributors

Preeti P Doshi MD FRCA FIPP
Consultant and In-charge
Department of Pain Management
Jaslok Hospital and Research Centre
Mumbai, Maharashtra, India
Email id: preetipd@gmail.com

Maulik S Doshi MD DM
Deputy General Manager
Department of India Clinical Research
Sun Pharma Laboratories Limited
Vadodara, Gujarat, India
Email id: maulik.doshi@sunpharma.com

Ramon Go MD
Fellow in Pain Medicine
Department of Anesthesiology, Pain Medicine
Weill Cornell Medicine-New York
Presbyterian Hospital
New York, New York, United States
Email id: rmg9014@nyp.org

Gerard Grahemsen MD
Physician Assistant
Department of Manhattan Spine and Pain Medicine
New York, New York, United States

Ashish Gulve FFPMCAI DPMed FCARCSI MD DNB
Consultant
Department of Pain Management
James Cook University Hospital
Middlesbrough, United Kingdom
Email id: ashishgulve@nhs.net

Shamim Haider MD FRCA FFPMRCA
Consultant
Department of Pain Medicine and Anesthesia
Colchester University Hospital NHS Trust
Colchester, United Kingdom
Email id: Dr.sh.haider@gmail.com

JD Hoppenfeld MD
Southeast Pain Care at Morehead,
Medical Plaza
Charlotte, North Carolina, United States
Email id: jhoppenfeld@hotmail.com

Abhinay M Huchche MD DM
Junior Consultant, Department of Neurology
Bombay Hospital Institute
Mumbai, Maharashtra, India
Email id: abhinayhuchche16@gmail.com

John Hughes FFPMRCA FRCA
Consultant, Department of Pain Management
James Cook University Hospital
Middlesbrough, United Kingdom
Email id: John.Hughes@stees.nhs.uk

PN Jain MD MNAMS FICA
Professor and Head
Department of Anesthesiology, Critical Care and Pain
Tata Memorial Centre
Mumbai, Maharashtra, India
Email id: pnj5@hotmail.com

Subhash Jain MD FIPP
Senior Attending Physician
Beth Israel Hospital
Medical Director
Institute for Pain and Palliative Care
New York, New York, United States
Email id: sjain@nycpain.com

Muralidhar Joshi MD DNB
Director
Pain Management Centre, Virinchi Hospitals
Hyderabad, Telangana, India
Email id: drmuralidharjoshi@gmail.com

Shirish Kataria DMRE
Consultant, Department of Radiology
Gurunanak Hospital
Mumbai, Maharashtra, India
Email id: shirishkataria@gmail.com

Jasmeen Kaur MD DNB
Senior Resident
Department of Anesthesiology, Critical Care and Pain
Tata Memorial Hospital
Mumbai, Maharashtra, India
Email id: drjasmeenkaur@gmail.com

Satish V Khadilkar MD DM DNBE FIAN FICP
Professor
Department of Neurology
Grant Medical College and Sir J J Group of Hospitals
Mumbai, Maharashtra, India
Email id: khadilkarsatish@gmail.com

Mansukhani A Khushnuma MBBS
Head
Department of Clinical Neurophysiology
Bombay Hospital and Medical Research Centre
Mumbai, Maharashtra, India
Email id: kilom@hotmail.com

Kailash M Kothari MD
Director
Department of Pain Management
Pain Clinic of India Pvt. Ltd.
Mumbai, Maharshtra, India
Email id: drkothari@yahoo.com

Makarand M Kulkarni MD
Consultant, Department of Radiology
Lilavati Hospital and Research Centre
Mumbai, Maharashtra, India
Email id: makarand_kul@yahoo.com

Kyriacos Kyriakides BSc MBChB FRCA FFPMRCOA
Consultant
Department of Anesthesia, Pain Management and Critical Care
Bradford Teaching Hospitals NHS Foundation Trust
Bradford, United Kingdom
Email id: Kyriacos.Kyriakides@bthft.nhs.uk

Thomas P Lione
Chief Resident, Department of Physical Medicine and Rehabilitation
Hofstra Northwell School of Medicine
Manhasset, New York, United States
Email id: tom.lione@gmail.com

Madhuri A Lokapur MD DA FIPP
Consultant
Department of Pain and Palliative Care
Jehangir Hospital
Pune, Maharashtra, India
Email id: madhulok@yahoo.com

Nilesh M Lokeshwar MD DM
Consultant
Department of Medical Oncology
Asian Institute of Oncology
Mumbai, Maharashtra, India
Email id: nileshlok@yahoo.com

Salil A Mehta MS DNB
Consultant
Department of Ophthalmology
Lilavati Hospital
Mumbai, Maharashtra, India
Email id: drsalilmehta@gmail.com

Neel Mehta MD
Medical Director of Pain Medicine
Department of Anesthesiology, Pain Medicine
Weill Cornell Medicine-New York Presbyterian Hospital
New York, New York, United States
Email id: nem9015@med.cornell.edu

Vivek Mehta FRCA MD FFPMRCA
Consultant and Director
Boyle's Department of Anesthesia and Pain Medicine
St Bartholomew's Hospital
London, United Kingdom
Email id: vivek.mehta@mac.com

Rob Naber PT OCS SCS ATC
President and CEO
Physiotherapy of Los Gatos
Los Gatos, California, United States
Email id: robnaber@ptoflosgatos.com

Yashwant L Nankar MD
Associate Professor
Department of Anesthesia and Pain Management
Bharati Hospital and Medical College
Pune, Maharashtra, India
Email id: dr.ylnankar@gmail.com

Annu Navani MD
Medical Director
Department of Degenerative Medicine
Comprehensive Spine and Sports Center
Campbell, California, United States
Email id: anavani@spineandsportsctr.com

Contributors

Selaiman Noori MD
Resident
Department of Anesthesiology,
Pain Medicine
Weill Cornell Medicine-New York Presbyterian Hospital
New York, New York, United States
Email id: sen9009@nyp.org

Vibhay Pareek MD
Fellow Resident
Department of Radiation Oncology
Jupiter Hospital
Thane, Maharashtra, India
Email id: vibhay@hotmail.com

Juhi J Parmar MSc
Clinical Psychologist
Department of Psychology
Mindtemple
Mumbai, Maharashtra, India

Pallavi B Patil DNB
Clinical Associate
Department of Nuclear Medicine
Lilavati Hospital
Mumbai, Maharashtra, India
Email id: pallavipatil.nm@gmail.com

Krishna Poddar MD FIPM
Director
Kolkata Pain Clinic
Senior Consultant
Department of Pain Management
Fortis Hospital and Bellevue Hospital
Kolkata, West Bengal, India
Email id: drpoddark@yahoo.co.in

Kavita Poply FRCA FCARCSI FFPMRCA
Pain Fellow
Boyle's Department of Anesthesia and Pain Medicine
St Bartholomew's Hospital
London, United Kingdom
Email id: kavitapoply@doctors.org.uk

K Ravishankar MD
Consultant-in-charge
The Headache and Migraine Clinics
Jaslok and Lilavati Hospitals
Mumbai, Maharashtra, India
Email id: dr.k.ravishankar@gmail.com

Saroj M Sanghavi DPT MIAP
Physiotherapist
Mumbai, Maharshtra, India
Email id: sarojsanghavi@hotmail.com

Dakshesh M Sanghavi PT MS DPT
Rehabilitation Coordinator and Administrator
Department of Physical Medicine and Rehabilitation, Jamaica Hospital Medical Center
Flushing Hospital Medical Center
New York, New York, United States
Email id: Dsanghav.flushing@jhmc.org

Manohar L Sharma MD MSc FFPMRCA
Clinical Director
Department of Pain Medicine
The Walton Centre for Neurology and Neurosurgery NHS Foundation Trust Liverpool,
England, United Kingdom
Email id: manoharpain@yahoo.co.uk

Anil K Sharma MD DABPM
Director of Pain Management
Monmouth Medical Center
Shrewsbury, New Jersey, United States
Email id: anilsharma1000@gmail.com

Harish K Shetty DPM MD
Consultant Psychiatrist
Dr L H Hiranandani Hospital
Mumbai, Maharashtra, India
Email id: harish139@yahoo.com

Shrradha V Sidhwani MA
Clinical Psychologist and REBT Practitioner
Department of Psychology
Mindtemple
Mumbai, Maharashtra, India

Madhu B Singla MD
Senior Resident, Department of Neurology
Bombay hospital
Mumbai, Maharashtra, India
Email id: madhusingla58@yahoo.com

Urmila M Thatte MD DNB PhD FAMS
Professor and Head
Department of Clinical Pharmacology
Seth Gordhandas Sunderdas Medical College
Mumbai, Maharashtra, India
Email id: urmilathatte@kem.edu

John A Titterington MBChB FRCA
Advanced Pain Trainee
Department of Anesthesia and Pain Medicine
Bradford Teaching Hospitals NHS Foundation Trust
Bradford, West Yorkshire, United Kingdom
Email id: john.titterington@bthft.nhs.uk

Surbhi C Trivedi MD DNB
Consultant Psychiatrist
Dr L H Hiranandani Hospital
Mumbai, Maharashtra, India
Email id: surbhit_21@yahoo.com

Lakshmi C Vas MD
Director
Ashirvad Institute for Pain Management and Research
Mumbai, Maharashtra, India
Email id: lakshmi@paincareindia.com

Sunil A Waghmare MD DMRE
Consultant
Department of Radiology
Om Sai Superspeciality Hospital Pvt Ltd
Mumbai, Maharashtra, India
Email id: prati.sunil@gmail.com

PREFACE TO THE SECOND EDITION

We are very delighted to present the second edition of our book titled "Symptom Oriented Pain Management", first published in 2012.

We are also basking in the glory of our earlier books titled "Interventional Pain Management – A Practical Approach" 2009, 2016; "Symptom Oriented Pain Management-2012"; and "World Clinic Anesthesia, Critical Care, & Pain: Pain Management-2012". We express our heartfelt gratitude to the readers for their tremendous response and many valuable comments and suggestions.

We have picked up one of the most important suggestion—the urgent need for a comprehensive and practical book about various types of pain and how to tackle them. Chronic pain as a complex symptom (now also a Disease) has a variety of facets which at times makes it difficult to manage.

Pain physicians often face the dilemma of how to reach to a correct diagnosis starting from a particular symptom such as backache, headache, neck pain, neuropathic pain, ischemic pain, or cancer pain. It is mandatory for pain physicians to understand and learn techniques to accurately diagnose the etiology and mechanisms of pain which facilitates appropriate management with pharmacotherapy and where-ever necessary with the right interventional procedure.

There are many books by eminent authors which provide excellent theoretical and other aspects of pain and its management. There was a need for a comprehensive book to help pain physicians reach a diagnosis to facilitate management with maximum pain relief. We always believed in bringing out quality book at affordable cost.

We have, through this book, sincerely attempted to help pain physicians reach a correct diagnosis and treat patients in a simplistic manner and aspire to achieve "total pain relief" for their patients.

We express our heartfelt gratitude to all contributors in this book for their invaluable support to make this herculean task easy.

Dwarkadas K Baheti
Sanjay Bakshi
Sanjeeva Gupta
Raghbir Singh P Gehdoo

PREFACE TO THE FIRST EDITION

We are very delighted to present our second book titled Symptom Oriented Pain Management.

We are basking in the glory of our first book titled "Interventional Pain Management - A Practical Approach". We express our heartfelt gratitude to the readers for their tremendous response and many valuable comments and suggestions.

We have picked up one of the most important suggestion about the urgent need of a comprehensive and practical book about various types of pain and how to tackle them. Chronic pain as a symptom (now also a disease) has a variety of facets which at times makes it difficult to manage.

Pain physicians often face dilemma of how to reach correct diagnosis of a particular symptom such as backache, headache, neck pain, neuropathic pain, ischemic pain and cancer pain.

It is mandatory for pain physician to learn techniques to accurately diagnose the etiology and mechanisms of pain which facilitates appropriate management with pharmacotherapy and where necessary the correct interventional procedure.

There are many books by eminent authors which provide excellent theoretical and other aspects of pain. There was a need for a comprehensive book to help pain physicians reach a diagnosis to facilitate management with maximum pain relief.

We have through this book sincerely attempted to help pain physicians to treat patients in simplistic manner and tips to reach a correct diagnosis and aspire to achieve "Total Pain Relief" for their patients.

We express our heartfelt gratitude to all contributors in this book for their invaluable support to make this herculean task easy.

Dwarkadas K Baheti
Sanjay Bakshi
Sanjeeva Gupta
Raghbir Singh P Gehdoo

CONTENTS

SECTION 1: BASICS

1. **Pain Management: A Historical Perspective** — 3
   Vasumathi M Divekar

2. **Acute Pain** — 6
   Gerard DeGregoris III

3. **Acute Turn to Chronic: Causes, Prevention, and Management** — 10
   Ramon Go, Neel Mehta

4. **Chronic Pain** — 19
   Neel Mehta, Timothy Connolly

5. **Interpretation of Blood Levels of Drugs Used in Chronic Pain Management** — 27
   Urmila M Thatte, Maulik S Doshi

SECTION 2: CLINICAL EXAMINATION AND EVALUATION

6. **Clinical Examination and Evaluation of Cervical Spine** — 43
   Vivek Mehta, Kavita Poply

7. **Clinical Examination and Evaluation of Lumbar Spine** — 52
   Steve M Aydin

SECTION 3: UNDERSTANDING IMAGING MODALITIES FOR PAIN PATIENT

8. **Interpretation of X-ray Spine** — 61
   Muthusamy Chandramohan

9. **Interpretation of Computer Tomography Scans for Interventional Pain Treatment Procedures** — 71
   Sunil A Waghmare

10. **Magnetic Resonance Imaging in Pain Management** — 83
    Makarand M Kulkarni

11. **Role of Electrodiagnosis in the Management of Neck and Back Pain** — 100
    Mansukhani A Khushnuma

12. **Bone Mineral Density: Interpretation, Treatment, and Prevention** — 109
    Shirish Kataria

SECTION 4: CERVICAL/NECK PAIN

13. **Headache: Causes and Treatment Modalities** — 123
    K Ravishankar

14. **Trigeminal Neuralgia: Causes and Treatment** — 132
    Manohar L Sharma

15. **Cervical Radiculopathy Pain and Its Management** — 146
    Ganesan Baranidharan

16. **Cervical Facet Joint Pain and Its Management** — 152
    Sherdil Nath

17. **Cervical Diskogenic Pain and Its Management** — 157
    Anil K Sharma

SECTION 5: LOW BACK PAIN

18. **Focal Back Pain and Its Management** — 163
    Sanjeeva Gupta, Shamim Haider, John A Titterington

19. **Lumbar Facet Joint Pain Syndrome** — 172
    Sanjay Bakshi, Gerard Grahemsen

20. **Lumbar Spinal Stenosis** — 180
    Steve M Aydin, Thomas P Lione

21. **Lumbar Diskogenic Back Pain** — 187
    Selaiman Noori, Sudhir Diwan, Neel Mehta

22. **Sacroiliac Joint Pain Syndrome and Its Management** — 198
    Andrew R Cooper

23. **Coccygodynia and Its Pain Management** — 204
    Yashwant L Nankar

24. **Piriformis and Iliopsoas Pain Syndromes and Its Pain Management** — 208
    Dwarkadas K Baheti

SECTION 6: UROGENITAL AND PELVIC PAIN

25. **Nonmalignant Urogenital Pain Management** — 217
    Ashish Gulve, John Hughes

26. **Chronic Nonmalignant Pelvic Pain** — 233
    Kyriacos Kyriakides

SECTION 7: CANCER PAIN

27. **Head and Neck Cancer Pain Management** — 241
    Manohar L Sharma

28.	**Breast Cancer: Pain and Its Management** *PN Jain*	248
29.	**Carcinoma Lung: Pain and Its Management** *Arun K Bhaskar*	252
30.	**Upper Abdominal Malignancy: Pain and Its Management** *Dwarkadas K Baheti*	264
31.	**Malignant Pelvic Pain and Its Management** *Subhash Jain*	270
32.	**Metastatic Bone Pain Management** *Raghbir Singh P Gehdoo, Jasmeen Kaur*	281

SECTION 8: NEUROPATHIC PAIN

33.	**Neuropathic Pain: Approach, Pathophysiology, and Management** *Satish V Khadilkar, Abhinay M Huchche, Nahush P Dilip, Madhu B Singla*	297

SECTION 9: ISCHEMIC PAIN

34.	**Peripheral Vascular Disease: Causes and Pain Management** *Kailash M Kothari*	309

SECTION 10: MYOFASCIAL PAIN

35.	**Management of Myofascial Pain** *Kritika M Doshi*	323
36.	**Fibromyalgia: Causes and Pain Management** *Muralidhar Joshi*	332

SECTION 11: SCAR PAIN

37.	**Post-herniorrhaphy Pain and Its Management** *Lakshmi C Vas*	341
38.	**Post-coronary Artery Bypass Grafting Scar Pain and Its Management** *Madhuri A Lokapur*	353

SECTION 12: CHALLENGING PAIN

39.	**Complex Regional Pain Syndrome: Where We Stand?** *Samyadev Datta*	359
40.	**Phantom Limb Pain: Causes and Pain Management** *JD Hoppenfeld*	372
41.	**Postherpetic Neuralgia: Causes and Pain Management** *Charles Daknis*	377

42. Post-laminectomy Pain and Its Management 383
    Preeti P Doshi

43. Restless Leg Syndrome: Causes and Pain Management 395
    Dwarkadas K Baheti

44. Calciphylaxis and Its Pain Management 400
    Krishna Poddar

45. Regenerative Medicine for Spine and Orthopedic Conditions 407
    Annu Navani, Joshua D Chrystal

SECTION 13: PHYSIOTHERAPY

46. Role of Physiotherapy in Treatment of Patients
    with Spinal Pain During the Acute/Inflammatory Phase 423
    Rob Naber

47. Role of Physiotherapy in Treatment of Spinal Pain
    During Subacute/Reparative Phase 437
    Neeraj D Baheti

48. Physiotherapy in Management of Chronic Pain 448
    Saroj M Sanghavi, Dakshesh M Sanghavi

SECTION 14: PSYCHOTHERAPY

49. Role of Psychiatric Medications in Chronic Pain Management 459
    Harish K Shetty, Surbhi C Trivedi

50. Pain Psychology and Its Treatment Options 463
    Anjali M Chhabria, Shrradha V Sidhwani, Juhi J Parmar

SECTION 15: ALLIED THERAPY

51. Role of Radiation in Cancer Pain 473
    Krishna A Balkundi, Pallavi B Patil

52. Role of Chemotherapy in Cancer Pain Management 478
    Ashish V Bakshi, Nilesh M Lokeshwar, Vibhay Pareek

53. Oncosurgery and Cancer Associated Pain 485
    Deepak Chabbra

54. Management of Ophthalmic Pain 491
    Salil A Mehta

Index 499

PLATE 1

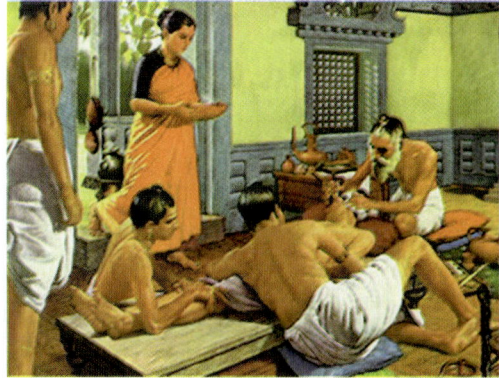

FIG. 1: Sushruta *(Chapter 1)*

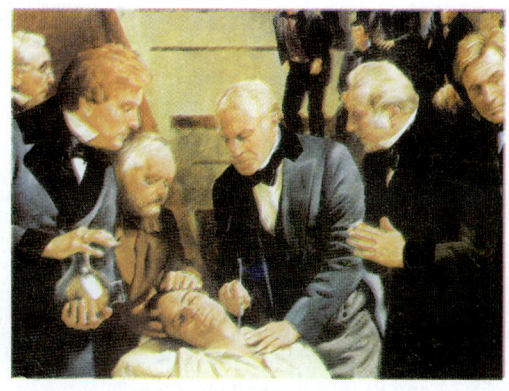

FIG. 3: Morton/ether *(Chapter 1)*

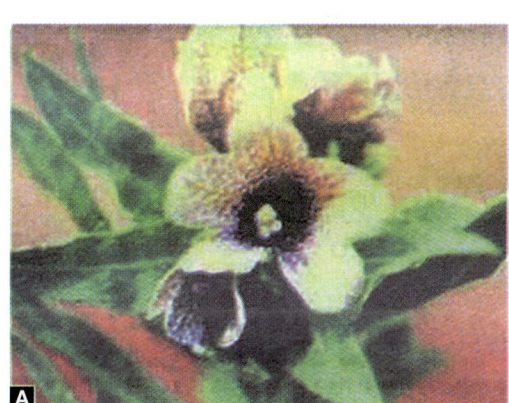
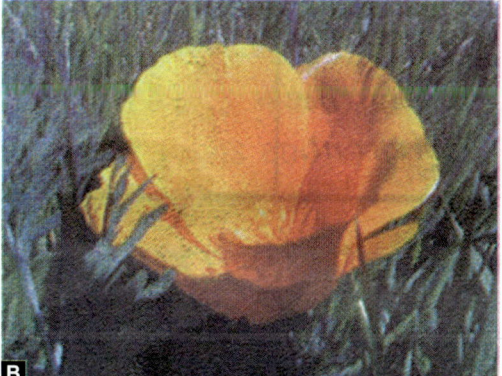

FIGS 2A and B: Selenium and wild lettuce *(Chapter 1)*

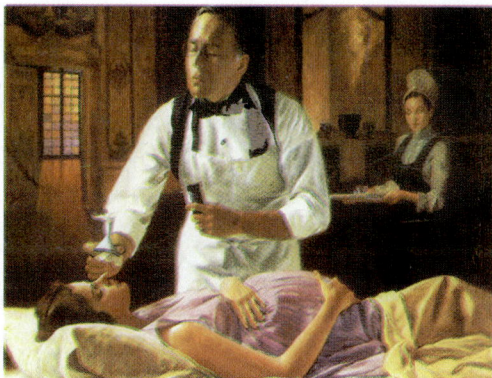

FIG. 4: Chloroform as labor analgesia for Queen Victoria *(Chapter 1)*

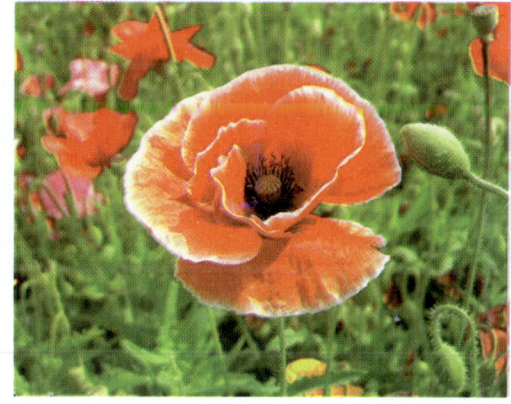

FIG. 5: Poppy (opium) flowers and buds *(Chapter 1)*

PLATE 2

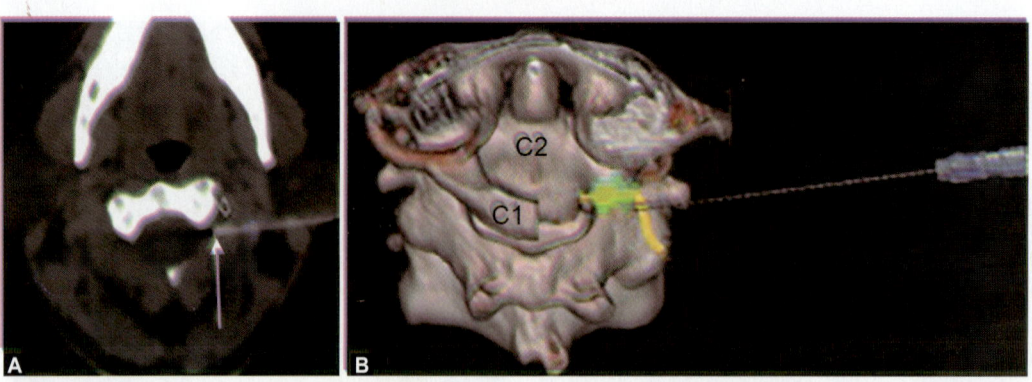

FIGS 2A and B: (A) Final position of needle at the level of C2 facet; (B) 3D scan depicting the needle position before infiltration *(Chapter 9)*

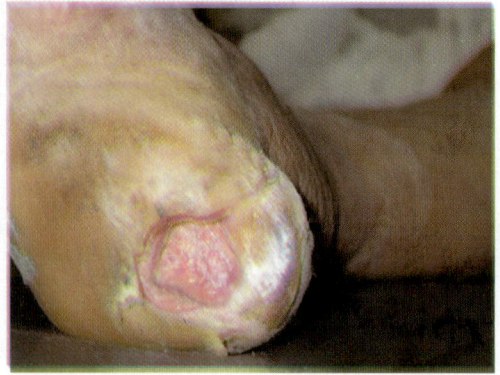

FIG. 10: Heel ulcer *(Chapter 11)*

PLATE 3

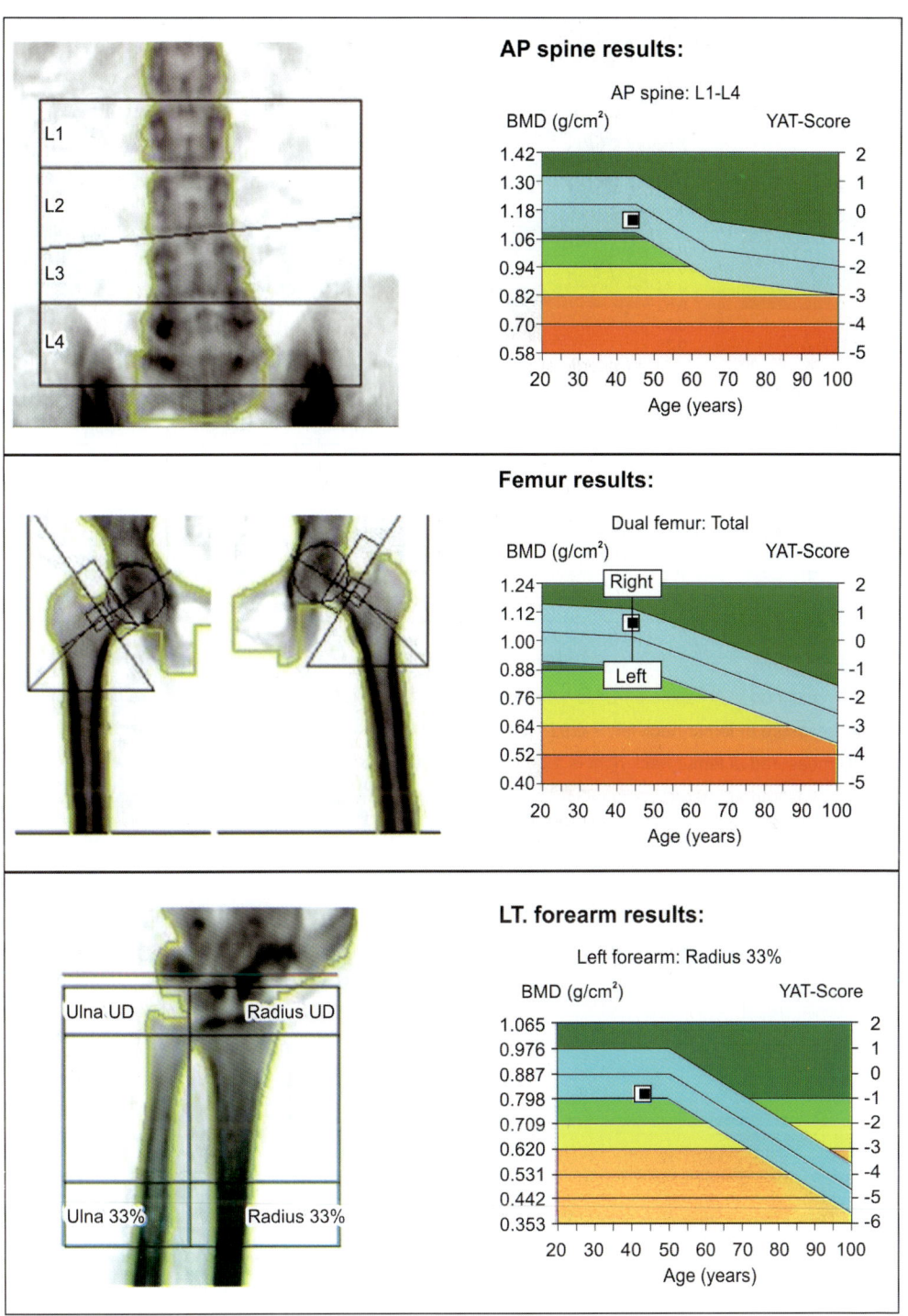

FIG. 3: Anterior-posterior spine, neck of femur and radius showing normal bone mineral density *(Chapter 12)*

PLATE 4

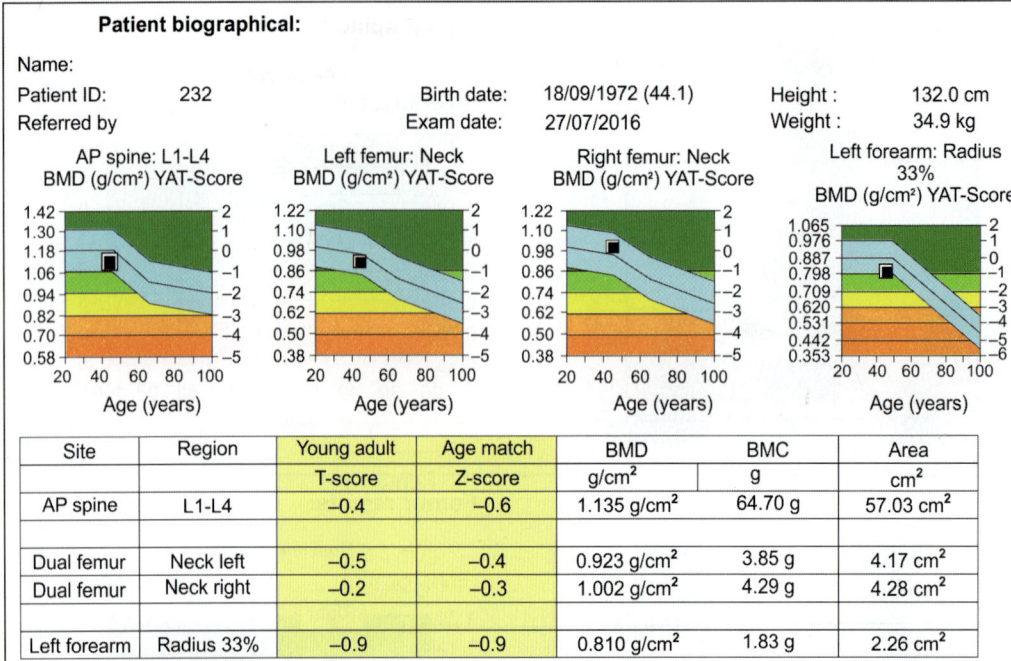

Patient biographical:

Name:
Patient ID: 232
Referred by
Birth date: 18/09/1972 (44.1)
Exam date: 27/07/2016
Height: 132.0 cm
Weight: 34.9 kg

Site	Region	Young adult T-score	Age match Z-score	BMD g/cm²	BMC g	Area cm²
AP spine	L1-L4	−0.4	−0.6	1.135 g/cm²	64.70 g	57.03 cm²
Dual femur	Neck left	−0.5	−0.4	0.923 g/cm²	3.85 g	4.17 cm²
Dual femur	Neck right	−0.2	−0.3	1.002 g/cm²	4.29 g	4.28 cm²
Left forearm	Radius 33%	−0.9	−0.9	0.810 g/cm²	1.83 g	2.26 cm²

Assessment:

The BMD measured at AP spine L1-L4 is 1.135g/cm² with a T-score of −0.4 is normal. Fracture risk is low.

The BMD measure at femur neck left is 0.923 g/cm² with a T-score −0.5 is normal. Fracture risk is low.

The BMD measured at femur neck right is 1.002 g/cm² with a T-score 0.2 is normal. Fracture risk is low.

The BMD measured at forearm radius 33% is 0.810 g/cm² with a T-score −0.9 is normal. Fracture risk is low.

World Health Organization (WHO) criteria for osteoporosis
Normal: T-score at or above −1 SD
Osteopenia: T-score between −1 and −2.5 SD
Osteoporosis: T-score at or below −2.5 SD

FIG. 4: Normal bone mineral density *(Chapter 12)*

PLATE 5

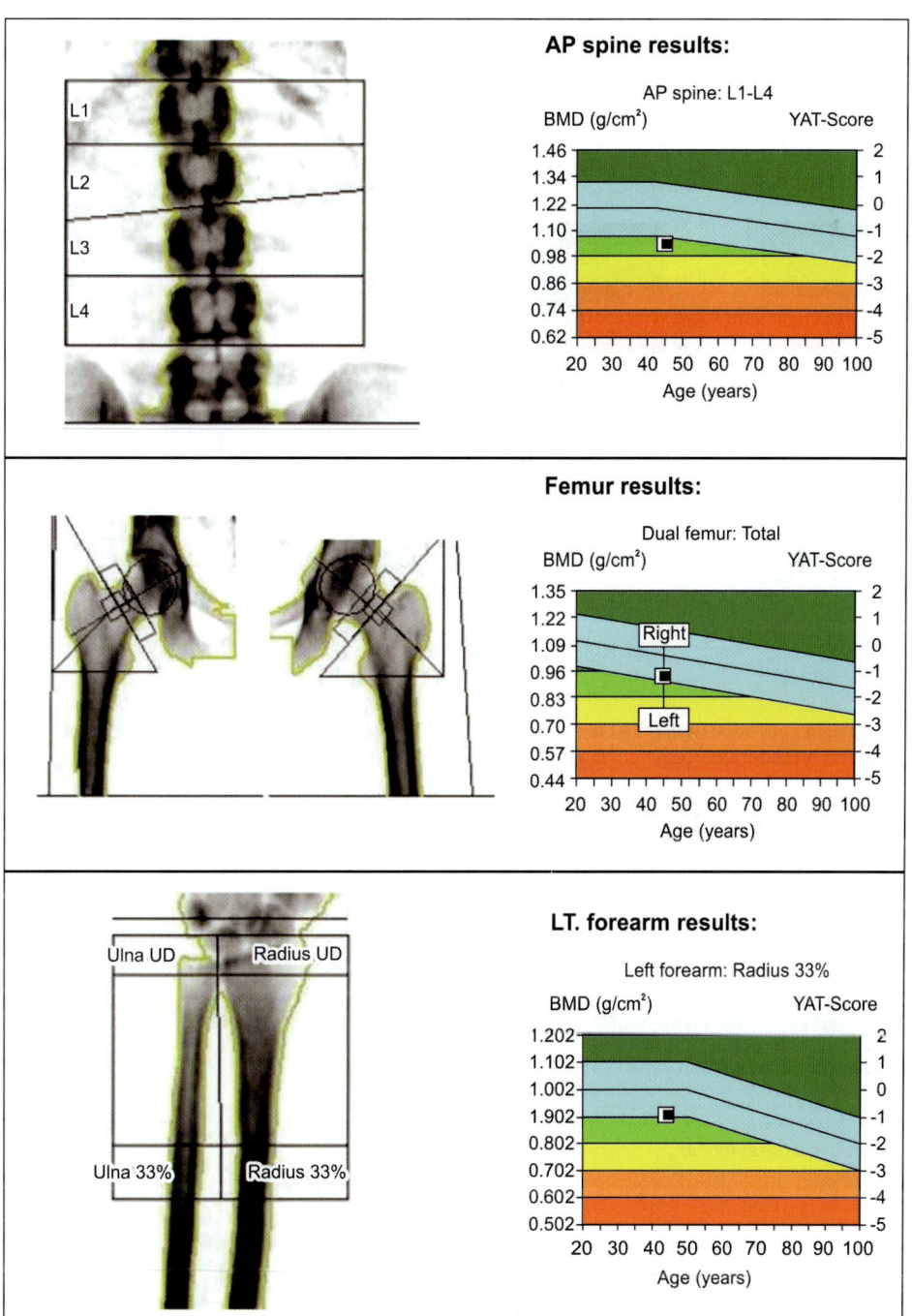

FIG. 5: Anterior-posterior spine, neck of femur, and radius showing osteopenia *(Chapter 12)*

PLATE 6

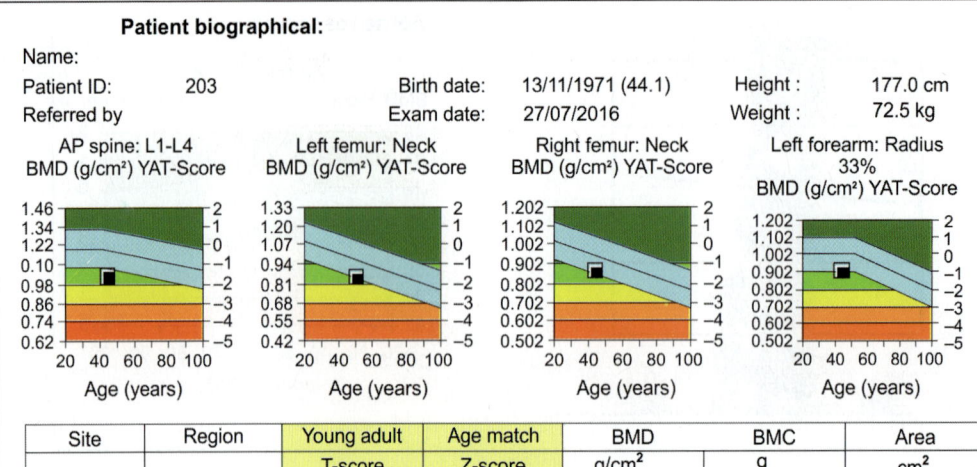

Patient biographical:

Name:						
Patient ID:	203		Birth date:	13/11/1971 (44.1)	Height:	177.0 cm
Referred by			Exam date:	27/07/2016	Weight:	72.5 kg

AP spine: L1-L4
BMD (g/cm²) YAT-Score

Left femur: Neck
BMD (g/cm²) YAT-Score

Right femur: Neck
BMD (g/cm²) YAT-Score

Left forearm: Radius 33%
BMD (g/cm²) YAT-Score

Site	Region	Young adult T-score	Age match Z-score	BMD g/cm²	BMC g	Area cm²
AP spine	L1-L4	−1.5	−1.3	1.035 g/cm²	52.51 g	50.72 cm²
Dual femur	Neck left	−1.7	−1.1	0.853 g/cm²	4.25 g	4.98 cm²
Dual femur	Neck right	−1.4	−0.8	0.887 g/cm²	4.31 g	4.86 cm²
Left forearm	Radius 33%	−1.0	−1.0	0.904 g/cm²	2.35 g	2.60 cm²

Assessment:

The BMD measured at AP spine L1-L4 is 1.035 g/cm² with a T-score of −1.5 is considered moderately low. Fracture risk is moderate. Treatment is advised if there are other risk factors.

The BMD measured at AP spine L1-L4 is 0.853 g/cm² with a T-score of −1.7 is considered moderately low. Fracture risk is moderate. Treatment is advised if there are other risk factors.

The BMD measured at AP spine L1-L4 is 0.887 g/cm² with a T-score of −1.4 is considered moderately low. Fracture risk is moderate. Treatment is advised if there are other risk factors.

The BMD measured at forearm radius is 0.904 g/cm² with a T-score of −1.0 is considered moderately low. Fracture risk is moderate. Treatment is advised if there are other risk factors.

> World Health Organization (WHO) criteria for osteoporosis
> Normal: T-score at or above −1 SD
> Osteopenia: T-score between −1 and −2.5 SD
> Osteoporosis: T-score at or below −2.5 SD

FIG. 6: Osteopenia *(Chapter 12)*

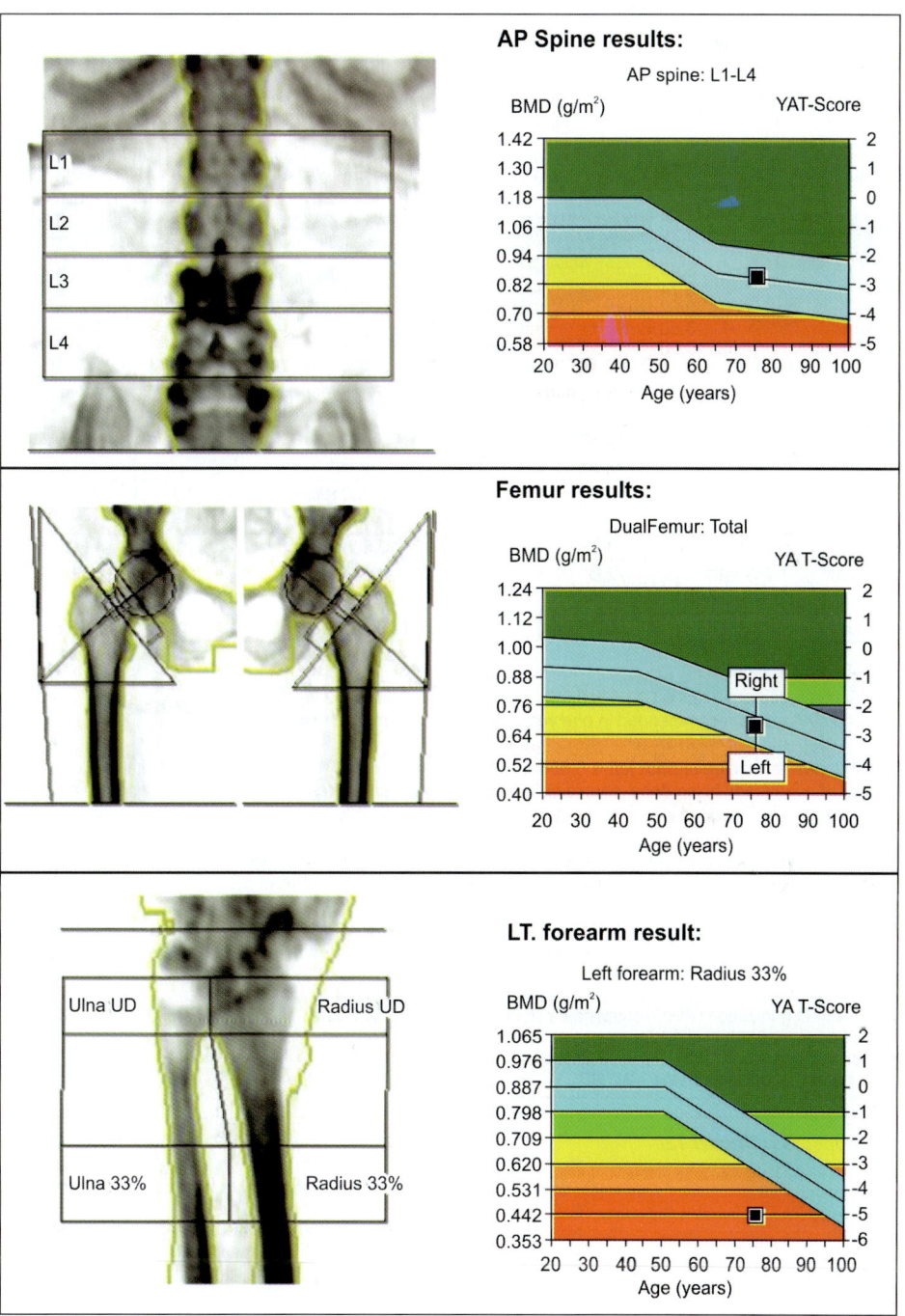

FIG. 7: Anterior-posterior spine, neck of femur and radius showing osteoporosis *(Chapter 12)*

PLATE 8

Patient biographical:

Name:
Patient ID: 155
Referred by

Birth date: 18/09/1940 (75.8)
Exam date: 28/07/2016

Height: 132.0 cm
Weight: 34.9 kg

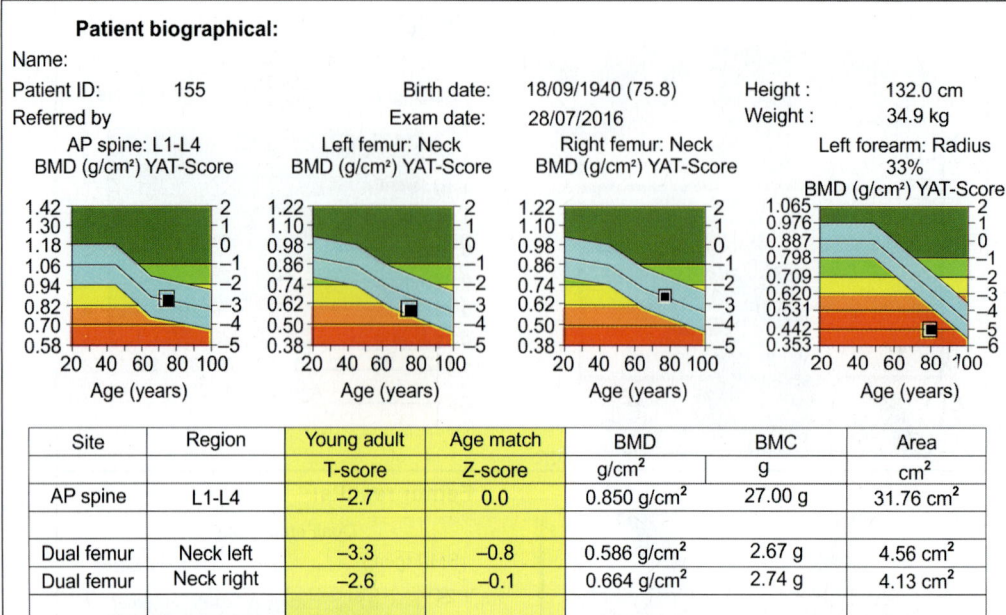

Site	Region	Young adult T-score	Age match Z-score	BMD g/cm²	BMC g	Area cm²
AP spine	L1-L4	–2.7	0.0	0.850 g/cm²	27.00 g	31.76 cm²
Dual femur	Neck left	–3.3	–0.8	0.586 g/cm²	2.67 g	4.56 cm²
Dual femur	Neck right	–2.6	–0.1	0.664 g/cm²	2.74 g	4.13 cm²
Left forearm	Radius 33%	–5.1	–2.7	0.438 g/cm²	2.94 g	2.14 cm²

Assessment:

The BMD measured at AP spine L1-L4 is 0.850 g/cm² with a T-score of –2.7 is low. Fracture risk is high. A follow-up DXA test is recommended in one year to monitor response to therapy.

The BMD measured at femur neck left is 0.586 g/cm² with T-score of –3.3 is markedly low. Fracture risk is high. Treatment, if not already being done, should be started. A follow-up DXA test is recommended in one year to monitor response to therapy.

The BMD measured at femur neck right is 0.664 g/cm² with a T-score of –2.6 is low. Fracture risk is high. A follow-up DXA test is recommended in one year to monitor response to therapy.

The BMD measured at forearm radius 33% is 0.438 g/cm² with a T-score of –5.1 is severely low. Fracture risk is high. Treatment, if not already being done, should be started. A follow-up DXA test is recommended in one year to monitor response to therapy.

World Health Organization (WHO) criteria for osteoporosis
Normal: T-score at or above –1 SD
Osteopenia: T-score between –1 and –2.5 SD
Osteoporosis: T-score at or below –2.5 SD

Fig. 8: Osteoporosis *(Chapter 12)*

PLATE 9

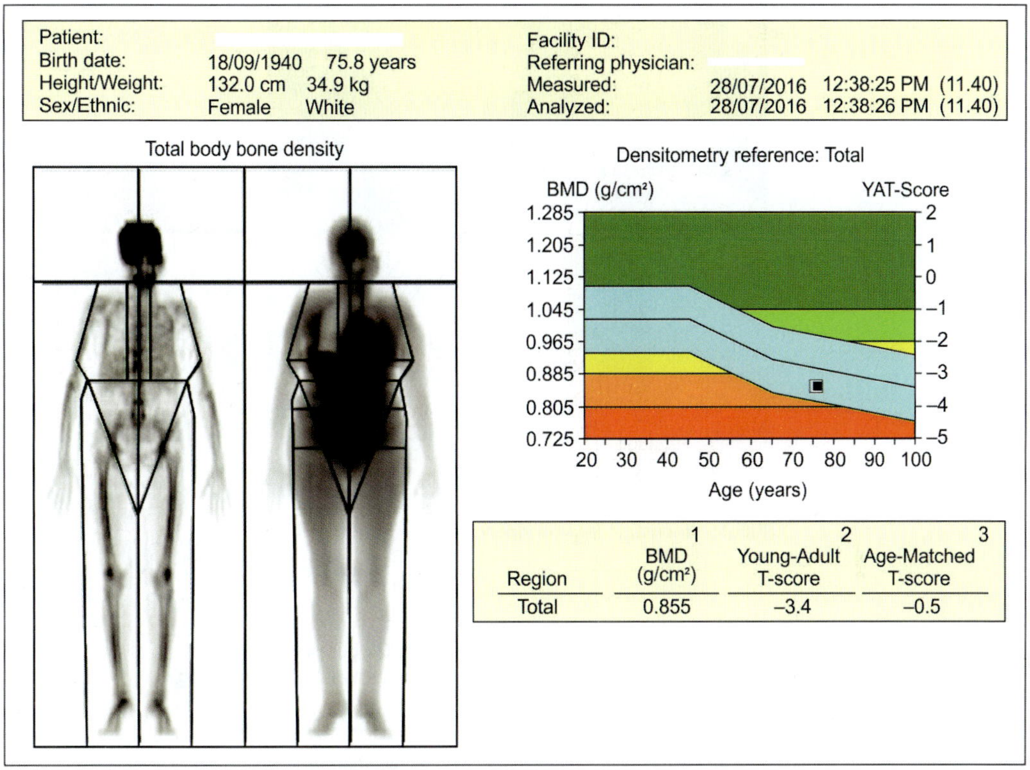

FIG. 9: Whole body scan showing osteoporosis *(Chapter 12)*

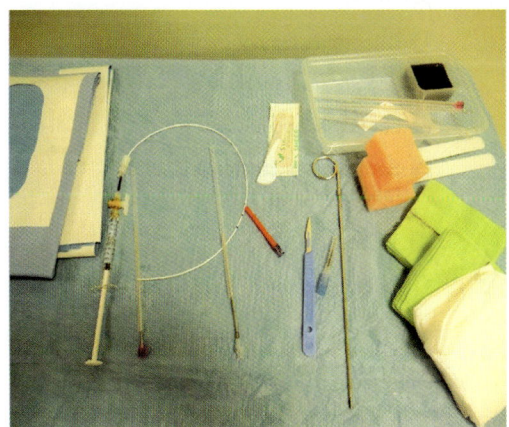

FIG. 8: Equipment set up for balloon microcompression (note a guard on the catheter) *(Chapter 14)*

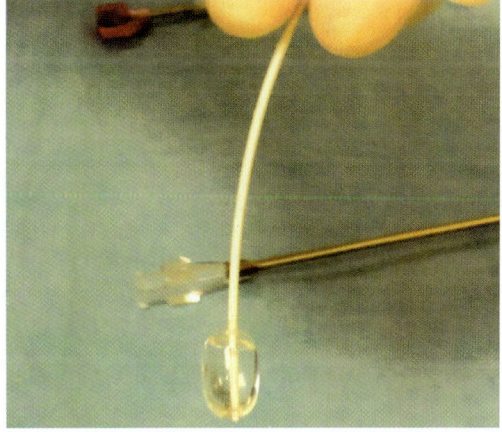

FIG. 9: Balloon being de-aired as it has air at the moment and if inflated with air the compression on ganglion is ineffective *(Chapter 14)*

PLATE 10

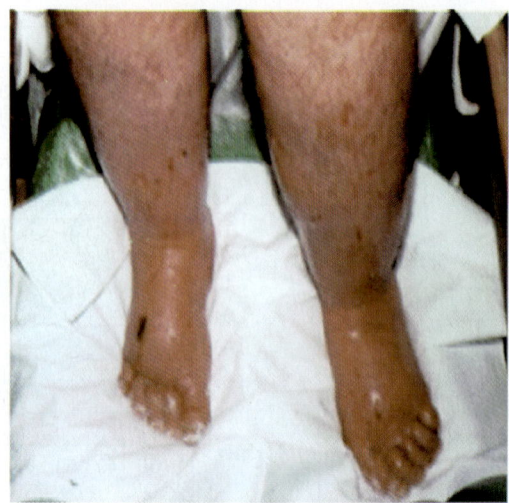

FIG.1: Vincristine legs *(Chapter 31)*

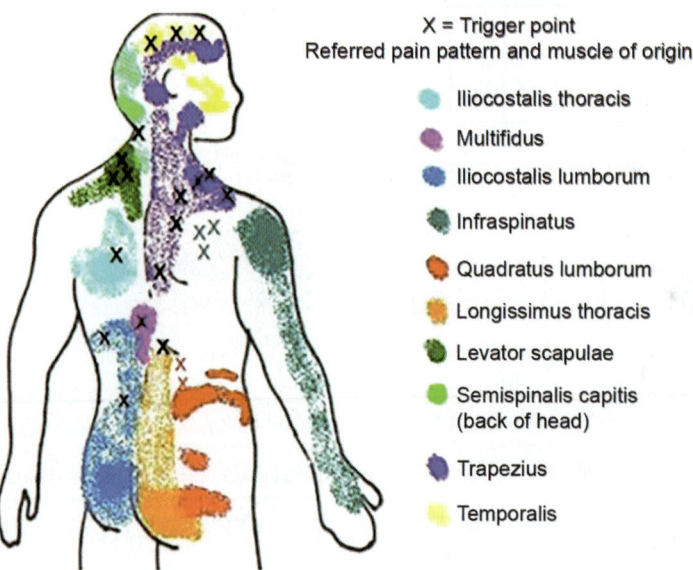

FIG. 2: Various tender points with the areas of referred pain *(Chapter 35)*

PLATE 11

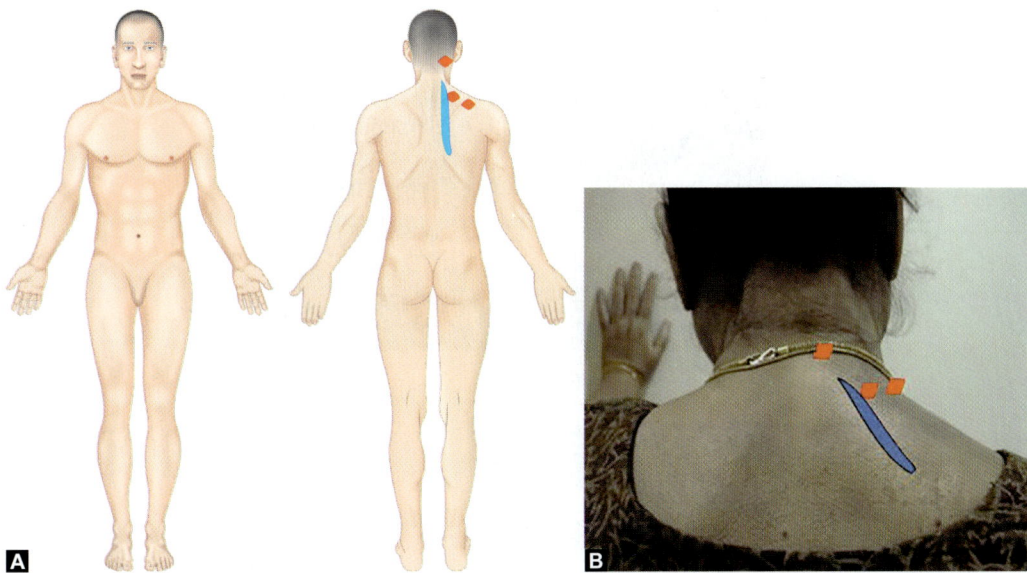

FIGS 3A and B: (A) Line diagram showing Red: Trapezius trigger ares, Blue: levator scapulae trigger point; (B) Patient with visible taut, levator scapulae, trigger point; Taut muscle band visible. referred pain to head, weakness restricted ROM *(Chapter 35)*

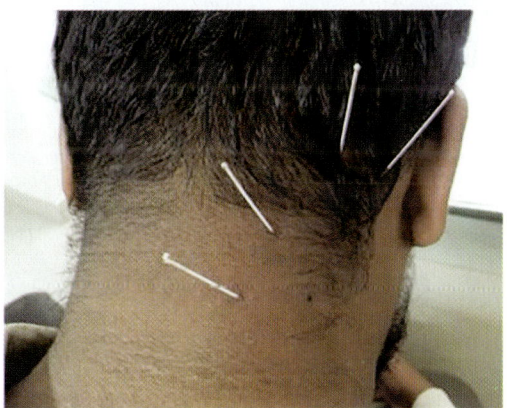

FIG. 5: Dry needling for upper trapezium trigger *(Chapter 35)*

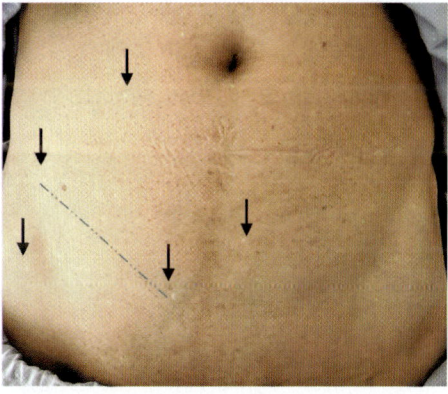

FIG. 6: KD Spots on abdominal dermatomes *(Chapter 35)*

PLATE 12

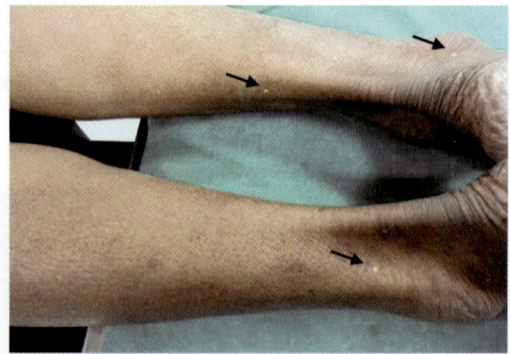

FIG. 7: KD spots *(Chapter 35)*

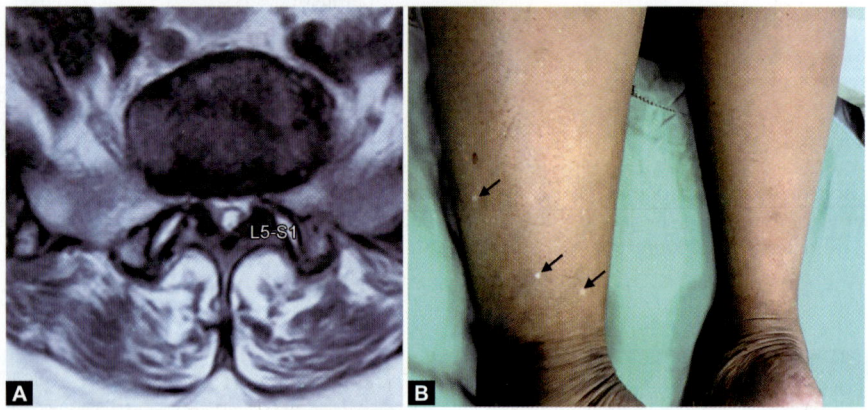

FIGS 8A and B: KD Spots, MRI of L5-S1 *(Chapter 35)*

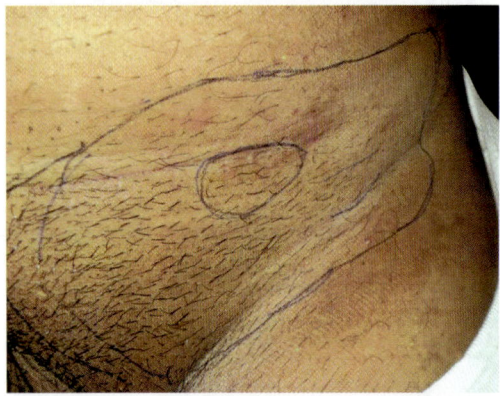

FIG. 1: Pain distribution in a patient with post-hernioplasty pain (laparoscopic). He had maximum pain (8–9/10 NRS) and allodynia in the small circular area marked next to the surgical scar. The surrounding areas including the root of penis and scrotum had pain of 6–7/10 NRS *(Chapter 37)*

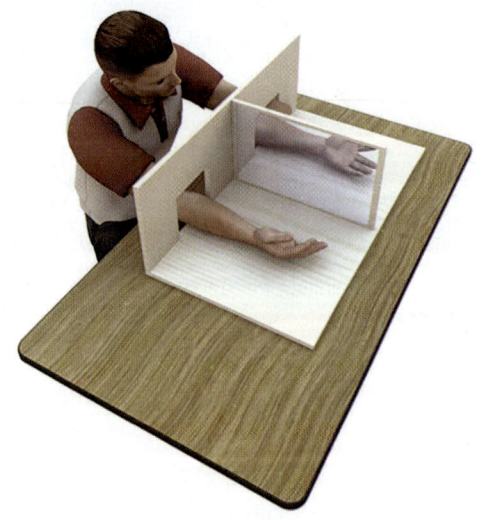

FIG. 2: Mirror image *(Chapter 40)*

PLATE 13

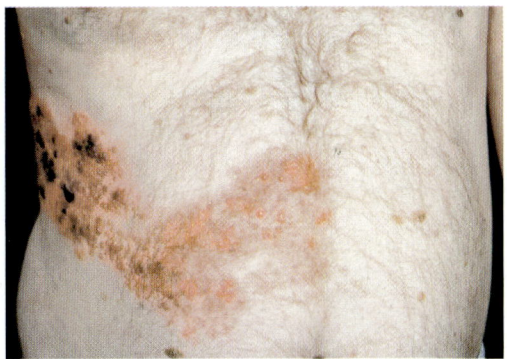

FIG. 1: Thoracic dermatome *(Chapter 41)*
Source: Mayo Clin Proc. 2009; 84(3):274–80.

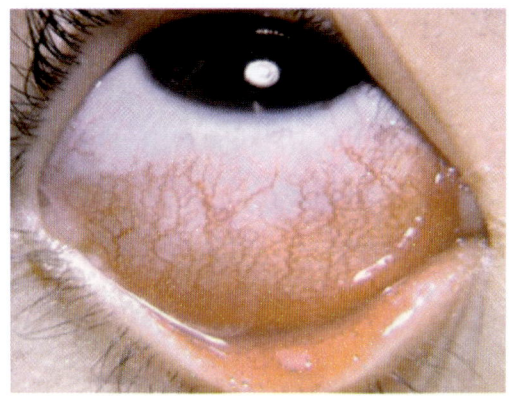

FIG. 4: Mucopurulent conjunctivitis *(Chapter 41)*

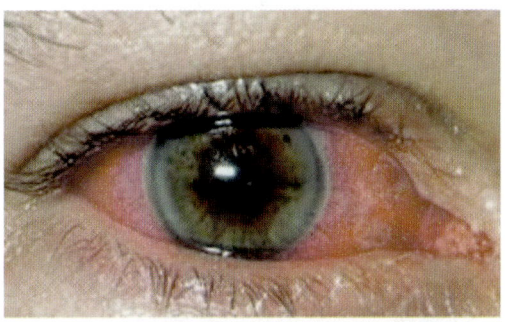

FIG. 2: Anterior uveitis inflammation of the middle layer of the eye, including the iris *(Chapter 41)*

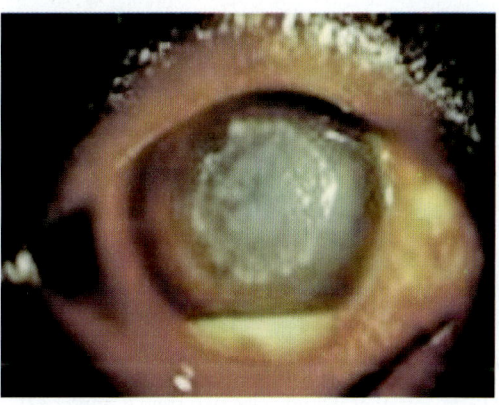

FIG. 5: Keratitis inflammation of the cornea *(Chapter 41)*

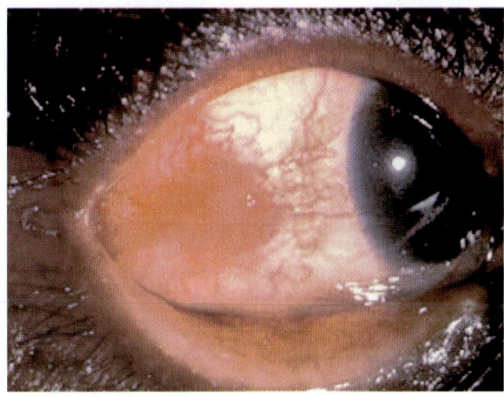

FIG. 3: Episcleritis inflammation of the sclera *(Chapter 41)*

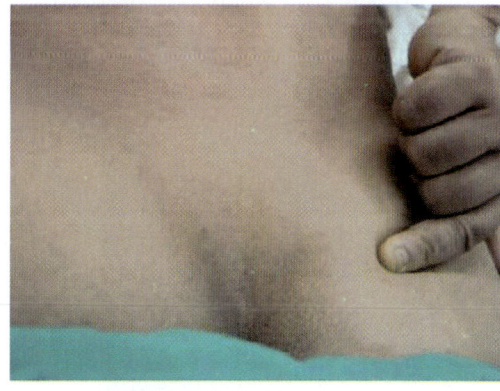

FIG. 2: Fortin finger test for sacroiliac joint mediated pain *(Chapter 42)*

PLATE 14

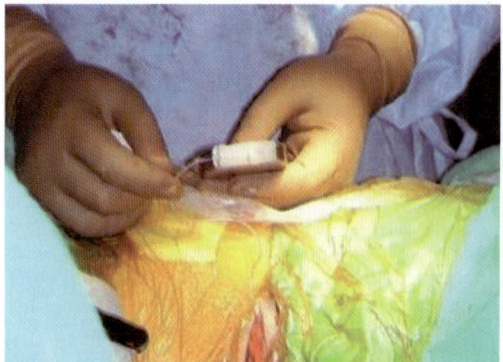

FIG. 7: Subcutaneous implantable pulse generator *(Chapter 42)*

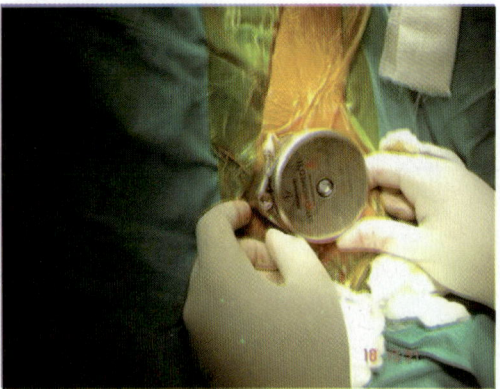

FIG. 8: Intrathecal drug delivery system *(Chapter 42)*

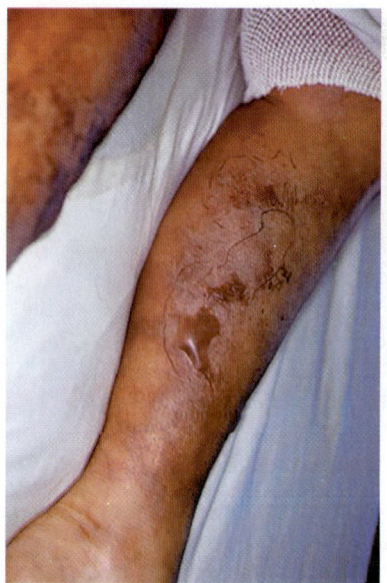

FIG. 2: Calciphylactic lesions at side of leg *(Chapter 44)*

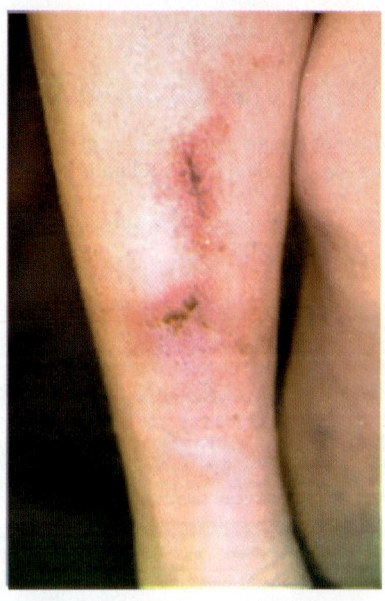

FIG. 3: Calciphylactic lesions at arm *(Chapter 44)*

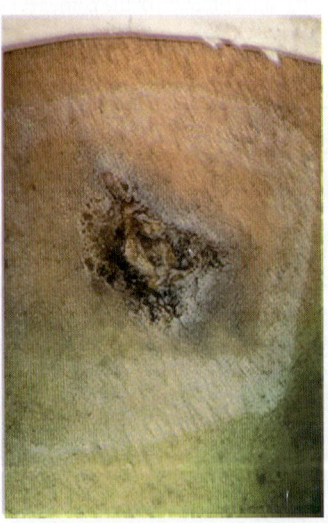

FIG. 1: Nonhealing necrotic ulcer over leg *(Chapter 44)*

PLATE 15

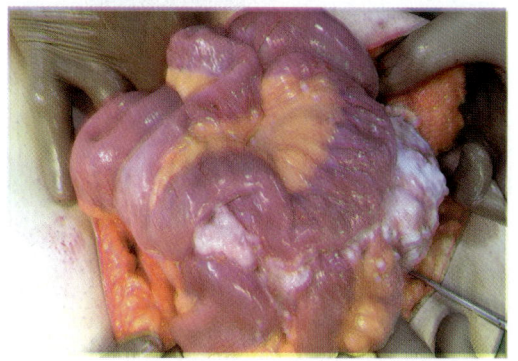

FIG. 1: Intraoperative photograph of a patient with advanced peritoneal carcinomatosis. Palliative major bowel resection was done for large mesenteric tumor deposits involving multiple small bowel loops causing obstruction *(Chapter 53)*

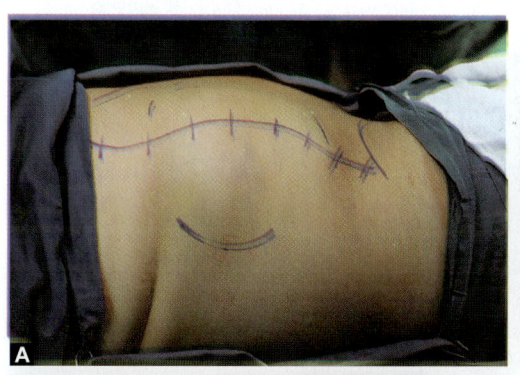
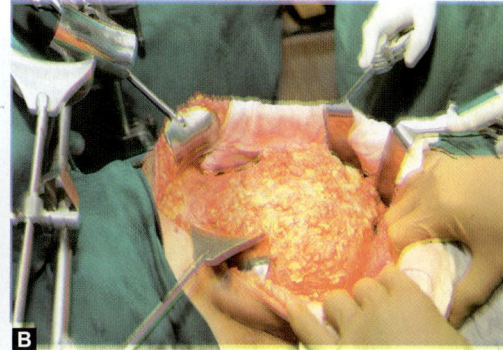
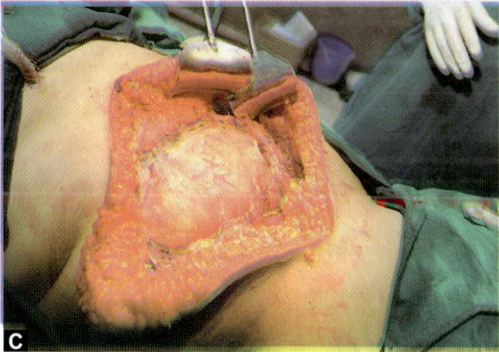

FIGS 2A to C: (A) Patient with a recurrent and metastatic hepatocellular carcinoma planned for palliative surgery; (B) Palliative resection of extra-abdominal tumor done for compression symptoms; (C) Abdominal wall reconstruction after tumor excision *(Chapter 53)*

PLATE 16

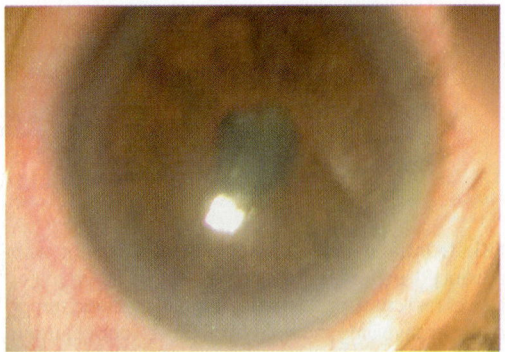 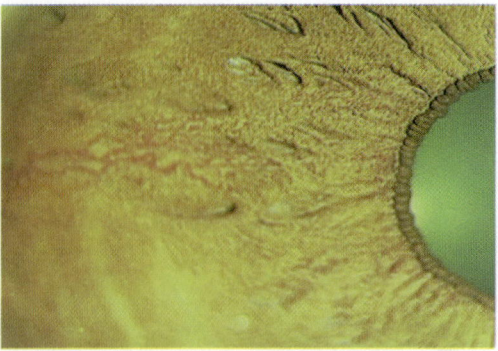

FIG. 1: Color photograph showing a congested painful eye with advanced neovascular glaucoma. extensive neovascularizaration of the iris is seen *(Chapter 54)*

FIG. 2: Color photograph showing new vessels on the iris *(Chapter 54)*

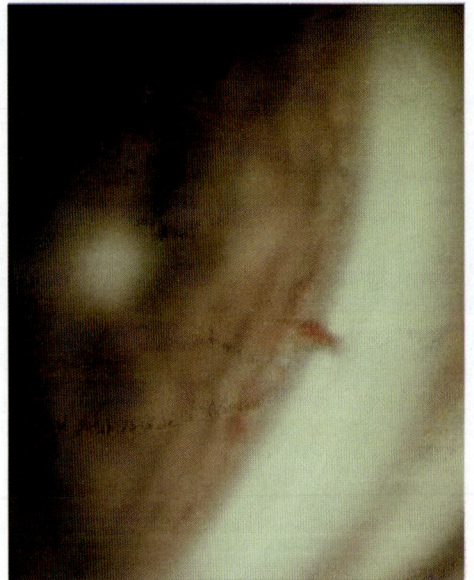

FIG. 3: Photograph of the angle showing new vessels of the angle *(Chapter 54)*

SECTION 1

Basics

CHAPTER 1

Pain Management: A Historical Perspective

Vasumathi M Divekar

"Farther we look back, further we can see"—Sir Winston Churchill

INTRODUCTION

Pain as a specialty is over half a century old. It is defined as a "discipline of medicine devoted to the diagnosis and treatment of pain related disorders". Pain is as old as humankind. Hippocrates first mentioned the brain as the center of sensation (over 2000 BC). Descartes (1700s) described nerves as tubes containing threads connecting the skin to the brain. From being a curse in ancient times, it has become the sixth sense.

HISTORICAL ASPECT

The first mention of pain relief in western literature (Thomas Schuman) is of Sushruta (500 BC) for surgical operations; it was achieved by opium, wine or Indian hemp (Fig. 1). In a chronicle "Bhoj Prabandh", Raja Bhoj (527 AD) mentions use of a concoction "Sammohini" for pain relief. For labor analgesia strong wines, inhalation of burnt mohini flowers, opium and marijuana (bhang) were used (Vagabhatta 400 AD). In Europe cold water, mandrake roots, solanium, and wild lettuce were used (Figs 2A and B). In the 16th-17th centuries hypnotism and mesmerism were practiced, made famous by James Esdaile in Calcutta (1845).

ROLE OF MEDICATION

With the discovery of ether, (1847—Morton) (Fig. 3) chloroform (Fig. 4) and cocaine a local anesthetic (1888—Bier), Esters and amides for local anesthesia revolutionized into nerve blocks and nerve lysis. In the early 20th century analgesics were synthesized. Twilight sleep was used in labor analgesia (1902—Van Steinbuchel) with an injection of morphine and scopolamine abandoned after 30 years! "Gwathmey analgesia" advocated a mixture of morphine, magnesium sulfate and ether in olive oil, alcohol and quinine. This was supposed to be harmless at that time! Inhalation agents like Trilene, Penthrane and Entonox ($N_2O + O_2$) had their days.

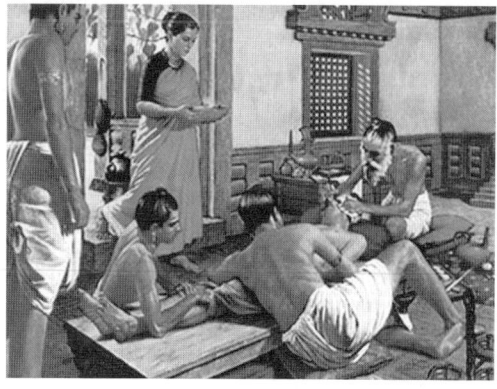

FIG. 1: Sushruta *(For color version, see Plate 1)*

Section 1: Basics

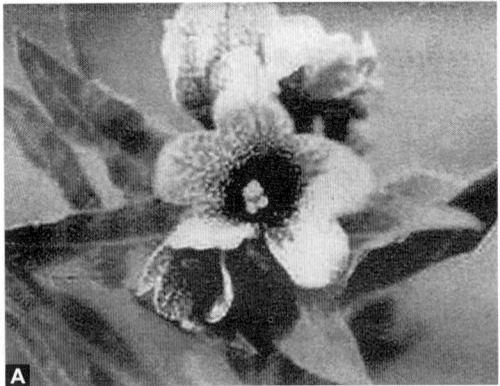
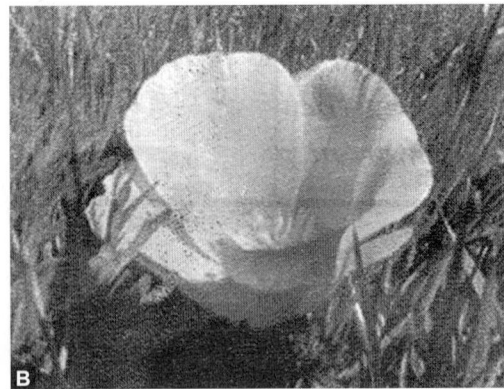

FIGS 2A and B: Selenium and wild lettuce *(For color version, see Plate 1)*

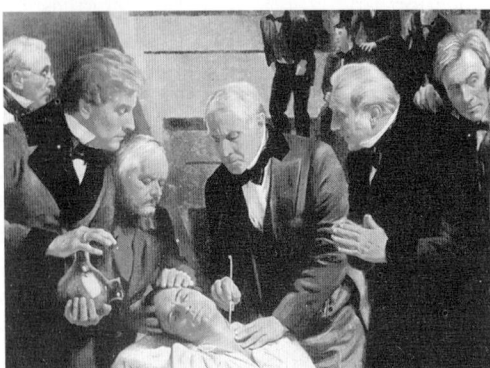

FIG. 3: Morton/ether *(For color version, see Plate 1)*

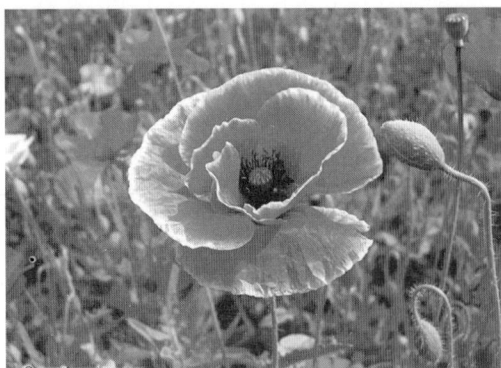

FIG. 5: Poppy (opium) flowers and buds *(For color version, see Plate 1)*

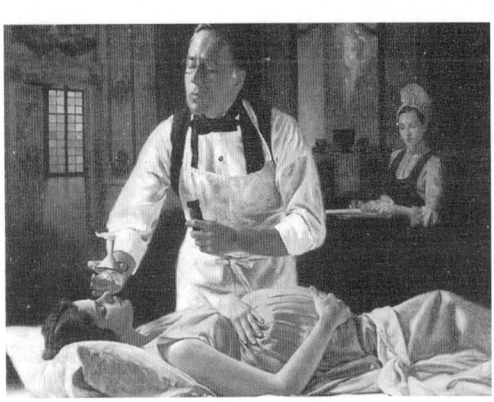

FIG. 4: Chloroform as labor analgesia for Queen Victoria *(For color version, see Plate 1)*

Morphine has a special place in pain relief. First used as an addiction; brought wealth to the British in India and two Sino-British wars (Fig. 5). Banned in India on February 26, 1950 in article 47 of the constitution of India except for medicinal purposes, however oral morphine was banned. Now, new licensing regulation has been enforced since 1998.

Melzack and Wall's "Gate Control Theory" opened up new avenues for pain management. N-methyl-D-aspartate (NMDA) receptor antagonists, opiate receptors in spinal cord and also discovery of endorphins, enkephalins (1970) contributed to the understanding and advances in pain relief.

Neuropathic pain syndrome was first recognized during the American Civil War (1864—Dr Mitchell) as "causalgia", later reviewed and managed by Dr Bowsher D (1991). Neuropathic pain was defined as "pain arising as a direct consequence of a lesion or disease affecting the somatosensory system", referred to by some as "deafferentation pain". Regional pain syndrome was conceptualized in 1994.

Electricity and pain relief—natural sources like electric fish and static electricity from amber were used in ancient times! Man-made electricity as electrostatic generators (1672); electro-acupuncture (1823) and peripheral nerve stimulators were in use and later banned in the US because of misuse and again revived with spinal cord stimulation by Sheeley (1967), and stereotaxic surgery for central pain syndrome (1970s).

An array of new drugs have been synthesized—opiates, opioids, nonsteroidal anti-inflammatory drugs (NSAIDs), NMDA receptor antagonists, gabapentine; pregabalin, adjuvants like tricyclic antidepressants, steroids, and antiepileptics. These have helped in supportive treatment. Neurolytic drugs like alcohol, phenol, etc. were introduced as a last resort in cancer pain (1970s).

Regional blocks (spinal and epidural) and peripheral as well as sympathetic nerve blocks have revolutionized pain management. A series of procedures and gadgets have revolutionized pain relief like fluoroscopy, radiofrequency ablation (1970s), a quarter century of percutaneous interventions have been introduced. Spinal endoscopy and myelos-copy (1931—Burmann). Endoscopy with rigid arthroscope and recognition of bands in the epidural space (1985—Bloomberg). Koki Simoji introduced the flexible fiberscope for subarachnoid and epidural visualization (1991).

Cancer pain needs a special mention, these patients need pain relief, palliative care, perhaps "end-of-life" care. This program has been adopted by some states in India (Kerala and Maharashtra). The World Health Organization introduced the "three-step analgesia ladder" in the treatment of cancer pain. Recent advances in drug delivery systems, e.g. percutaneous patches of opioids, etc. have alleviated the suffering of cancer patients.

Recent advances in drug delivery systems like percutaneous patches, analgesics, psycho-therapy, radiation, chemotherapy or hormonal therapy and in extreme cases neurosurgery. However, there are many issues to be tackled, such as addiction, tolerance, depression and toxicity. Newer procedures and medications have made it possible for precise diagnosis, location and ablation of pain sources and created the modern pain physician.

CONCLUSION

It is highly important to know historical aspects to understand pain better and it definitely helps in clinical practice.

BIBLIOGRAPHY

1. Bowsher D. Neuropathogenic pain syndromes and their management. Br Med Bull. 1991;47(3):644-66.
2. Bennett I. Spinal cord stimulation. In: Bennett MI (Ed). Neuropathic Pain, 2nd edition. London: Oxford University Press; 2010. p. 161.
3. Keys TE. The History of Surgical Anaesthesia. New York: Schuman; 1945. pp. 84, 110, 111.
4. Melzack R, Wall PD. Pain Mechanisms: a new theory. Science. 1965;50(3699):971-9.
5. Simpson BA. Electrical stimulation and relief of pain. In: Simpson BA (Ed). Pain Research and Clinical Management. Amsterdam: Elsevier; 2003.
6. Souvenir—Centenary of the Afzal Gunj Hospital and Diamond Jubilee Osmania Hospital, Hyderabad; 1988.
7. Souvenir—III Joint Indo-US Anaesthesiology—update cum workshop. New Delhi; 1994. p. 15.
8. Sushruta Samhita. Ayurveda. 500 BC.
9. World Health Organization. Analgesic Ladder for Pain Management. Geneva: WHO; 1986.

CHAPTER 2

Acute Pain

Gerard DeGregoris III

INTRODUCTION

The International Association for the Study of Pain (IASP) has defined pain as "an unpleasant sensory and emotional experience associated with actual or potential tissue damage, or described in terms of such damage".[1] By the insertion of the "or" conjunction in the latter part of the sentence, the IASP authors provided that actual tissue damage is not a prerequisite for a patient's symptoms to be classified as pain. While not universally accepted, this working definition is the one which is usually used in peer-reviewed journals and subspecialty textbooks.[2]

ACUTE PAIN

Pain is frequently divided into categories based on several factors, among these is the interval between the onset of pain and the present time.[1] Acute and chronic pain intervals were not explicitly defined in the IASP manuscript, but are nevertheless an important component of the patient history. While no clear consensus exists, the most frequently cited times to divide acute pain from chronic pain are 3 months and 6 months.[2] Acute pain has been further described as "pain elicited by the injury of bodily tissues and activation of nociceptive transducers at the site of local tissue damage". This local damage not only depolarizes nociceptors, but may also alter the response characteristics (for example the resting membrane potential or the expression of surface proteins) and their connections to the central nervous system and autonomic nervous system.[2] Generally speaking, a state of acute pain exists for a limited time and abates when the underlying pathology resolves or tissue damage is repaired.

Cause and Mechanism of Acute Pain

Pain is frequently triggered by injury or disease and can be caused by damage to peripheral tissues or the nervous system itself, as with diabetic neuropathy, spinal cord injury or stroke.[3] The proximate causes of acute pain are widespread, but those most commonly studied include pain due to skeletal trauma and surgery.[3] A wide variety of traumatic insults cause acute pain by a well-studied (but not completely understood) pathway. Tissue damage sets off a variety of responses which serve to meet several timely goals, including mobilizing the body's resources to fight infection, limiting further bodily damage including blood loss, and initiating repair.[4] This tissue damage is usually first detected by nociceptors, which are the primary afferent endings of nerves that transmit pain information to the spinal cord. Nociceptors are distributed at varied concentrations throughout the skin, muscle, joints and visceral organs. Certain nociceptors are specific to one kind of threat, such as heat, or pressure, but most are polymodal, activated by a variety of potentially damaging environmental conditions.[5,6] In order for a stimulus to be perceived as pain, a chain of five events must occur, as illustrated in Flowchart 1.

Each of these five steps in the acute pain pathway represents an opportunity to intervene and ameliorate the experience of pain. When tissues are damaged locally, epithelial cells, mast cells, and macrophages release inflammatory molecules such as adenosine triphosphate, nerve growth factor, tumor necrosis factor alpha, bradykinin, prostaglandin E2, serotonin and protons. Nociceptors react to cellular damage by responding to these chemical irritants.[5] After nociceptor signal transduction, an action potential is generated that must then propagate down the axon of the first order neuron.[2] Voltage gated sodium channels are responsible for the upstroke of the action potential and its propagation down the nerve fiber of interest. The axons of nociceptors come in several distinct varieties, classified by their physical characteristics including their conduction speed and presence or absence of myelin sheathing.[7] Two general pathways of ascending acute pain have been described. The first is known as physiological pain and uses A-delta fibers which are myelinated, fast-conducting fibers. These are typically related to high threshold thermoreceptors and mechanoreceptors. Note that not all A-delta fibers transmit pain, but it is thought that 50% or more of the body's A-delta fibers are involved in pain transmission. The rest are responsible for mechanical and nonpainful thermal input.[7] A-delta fibers enter the dorsal horn of the spinal cord and synapse in Rexed laminae I, V, and X. They typically convey sharp and well localized pain symptoms of short duration.[7]

A second, parallel pain pathway conveys what is known as pathophysiological pain and is carried by C fibers. These fibers are unmyelinated and conduct impulses much slower. They can convey mechanical, chemical and thermal stimuli and synapse at Rexed laminae II and III (the substantia gelatinosa of the dorsal horn) in the spinal cord.[7] They may produce such responses as muscle spasm, rigidity, or guarding. Stronger stimuli result in a proportional increase in the rate of neuron firing.[6] Once this action potential reaches the synapse of the second order neuron, several events occur, usually culminating in voltage gated calcium channels allowing for calcium influx into the cell. Following this calcium influx, neurotransmitters are released into the synapse to activate the second order neuron in the spinal cord. These second order neurons in turn ascend via the spinothalamic tracts in the spinal cord to activate third order neurons in the thalamus including the posterior thalamic nuclei (including the ventral posterolateral nucleus and ventral posteromedial nucleus).[7,8] Indeed this is probably an oversimplification, as other pathways have also been described in the ascending pain pathway including the spinoreticular tract, the spinocervicothalamic tract, the postsynaptic dorsal column fibers,

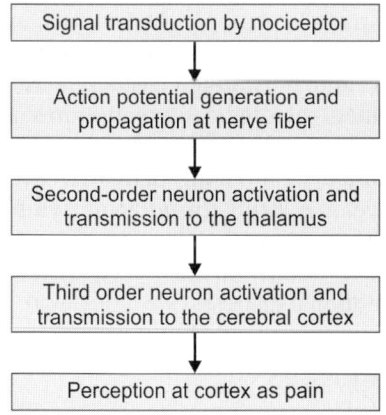

Flowchart 1: Five steps by which stimuli result in the perception of pain

and the visceral nociceptive tracts.[9] These tracts also ascend and then project into a wide variety of areas in the cerebral cortex. These areas have rich connections with each other and to areas of the brain responsible for past experience and behavior generation. Together their interaction can create the somatic and emotional experience of pain.[10]

Rationale for Treatment of Acute Pain

Expert opinion and scientific studies suggest that prolonged acute pain can lead to both peripheral and central sensitization that conspire to synergistically exacerbate pain perception.[4] Recent literature across several disciplines has suggested that acute pain can cause prolonged neurohumoral changes[11] as well as clinically observable changes that can lead to physical harm[12] chronic pain[13-15] and negatively impact patient's quality of life.[3] The potential for long-term harm caused by acute pain has been described in children[16] as well.

Among the best reasons for the aggressive treatment of acute pain is to possibly prevent the progression of acute pain to chronic pain. The traditionally held belief that acute and chronic pain are discrete entities is now disputed.[12] Basic science research has shown that changes in gene expression after exposure to pain occur remarkably quickly, perhaps within as little as 20 minutes of injury.[12] The activation of peripheral nociceptors can lead to peripheral and occasionally central sensitization to pain. This process then lowers the threshold for subsequent stimuli to activate the pain pathway, whereby increasingly less innocuous stimuli will become interpreted as painful.[4]

Animal research studies of chronic pain have uncovered long-term behavioral changes within approximately 24 hours after noxious interventions such as transient nerve ligation. Human data support these observations as well. Indeed, neonates have been found to have weeks of local sensitivity to heel touch after heel lancing[17] and infant circumcision has been found to correlate with an exaggerated response to preventative inoculation several months later.[18]

Data also exist to suggest that good control of acute pain produces measurable longer term benefits. In adults, aggressive pain control after radical prostatectomy was shown to lower analgesic requirements and improves functional status for several months after surgery.[19] The long-term harm that can follow from acute pain has served to motivate physicians to develop more aggressive protocols for managing acute pain. Prophylactic treatment of pain by paravertebral nerve block has been shown to reduce the prevalence of chronic pain at 1 year after breast surgery.[20] Other pain alleviating modalities have also been shown to decrease the incidence of postsurgical chronic pain.[21]

The consequences of acute pain extend beyond the development of chronic pain. The effect of acute pain has been found to adversely affect patients' overall quality of life after various surgical procedures including prostatectomy, total hip replacement and total knee replacement.[3] Uncontrolled acute surgical pain has also been shown to have deleterious effects on sleep and activity level.[22]

CONCLUSION

Acute pain is among the most common reasons that patients utilize the health care system, and it is widely regarded as a top component of medical expenditures and a cause of human suffering. Early aggressive care aimed at reducing pain may decrease the development of chronic pain syndromes and may ameliorate other problems including decreased quality of life, sleep disturbance and emotional distress.

REFERENCES

1. ISAP. (1994). ISAP taxonomy. [online] Available from http://www.iasp-pain.org/Taxonomy [Accessed December 2016].

2. Bonica JJ. The Management of Pain, 2nd edition. Philadelphia: Lea & Fabiger; 1990.
3. Sinatra R. Causes and consequences of inadequate management of acute pain. Pain Med. 2010;11(12):1859-71.
4. Voscopoulos C, Lema M. When does acute pain become chronic? Br J Anesth. 2010;105(Suppl 1):i69-85.
5. Gold M, Gebhart G. Peripheral pain mechanisms and nociceptor sensitization. In: Fishman SM, Ballantyne JC, Rathmell JP (Eds). Bonica's Management of Pain, 4th edition. Philadelphia: Lippincott Williams & Wilkins; 2009. pp. 25-34.
6. Gold M. Ion channels: recent advances and clinical applications. In: Flor H, Kaslo E, Dostrovsky JO (Eds). Proceedings of the 16th World Congress on Pain. Seattle: IASP Press; 2006. pp. 73-92.
7. Serpell MG, Makin A, Harvey A. Acute pain physiology and pharmacological targets: the present and future. Acute Pain. 1998;1(3):31-47.
8. Serpell M. Anatomy, physiology and pharmacology of pain. Anaesth Intensive Care Med. 2005;6(1):7-10.
9. Besson JM. The neurobiology of pain. Lancet. 1999;353(9164):1610-5.
10. Loeser JD, Melzack R. Pain: an overview. Lancet. 1999;353(9164):1607-9.
11. Dunwoody CJ, Krenzischek DA, Pasero C, Rathmell JP, Polomano RC. Assessment, physiological monitoring, and consequences of inadequately treated acute pain. J Perianesth Nurs. 2008(1 Suppl):S15-27.
12. Carr DB, Goudas LC. Acute pain. Lancet. 1999;353(9169):2051-8.
13. Joshi GP, Ogunnaike BO. Consequences of inadequate postoperative pain relief and chronic persistent postoperative pain. Anesthesiol Clin North America. 2005;23(1):21-36.
14. Fassoulaki A, Melemeni A, Staikou C, Triga A, Sarantopoulos C. Acute postoperative pain predicts chronic pain and long-term analgesic requirements after breast surgery for cancer. Acta Anaesthesiol Belg. 2008;59(4):241-8.
15. Katz J, Jackson M, Kavanagh BP, Sandler AN. Acute pain after thoracic surgery predicts long-term post-thoracotomy pain. Clin J Pain. 1996;12(1):50-5.
16. Taddio A, Chambers CT, Halperin SA, Ipp M, Lockett D, Rieder MJ, et al. Inadequate pain management during routine childhood immunizations: the nerve of it. Clin Ther. 2009;31:S152-67.
17. Fitzgerald M, Millard C, McIntosh N. Cutaneous hypersensitivity following peripheral tissue damage in newborn infants and its reversal with topical anaesthesia. Pain. 1989;39(1):31-6.
18. Taddio A, Nulman I, Koren BS, Stevens B, Koren G. A revised measure of acute pain in infants. J Pain Symptom Manage. 1995;10(6):456-63.
19. Carr DB. Preempting the memory of pain. JAMA. 1998;279(14):1114-5.
20. Kairaluoma PM, Bachmann MS, Rosenberg PH, Pere PJ. Preincisional paravertebral block reduces the prevalence of chronic pain after breast surgery. Anesth Analg. 2006;103(3):703-8.
21. Tasmuth T, Kataja M, Blomqvist C, Smitten KV, Kalso E. Treatment-related factors predisposing to chronic pain in patients with breast cancer a multivariate approach. Acta Oncologica. 1997;36(6):625-30.
22. Pavlin DJ, Chen C, Penaloza DA, Buckley FP. A survey of pain and other symptoms that affect the recovery process after discharge from an ambulatory surgery unit. J Clin Anesth. 2004;16(3):200-6.

Acute Turn to Chronic: Causes, Prevention, and Management

Ramon Go, Neel Mehta

INTRODUCTION

The transformation of acute pain to chronic pain can be debilitating and frustrating to both patients and physicians. In the surgical population, the development of a chronic pain syndrome after a procedure can cause poor patient satisfaction and strain the patient-physician relationship especially when this potential complication is not discussed prior to the surgical procedure.[1] The development of chronic postsurgical pain (CPSP) has been associated with annual direct patient cost of $12,000, and $30,000 for indirect cost.[2] This totals to over $600 billion a year in the United States. Although the development of chronic pain postoperatively such as phantom limb pain syndrome has been described for centuries, the research behind developing chronic pain from acute pain is still in its infancy. It appears that the transition from acute to chronic pain is a multifactorial process involving surgical technique, environmental factors, and genetics. The mechanism and risk factors for developing chronic pain, along with prevention strategies and management are discussed in this chapter.

CHRONIC POSTSURGICAL PAIN

From an evolutionary standpoint, a hyperalgesic limb may prevent the exacerbation of an underlying injury and allow for healing.[3] However, when this mechanism persists, a debilitating chronic neuropathic pain may result. CPSP is defined as pain that persists greater 2 months after surgery. Macrae and Davies also add to the definition by requiring other causes of pain to be excluded, along with preexisting pain syndrome prior to surgical procedure.[4] CPSP has been shown to occur at a rate of 10-50% of postsurgical patients. This wide range may be due to the heterogeneity of patient populations, surgical procedures, anesthetic choices, and data collection and interpretation (Table 1). Of the patients who develop CPSP, 2-10% may experience severe chronic pain. Surgical procedures associated with high rates of chronic pain development include mastectomy, inguinal hernia and thoracotomy. A prospective study performed by Thomas et al. in 91 patients undergoing

TABLE 1: Surgical procedures and prevalence rates of developing postsurgical pain syndrome[6]

Procedure	Prevalence
Breast surgery	22–35%
Thoracotomy	11–52%
Cholecystectomy	21%
Limb amputation	5–50%
Hip	7–13%
Laparoscopic hernia repair	15% at nine months

orthopedic procedures showed that female patients and younger patients were also more likely to report higher pain scores and lower patient satisfaction.[5]

RISK FACTORS FOR DEVELOPING CHRONIC POSTSURGICAL PAIN

Preoperative and Postoperative Pain

The severity of preoperative or presurgical pain has been associated with an increased risk of developing CPSP. Specifically, in the phantom limb pain literature, multiple studies have demonstrated preamputation pain as a risk factor for developing phantom limb pain. The severity of the postsurgical pain has been associated with the development of chronic pain.[6] More severe the pain higher, the likelihood of CPSP. In a 2-year prospective study performed by Hanley et al. the intensity of acute postamputation pain within the first five postoperative days was the only significant predictor of chronic phantom limb pain at 6 months and 12 months after the surgical procedure.[7] This suggests that the increased activity of nociceptors in the immediate postoperative period is a critical time period for pain management. Under treating the patient's pain may also play a role in the development of chronic pain as the severity of pain would increase with poor pain control. Hence, aggressive pain control in the immediate postoperative period has shown to be protective in the development of CPSP.[1] Trauma resulting in severe acute pain may also play a role as nearly 50% of surgical amputees are likely to develop phantom limb pain.[8]

Surgical Types

They have been associated with different risks of CPSP given in Table 1. This may be related to the different nerves injured at specific surgical sites. The development of postmastectomy pain syndrome has been associated with more extensive surgical procedures. Mastectomy only patients were less likely than mastectomy with reconstruction to report postmastectomy pain 1 year after surgery.[9] Breast reconstruction when added to mastectomy also increases the length of surgery which on its own has been shown to increase the risk of developing chronic pain.[10] Laparoscopy has also been shown to lower the risk of developing CPSP when compared to open inguinal hernia repair. The extent and type of the surgery incision also affects the risk of CPSP, the larger the incision, the higher the risk of CPSP. Patients receiving Pfannenstiel incision have been observed to develop chronic abdominal pain from injury of iliohypogastric nerves.[11] Multiple factors may play a role as the interplay of each factor often occurs, as a long surgical time, extensive surgical procedure, and nerve injury may all be intertwined within one procedure. Radiation along with chemotherapy has also been found to be a risk factor for developing post-mastectomy pain.[12]

GENETICS

An exciting area of research in the development of chronic pain from acute pain is the role of genetics and environment. Genetics may explain up to 70% of the variability in experiencing pain among different patients.[2] Diminished pain sensation is observed in patients with mutant hereditary sensory neuropathy type 1 (*HSN1*) gene.[13] Different polymorphisms to the catechol-O-methyltransferase (COMT) enzyme may show different phenotype depending on the function of COMT, which is involved in the degradation of catecholamines such as dopamine, epinephrine and norepinephrine. Mutation resulting in increased enzyme function may result in lower response to opioids resulting in higher pain scores and negative patient although an allele has been found in which an increased activity of the enzyme resulted in lowered pain sensitivity.[13,14] Disease states such as fibromyalgia syndrome, migraine headaches, irritable bowel syndrome and irritable bladder, and Raynaud's syndrome have also been associated with the development of CPSP and may provide a link to susceptibility genes.[15] A table of genes associated with pain perception is given in Table 2. More research is needed to identify the role of susceptibility genes to identify patients at risk of developing chronic pain after an acute pain episode.

Twin studies also suggest that genetics alone is not solely responsible for the development of chronic pain.[16] The modification of gene expression by environmental factors may explain the discordance of monozygotic twin studies.[17,18] Chromatin is wrapped around histones and genes are regulated by acetylation and deacetylation of the histone proteins. The expression of opioid receptors has been shown to be highly regulated by this process. Histone deacetylase has become a potential drug target. Valproic acid, an antiepileptic drug, has been shown to inhibit histone deacetylation.[16]

NERVE INJURY

Extensive studies have shown that nerve injury results in the development of a chronic neuropathic pain syndrome and may explain many cases of CPSP. Animal models for neuropathic pain syndromes are often created by intentionally injuring a peripheral nerve, i.e. ligation of the sciatic nerve. This results in a hyperalgesic response and guarding behavior to the affected limb by the animal.[19] Although not all surgical procedures require cutting of nerves, the placement of retractors required for surgical exposure may result in the compression or stretch of nervous tissue may explain nerve injury. Nerves most likely to be injured for

TABLE 2: Genes implicated in human pain variability and the protein encoded

Increased pain sensitivity		
Gene	Protein affected	Phenotype
KCNS1	Voltage gated potassium ion channel	Increase sciatica pain and phantom limb pain
SCN9A	Voltage gated sodium ion channel	Chronic burning pain, phantom limb pain
ADRB2	Beta-2-adrenergic receptor	Risk for widespread body pain
IL6	Interleukin 6	Pain from endometriosis
CACNG2	Voltage-gated calcium ion channel	Post mastectomy pain
HTR2A	Serotonin receptor	Increased post-surgical pain
Decreased pain sensitivity		
Genes	Protein affected	Phenotype
COMT	Catechol-0-methyltransferase	Decreased or increased pain perception
OPRM1	OPRM1: opioid receptor mu 1	Decreased pain perception
TRPV1	Transient receptor potential vanilloid 1	Decreased thermal pain sensitivity
MC1R	Melanocortin 1 receptor	Decreased pain perception
GCH1	GTP cyclohydrolase	Decreased post-surgical pain
CACNA2D3	Voltage-gated calcium ion channel	Decreased thermal pain sensitivity

Source: Adapted from Young EE, Lariviere WR, Belfer I. Genetic basis of pain variability: recent advances. J Med Genet. 2012;49(1):1-9.

Chapter 3: Acute Turn to Chronic: Causes, Prevention, and Management

TABLE 3: Nerves likely to be injured along with surgical procedure are shown[11]

Surgical procedure	Nerves likely to be injured
Mastectomy	Lateral pectoral, medial pectoral, intercostal
Thoracotomy	Intercostal
Herniorrhaphy	Ilioinguinal
Cesarean section	Ilioinguinal, iliohypogastric

different surgical procedures are given in Table 3. Modifications to surgical procedure to avoid nerve injury may prevent some forms of CPSP as not all cases of CPSP are associated with specific nerve injury.

PSYCHOSOCIAL

Both mental and emotional states of the patient have been shown to play a significant role in the development of chronic pain.

Peters et al. performed a large study of 625 patients for elective surgery and found that fearful and pessimistic attitudes prior to surgery, resulted in patients who were more likely to develop high pain scores, poor recovery and poor quality of life 6 months after the surgical procedure.[10]

Catastrophizing is a maladaptive coping strategy in which the patient has unrealistic beliefs that the current situation will lead to worse pain outcomes and an exaggerated negative state. Catastrophizing is noted to be the most significant psychiatric behavior predictive of poor pain control. Other risk factors associated with developing CPSP include social support, neuroticism, and preoperative anxiety. When patients are provided excessive empathy from family members in which the patient obtains secondary gain, the incidence of pain behavior may also increase.[19] Providing education and consistent information on expectations of surgery have been found to reduce catastrophizing and patient distress. A summary of risk factors for the development of CPSP are shown in Box 1.

> **Box 1: Risk factors for the development of chronic postsurgical pain (CPSP)**
> - Age
> - Female gender
> - Preoperative pain score
> - Postoperative pain score
> - Surgical type
> - Adjuvant therapy: radiation, chemotherapy
> - Genetics
> - Nerve injury
> - Psychosocial and mood factors
>
> *Source:* Adapted from Voscopoulos C, Lema M. When does acute pain become chronic? Br J Anaesth. 2010;105 (Suppl 1):i69-85.

PATHOPHYSIOLOGY OF CHRONIC PAIN

Neuroplasticity

It is the remodeling of neuronal cytoarchitecture creating new neural pathways. This mechanism allows humans to adapt to their environment, thinking and emotions. Neuroimaging studies of patients with chronic pain display functional, anatomical and chemical changes in the central nervous system. The prefrontal gyrus and nucleus accumbens have been shown to have increased synchrony in patients who develop a chronic pain syndrome from an acute pain episode.[20] When peripheral lesions during an acute pain process continue to send impulses to the spinal cord, inhibitory interneurons responsible for modulating this signal wane, while glial cells increase neuronal synapses resulting in the intensification of pain signals.

Peripheral and Central Sensitization

The underlying mechanism in which the theory of the development of chronic pain from acute pain may be divided into two components, peripheral and central sensitization. Free nerve ending C fibers are stimulated causing a cascade of neural firing to the spinal cord. Peripheral nociceptors are then exposed to inflammatory products such as K^+, H^+ ions, prostaglandins (and cytokines, such as interleukin 6 (IL-6), IL-8, and tumor necrosis factor alpha (TNF-α), resulting in a decrease of threshold of nociceptors. Peripheral sensitization ultimately results in increased nociceptors such as transient receptor potential vanilloid 1 (TRPV1). Fifteen percent of human peripheral nociceptor receptors are considered dormant. With resultant inflammation and expression of the receptors to the periphery, a substantial increase in pain is perceived.[3] It is unclear if and when these receptors eventually become deactivated or resorbed into the cell.

Central sensitization is the process by which an increased activity and response to pain occurs after exposure to a noxious stimulus. Central sensitization occurs within the central nervous system resulting in secondary hyperalgesia. It is believed that ongoing uncontrolled pain from continuous nociception results in wide dynamic range (WDR) neurons, located at the dorsal horn, to sprout abnormal connections to the postsynaptic membrane. This results in the widening of the WDR neuronal field and lowering of the threshold for activation. These excess connections result in increased N-methyl-D-aspartic acid (NMDA) receptors, making the NMDA-antagonist ketamine an excellent candidate for the treatment of chronic pain.[3]

Transient receptor potential vanilloid 1 is a canonical member of a superfamily of TRP ion channels and is a nonselective calcium channel.[21] TRP channels have been found to be ubiquitous among different cells. The naked mole rat have been found to lack TRPV1 resulting in loss of heat and low pH transduction.[22] TRPV1 has been found to be upregulated in neuropathic pain syndromes along with the proinflammatory pathway of protein kinase C epsilon. The utilization of capsaicin to activate TRPV1 has been used to treat chronic pain syndromes. However, the use limited studies are available in the prevention in the upregulation of TRPV1 to prevent the development of chronic pain. Multiple compounds have been found to either activate or inhibit TRPV1 but at this time, few are in clinical practice.[23]

PREVENTION AND MANAGEMENT

The treatment of chronic pain involves a multimodal and often multidisciplinary approach. Preemptive analgesia is the introduction of analgesic therapy prior to noxious stimuli such as surgical incision. With surgical stimulation resulting in tissue damage both mechanisms of peripheral and central sensitization are activated. The goal of preemptive analgesia is to prevent this sensitization process by decreasing the nociceptive barrage. The mechanism for sensitization has not been fully elucidated but the underlying mechanism is the overstimulation of spinal neurons results in sensitization. Patients with risk factors as discussed earlier, need to be identified and interventions must be considered throughout the entire perioperative period to mitigate the development of CPSP. The perioperative surgical home may be able to implement this framework.

Animal studies have shown that preemptive analgesia may prevent the development of chronic pain. Animals models have shown that infiltration with local anesthetic prevents central sensitization.[24] Several meta-analyses have been published concerning preemptive analgesia with mixed results. Patient and surgical heterogeneity, along with the many different types of preemptive analgesia used may play a role in the inconsistency of outcomes. At this time, it is unclear which medications or interventions, and for which surgical procedures will be most likely to be effective in the prevention of the development of CPSP.

Preemptive analgesia encompasses multiple interventional measures. They may be divided into pharmacological and procedural interventions. Pharmacological preemptive analgesia involves the use of agents taken preoperatively to decrease the risk of severe postoperative pain and may subsequently decrease opioid consumption. Agents commonly used include nonsteroidal anti-inflammatory drugs (NSAIDs), gabapentinoids, and ketamine.

Steroidal and Nonsteroidal Anti-inflammatory Drugs

Inflammatory mediators and cytokines have been linked to the causation of the development of chronic pain and the use of anti-inflammatory agents appears to attenuate the development of chronic pain. During a noxious stimulus in which cell membranes are damaged, cyclooxygenase 2 (COX-2) converts arachidonic acid from the lipid bilayer to prostaglandin E2 (PGE2), a molecule that further mediates the noxious environment and promotes signal transduction. COX-2 ultimately promotes further sensitization and plays a role in central sensitization.[3,25] Anti-inflammatory agents have been linked to the prevention of the development of chronic pain from noxious stimuli. Steroidal and NSAIDs comprise this class of agents. Currently, there are more than 20 different NSAIDs with multiple modes of administration to a patient. COX-1 enzyme creates prostanoids that promote protection of the gastric mucosa, while COX-2 promotes the production of inflammatory agents, thromboxanes and prostaglandins. Inhibition of COX-2 decreases the extent of the inflammatory process and decreases pain. Two commonly used NSAIDs are celecoxib a COX-2 inhibitor and ibuprofen a nonselective COX-1 and COX-2 inhibitor. The use of both selective and nonselective COX-2 inhibitors to limit the inflammatory process as a preemptive analgesia however has yielded mixed results.[25,26]

Lakjda et al. published a double-blinded placebo-controlled study in 1997, investigating the effect of ibuprofen 400 mg administration prior surgical procedure, 2 hours after surgical procedure, followed by every 8 hours.[27] A follow-up at 6 months showed no difference in the development of CPSP in the placebo group. Celecoxib at a low dose of 200 mg was shown to be superior than ibuprofen at 600 mg in controlling postsurgical pain.[26] Overall, the evidence for NSAIDs as preemptive analgesia are mixed, likely due to the heterogeneity of the studies. Often times, NSAIDs are not used as the sole drug for analgesia. Combining an NSAID with low dose tramadol was found to decrease the transition of acute low back pain to chronic pain. Further investigation is needed to assess the role of NSAIDs and CPSP.

The administration of steroid into the epidural space to treat disc herniation is a long standing and common practice. Radiculopathy from an inflamed nerve root is targeted using an interlaminar or transforaminal approach. The utility of steroids in radicular low back pain appear to be limited by route of administration. A targeted injection of steroid into the epidural space minimizes side effects of steroid. Furthermore, in a study performed in patients with acute low back pain, oral prednisone at 50 mg daily for 5 days to treat acute low back pain was no better than placebo with respect to pain scores and patient activity.[28]

Gabapentinoids

Gabapentinoids are derivatives of γ-aminobutyric acid (GABA) and targets the α2-subunit of presynaptic voltage-dependent calcium channels and classified as anticonvulsants. The mechanism of function involves decreased glutamate release in the presynaptic junction, causing an attenuation in excitation. Gabapentinoids have been shown to decrease postoperative pain scores and opioid consumption. The two most commonly used are gabapentin and pregabalin. Gabapentin has been shown to be safe and effective as an agent for preemptive analgesia. The optimal dose of gabapentin has not been fully elucidated but a study by Schmidt et al. recommend a dose of 1,200 mg administered orally 2 hours prior to surgery and 300 mg three times a day in the postoperative period. Lower doses at 600 or 900 mg of gabapentin preoperatively have also shown some appears to be a safe and effective dose.[29] If not administered preoperatively, a dose of gabapentin postoperatively may still confer benefit as shown in a recent Cochrane review.[30] In a large randomized, placebo-controlled, double-blind trial of pregabalin administered prior to total knee arthroplasty (TKA) and during the immediate postoperative period, 0% of patients with pregabalin developed neuropathic pain while about 9% of the placebo group developed neuropathic pain at 2 months.[31] This study was limited to patients for TKA and may limit its applicability to other patient populations. Gabapentinoids are generally well tolerated although side effects do occur, which include sedation, dizziness and confusion. These side effects may be more likely during the postoperative period when administered as preemptive analgesia.[29]

Ketamine

Ketamine is an NMDA receptor antagonist with both anesthetic and analgesic properties and has been shown to provide excellent analgesic benefits for neuropathic pain syndromes at low doses. Ketamine also enhances the descending inhibitory pathway and may also have anti-inflammatory properties.[32] Along with NMDA antagonism, animal studies have shown some effect on the μ-opioid receptors.[33] Low dose (0.5 mg/kg) ketamine bolus to surgical incision have been shown to decrease postoperative pain scores at rest and movement, and decrease opioid consumption with minimal hemodynamic effects. An intraoperative ketamine infusion of 0.25 mg/kg/h after the bolus administration has also been recommended. The optimal dose and duration of ketamine remains to be elucidated.

Mechanistically, ketamine would seem to be an excellent candidate to prevent chronic pain as it targets the "windup" phenomenon of the WDR neurons. However, there are a limited number of studies that investigate the efficacy of ketamine as a preemptive mode of analgesia to prevent the development of chronic pain. A randomized, double-blinded, placebo-controlled clinical trial by Duale et al. in which thoracotomy patients were randomized to perioperative ketamine infusion versus normal saline for 24 hours showed no difference in the incidence of post-thoracotomy pain syndrome at 6 weeks and 4 months after surgery.[34] Currently there are multiple protocols for ketamine infusions. Significant heterogeneity exists among perioperative ketamine studies. Further studies are needed to determine optimal patient/surgical population and ketamine regimen. However, it is also important to keep in mind that glutamate also activates not only NMDA receptors but α-amino-3-hydroxy-5-methyl-4-isoxazolepropionic acid (AMPA) receptor and metabotropic glutamate receptor 5 (mGluR5), which ketamine does not antagonize.[3]

Regional Anesthesia

The utility of regional anesthesia to prevent the development of CPSP has been promising. A Cochrane review of 23 randomized control trials comparing regional anesthesia and general anesthesia in preventing the development of CPSP at 6 months and 12 months postprocedure, showed that epidural anesthesia prevented the development of CPSP in patients who underwent thoracotomy. The study also favored paravertebral blocks for the prevention of CPSP in patients who received mastectomy.[35] This large-scale study signifies the importance of preemptive analgesia using regional anesthetic technique. More studies are needed for other surgical procedures although the principal theory of preventing central sensitization by preventing nociceptive input into the central nervous system may be applicable to other postsurgical pain syndromes.

CONCLUSION

Chronic pain costs the US health care system more than cancer, coronary artery disease, and diabetes management.[36] According to the Center for Disease Control, nearly 50 million surgical procedures were performed in 2009. The development of chronic pain from acute pain remains to be a complex, multifactorial, and costly phenomenon. More research is needed in understanding the transition of acute to chronic pain along with preventative measures. If the development of chronic pain can be prevented by aggressively treating acute pain or utilizing preemptive measures, then the burgeoning of this patient population may be controlled, subsequently help alleviate further consequences such as opioid dependence/addiction, poor patient quality of life, and lost productivity. It is critical for physicians to provide measures to prevent the transformation of acute pain to chronic pain. Such measures are needed prior to the surgical insult as in the case of preemptive analgesia thus requiring active thinking in the preoperative period. The perioperative surgical home may play a significant role in implementing a framework to identify patients at risk for developing CPSP. A personalized approach to perioperative pain management due to the emerging role of genetics in CPSP may also be seen in the future.

REFERENCES

1. Reddi D. Preventing chronic postoperative pain. Anaesthesia. 2016;71(Suppl 1):64-71.
2. Clarke H, Katz J, Flor H, Rietschel M, Diehl SR, Seltzer Z. Genetics of chronic post-surgical pain: a crucial step toward personal pain medicine. Can J Anaesth. 2015;62(3):294-303.
3. Voscopoulos C, Lema M. When does acute pain become chronic? Br J Anaesth. 2010;105(Suppl 1):i69-85.
4. Crombie IK, Davies HT, Macrae WA. Cut and thrust: antecedent surgery and trauma among patients attending a chronic pain clinic. Pain. 1998;76(1-2):167-71.
5. Thomas T, Robinson C, Champion D, McKell M, Pell M. Prediction and assessment of the severity of postoperative pain and of satisfaction with management. Pain. 1998;75(2-3):177-85.
6. Macrae WA. Chronic pain after surgery. Br J Anaesth. 2001;87(1):88-98.
7. Hanley MA, Jensen MP, Smith DG, Ehde DM, Edwards WT, Robinson LR. Preamputation pain and acute pain predict chronic pain after lower extremity amputation. J Pain. 2007;8(2):102-9.
8. Nikolajsen L, Jensen TS. Phantom limb pain. Br J Anaesth. 2001;87(1):107-16.
9. Wallace MS, Wallace AM, Lee J, Dobke MK. Pain after breast surgery: a survey of 282 women. Pain. 1996;66(2-3):195-205.
10. Peters ML, Sommer M, de Rijke JM, Kessels F, Heineman E, Patijn J, et al. Somatic and psychologic predictors of long-term unfavorable outcome after surgical intervention. Ann Surg. 2007;245(3):487-94.
11. Kuponiyi O, Alleemudder DI, Latunde-Dada A, Eedarapalli P. Nerve injuries associated with gynaecological surgery. Obstet Gynaecol. 2014;16(1):29-36.
12. Niraj G, Rowbotham DJ. Persistent postoperative pain: where are we now? Br J Anaesth. 2011;107(1):25-9.
13. Young EE, Lariviere WR, Belfer I. Genetic basis of pain variability: recent advances. J Med Genet. 2012;49(1):1-9.
14. Zubieta JK, Heitzeg MM, Smith YR, Bueller JA, Xu K, Xu Y, et al. COMT val158met genotype affects mu-opioid neurotransmitter responses to a pain stressor. Science. 2003;299(5610):1240-3.
15. Neil MJ, Macrae WA. Post Surgical Pain—The Transition from Acute to Chronic Pain. Rev Pain. 2009;3(2):6-9.
16. Buchheit T, Van de Ven T, Shaw A. Epigenetics and the transition from acute to chronic pain. Pain Med. 2012;13(11):1474-90.

17. Javierre BM, Fernandez AF, Richter J, Al-Shahrour F, Martin-Subero JI, Rodriguez-Ubreva J, et al. Changes in the pattern of DNA methylation associate with twin discordance in systemic lupus erythematosus. Genome Res. 2010;20(2):170-9.
18. Kiguchi N, Kobayashi Y, Maeda T, Fukazawa Y, Tohya K, Kimura M, et al. Epigenetic augmentation of the macrophage inflammatory protein 2/C-X-C chemokine receptor type 2 axis through histone H3 acetylation in injured peripheral nerves elicits neuropathic pain. J Pharmacol Exp Ther. 2012;340(3):577-87.
19. Katz J, Seltzer Z. Transition from acute to chronic postsurgical pain: risk factors and protective factors. Expert Rev Neurother. 2009;9(5):723-44.
20. Apkarian AV, Baliki MN, Farmer MA. Predicting transition to chronic pain. Curr Opin Neurol. 2013;26(4):360-7.
21. Holzer P, Izzo AA. The pharmacology of TRP channels. Br J Pharmacol. 2014;171(10):2469-73.
22. Malek N, Pajak A, Kolosowska N, Kucharczyk M, Starowicz K. The importance of TRPV1-sensitisation factors for the development of neuropathic pain. Mol Cell Neurosci. 2015;65:1-10.
23. Carnevale V, Rohacs T. TRPV1: A Target for Rational Drug Design. Pharmaceuticals (Basel). 2016;9(3).
24. Coderre TJ, Vaccarino AL, Melzack R. Central nervous system plasticity in the tonic pain response to subcutaneous formalin injection. Brain Res. 1990;535(1):155-8.
25. Inage K, Orita S, Yamauchi K, Suzuki T, Suzuki M, Sakuma Y, et al. Low-Dose Tramadol and Non-Steroidal Anti-Inflammatory Drug Combination Therapy Prevents the Transition to Chronic Low Back Pain. Asian Spine J. 2016;10(4):685-9.
26. Costa FW, Esses DF, de Barros Silva PG, Carvalho FS, Sá CD, Albuquerque AF, et al. Does the Preemptive Use of Oral Nonsteroidal Anti-inflammatory Drugs Reduce Postoperative Pain in Surgical Removal of Third Molars? A Meta-analysis of Randomized Clinical Trials. Anesth Prog. 2015;62(2):57-63.
27. Lakdja F, Dixmérias F, Bussières E, Fonrouge JM, Lobéra A. [Preventive analgesic effect of intraoperative administration of ibuprofen-arginine on postmastectomy pain syndrome]. Bull Cancer. 1997;84(3):259-63.
28. Eskin B, Shih RD, Fiesseler FW, Walsh BW, Allegra JR, Silverman ME, et al. Prednisone for emergency department low back pain: a randomized controlled trial. J Emerg Med. 2014;47(1):65-70.
29. Schmidt PC, Ruchelli G, Mackey SC, Carroll IR. Perioperative gabapentinoids: choice of agent, dose, timing, and effects on chronic postsurgical pain. Anesthesiology. 2013;119(5):1215-21.
30. Straube S, Derry S, Moore RA, Wiffen PJ, McQuay HJ. Single dose oral gabapentin for established acute postoperative pain in adults. Cochrane Database Syst Rev. 2010(5):CD008183.
31. Buvanendran A, Kroin JS, Della Valle CJ, Kari M, Moric M, Tuman KJ. Perioperative oral pregabalin reduces chronic pain after total knee arthroplasty: a prospective, randomized, controlled trial. Anesth Analg. 2010;110(1):199-207.
32. Niesters M, Martini C, Dahan A. Ketamine for chronic pain: risks and benefits. Br J Clin Pharmacol. 2014;77(2):357-67.
33. Sarton E, Teppema LJ, Olievier C, Nieuwenhuijs D, Matthes HW, Kieffer BL, et al. The involvement of the mu-opioid receptor in ketamine-induced respiratory depression and antinociception. Anesth Analg. 2001;93(6):1495-500, table of contents.
34. Duale C, Sibaud F, Guastella V, Vallet L, Gimbert YA, Taheri H, et al. Perioperative ketamine does not prevent chronic pain after thoracotomy. Eur J Pain. 2009;13(5):497-505.
35. Cheng GS, Ilfeld BM. An Evidence-Based Review of the Efficacy of Perioperative Analgesic Techniques for Breast Cancer-Related Surgery. Pain Med; 2016.
36. Gaskin DJ, Richard P. The economic costs of pain in the United States. J Pain. 2012;13(8):715-24.

CHAPTER 4

Chronic Pain

Neel Mehta, Timothy Connolly

DEFINITION

While acute nociceptive pain serves as a biologically necessary marker of inflamed or damaged tissue, chronic pain fails to serve physiologic purpose and can be thus defined as overwhelmingly pathologic in nature. Chronic pain is devoid of the innate adaptive and protective functions intrinsic to acute pain. The underlying pathology, if accompanying the symptomatic chronic pain patient, frequently cannot fully explain the presence nor severity of the patient's pain.

Chronic pain is a multifaceted disorder comprised of physical, psychological, and social components. The extensive variability in symptoms and severity compounds the difficulty in the therapeutic approach. Chronic pain has been defined in contemporary literature as unresolving pain lasting for a period of time longer than 3 to 6 months.[1-3] A more encompassing definition, presented by Merskey had defined chronic pain as simply that which persists beyond the duration of underlying tissue damage.[4] The benefit gained by the latter definition is in bypassing the dilemma of holding a largely variable disease process to such objective temporal constraints. The definition presented by the American Society of Anesthesiologists (ASA) analogously follows Merskey in citing chronic pain to be "beyond the expected temporal boundary of tissue injury and normal healing, and adversely affecting the function or well-being of the individual".[5]

The impediment to descriptions intentionally devoid of explicit time constraints lies in the determination of when it becomes appropriate to address the afflicted patient as suffering from chronic pain. The distinction between acute and chronic pain has no clear watershed moment, and it is this ambiguity that compounds on the therapeutic challenge. The evolution of acute into chronic pain is complex with both physiologic, psychological and social aspects. The elusive nature of pain lies within the fact that it's perceived quality and severity is influenced by the context in which it is experienced.

A painful stimulus interferes with the patient's conscious thought processes, evolutionarily designed to draw focus towards a perceived threat to the individual's well-being. While serving a beneficial adaptive purpose in the acute state, the psychological, social and behavioral consequences of such perpetual cognitive interference can lead to detrimental outcomes for the suffering patient. The impact of the patient's condition can take a substantial toll on not only their well-being, but on their emotional health, profession, and personal relationships. The challenges of chronic pain translate correspondingly to the practitioner, with requirements similar to any chronic disease such as diabetes and congestive heart failure. This may include resource intense treatments, a need for further guidelines and algorithms, and a variety of ailments.

Chronic pain can be involve ereliance on the patient's given description of their pain, owing to the personal and subjective experiences of their affliction. Chronic pain is distinctive from most all other disease processes in it's multicomponent nature. In addition to the principal sensory and discriminative component, localizing location and severity, there will often be affixed affective, emotional and even cognitive elements. Thus unequivocal terminology is a necessity to best determine the likely etiology and most efficacious path for treatment. As seen in the acute pain chapter, there are several overlapping features and decscriptors.

- Nociceptive pain: Pain attributable to trauma or noxious stimuli. Physiologic in nature
- Neuropathic pain: Pathologic constitution. pain due to prior nerve injury, thought secondary to peripheral and central reorganization
- Inflammatory pain: Pain attributable to tissue injury without neural component. Can be categorized as physiologic or pathologic
- Allodynia: Pain secondary to a stimulus containing no intrinsic painful properties
- Hyperalgesia: Disproportionately elevated perception of pain in response to a noxious stimulus.

PREVALENCE

Chronic pain is one of the most common healthcare afflictions, affecting anywhere between 20 and 37% of the world's population.[6] The Institute of Medicine (IOM) estimates the prevalence of chronic pain conditions to afflict more than 116 million individuals within the United States alone, and constitutes a patient population larger than cardiac disease, cancer and diabetes combined.[7] The etiologies of specific ailments attributed to these chronic pain conditions were largely musculoskeletal pain, with low back pain comprising the most common identifiable cause. According to a 2008 National Health and Nutrition Examination Survey (NHANES), the estimated prevalence of back pain within the population was 10.1%. This was followed by pain localized to the lower extremities, affecting 7.1% of patients, the upper extremities (4.1%), and lastly by those with pain due to headaches (3.5%).[8] About 19% of adults in the United States report persistent pain throughout their daily lives,[9] with more than 126 million US adults afflicted by a pain condition within the past 3 months.[10]

Epidemiological studies into the prevalence and trends of chronic pain provide necessary data to begin to formulate the appropriate treatment modalities for these patients. This is important in not only understanding the etiology of chronic pain patients within the developed world, but the developing world as well. The Global Burden of Disease Study compiled data on global injuries and diseases for 188 countries between 1990 and 2013, utilizing the metric of years lived with disability (YLDs). Chronic pain conditions comprised half of the top 10 leading causes of global YLDs, with marked consistency noted across most all nations. Lower back pain was found to be the overwhelmingly preeminent contributor, with over 72 million YLDs attributed.[11] Lower back pain was found to be the leading cause of YLDs in 86 of the 188 nations, and either the second or third leading cause for an additional 61 countries. Over 34 million YLDs were as a result of neck pain, nearly 29 million YLDs due to chronic migraines, and 22.6 million YLDs caused by chronic musculoskeletal pain secondary to disorders such as shoulder pain, hip, and joint disease, as well as arthritis. These conditions often affect women more than men, with an increasing prevalence for both genders seen with increasing age appreciated in the literature

However, there are limitations with these studies.

These studies are often faced with the difficult task of a multitude of confounders. Chronic pain is known to have an increasing prevalence within the population as age increases, however, proper evaluation of the true etiology of pain becomes difficult with the concomitantly rising incidence of multimorbidity in this age group. Whereas moderate to severe pain has been found to only affect approximately 5% of children and adolescents, up to 44% patients 65 years of age and greater are afflicted by some form of chronic pain.[12,13] The difficulty becomes in appropriately addressing the primary cause of the chronic pain in the setting of additional effects of disease interactions.

ECONOMICS

The economic impact of patients with chronic pain conditions constitute a significant cost to the healthcare system as a whole. In the United States, the annual cost of treating conditions rooted in pain has been found to be higher than heart disease, cancer and diabetes.[14] In an analysis of more than 20,000 individuals between 2008 to 2010 the IOM found the mean yearly health care spending on patients with severe pain to be nearly $9,000 more than for those without pain. The direct healthcare costs related to pain conditions were found to be between $261 and $300 billion annually.[15] The substantial impact of direct costs to the pain patient and healthcare system are significantly augmented when accounting for factors that consider the harm done to the productivity of the individual. The estimated losses due to days of work missed ranges between $11.6 and $12.7 billion. Up to $96.5 billion is lost due to individual hours of lost productivity, and between $190.6 and $226.3 billion attributed to a compensatory decline in wages. When accounting for the whole fiscal scope impacted by chronic pain, the estimated healthcare cost within the United States alone can range from $560 to $635 billion.[16]

Pain conditions are one of the most common afflictions resulting in lost productive time and work hours. Data from the American Productivity Audit estimates a loss of over $61 billion each year due to lost productive time from pain-associated conditions, accounting for 12.7% of individuals comprising the United State workforce.[17] The impact on the workforce and increasing economic consequences pose a significant public health challenge. Recent years continue to show the demographic proportion of older adults within the global population progressively increasing in most all nations. The continued rise in an aging population come following a multitude of advancements in healthcare and comprehensive gains in life expectancy.[18] This can lead to increasing costs for something as common as low back pain, P with decreased compensation for affected patients.[19] Furthermore, Iit is estimated that up to 20% of all primary care visits are secondary to pain conditions.[20]

CLASSIFICATION

Establishing a taxonomy to best classify the array of disorders that comprise chronic pain is intrinsic to the proper evaluation of the patient. A comprehensive model for diagnosis will optimize the understanding of the disorder and lay the necessary groundwork towards the path of optimal treatment. Constructing a model to accurately diagnose between related disorders is an established and familiar concept within the medical field, yet the multifaceted nature of chronic pain has separated it from other fields. Restrictive "cause-and-effect" models of diagnosis are essential to the many disorders that require identification of a solitary etiology, yet cannot successfully capture disease states with such multitudinal origins.

Chronic pain is traditionally preceded with the qualifying description of malignant or nonmalignant pain. Pain secondary to cancerous origins more accurately represents an ongoing collection of nociceptive stimuli, classically more analogous to acute pain than chronic pain. Chronic pain due to noncancerous origins is more aptly described in this sense, as the converse term "benign" chronic pain beguiles a misleading and incorrect terminology in describing the potentially debilitating conditions that fall within its domain.

While there are several methods of categorizing chronic pain from noncancerous origins, an encompassing classification consists of chronic pain due to inflammation, musculoskeletal pain, neuropathic pain, chronic headache pain, and chronic recurrent pain. The latter comprises chronically resurgent pain secondary to acute injury to tissue, such as osteoarthritis and sickle cell disease.

The current framework for chronic pain conditions, as according to the International Association for the Study of pain (IASP), has grouped the multiple etiologies of pain conditions into seven separate categories. These include chronic musculoskeletal pain, chronic visceral pain, chronic headache and orofacial pain, chronic posttraumatic and postsurgical pain, neuropathic pain, cancer pain, and chronic primary pain. The IASP has successfully collaborated with the World Health Organization (WHO) and begun the integration of this subcategorization of chronic pain conditions into the 11th revision of the WHO's International Classification of Diseases (ICD-11).[21] The IASP task force has placed forth a classification system of coding chronic pain as a distinct diagnosis in itself. The new ICD category for chronic pain as a panoptic heading for its family of disease is subcategorized by perceived anatomic location, etiology, or affected system. Each of the seven categories are built upon content models in the description of the clinical characteristics of their respective branch of chronic pain conditions, with inclusion for psychosocial factors as well as number of modifiable variables to constitute pain quality and severity. This approach significantly improves the approach to chronic pain conditions, in that it is recognized as the distinct clinical disease process it is, rather than the outcome or result of other clinical conditions.

CAUSES

While the detailed explanation of each of the chronic pain conditions is beyond this chapter and is gone into more detail elsewhere in this book, it is useful to broadly mention and categorize the causes as follows:
- Anatomic
  - Headache
  - Craniofacial
  - Neck and upper extremity
  - Lower back pain
  - Abdominopelvic
  - Lower extremity pain
- Widespread/neuropathic
  - Fibromyalgia
  - Complex regional pain syndrome
  - Diabetic neuropathy
  - Post-stroke
  - Spinal cord injury
  - Multiple sclerosis
- Cancer.

ETIOLOGY

The acute pain pathway evolved as a protective biologic mechanism in order to identify real or potential tissue damage an injury. Peripheral nociceptive fibers, when triggered by a noxious stimulus, will send afferent signals towards the spinal cord, where they synapse within the dorsal horn. The afferent peripheral fibers consist of myelinated A-delta fibers, which constitute the rapid, sharp initial pain sensed by the individual, as well as unmyelinated C-fibers, mediating the slow burning pain persisting at the site of original injury. The afferent impulse travels the ascending projections of the anterior portion of the spinothalamic tract (STT) following synapse with respective neurons in lamina IV-V. Once projected to the second order neurons, the impulse ascends after crossing midline at the anterior white commissure. Second order neurons then project the impulse into the thalamus.

It is important to note that normal physiology of transmitting input from peripheral nociceptors to second order neurons Is mediated by cellular depolarization resulting in an action potential propagating towards the higher order neural pathways. These synaptic transmissions propagated between nociceptors and dorsal horn neurons serve a physiological function to protect from an identified noxious stimulus with eventual return to a set baseline. Continued or prolonged excitation of peripheral nociceptors can permit for a pathologic increase in subsequent output and for a markedly longer window of time the individual will be afflicted by the original insult.

A novel approach to the concept depicting the means by which sensory information is processed at the spinal cord was first proposed in 1965 by Ronald Melzack and Patrick Wall.[22] They postulated a gate-control theory as a means of describing a physiological mechanism by which psychological factors could mediate the perception of pain. They described a model in which all pain signals and information must pass through a "gate" in or near the substantia gelatinosa if the spinal cord in which only particular impulses would be allowed to transmit to the brain. This would, in turn, relay transmission of pain signals to the brainstem and cerebral cortex. This narrow gate, therefore, would be one that can open and close, thereby modulating the sensation of pain. They described pain, therefore, to not simply be a direct result of activation of receptor neurons, but rather a modulated perception through interactions amongst different neurons. In the absence of a noxious stimulus, inhibitory interneurons sit at the substantia gelatinosa blocking activation of projection neurons connecting to the brain. With a painful stimulus, signals carried by the peripheral afferent A-delta and C fibers will activate projection neurons connecting to the brain, as well as inhibit the attempt of inhibitory cells to block the output of the projection neuron that connects with the brain, thus "opening" the gate. Peripheral pain is then successfully transmitted to the spinal cord, hypothalamus, and cerebral cortex. Conversely, however, collateral projections from proprioceptive myelinated fibers will activate the inhibitory cells, leading to subsequent inhibition of noxious signal transmission. This mode of transmission thus closes the gate and limits pain stimuli from reaching the higher nervous system centers. This theory can be appreciated clinically with appreciable lessening of pain following the application of pressure over a site of acute injury.

Melzack and Wall additionally postulated the important concept of similar gating mechanism within nerve fibers originating from the thalamus and cortex and transmitted to the descending spinal tracts. Influence from cerebral and brainstem centers regulating concept and emotion can thus influence the intensity and volume of pain signals. The inhibitory effects of these impulses originate principally from periaqueductal grey matter (PAG) within the midbrain and raphe nucleus magnus (RNM) of the medulla. Neurotransmitters released from these sites produce activation of the inhibitory interneurons within the substantia gelatinosa, and thus reduce the transmission of pain. The perceptual notion of pain is, therefore, best conceptualized by not merely a transmission of a noxious stimulus, but a dynamic modulation depending on the individual's cognitive and emotional experience. Analogous to the functional alterations and neuroplastic changes seen of sensitized peripheral nociceptors, plasticity and "central sensitization" of the higher order nervous system with corresponding functional alterations in clinical pain modulation is an intrinsic perpetrator to many chronic pain disorders.[23]

While the role of plasticity in the reorganization of neural function has been long established, only recently have we been able to demonstrate a corresponding effect in the reorganization of neural structure. The rapid technological advances of recent years has provided innovative advancements in the approach to understanding the pathophysiology of chronic pain.

Recently, functional magnetic resonance imaging (fMRI) has shown chronic clinical pain conditions are often associated with decreased baseline activity or decreased stimulus related activity in the thalamus.[24] These studies have demonstrated patterns of altered brain function and neurochemistry[25] with the potential to not only identify markers and sequences of chronic pain but another approach for treatment.

SOCIAL AND PSYCHOLOGICAL IMPACT

The psychological effects of pain are well known to all individuals afflicted by an acute painful experience during the course of their lives. The predominating focus of the mind becomes engrossed by the foci of pain, detracting away from work, family, friends and interests. The return to a normal state of being intrinsically depends on the resolution of the painful stimulus over time. Patients suffering from pain devoid of such resolution will consequently and almost inevitably suffer a similarly prolonged course of social and psychological harms. The persistence of pain is wrought with changes in personality; distress from prolonged suffering results largely in a predictable withdrawal and depression with lapses in previously held personal goals and responsibilities. It is paramount for the practitioner to appreciate the multifaceted nature of chronic pain, with cognizance given to the interdependent fibers required for the generation of chronic pain.

There has been a progressive evolution over the past several decades in creating the modern comprehensive model of chronic pain. The traditional biomedical model of health, derived from Louis Pasteur's germ theory, conceptualizes illness as purely biologic factors devoid of environmental, psychological, or social components. While the biomedical model has demonstrated great efficacy in the diagnosis and treatment of innumerous disease processes, such a restrictive model has failed to fully depict the domain of chronic pain. The absence of an algorithmic structure predictively demonstrating clear cause-and-effect pathology obligates a multimodal approach in modeling this disease.

Pain is both variable and modifiable, not only by medical or physical interventions, but by the patients themselves. The cognitive and emotional impact of pain on the individual heavily dictates the severity of its subjective nature. Even before the turn of the 20th century, Sir William Osler advocated physicians to "...care more particularly for the individual patient than for the special features of the disease."[26] Similar nociceptive stimuli will yield markedly variable perceived attributes of pain depending on the individual, their culture, and personal experiences. It is important to identify and understand the separate entities of nociceptive stimuli and the perception of pain. There is a remarkably vast gradient in the correlation between these two values. The development of chronic pain leads to a continual focalization of the mind towards the perceived noxious stimulus. The predominant majority of the patient's consciousness is unremittingly centralized around the painful sensation.

Patients attach meaning to pain, the variable nature of which will greatly influence the degree and quality of their expressed pain.

Patients with chronic pain who report to their primary care vs those who seek out pain specialists may have starkly different perceptions of both their level of distress and perceived severity of their illness.

This pain can lead to a cycle of psychological attributes which can feed into a cycle of perceived pain. The treatment should focus of directing the patient to focus on gaining "better control" of pain, encouraging "manageable pain" rather than feeding into cycle of failed treatments that lack ability to cure multifaceted roots.

CONCLUSION

Much work needs to be done to further research understanding of causes and treatment of chronic pain. Physicians must address patients of the current world, with many presenting already marred by attempts at self-education or self-diagnoses that have become exponentially available through virtual libraries and online communities.

These include use of proper education and explanations as a tool to ease any of these anxieties or psychologic factors augmenting their perceived pain.

REFERENCES

1. Merskey H, Bogduk N. Classification of chronic pain. 2nd ed. Seattle: IASP Press, 1994. p. 1
2. Treede R-D, Rief W, Barke A, et al. A classification of chronic pain for ICD-11.Pain. 2015;156(6):1003-7.
3. Bonica, John J. Bonica's Management of Pain. Eds. Scott Fishman, Jane Ballantyne, and James P. Rathmell. Lippincott Williams & Wilkins, 2010
4. Merskey, Harold Ed. Classification of chronic pain: Descriptions of chronic pain syndromes and definitions of pain terms. Pain (1986).
5. "Practice Guidelines for Chronic Pain Management." Anesthesiology 112.4 (2010): 810-33.
6. Tsang, Adley, et al. Common chronic pain conditions in developed and developing countries: gender and age differences and comorbidity with depression-anxiety disorders. J Pain. 2008;9(10):883-91.
7. Institute of Medicine (US). Committee on Advancing Pain Research, Care, and Education. Relieving pain in America: A blueprint for transforming prevention, care, education, and research. National Academies Press, 2011.
8. Hardt J, Jacobsen C, Goldberg J, et al. Prevalence of chronic pain in a representative sample in the United States. Pain Med 2008; 9:803.
9. J. Kennedy, J.M. Roll, T. Schraudner, S. Murphy, S. McPherson Prevalence of persistent pain in the U.S. adult population: New data from the 2010 National Health Interview Survey J Pain. 2014;15:979-84.
10. Nahin, Richard L. Estimates of pain prevalence and severity in adults: United States, 2012. J Pain. 2015;16(8):769-80.
11. Vos, Theo, et al. Global, regional, and national incidence, prevalence, and years lived with disability for 301 acute and chronic diseases and injuries in 188 countries, 1990–2013: a systematic analysis for the Global Burden of Disease Study 2013. Lancet. 386.9995 (2015): 743-800.
12. Groenewald CB, Essner BS, Wright D, Fesinmeyer MD, Palermo TM. The economic costs of chronic pain among a cohort of treatment-seeking adolescents in the United States. J Pain. 15(9), 925–933 (2014)
13. Scherer, Martin, et al. Association between multimorbidity patterns and chronic pain in elderly primary care patients: a cross-sectional observational study. BMC family practice 17.1 (2016): 1
14. Institute of Medicine (IOM). Relieving pain in America: a blueprint for transforming prevention, care, education, and research. Washington, DC: The National Academies Press, 2011.
15. Gaskin, D. J., and P. Richard. The Economic Costs of Pain in the United States. J Pain. 2012;13(8):715-24.
16. Institute of Medicine (IOM). Relieving pain in America: a blueprint for transforming prevention, care, education, and research. Washington, DC: The National Academies Press, 2011.
17. Stewart, Walter F, et al. Lost productive time and cost due to common pain conditions in the US workforce. Jama 290.18 (2003): 2443-2454.
18. Patel, Kushang V., et al. Prevalence and impact of pain among older adults in the United States: findings from the 2011 National Health and Aging Trends Study. Pain. 2013;154(12):2649-57.
19. Martin, Brook I, et al. Expenditures and health status among adults with back and neck problems. JAMA. 299.6 (2008): 656-64.
20. Mäntyselkä P, Kumpusalo E, Ahonen R, Kumpusalo A, Kauhanen J, Viinamäki H, Halonen P, Takala J. Pain as a reason to visit the doctor: a study in Finnish primary health care. Pain. 2001;89:175-80.

21. Treede, Rolf-Detlef, et al. "A classification of chronic pain for ICD-11." Pain156.6 (2015): 1003-7.
22. Melzack R, Wall PD. Pain mechanisms: A new theory. Science. 1965; 150:971-5.
23. Tracey, I. Imaging pain. Brit J Anaest. 2008;101(1) :32-9.
24. Apkarian, A. Vania, et al. Human brain mechanisms of pain perception and regulation in health and disease. Eur J Pain. 2005;9(4):463-3.
25. Harris, Richard E, et al. Pregabalin rectifies aberrant brain chemistry, connectivity, and functional response in chronic pain patients. J Am Soc Anesthesiol.2013;119(6): 1453-64.
26. Osler W. Address to the students of the Albany Medical College. Albany Medical Annals, 1899;20:307-9

CHAPTER 5

Interpretation of Blood Levels of Drugs Used in Chronic Pain Management

Urmila M Thatte, Maulik S Doshi

INTRODUCTION

Lance Armstrong (the American cyclist) once said "pain is temporary. It may last a minute, or an hour, or a day, or a year, but eventually it will subside and something else will take its place. If I quit, however, it lasts forever". Yet, the quest for the relief of pain has been known to man since time immemorial. And though the perception of and response to pain will vary, the desire for relief is universal.

All through history, man has searched for ways to relieve pain. From chewing the willow bark to modern pharmaceutical, the history of pain a pill is long and interesting. Yet, according to the World Health Organization, around 80% of the world's population does not have adequate access to pain relief today.[1] This chapter discusses the principles underlying therapeutic drug monitoring of pain medications.

GENERAL PRINCIPLES OF THERAPEUTIC DRUG MONITORING

The International Association of Therapeutic Drug Monitoring and Clinical Toxicology defines therapeutic drug monitoring (TDM) as "a measurement made in a laboratory of a parameter which, with appropriate interpretation, will directly influence prescribing procedures".[2]

Why? (Table 1)

Overall, the recommended dose of a drug is used as a basis for positive clinical outcome. However, this dose is recommended for the general population while in the clinic the physician treats the individual patient and

TABLE 1: Indications for therapeutic drug monitoring

• Drugs with low therapeutic index (antiepileptics, antidepressants like TCAs, etc.)
• Monitoring of special populations (children, elderly and pregnant female)
• Patients with hepatic or renal insufficiency
• Poisoning (e.g. paracetamol)
• To document interactions (St John's Wort and amitriptyline and methadone)
• To monitor drug compliance
• In absence of simple and clear clinical parameter available to evaluate the clinical efficacy (analgesics, antidepressant and antiepileptics)
• If there is large intra-and interindividual variability and unpredictability of the pharmacokinetic parameters
• Routine
• Nonresponders

not the population. In such cases, measuring the plasma concentration of a drug can help the physician to provide a better standard of care to the patients by maximizing efficacy and minimizing side effects.

Indications for the TDM (TABLE 1)

The concentration of a drug at the effector site would truly relate to the clinical response or toxicity. However, this concentration is not practically measurable. Therefore, plasma (or any other appropriate body fluid, like saliva) concentration is measured which reflects the concentration at effector site. Plasma concentration, therefore, can predict the clinical outcome and we can tweak this concentration to suit our requirements by modifying the dose. This is especially true when drugs do not have a classical response that is easily measured (no objective parameter to monitor clinical effect), e.g. anti-convulsant effect. This, then, is the crux of TDM. We do not do blood concentration measurements for all drugs. However, when a drugs has a low therapeutic index (antiepileptics, antidepressants like TCAs, etc.), i.e. the "safe" range of concentration in which we can keep a drug in the plasma is narrow, TDM becomes especially useful. If concentrations are in the higher range we can reduce the dose before debilitating side effects occur. Monitoring is especially useful in special populations (children, elderly and pregnant female), patients with hepatic or renal insufficiency, when multiple medications are being taken to avoid drug interactions (e.g. St. John's Wort and amitriptyline and methadone). Variability in drug clearance-in such patients (relevant for TCAs and antiepileptics) can have serious, even life-threatening consequences. As measuring pharmacokinetic parameters like clearance can be challenging in routine clinical practice, measuring the plasma drug concentration and/or genotyping the patient is useful to predict drug response. Sometimes TDM is useful to monitor compliance routinely and also to assess why a person is not responding (e.g. is it due to change in brand leading to altered bioavailability causing a diminished response?). Poisoning or overdose is also an indication for TDM.

Genetic polymorphisms in drug metabolizing enzymes (like CYP2C9 and CYP2C19) and drug transporter systems (e.g. ABCB1) is a very important cause for interindividual variations (Table 2) in drug response and TDM can help in terms of optimizing dosing schedules in such cases. In a study, conducted in our department, we found that TDM is more cost effective than pre-prescription genetic screening (CYP2C9 genetic polymorphism) in predicting toxicity of phenytoin.[3] A number of drugs (e.g. antidepressants and antiepileptics) act through a number of mechanisms and at

TABLE 2: Sources of variability in drug response[4,5]

Host factors	Drug factors
Demographic: Age, gender, weight	Drug-drug interactions
Health status: Comorbid conditions (hepatic, renal insufficiency, GI disturbances, thyroid, cardiac diseases)	Drug-food interactions
Genetic make-up	Formulations (immediate release, sustained release, etc.)
Phenotypic differences.	Physical properties (powder, hydrophillcity, nature of excipient, etc.)
Ethnicity Circadian effects	Route of administration

different biological sites (e.g. sodium valproate).[6] Hence, they produce different biological actions at different plasma concentrations.[7, 8] For example, tricyclic antidepressants inhibit norepinephrine reuptake (leading to an antidepressant effect) at the lowest concentrations. As plasma concentrations increase antihistaminic effects are seen (leading to sedation), followed by? Adrenergic blocking effects resulting in orthostatic hypotension, anticholinergic effects like dry mouth, constipation, serotonin reuptake blockade (exerting antidepressant effects) and finally inhibition of sodium conductance (leading to CNS and cardiotoxicity).[7-9] In such cases, when we are targeting specific actions (or avoiding certain side effects) it is useful to know the concentrations we have achieved so as to adjust the dosage.

For a number of drugs, the early stages of mild toxicity developed due to excessive plasma concentration may be clinically 'silent' (e.g. slowing of intracardiac conduction by TCAs) or can mimic worsening of a condition for which the drug was prescribed (e.g. insomnia and anorexia from a serotonin reuptake inhibitor). In such cases, TDM can help the clinician to optimize the dose and avoid toxicity. Drugs that are more than 80% plasma protein bound are good candidates for drug monitoring.[10] Anticonvulsants, such as phenytoin, carbamazepine and valproic acid, antidepressants such as TCAs and venlafaxine, opioids like methadone and buprenorphine are strongly protein bound drugs and, therefore, amenable to TDM.

Why Not?

There are times when TDM is not useful or is unnecessary. For example, if the effect or toxicity of a drug is not predictably related to its plasma concentration TDM has no value. Further, if dosage does not need to be individualized (high safety margins) TDM is not important.

How and when?

When drugs levels are requested by physicians for any of the above indications, for best results, blood (which is still the most popular biological fluid used for TDM: Others like saliva often present inherent methodological challenges and plasma concentrations most closely reflect the concentration at the site of action) is collected when the drug is expected to have achieved steady state concentrations at trough levels. Both these aspects are relevant to the best interpretation of results. Steady state concentration is the concentration when drug elimination equals to drug availability. Measuring drug levels at steady state allows for predicting of the dosage mathematically. The least variable point in the dosing interval is trough concentration (just prior to the next dose) and hence, this is preferred as the time point of collection. The reason we use this time point is that sometimes after the oral dose very high concentrations are achieved (e.g. after an oral dose, the levels of digoxin are often 2 ng/mL which is a toxic value), but no toxicity may occur.

Importantly, when drug toxicity is suspected and levels are ordered, any time point would be relevant as the level should at all times be below the toxic range.

In the Laboratory[11]

The laboratory will measure the drugs levels using the most appropriate analytical technique. The choice of the technique depends on the characteristics of the drug to be measured, the sensitivity, specificity and precision desired and the cost. The most common method used is the high performance liquid chromatography (HPLC) or more recently Liquid chromatography with mass spectrometry (LC-MS-MS). As a clinician it is important to ensure that the laboratory is maintaining appropriate quality assurance measures for this estimation as your clinical decisions will depend on the result given to you. Both internal and external quality control tests are run by laboratories to ensure that the best results are obtained.

Cost-effectiveness of TDM

The optimal use of TDM can lead to huge savings in terms of health resources, time and money. The potential savings include following costs:[12]
- Failed treatment because the dose was inadequate or too high
- Manpower and other resource utilization during a prolonged dose titration based on clinical response
- Treatment for adverse effects related to excessive plasma drug concentrations.

TDM OF CHRONIC PAIN MEDICATIONS

The clinical pharmacokinetic parameters of chronic pain medications namely are antiepileptics, antidepressants, opioids, and NSAIDs.

Antiepileptic Agents

The antiepileptics have been used in the management of neuropathic pain since five decades. They depress abnormal and excessive neuronal discharges and thus raise the threshold for neural impulse propagation. The older agents (phenytoin and carbamazepine) have been largely replaced due to the introduction of many newer, better-tolerated, and safer antiepileptic drug like gabapentine and lamotrigine.[13-15]

Gabapentin[14-19]

The efficacy of the GABA analog gabapentin in the treatment of painful diabetic neuropathy[20] (comparable to amitriptyline), post herpetic neuralgia and direct peripheral nerve injuries has been established over the last few years. There are case reports on its treatment benefit in various types of neuropathic pain states including headache and many others. The mechanism by which gabapentin exerts its benefits in neuropathic pain is not fully clear. Although earlier it was believed that central actions [enhanced inhibitory input of GABA-mediated pathways (thus reducing excitatory input levels), antagonism of NMDA receptors and antagonism of central voltage dependent L-type Ca^{2+} channels] underpinned its effects it pain, gabapentin has been shown to inhibit ectopic discharge activity from injured peripheral nerves.

The most common side effects are drowsiness, somnolence, ataxia, nausea, and fatigue. These side effects are usually self-limited and subside after a couple of weeks allowing gradual dose escalation. Recent case reports have suggested that gabapentin may cause reversible acute renal allograft dysfunction and Stevens–Johnson syndrome. Gabapentin can possibly unmask myasthenia gravis, and, therefore, should be used with caution in patients with this disease. The usual oral starting dose is 100–300 mg at bedtime, which can be gradually increased to 1200 mg/day (split into three doses) over 30–60 days. Some patients may require up to 3600 mg/day or more for clinical benefits. Gabapentin is actively absorbed via the L amino acid transporter system. There can a wide variation between patients in the absorption of gabapentin, though the within subject variability is small. As the carrier-dependent transport for gabapentin is saturable, its bioavailability varies inversely with the dose. The bioavailability of a 300 mg dose is approximately 60%, while that of a 600 mg dose is only 40%, and this further decreases to 35% at steady state with doses of 1600 mg three times daily. Peak plasma levels (C_{max}) of gabapentin of 2.7–2.99 mg/mL are achieved 3–3.2 hours after ingestion of a single 300 mg capsule. As a result of the dose-dependent saturable absorption of gabapentin, the C_{max} increases less than threefold when the dose is tripled from 300–900 mg. Twenty percent of plasma concentrations are achieved in the CSF, and have been estimated to range between 0.09 and 0.14 µg/mL. Brain tissue concentrations are almost 80% of the plasma level. Gabapentin is not metabolized in humans and is eliminated unchanged in the urine. It undergoes first-order kinetic elimination and renal impairment decreases gabapentin elimination in a linear fashion with a good correlation with creatinine clearance. As it is removed by hemodialysis, patients in renal failure must receive their maintenance dose after each dialysis. The elimination half-life of gabapentin is between 4.8 hours and 8.7 hours. Unlike other anticonvulsant drugs, it does not induce or inhibit hepatic microsomal enzymes.

Plasma drug monitoring is useful for dose individualization, and a therapeutic range of 2–15 μg/mL has been recommended.

Lamotrigine

Primarily developed as an anticonvulsant, lamotrigine has been shown to have efficacy in the treatment of trigeminal neuralgia, migraine headache and painful diabetic neuropathy.[21] It is an inhibitor of voltage gated Na^+ channels, suppresses excitatory glutamate release and inhibits serotonin reuptake thereby increasing its concentration in the synapse. Side effects include dizziness, diplopia, drowsiness, and rash. The rash occurs in up to 10% of patients. Dosing is started at 25–50 mg/day and increased by 50 mg/day per week until analgesia is reached or to a maximum of 900 mg/day administered twice or thrice a day.

Carbamazepine

Carbamazepine was introduced by Blom in the early 1960s and has now become the primary agent for treatment of trigeminal and glossopharyngeal neuralgia.[22-24] The efficacy of this medication in trigeminal neuralgia and other lancinating pain has been shown in three well designed double blind, placebo controlled crossover studies. It is also effective for lightning tabetic pain associated with bodily wasting. Most patients with neuralgia benefit initially, but only 70% obtain lasting relief. The effect appears to be mediated by a slowing of the rate of recovery of voltage-activated Na^+ channels from inactivation. Adverse effects have required discontinuation of medication in 5–20% of patients. The starting dose is 200 mg twice a day, with the effective dose ranging from 400 to 1000 mg/day. During long-term therapy, the more frequent untoward effects of the drug include drowsiness, vertigo, ataxia, diplopia, and blurred vision. Aplastic anemia can occur in 1:200,000 patients, more commonly a reversible leukopenia and thrombocytopenia can be seen.

It significantly induces the P450 cytochrome system thereby increases phenytoin metabolism. Phenobarbital, phenytoin, and valproate may increase the metabolism of carbamazepine by inducing CYP3A4. Unfortunately, unlike with phenytoin, there is no simple relationship between the dose of carbamazepine and concentrations of the drug in plasma. The therapeutic range of plasma concentrations for antiseizure therapy also serves as a guideline for its use in neuralgia.[25]

Therapeutic concentrations are reported to be 4 to 12 μg/mL, although considerable variation occurs. Side effects referable to the CNS are frequent at concentrations above 9 mg/mL.

Phenytoin

In the 1970s several trials were completed to evaluate the efficacy of phenytoin in painful diabetic neuropathy with mixed results. It is also described to be useful in trigeminal neuralgias although carbamazepine has replaced phenytoin in this indication by and large.

The usual dose of phenytoin in painful diabetic neuropathy is 200 to 400 mg/day. The desired therapeutic range for phenytoin is 10–20 μg/mL. The values below 10 μg/mL are considered sub-therapeutic and dose may have to be increased while those above 20 μg/mL are considered as potentially toxic and dose must be reduced. It is important to note that in our populations, these cut-offs may be lower, with control achieved at concentrations of 8 or 9 μg/mL.

The most common side effects are nausea, diplopia, dizziness, confusion, gingival hyperplasia, and rarely Stevens-Johnson syndrome. It also induces the P450 system.

Tiagabine and Vigabatrin

A gamma-aminobutyric acid (GABA) reuptake inhibitor and a GABA metabolism inhibitor respectively with future potential for the treatment of painful conditions.[26]

The clinical pharmacokinetic parameters of anti-epileptic drugs are given in Table 3.

Antidepressants, Tricyclic antidepressants, together with anticonvulsants, are considered to be first-line drugs for the treatment of neuropathic pain. Anti-depressants are analgesic in patients with chronic pain and no concomitant depression, indicating that the analgesic and antidepressant effects occur independently. The analgesia induced by these drugs seems to be centrally mediated but consistent evidence also indicates a peripheral site of action.

Most evidence in the form of RCTs is available for the tricyclic antidepressants (amitriptyline, doxepin, imipramine, nortriptyline and desipramine) as well as selective nor epinephrine inhibitor (SNRI) (venlafaxine, bupropion and duloxetine) to a lesser extent to selective serotonin reuptake inhibitors such as paroxetine, citalopram, or fluoxetine. Despite of availability of a wide range of medications the practical application of these drugs has often proven difficult primarily due to pharmacokinetic and pharmacodynamic variability and therefore use of TDM is recommended for this group of drugs.

Tricyclic Antidepressants

Tricyclic antidepressants (TCAs) were the mainstay of antidepressant pharmacotherapy for over 30 years. They are the most studied antidepressants for the treatment of neuropathic pain.[27] According to chemical structure, they inhibit the reuptake of serotonin and norepinephrine at the synapse differentially. For example, the tertiary amines (e.g. amitriptyline, doxepin, imipramine) are more effective than secondary amines, inhibit serotonin to a greater degree than norepinephrine while the secondary amines (e.g. desipramine, nortriptyline) have more pronounced effects on norepinephrine.[27-29] Binding to opioid receptors and antagonism at the N-methyl-D-aspartate-receptors has been reported for tricyclic antidepressants, but their binding is probably too low to be relevant in humans at therapeutic drug concentrations. It has been shown that TCAs block sodium channels in neuronal tissue, causing blockade of the open and inactivated channel state at therapeutic drug concentrations. Tricyclic antidepressants seem also to block voltage-dependent calcium channels. The side effects occurring according to concentration of drugs are weight gain, anticholinergic effects, orthostatic hypotension, cardiovascular effects, and lethality in overdose suggesting

TABLE 3: Clinical pharmacokinetic parameter of antiepileptic drug which may be used in pain

Antiepileptic	Antiepileptic range (µg/mL)	Toxic concentrations	Half life (h)	T_{max} (h)
Carbamazepine	4–12	>12	15	4–8
Phenytoin	10–20	>20	12–36	6–18
Vigabatrin	1–36	-	5–8	1
Tiagabine	10–100 µg/L	-	7–9	0.5–2
Gabapentin	2–15	-	5–7	2–3
Lamotrigine	3–14	-	13.5	1–3

a TDM is recommended at least in more vulnerable populations like the elderly. Thus, as the TCAs demonstrate complex pharmacodynamics with multiple biological activities and substantial interpatient variability in drug clearance due largely to their dependence on the genetically polymorphic, CYP2D6 for their metabolism, they are very amenable to TDM.

In general, the optimal plasma concentration for therapeutic response is 100 to 300 µg/mL for tertiary amine tricyclics and 50 to 150 µg/mL for secondary amine tricyclics.

Selective Serotonin Inhibitor and Serotonin Noradrenaline Reuptake Inhibitors[30]

The selective serotonin reuptake inhibitors (SSRIs) (fluoxetine, paroxetine, citalopram, escitalopram, sertraline and fluvoxamine) are non-tricyclic drugs which inhibit serotonin reuptake without action on noradrenaline reuptake. Fluoxetine has been reported to block sodium channels, but apparently the blockade is different than the sodium channel blockade of tricyclic antidepressants.

Bupropion, another second generation non-tricyclic antidepressant, is a noradrenaline and dopamine reuptake inhibitor without postsynaptic effects.

Serotonin noradrenaline reuptake inhibitors such as venlafaxine, milnacipran and duloxetine cause a balanced inhibition of serotonin and noradrenaline. These drugs are sometimes called balanced inhibitors of serotonin and noradrenaline. For venlafaxine, the balance *in vivo* depends on the drug dose or concentration. Venlafaxine has no postsynaptic effects but it blocks sodium channels although the characteristics of the blockade are different from that of tricyclic antidepressants. Duloxetine is itself a potent balanced inhibitor of serotonin and noradrenaline reuptake with no significant effect on a range of postsynaptic receptors or sodium channels.

In all these drugs, TDM is not part of management strategy as they have a wide therapeutic range. However, due to biological variability, compliance issues TDM may be performed in specific situations including nonresponders and when agents likely to interact with these drugs also have to be used which may impact the levels. The therapeutic concentration for most SSRIs is 40–500 ng/mL and for SNRI (venlafaxine) is 20–200 ng/mL.

Opioids

Opioids are the mainstay of pain treatment. The term "opiate" refers to compounds structurally related to products found in opium (derived from interpretation of Blood "opos", Greek for "juice"). Opioids are agents regardless of structure that have functional and pharmacological properties of an opiate. The pharmacology of all the opioids that form the mainstay of management of many clinical conditions associated with pain is too extensive to be covered in detail here.

Table 4 summarizes dosing data for opioids used clinically. Only some representative brand names are mentioned in the table–these are not in any way recommendatory. What will be discussed is the rational choice of an opioid and its dose, and whether and where TDM is recommended.

There is a wide interindividual variation in response to opioids. The minimal effective analgesic concentrations of morphine and pethidine vary by a factor of 5–10 among patients. A therapeutic strategy should be evolved that addresses:

- The pain state
- Minimizes adverse effects
- Accounts for variables that influence an individual's response to opioids analgesia. Importantly, TDM is not needed as a careful clinical follow-up of objective signs and subjective symptoms is sufficient for dosage titration.

Several factors can influence dose titration of opioids.[31-33]

TABLE 4: Dosing data for opioids used clinically[31]

Drug	Approximate equianalgesic oral dose	Approximate equianalgesic parenteral dose	Recommended starting dose (Adult> 50 kg)		Recommended starting dose (adult<50 kg)	
			Oral	Parenteral	Oral	Parenteral
Opioid agonist						
Morphine (MORF SR-tab)	30 mg, q 3–4 h (round-10 mg q 3–4 hr the- clock dosing) 60 mg q 3–4 h (single dose or intermittent dosing)		15 mg q 3–4 hr	5 mg q 3–4 hr	0.3 mg/kg q 3–4 hr	0.1 mg/kg q 3–4 hr
Codeine (PHENSEDYL liquid)	130 mg q 3–4 hr	75 mg q 3–4 hr	30 mg q 3–4 hr	30 mg q 2 hr (intramuscular/ subcutaneous)	1 mg/kg q 3–4 hr	Not recommended
Hydrocodone (CARDIAZOL DICODID liquid)	7.5 mg q 3–4 hr	1.5 mg q 3–4 hr	4 mg q 3–4 hr	1 mg q 3–4 hr	0.06 mg/kg q 3–4 hr	0.015 mg/kg q 3–4 hr
Pethidine	300 mg q 2–3 hr	100 mg q 3 hr	Not	50 mg q 3 hr recommended	Not	0.75 mg/kg q 2–3 hr recommended
Oxycodone (Not registered in India)	30 mg q 3–4 hr	Not available	10 mg q 3–4 hr	Not available	0.2 mg/kg q 3–4 hr	Not available

contd...

Chapter 5: Interpretation of Blood Levels of Drugs Used in Chronic Pain Management

contd...

Drug	Approximate equianalgesic Oral dose	Approximate equianalgesic Parenteral dose	Recommended starting dose (Adult > 50 kg)		Recommended starting dose (adult <50 kg)	
			Oral	Parenteral	Oral	Parenteral
Propoxyphene (CENTRIVON)	130 mg	Not available	65 mg q 4–6 hr	Not available	Not recommended	Not recommended
Tramadol (OPI-OT tab)	100 mg	100 mg	50–100 mg q 6 hr	50–100 mg q 6 h 5	Not recommended	Not recommended
Oxymorphone (Not registered in India)	Not available	1 mg q 3–4 hr	Not available	1 mg q 3–4 hr	Not recommended	Not recommended
Methadone (Not registered in India)	20 mg q 6-8 hr	10 mg q 6–8 hr	2.5 mg q 12 hr	2.5 mg q 12 hr	0.2 mg/kg q 12 h	0.1 mg/kg q 6–8 hr
Opioid agonist—antagonist or partial agonist						
Buprenorphine (ADDNOK)	Not available	0.3–0.4 mg q 6–8 hr	Not available	0.4 mg q 6–8 hr	Not available	0.4 mg q 6–8 hr
Butorphanol (BUTODOL)	Not available	2 mg q 3–4 hr	Not available	2 mg q 3–4 hr	Not available	Not available
Nalbuphine (NALFY)	Not available	10 mg q 3–4 hr	Not available	10 mg q 3–4 hr	Not available	0.1 mg/kg q 3–4 hr

These include:
- Pain intensity (increase dose according to intensity of pain)
- Type of pain state (neuropathic pain responds better to combination therapy than opioids alone)
- Chronicity/acuity of pain (dose to be varied according to need–in chronic states too there are often variations and the dose needs to be adjusted accordingly)
- Tolerance (e.g. a 10 mg oral dose of morphine is considered a high dose in a person not previously exposed, while a tolerant person will experience only mild sedation even with a 100 mg IV dose)
- Pharmacokinetic factors (Table 5)
- Availability of medication according to desired route of administration (prefer to use the least invasive route–oral, buccal or transdermal if available; IV useful in perioperative conditions and end of life situations, spinal delivery in chronic pain when adverse effects due to systemic administration are intolerable; chronic states prefer long acting agents that can be given once a day)
- Dose titration (based on response; choice based on pharmacokinetic characteristics and need of patient)
- Opioid rotation (it has been found in a retrospective study that in only 36% patients is the first dose of opioids effective. It was stopped due to side effects in 34% and for ineffectiveness in 34%. A second opioids is effective in 31%, the third in 40%, fourth in 56% and the fifth in 14%. Response to one opioids does not predict or influence response to other opioids. In principle, the first opioids should be given in increasing doses limited by adverse effects. Then opioids switch may be tried.
- Combination of opioids (not to combine agents with the same pharmacokinetic profile, opposing sites of action).

TDM for Opioids

As has been said, the cornerstone for opioid use in patients is clinical monitoring. The only situation when TDM is recommended is when methadone is used:[34]
- In doses more than 100 mg/day to prevent cardiotoxicity.

TABLE 5: Pharmacokinetic factors influencing opioids effects

Factor	Drugs	Effect
Prodrug or not -needs to metabolised into active drug by CYP26D	Codeine, hydrocodone, oxycodone	If activity of CYP206 is diminished the drugs will be ineffective (3% Indians have diminished activity)
Coadministration of drugs that inhibit CYP206 (e.g. SSRI)	Codeine, hydrocodone, oxycodone Methadone	Diminished activity High plasma concentrations and adverse effects free levels reduced
Protein binding ($_1$-acid glycoprotein is elevated in cancer)	Morphine, pethidine	–
Impaired renal function	Morphine, pethidine	Levels will rise leading to toxicity
COPD, sleep apnea, dementia, benign prostatic hypertrophy, unstable gait, pretreatment constipation	Opioids	Greater adverse effects

- In cases of treatment failure, i.e. persistence of withdrawal symptoms or intake of illicit opioids.
- Upon introduction of a comedication or during pregnancy.[35]
- On introducing a drug known to induce methadone clearance, a simple TDM of methadone before and after the introduction of the inducing agent can be helpful for adapting the dosage. This helps to diminish the patient's discomfort due to severe withdrawal symptoms.
- To quickly adapt the dosage. Without TDM, adaptation could take months because of the necessary slow dosage increase for fear of overmedication.
- To convince patients to increase their methadone dosage and avoid stopping comedication for withdrawal symptoms, as it has been described with antiviral drugs.
- Ensuring compliance.

Target values are 250 µg/L (for the (R) enantiomer) or 400 µg/L for the (R, S)-methadone.

Nonsteroidal Anti-inflammatory Drugs

Although Hippocrates used the willow bark the use was scientifically documented by Edward Stone in 1783. The chemist, Felix Hoffmann, at Bayer in Germany, synthesized a stable form of acetyl salicylic acid (ASA) to relieve his father's rheumatism. This compound later becomes the active ingredient in aspirin (the brand name given by Bayer) so named-"a" from acetyl, "spir" from Spiraea ulmaria (which yields salicin) and "in," a common suffix for medications.[36]

After aspirin a large number of drugs have been synthesized—together called the nonsteroidal anti-inflammatory drugs. They all act by blocking the COX2 enzyme and bring about their anti-inflammatory and analgesic effects. Recognizing that the major adverse effects of these drugs were due to blockage of constitutive COX1, selective COX2 inhibitors like celecoxib and etoricoxib were developed, but have never shown any efficacy advantage over the older NSAIDs.

The NSAIDs form a very important component in the pain management physician's repertoire. These drugs have a fairly large safety margin and by and large use is monitored clinically–the emergence of adverse effects limiting dose escalation or even use of a given agent.

The choice and dosing of NSAIDs is largely empirical but is guided by:
i. Therapeutic indication (rapid onset agents with a short duration of action preferred for acute inflammatory or post-traumatic pain while a longer duration of action may be preferred in chronic conditions like arthritis)
ii. Age of patient (older patients may require lower doses)
iii. Comorbidities (patients at risk for cardiovascular diseases should not be prescribed selective COX2 inhibitors)
iv. History of allergy
v. Drug's safety profile (naproxen and ibuprofen interfere with platelet inhibitory activity of low dose aspirin; use alternate drugs or give them separated by adequate interval)
vi. Drug interactions
vii. Costs
viii. Individual response (substantial differences have been noted in the way a person responds to an NSAID)
ix. Kinetic profile of the NSAID

- At least 3–4 half lives of the drug have to elapse before the effect of a dose change may become clinically evident
- The drug needs to achieve adequate concentrations in the synoviual fluid for it to start acting–some drugs achieve higher concentrations in synovial fluid than is measurable in the plasma.

Therapeutic drug monitoring is not the usual practice when NSAIDs are used. Overdose (Table. 6) is the most common indication for measuring drug levels of NSAIDs. Other indications for TDM are given below:

Salicylates[37]

i. Suspected dose-related drug toxicity
ii. Acute overdose

TABLE 6: Selected toxicokinetic parameters for analgesics monitoring[37]

Analgesics	Toxic dose	Toxic concentration
Salicylate (acetylsalicylic acid)	140 mg/kg (acute ingestion)	>300 mg/L
Diflunisal	7.5 g (adults)	800–1000 mg/L
Acetaminophen	140 mg/kg (acute ingestion)	150 mg/L[2]
Ibuprofen	>3 g or 100 mg/kg	200–500 mg/L
Naproxen	Variable	200–400 mg/L

iii. Chronic abuse
iv. Suspected noncompliance
v. Change in renal function, mental status, acid-base status, or pulmonary status in patients using salicylates chronically
vi. After the addition of a second drug that alters salicylate pharmacokinetics.

In the case of salicylate overdose, concentrations should be obtained initially and then every 2 hours after an acute overdose until a peak occurs, then every 4 to 6 hours thereafter until concentrations are less than 200 µg/mL (assuming unaffected acid-base and mental status).

Ibuprofen and Naproxen

- Suspected noncompliance
- Change in renal or hepatic function in a patient using these medications chronically.

Paracetamol[37]

Levels of paracetamol are only done after acute paracetamol overdose. A level at approximately 4 hours after ingestion allows for hepatotoxicity risk categorization via a Rumack nomogram plot. This initial concentration is followed by one additional concentration every 2 hours until a peak occurs if coingestants that would impair absorption or decrease gut motility are present (i.e. opioids or anticholinergic medications).

Issues in Special Populations

- Paracetamol crosses the placenta, placing the fetus at risk for hepatotoxicity after maternal overdose. Therefore, cord-blood concentrations may be indicated, if the child is delivered, to determine the need for antidote therapy.
- The free fraction of salicylate increases to 12% during pregnancy.
- Salicylates may displace bilirubin from plasma proteins in neonates, producing kernicterus.
- Alcoholics ingesting "upper" therapeutic doses (2.5-4 g) of acetaminophen may sustain hepatic necrosis. This may occur, in part, because of the induction of hepatic P450 CYP2E1 by ethanol, thus increasing the formation of the toxic metabolite NAPQI. Glutathione stores in the liver and other susceptible tissues may be diminished in alcoholic patients, rendering them more susceptible to the oxidant effect of NAPQI.

CONCLUSION

Medicines are the backbone of pain therapy irrespective of the cause of the pain. Using these medicines rationally rather than fashionably would be the need of the hour. Measuring blood levels can go a long way in helping achieve this aim.

REFERENCES

1. Taylor L. Access to pain killing drug is human right. Pharma times 2009. (cited on 20/1/11) Available from: http://www.opioids.com/pain killer/ painrelief.html.
2. Fishbain D, Cutler R, Rosomoff HL, et al. Evidence-based data from animal and human experimental studies on pain relief with antidepressants: A structured review. Pain Medicine. 2000;1:310-16.
3. Nee cf, Touw 2 DJ, Stolk LM. Therapeutic Drug Monitoring in Clinical Research. Pharm Med. 2008;22(4):235-44.

4. Hiemke C. Clinical utility of drug measurement and pharmacokinetics–therapeutic drug monitoring in psychiatry. Eur J Clin Pharmacol. 2008;64: 159-66.
5. Thakkar A. Is genotyping cost-effective for predicting phenytoin induced toxicity. (cited on 2011 January 19). Available from *http://www.kem.edu/ dept/clinical_ pharmacology/UG_awardwin.htm*.
6. Burke MJ, Preskorn SH. Therapeutic drug monitoring of Antidepressants. Clin Pharmacokinet. 1999;37(2):147-65.
7. Burke MJ, Preskorn SH. Short-term treatment of affective disorders using standard antidepressants. In: Watson SJ, editor. Psychopharmacology: CD-ROM. New York: Lippincott-Raven Press. 1999.
8. Richelson E. Pharmacology of antidepressants: Characteristics of the ideal drug. Mayo Clin Proc. 1994; 69:1069-81.
9. Bolden-Watson C, Richelson E. Blockade by newly-developed antidepressants of biogenic amine uptake into rat brain synaptosomes. Life Sci. 1993;52:1023-9.
10. Preskorn SH. Antidepressant drug selection: Criteria and options. J Clin Psychiatry. 1994;55(9 Suppl. A):6-22.
11. Dasgupta A. Clinical utility of free drug monitoring. Clin Chem Lab Med. 2002;40:986-93.
12. Touw DJ, Neef C, Thomson AH, Vinks AA. Cost-effectiveness of therapeutic drug monitoring: A systemic review. Ther Drug Monit Feb. 2005;27(1):10-7.
13. Eadie MJ. Therapeutic drug monitoring-antiepileptic drugs. Blackwell Science Ltd Br J Clin Pharmacol 52, 11S ± 20S.
14. Backonja M, Beydoun A, Edwards KR, et al. Gabapentin for the symptomatic treatment of painful neuropathy in patients with diabetes mellitus: A randomized clinical trial. JAMA. 1998;280:1837-42.
15. Rowbotham M, Harden N, Stacey B, Podolnick P, Magnus-Miller L. Gabapentin for the treatment of post-herpetic neuralgia: A randomized clinical trial. JAMA. 1998;280:1837-42.
16. Candis MM, Susan GL, Carol PS. Effects of gabapentin. compared to amitryptiline on pain in diabetic neuropathy. Diabetes. 1998;47:A374.
17. Ben-Menachem E, Persson LI, Hedner T. Selected CSF biochemistry and gabapentin concentrations in the CSF and plasma in patients with partial seizures after a single oral dose of gabapentin. Epilepsy Res Mar. 1992;11(1): 45-9.
18. BE Gidala, LL Radulovicb, S Krugera, P Ruteckia, P Michael. Inter and intra-subject variability in gabapentin absorption and absolute bioavailability. Epi Research. 2000;40(2):123-27.
19. Rose MA, Kam PCA. Gabapentin: Pharmacology and its use in pain management. Anesthesia. 2002;57(5):451-62.
20. Backonja M, Beydoun A, Edwards KR, et al. Gabapentin for the symptomatic treatment of painful neuropathy in patients with diabetes mellitus: A randomized clinical trial. JAMA. 1998;280:1837-42.
21. McCleane GJ. Lamotrigine in the management of neuropathic pain: A review of the literature. Clin Jnl Pain. 2000;16:321-26.
22. Nicol CF. A four years double-blind study of tegretol in facial pain. Headache. 1969;9:54-7.
23. Campbell FG, Graham JG, Zilkha KJ. Clinical trial of carbamazepine in trigeminal neuralgia. J Neurol Neurosurg Psychiat. 1966;29:265-7.
24. Killian JM, Fromm GH. Carbamazepine in the treatment of neuralgia. Use and side effects. Arch Neurol. 1968; 19:129-36.
25. Saudek CD, Werns S, Reidenberg MM. Phenytoin in the treatment of diabetic symmetrical polyneuropathy. Clin Pharmacol Ther. 1977;22:196-9.
26. Perucc E, Bialer M. The clinical pharmacokinetics of the newer antiepileptic drugs. Focus on topiramate, zonisamaide, and tiagibine. Clin Pharmcokinet. 1996;31:29-46.
27. Jackson KC, St. Onge EL. Antidepressant pharmacotherapy: Considerations for the pain clinician. Pain Pract. 2003;3:135-43.
28. Sharp J, Keefe B. Psychiatry in chronic pain: A review and update. Curr Psychiatry Rep. 2005;7:213-19.
29. Sharp J, Keefe B. Psychiatry in chronic pain: A review and update. Curr Psychiatry Rep. 2005;7:213-9.
30. Lundmark J, Bengtsson F, Nordin C, et al. Therapeutic drug monitoring of selective serotonin reuptake inhibitors influences clinical dosing strategies and reduces drug costs in depressed elderly patients. Acta Psychiatr Scand. 2000;101(5):354-9.
31. Yaksh TL, Wallace MS. Goodman and Gilman's. The Pharmacological Basis of Therapeutics, 12th edition. New York: McGraw Hill; Opioids, Analgesia, and Pain Management. 2011. pp. 481-525.
32. Dole VP. Implications of methadone maintenance for theories of narcotic addiction. JAMA. 1988;260:80-4.
33. Maxwell S, Shinderman M. Optimizing response to methadone maintenance treatment: Use of higher dose methadone. J Psychoactive Drugs. 1999;31:95-102.
34. Eap CB, Buclin T, Baumann P. Interindividual Variability of the Clinical Pharmacokinetics of Methadone Implications for the Treatment of Opioid Dependence. Clin Pharmacokinet. 2002;41(14):1153-93.
35. Pond SM, Kreek MJ, Tong TG, et al. Altered methadone pharmacokinetics in methadone-maintained pregnant women. J Pharmacol Exp Ther. 1985;233:1-6.
36. Grosser T, Smyth E, Fitzgerald GA.Goodman and Gilman's The Pharmacological Basis of Therapeutics, 12th edition. New York: McGraw Hill. Chapter 34, Anti-Inflammtory, Antipyretic and Analgesic Agents; Pharmacotherapy of Gout. 2011. pp. 959-1004.
37. White S, Wong SHY. Standards of laboratory practice: Analgesic drug monitoring. Clinical Chemistry. 1998; 44:1110-23.

SECTION 2

Clinical Examination and Evaluation

CHAPTER 6

Clinical Examination and Evaluation of Cervical Spine

Vivek Mehta, Kavita Poply

INTRODUCTION

Pain symptoms in the neck or shoulder are one of the most common musculoskeletal problems encountered by specialists in the clinic. Symptoms associated with cervical pain may either be localized to the cervical spine or more commonly may also include cervicogenic headache, shoulder/scapular/arm pain, neuropathic, radicular distribution including neurological symptoms, disturbances in sleep and effect on memory/concentration. Diagnosis is established by a comprehensive clinical history, detailed clinical examination, radiological investigations and performing interventional diagnostic local anesthetic blocks. This chapter will focus on history and clinical examination of a patient presenting with cervical symptoms.

CAUSES

Anatomical Considerations

Cervical spine consists of 7 vertebrae with the vertebral arch protecting the spinal cord and the spinous process along with transverse process providing attachment to muscles. Spinous process is absent at C1, hence the first palpable spinous process is of C2. There are eight cervical nerve roots with seven vertebrae. This is due to the first nerve root originating between the occiput and C1 vertebrae; this is C1 nerve root. Each nerve root arises above the corresponding vertebrae hence C8 originates between C7-T1 vertebrae. The vertebrae are in continuation with each other by the means of facet joints, a set of diarthrodial synovial joints with healthy innervations of sensory nerve supply. In contrast to the lumbar facet joints the cervical facets have a higher proportion of mechanoreceptors. Free and encapsulated nerve endings within these joints containing substance P and calcitonin gene-related peptide, and these joints are well innervated by the medial branches of the dorsal rami. Although there are 14 cervical facet joints, often the upper 4 thoracic facet joints are also included in the assessment. (Figs 1 to 4)

The superior facets of cervical spine face upward, backward, and medially; the inferior facets face downward, forward, and laterally. This arrangement helps in flexion and extension of spine a movement that involves sliding of these joints. Much of the movements are between C4-7 segments hence this is the area more likely to have degenerative changes. Intervertebral discs are present between the vertebrae contributing to 1/4th of the height of the cervical spine. There is no disc between occiput and the atlas, i.e. C0-C1 and Atlas and Axis C1-C2.

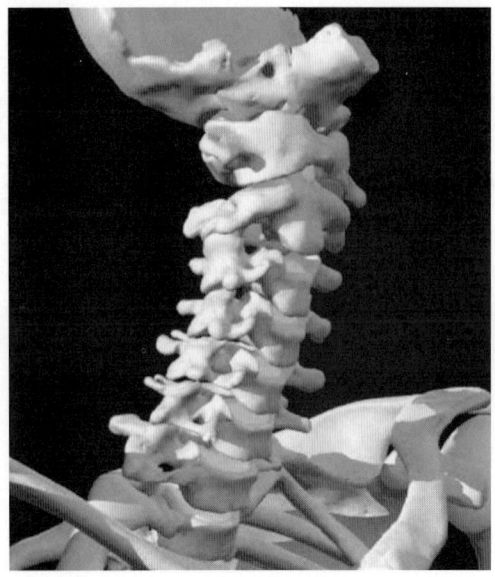

FIG. 1: Vertebrae (7), intervertebral discs (6), pairs of exiting nerve roots (8), cervical lordosis Occ-C7 averages 40°, most of the lordosis occurs at the C1-C2 segment

HISTORY

A comprehensive history about the nature of the symptoms would enable in assisting the examination and to arrive at a diagnosis. The following classification for neck pain and associated symptoms has been proposed.
- *Grade I neck pain*: No symptoms indicating serious pathology and minimal influence on daily activities.
- *Grade II neck pain*: No symptoms indicating serious pathology, but having influence on daily activities.
- *Grade III neck pain*: No symptoms indicating serious pathology, presence of neurological disorders such as decreased reflex, muscle weakness, or decreased sensory function.
- *Grade IV neck pain*: Indications of serious underlying pathology such as fracture, myelopathy, or neoplasm.

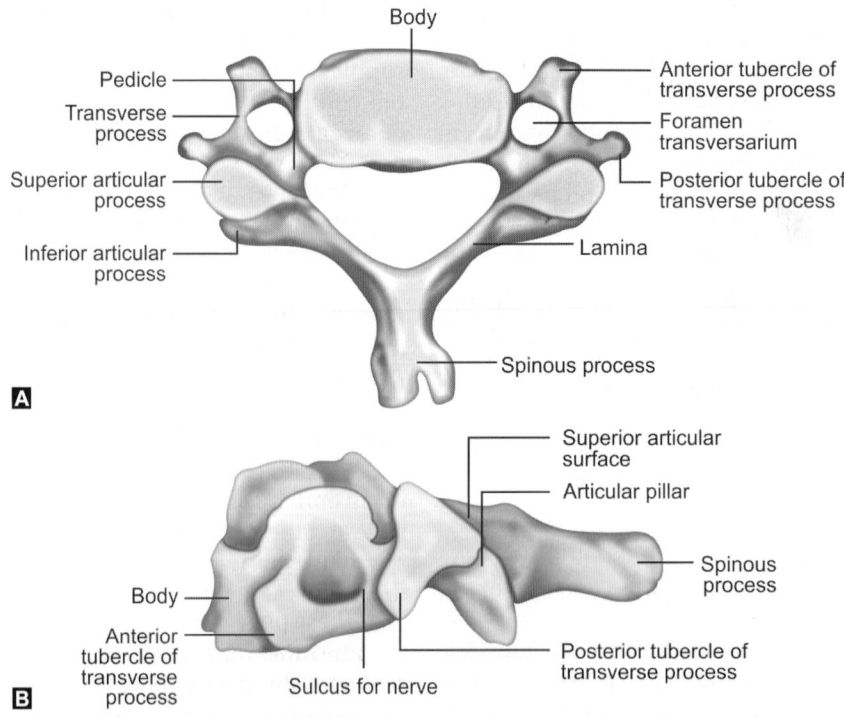

FIGS 2A and B: Cervical spine anatomy

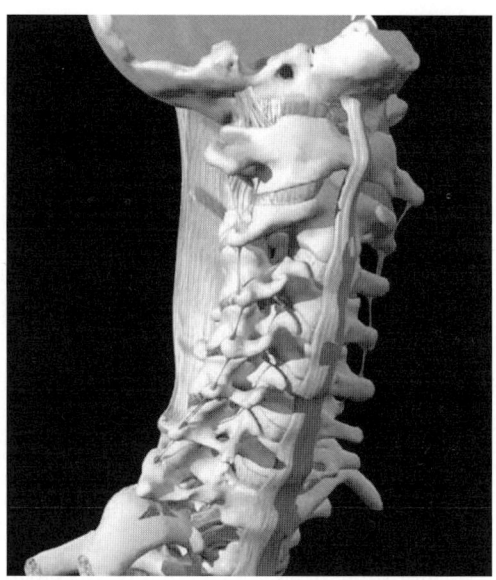

FIG. 3: The cervical spine also features a complex arrangement of ligaments to supplement its structure and mobility

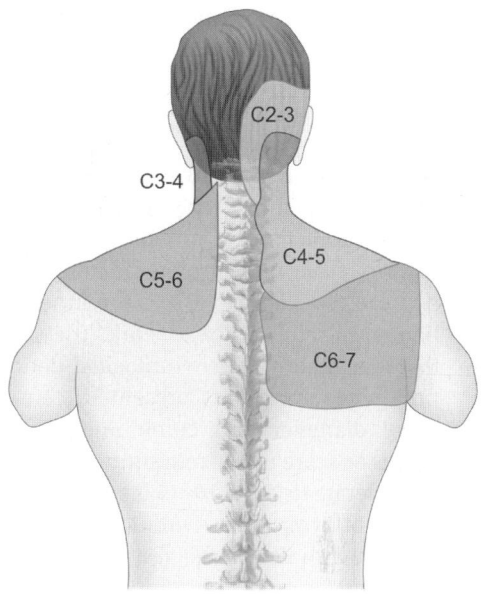

FIG. 5: The distribution of facet joint pain in cervical spine

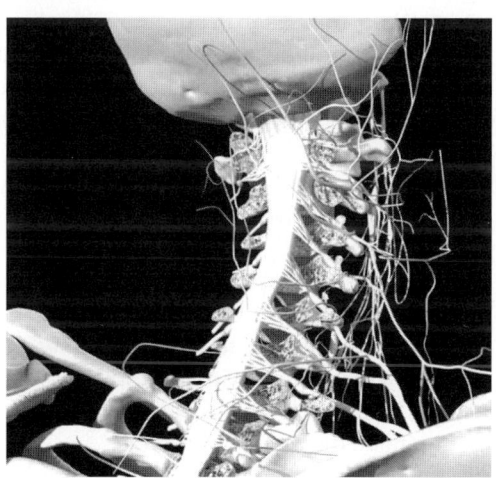

FIG. 4: Neural elements : 8 pair of cervical nerves Exit the spinal canal superior to the vertebrae for which they are numbered - C1 nerves exit the canal between Occ and C1, C2 nerves exit the canal between C1 and C2, C8 nerves exit the canal between C7 and T1

Besides routine medical history, the pain history should specifically focus on:

- Red flag symptoms need to be ruled out. Any history suggestive of malignancy, unexplained symptoms after the age of 50, continuous pain, independent of posture or movement, loss of weight, anorexia should be further investigated extensively.
- *Distribution of pain*: Paraspinal cervical tenderness is suggestive of facet joint disease. The pain symptoms may also radiate to upper limb or associated with headache with facet joint disease (Fig. 5).
- *Character of pain*: Burning, shooting pain with radiation to upper limb may be indicative of neuropathic involvement with nerve root irritation. Any numbness or tingling sensation may point towards neuropathic involvement. Any association with sleeping position—number of pillows are used and the type whether foam or feather. What type of mattress they use hard or soft. Does the patient "hug" the pillow or abduct the arms when sleeping? These positions can increase the stress on the lower cervical nerve roots.
- Severity of symptoms: The impact on activities of daily living, health quality and psychosocial impact needs to be

considered. Does patient avoid any particular movement or posture, what type of work patient is involved and does it involve standing or sitting in any particular position for a long period. Normally activities involving push and pull like cleaning, hovering may cause cervicothoracic joint problems. Watkins[1] severity scale of neurological injury can be used especially to assess the fitness of patient to return back to work. The scale includes grading for neurological deficit, time since symptoms presented, central canal diameter and combining all the scores as score of 6 is minimum risk, 6–10 is moderate risk and 10–15 is severe risk.

- Onset of symptoms: Duration of symptoms, in chronic myofacial syndrome pain is present for more than 3 months with the aches being more generalized with trigger points with no history of trauma. Any radicular symptoms would be associated with neuropathic origin. If there is suggestion of nerve root injury or irritation above C4 then the symptoms usually would not go down the arms however cervical radiculopathy often presents with both motor and sensory symptoms in upper limbs presenting as weakness, altered neurological examination. Cervical myelopathy or injury to spinal cord presents with additional symptoms in lower limbs such as weakness, paresthesia and incoordination of movements with or without sphincter disturbances. With radicular symptoms dermatomal distribution often correlates with the level of neuropathic origin. Bilateral symptoms usually indicate either systemic disorders (e.g., diabetes, alcohol abuse) that are causing neuropathies or central space-occupying lesions
- Mechanism of injury, whether it is trauma, stretching or overuse. Trauma can lead to whiplash injury,[2] stretching may be related to overuse or sustained postures which may result in thoracic outlet syndrome or an insidious onset in someone aged >55 years may indicate cervical spondylosis with osteoarthritis. Although spondylosis of spine is quite variable and can itself be present in patient as young as 25 years or in elderly but osteoarthritis changes usually does not present until 55 years of age.
- If there is any history of head injury then any loss of consciousness or unsteadiness should be noted.
- Headache: Cervical pain may be associated with occipital or suboccipital headaches, C1 headaches occur at the base and top of the head, whereas C2 headaches are referred to the temporal area. There is painful limitation of movement, associated abnormal head and neck postures with sub occipital or nuchal tenderness with sensory abnormalities in occipital and suboccipital areas. Sometimes the head position may alter headache, with some patients finding relief by placing hand or arm over head on the affected site (Bakody's sign), indicative of problems in C4/C5 area.
- Sympathetic association: Are there any sympathetic symptoms like ringing in the ears, dizziness, blurred vision, photophobia, rhinorrhea, sweating, lacrimation, and loss of strength. This can be related to injury to cranial nerves or sympathetic nerves in neck, which lies in the soft tissues of the neck anterior and lateral to the cervical vertebrae.
- Any change in voice or difficulty in swallowing: This can be neurological, mechanical or muscle in-coordination. Pain on swallowing may be indicative of soft-tissue swelling in the throat, vertebral subluxation, osteophyte projection, or disc protrusion into the esophagus or pharynx. In addition, swallowing becomes more difficult and the voice becomes weaker as the neck is extended.

EXAMINATION

A neuromusculoskeletal examination of cervical spine is done to evaluate neck pain. Examination of the cervical spine helps in assessing the level of injury or pathology involving either the cervical spine or upper limb.[3] Examination of cervical spine follows the routine practice of inspection, asking patient to perform range of movements, palpation of spine and in addition it involves examination of motor and sensory system.

Inspection

Examiner should watch for patient's gait as they walk into the examination room. They should be suitably undressed and even observing the patient while disrobing examiner should note the movement patterns of neck, shoulder and arms, even the facial expressions gives a clue regarding the intensity of pain.

Any abnormalities are noted and fully described. The examiner should note any muscle atrophy and fasciculation and, if either or both are present, describe their exact location and specific muscles involved.[4]

Look for head and neck posture: whether in midline, any tilt or deformity should be noted. Are there any postural compensation, weak muscles, and temporomandibular joint problems? Also look for trapezius neckline, should be equal on both sides. Inspect the shoulders for any asymmetry and also observe for any muscle spasm or atrophy.

Finally, the patient is inspected for unusual facial characteristics, involuntary movements, and deformities of the neck or rest of the body. The patient's eyes are inspected and special note taken of any eyelid drooping, abnormal pupillary contractions, or asymmetric facial characteristics.

Range of Movements

Examiner should note that the movements are smooth and painless. Also note any limitation of movement and/or pain on any particular movement. This examination involves active and passive movement assessment done in sitting position.

Active movements involve flexion, extension, side flexion and rotation of cervical spine. These movements can be repeated or combined. The range of movements involves assessment of the entire cervical spine assessing the facet joints, ligaments, joint capsules and intervertebral discs. With increasing age the range of movement will reduce except for movements at C1-C2 that actually increases. Always ask patient for the movement that elicits pain, this can be done at the end so that the background pain does not inhibit rest of the movements. During this assessment look for causes for limitation whether it is pain, spasm, stiffness or deformities. It is also possible to differentiate between upper and lower cervical movements i.e. the nodding head involving C1-C2 and rest the movements occurs at lower cervical level. If there is a limited movement, pressure can be applied to assess the maximum movement possible but taking into consideration that the patient is pain free and there are no signs of vertebral artery compression such as dizziness or feeling faint.

The maximum flexion (chin to chest) possible is 80-90° but even a two finger width between the chin and chest is acceptable. During flexion it is important to identify any prominence in the spinous process at C2, this indicates anterior subluxaton of the atlas and extreme caution should the taken in the rest of the examination of cervical spine.

To verify this subluxation examiner can perform Sharp Purser test, examiner should place one hand over patient's forehead and the thumb of the other hand is placed over the spinous process of axis to stabilize it. Ask patient to slowly flex the head and the examiner will press backward on the forehead. If the head slide backward during this movement, it is considered as a positive test.

Extension is normally around 70° and the plane of nose and forehead is almost horizontal.

Side flexion is around 30–40° both on the right and left side, here examiner should look for ear moving towards shoulders but exclude any shoulder elevation. Rotation movements are limited to around 70–90° with chin almost reaching plane of shoulder. Here the rotation and side flexion can be combined together. If in history patient had complained of pain on any particular movement or pain on maintaining a sustained posture or on repetition, then this should be simulated in examination.

If the examination of range of movements is not satisfactory then passive movements can examine the cervical spine. Here patient lies on his/her back and the examiner will take control of the head testing the flexion, extension, rotation and side flexion. The range of movement in supine is much greater than sitting position with greater improvement in side flexion from 45° to 75°. This increase range of movement is mainly due relaxed muscles which otherwise are working against gravity to support the head in sitting position.

In this way, the examiner ensures that the movement is as isometric as possible and that a minimal amount of movement occurs. If a neurological injury is suspected, the examiner must carefully assess for muscle weakness to determine the structures injured. If a severe neuropraxla or axonotmesis has occurred, there may be residual weakness even though muscle atrophy is not as evident.

Palpation of Spine

Palpation may elicit tenderness (Fig. 6). If so, its exact location and the amount of pressure needed to produce pain is noted. In addition, the patient's nonverbal response to palpation, such as withdrawal or facial grimaces, should be observed. During palpation the examiner should note any tenderness, trigger points, muscle spasm, or other signs and the symptoms that may indicate the source of the pathology. During palpation examiner should also note the skin and surrounding bony and

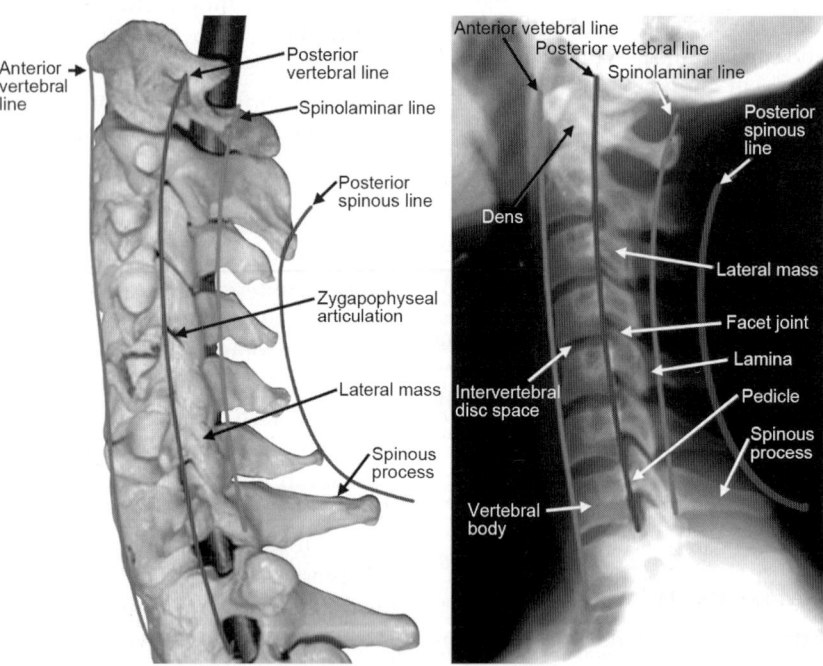

FIG. 6: Bony landmarks with comparison to X-ray

soft tissue structures on the anterolateral and posterior aspects of neck. Palpation can be performed in either supine or sitting position or prone if it is comfortable for patient. For palpation of posterior structures examiner stands behind and uses fingers of both hands to palpate the patient.

To begin the examiner would start palpation from midline on the posterior skull and run down until a dip that is external occipital protuberance. The mastoid process is also palpated as a part of examination. Following down the neck the examiner can feel the cervical spine and facet joints. After palpation of occipital protuberance the next prominent structure palpable in midline will be the spinous process of C2. The next structure which is most obvious are the C6 and C7 spinous process, however on deep palpation one can still feel the spinous process of C3, C4 and C5. The passive flexion and extension of neck will help in differentiating C6/C7 where C6 moves in and out but C7 remains stationary (Fig. 7). Also the movement between the spinous process can be palpated, even the movement between the cervical vertebrae can be established which can be normal or less or more mobile. The facet joint can be palpated 1.5 to 2.5 cm from midline although they are not felt as distinct structures but rather a hard bony mass under fingers. The muscles in the paraspinal region can be palpated for swelling, spasm, tenderness or any other pathology.

Palpation on the lateral aspect involves cervical transverse process, temporomandibular joints, mandible, parotid glands, lymph nodes and vessels. During examination the easier transverse process to palpate will be the C1, as examiner palpates the mastoid process and moves down and slightly anteriorly a hard bump felt which patient feels uncomfortable. The other transverse process can be felt on deep palpation if the patient is in relaxed position where the bone can be felt under the sternocleidomastoid muscle.

On the anterior aspect the structures palpated are hyoid bone, thyroid and cricoid cartilage. Hyoid is at the level of C2-3 whereas the thyroid is at C4-5 and cricoid is at C6. Anterior examination involves palpation of paranasal

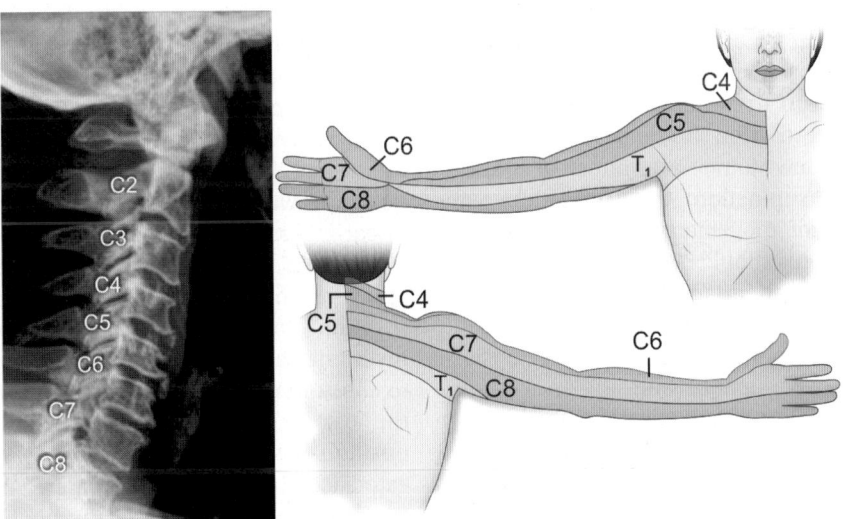

Nerve roots leave the spine between two corresponding vertebrae. The anatomical distribution of sensory disturbance/pain indicate the nerve root involved.

FIG. 7: Cervical nerve root sensory distribution

sinuses, first three ribs, sternocleidomastoid muscle and supraclavicular fossa. Examiner should palpate first three ribs and follow them posteriorly, ask patient to deep breathe and compare movements bilaterally. During palpation of supraclavicular fossa examiner should look for soft tissue swelling, bony tenderness.

Examination of Peripheral Joints

After assessment of cervical spine with resisted isometric movements the peripheral joints should be examined to look for any abnormality. These joints are examined bilaterally.

Temporomandiblular joints are examined by placing the fingers into patient ears and the pulp of finger will help to feel the movement of condyles of the joint. The examiner should observe patient during opening or closing of mouth and also watch for any deviation of movement. Pain or tenderness especially on closing mouth indicates posterior capsulitis.

Shoulder joints[5] are examined in each arm for abduction, active elevation through forward flexion and elevation through the plane of the scapula (SCAPTION). In addition, the examiner quickly tests medial and lateral rotation of each shoulder with the arm at the side and with the arm abducted to 90º Any pattern of restriction should be noted.

The elbow joints examined in flexion, extension, supination, and pronation. Any restriction of movement or abnormal signs and symptoms should be noted. The wrist and assessment, patient actively performs flexion, extension, and radial and ulnar deviation of the wrist. Active movements (flexion, extension, abduction, adduction, and opposition) are performed for the fingers and thumb.

Following examination of joints examine for muscle power and possible neurological weakness originating from the nerve roots in the cervical spine by testing the myotomes. The myotomes are tested by resisted isometric contractions with the joint at or near the resting position. Here patient is comfortable seated and instructed to resist any movement so that an isometric contraction is obtained. The contraction should be held for at least 5 seconds so that the weakness can be noted.

NEUROLOGICAL EXAMINATION

Examination of Myotomes

C1-C2 myotome: With the head slightly flexed examiner applies pressure on forehead while supporting patient with a hand between scapulae.

The *C3 myotome* is examined by placing one hand above patient ear and apply a side ward force while stabilizing patient with a hand on opposite shoulder.

The *C4 myotome* is examined by asking patient to elevate the shoulder and then to resist the examiner from pressing down.

C5 myotome is assessed by asking patient to abduct the shoulders to around 75º with elbow flexed to 90º and forearm pronated. Here patient is instructed to resist examiner from pressing down on humerus.

C6 and C7 myotome: Examiner will assess elbow flexion and extension with arm on side and elbow flexed to 90⁰ elbow flexors and extensors are represented by C6 & C7 myotomes respectively. The wrist movements are tested in flexion, extension and ulnar deviation with the patient's arms by side and forearm pronated.

C8 and T1 myotome: The examiner will apply downward force to test extensor (C6 myotome) and upward force for flexors (C7 myotome) and lateral force radially deviated to check ulnar deviation (C8 myotome) while the patient's attempts to maintain neutral position. Also patient is examined for thumb extension (C8 myotome) where examiner applies force to bring the thumb back into flexion. The intrinsic muscles of hand (T1 myotome) are examined where patient tries to hold a piece of paper between finger with examiner trying pull the paper away or else patient abducting finger with examiner adducting isometrically.

Sensory and Motor Examination

If an upper motor neuron lesion is suspected then Babinski's reflex should be checked along with Hoffman's sign. To test for Hoffmann's sign, the examiner holds the patient's middle finger and briskly flicks the distal phalanx. A positive sign is noted if the interphalangeal joint of the thumb of the same hand flexes.

Sensory examination involves checking the dermatome pattern of the various nerve roots as well as the sensory distribution of the peripheral nerves. It is important to check for differences between two sides. The dermatomal distribution varies from patient to patient and they tend to overlap each other. So it is difficult to map each dermatome separately hence examiner tests sensation by sensory scanning examination. This scanning can be done by running relaxed hands over the patient's head (sides and back); down over the shoulders, upper chest, and back; and down the arms, being sure to cover all aspects of the arm. If there is any difference noted then a specific sensory test can be conducted with pin, cotton or brush to map out the specific sensory area.

As the nerve roots and spinal cord are in close relation to bony and other soft tissue structures, there can be a referred pain related to these structures. In the cervical spine complex structures like the intervertebral discs, facet joints, joint capsules, ligaments can refer pain to other segments of neck (dermatomes) or to the head, the shoulder, the scapular area, and the whole of the upper limb.

The examination is completed by eliciting the biceps C5-6, the brachioradialis C5-6, the triceps C7-8 and the jaw jerk (cranial nerve 5) reflexes. For eliciting biceps reflex and jaw jerk examiner will place the thumb on the tendon. The brachioradialis and triceps reflexes are tested by directly tapping the tendon or muscle.

CONCLUSION

The understanding of neuroanatomy and its correlation with affected deramatome is necessary in management of cervical pain. On top of it the detailed history; through clinical and neurological examination; and interpretation of X-ray, CT and MRI of cervical spine will help in pin pointing of clinical diagnosis and the management of pain in these patients.

REFERENCES

1. Watkins RG. Neck injuries in football. The Spine in Sports. St Louis, Mosby year book Inc, 1996.
2. Foreman SM, Croft AC. Whiplash Injuries: The Cervical Acceleration/Deceleration Syndrome. Baltimore, Williams and Wilkins. 1988.
3. Bradley JP, Tibone JE, Watkins RG. History, examination and diagnostic tests for neck and upper extremity problems. The Spine in Sports. St Louis, St Louis, Mosby Year Book Inc, 1996.
4. Magarey ME. Examination of the Cervical Spine. In: Grieve GP (Ed). Modern Manual Therapy of the Vertebral Columa. Edinburgh, Churchill Livingstone, 1986.
5. Wells P. Cervical dysfunction and shoulder problems. Physiotherapy. 1982; 68:66-73.

SUGGESTED READINGS

1. Bateman JE. The Shoulder and Neck. Philadelphia WB. Saunders Co, 1972.
2. Beggsl. Radiological Assessment of Degenerative Diseases of the Cervical Spine. Semin Orthop. 1987;2: 63-73.
3. Bland JH. Disorders of Cervical Spine. Philadelphia WB. Saunders Co, 1994.
4. Bonica. JJ. The Management of Pain. Philadelphia; Lea and Febiger, 1953.
5. Cervical spine, orthopedic physical assessment. 1997. pp. 101-51.
6. Evaluation and treatment of cervical spine Injuries. Clincal Sports Medicine. 1995;691. pp. 701.
7. Examination of Neck. Orthopedica Essentials of Diagnosis and treatment. Churchill Livingstone, 1994.
8. Functional human anatomy. Philadelphia; Lea and Febiger, 1973.
9. Physical examination of the musculoskeletal system. Chicago, Year Book Medical Publishers, 1987.
10. Radiologic Evaluation of Cervical Spine. Injuries Spine. 1988;12: 742-7.

CHAPTER 7

Clinical Examination and Evaluation of Lumbar Spine

Steve M Aydin

INTRODUCTION

Low back pain or lumbar pain is one of the most common complaints that patients will have. Its lifetime prevalence is more than 70% in most countries, and is one of the most common reasons for disability in people under the age of 45.[1] About 60–80% of the population experience an event of low back pain, and therefore, has shown to be an impact on both the social and economic arms of medical systems.[2] When patients present with symptoms of low back pain, a formal history and physical examination should be performed.

A history is taken to determine the mechanism of injury. Patients will often be physically examined with provocation tests to determine the driver of the pain as well. Diagnostic work up can be done with imaging and electrodiagnostics testing. Most often, patient will improve with conservative treatment and education. However, more refractory cases will require further work-up and more interventional treatments.[3]

The goal of treatment is to decrease pain, improve function, prevent further events, and educate the patient. Most events are self limiting, however, patients who have experience one episode of back pain, are at a higher risk for repeat episodes. Proper diagnosis and work-up are important during evaluation to exclude life threatening conditions by the identification of "red flag" symptoms.[4]

CAUSES

The majority of back pain episodes will be benign and may not have a definitely diagnosed cause. Most cases will be diagnosed as mechanical low back pain. However, it is important to be aware of the syndromes which can be diagnosed by history and physical examination, as well as the cases which is potentially life threatening.

Presentations where the symptoms are local, mechanical, and musculoskeletal will often resolve with conservative treatments. This will be the largest number of patients seen and evaluated. The diagnosis that falls into this group of symptoms is of myofascial pain syndrome, intervertebral disk disease, lumbar radicular syndrome, herniated lumbar disk, lumbar facet syndrome, lumbar spinal stenosis, and internal disk disruption.[5]

The biomechanics of the lumbar spine shows that certain activities, positions, and movements place the spine at higher risk for injury. The lumbar spine is made up of anterior and posterior elements. The anterior elements include the vertebral body, and the intervertebral disks. The posterior elements consist of the facets, the lamina, pedicles, spinous process and transverse process.[6] The greatest amount of force is placed on the lumbar spine in the seated and flexed position. Many mechanisms of injury are usually coupled with history of leaning forward, twisting, and picking upon an object.[7] These motions all place added stress onto the structures of the spine and puts them at risk for injury, and hence resulting in pain.[8]

SIGNS AND SYMPTOMS

Low back pain can often be a complex puzzle when looking for the pain generator. One of the most helpful ways in finding the cause of pain is determining the generator, or provoking the pain with movement, or diagnostic tests. About 85% of the diagnosis is made from the history the patient presents with. Features to pay attention to are the location, quality, duration, timing, severity, alleviating and aggravating factors.[9]

Symptoms can present as localized pain in the lower lumbar region, and may occur with referred pain into one side over the other. Radiation of pain may occur into the buttock or leg(s). Special attention should be given to how the pain develops if it was insidious or was there a specific event. "Red flag" symptoms should be given special attention. These are symptoms that would require more urgent attention and further investigation. History of trauma, pain worse in a laying supine position, evening pain, history of cancer, history of systemic illness or infection, loss of muscle tone, strength, or bowel and bladder control.[4]

Mechanical back pain may present as mostly lower lumbar pain with components of buttock pain. Where back pain with leg pain would present mostly with symptoms in the leg in a dermatomal pattern. Concern for spinal malignancy, infection, fracture, or instability should be present when history correlates. The malignancy should be with the previous history of cancer, weight loss, failure of improvement after one month of conservative treatment, sedimentation rate greater than 50, and/or pain when in the supine position. Infection is a concern with previous infection history, fevers, vertebral tenderness, and history of intravenous drug abuse.[6,9]

A better understanding of the patient's pain can be further attained with history and questioning about how the patient feels the pain has affected his function and what the patient thinks is the cause of his pain. This may facilitate a more comprehensive evaluation to the patient's signs and symptoms.[9]

CLINICAL EXAMINATION

Physical examination is a crucial portion of the evaluation in trying to determine the driver of the patient's pain. The examination can be split up into components to allow for a comprehensive overview of the lumbar spine. This includes observation (static, dynamic, gait, posture), palpation, range of motion (lumbar and extremities), neurologic examination (sensation, reflexes, and motor strength), and provocative testing.[10]

Observation should include both static and dynamic examination. The skin, posture, muscle mass, and bone structure should be commented on. The curve of the lumbar spine should be examined in a standing position, as well as in a seated position. Observation of the curve should be monitored in the dynamic flexion and extension motions as well. The gait should also be observed and monitored to give clues into antalgic problems, compensatory movements, and general motion of the body in relation to the kinetic chain.[11]

Palpation should then be done to the lumbar spine region, specifically the spinous process and paraspinal muscle. This should be done in the standing upright position, standing in lumbar flexion, and prone positions. This will help appreciate any spasm, tenderness, scoliosis or palpable vertebral step off.[12]

Range of motion of the lumbar spine, torso and lower extremity joints should be checked. While examining range of motion, observations of full range of motion, functional range of motions, and painful range of motion should be considered. The passive, assisted, or active range of motions may all be examined. Normal lumbar flexion ROM is considered to be 40º to 60º of motion at the lumbar spine. Many times, patients may compensate with the rotation at the hips and pelvis. Lumbar extension is considered normal at 20º–35º (Fig. 1). Lateral flexion can reach 15º–20º in nonpainful movement.[12,13]

The neurological examination done on the lower extremities may provide direction into a diagnosis, especially in the cases where symptoms are coupled with lumbar pain with lower extremity pain. When paresthesia, numbness/tingling, or weakness is present in the lower limbs, consideration for proximal nerve impingement should be considered. The sensation to pin, light touch, and vibration should be done. Motor strength testing should be done at the key muscles and graded; hip flexors, knee extensors, ankle dorsi flexors, ankle plantar flexors, and long toe extensors.

The attention to the reflexes should also be taken, and rated. The patellar, hamstring, and Achilles' reflexes should be compared bilaterally. Attention for upper motor responses, such as a Babinskis' reflex, spasticity or clonus should also be given. The synthesis of the findings on physical examination and neurologic examination will help determine diagnostic impressions as well as treatment plans.[12-14]

The provocative testing may be helpful in determining the pain driver that a patient may have. Special attention to the supine and/or seated straight leg raise is often used to determine, if nerve root irritation could be present in the lower lumbar segment (Fig. 2). The reverse straight leg raise may be used to determine impingement of upper lumbar nerve. A sphinx test is used to load the facets and posterior elements of the lumbar spine, and may determine a facet mediated pain driver (Fig. 3). The Gaenslen's and FAbERs test can be used to look at the presence of sacroiliac joint dysfunction, or hip driven pain (Fig. 4). A FAdIRs (flexion, adduction, internal rotation) test can be used to look at piriformis muscle as a cause of pain.[15]

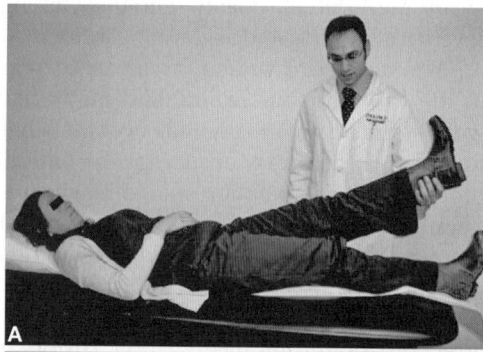

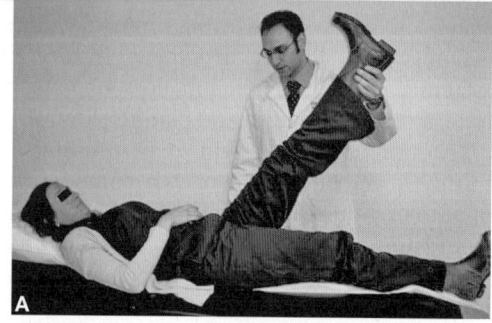

FIG. 2: Straight leg raise done in the supine position. Initially started at 20° of hip flexion, and then raised slowly to about 70° to 80° of hip flexion, while maintaining knee extension

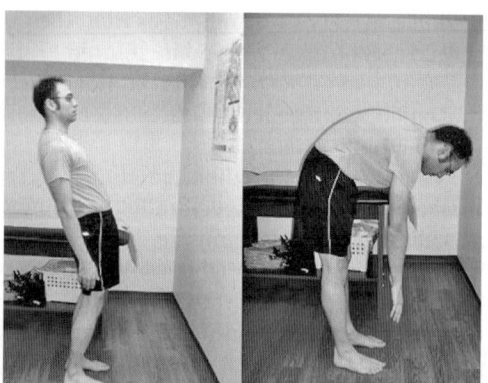

FIG. 1: Range of motion of the lumbar spine. Extension and flexion are shown

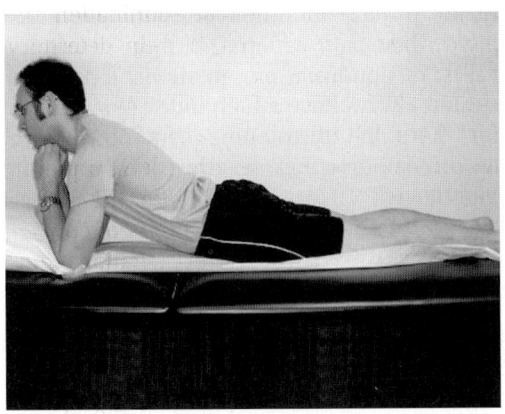

FIG. 3: This shows the sphinx test, which will load the lumbar facets joint

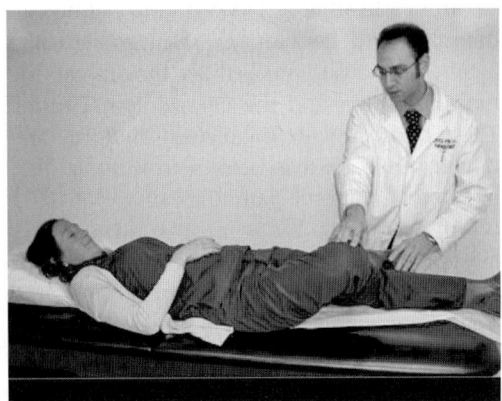

FIG. 4: The FAbERs test, bring the hip into a position of flexion, abduction, and external rotation which will load the hip joint

The straight leg raise is done while the patient is in the supine or seated position. In the supine position, the leg is maintained in extension at the knee, and then raised to 20° of flexion at the hip (Fig. 4). The range for pain and nerve root irritation should be noted from 20° to 70°. A positive test is noted when the patient notes a radicular pattern and concordant pain down the leg.[15]

The FAbERs test (flexion, abduction, external rotation) is done to evaluate for hip pathology. This maneuver is done in the supine position, while flexing the hip, then abducting, followed by external rotation. This loads the hip joint, and will elicit a pain in the groin area when hip pathology is present. A FAdIRs test, looks at the piriformis area, and is performed in a similar fashion as the FAbERs test; however it is done with the hip in flexion, adduction and internal rotation (Fig. 4).[15]

Sphinx test is performed with the patient in the prone position, and which then extends the lumbar spine, by pushing up off the table with his arms. This will load the lumbar facets (Fig. 3).

A Gaenslen's test looks at the SI joint. It is a provocative maneuver where the patient is supine, and the contralateral leg is off the table toward the floor, and the ipsilateral leg is flexed at the hip and flexed at the knee and brought toward the torso. The pain in the SI joint region would be noted and would be a positive test.[16]

The summation of all the findings on physical examination should be coupled with the history taken. The combination of the findings will help determine a treatment and diagnostic plan of action for the patient.

INVESTIGATIONS

The imaging studies may be ordered as a case basis. When symptoms of radiculopathy or red flag symptoms are present, further imaging may be required. The studies available include radiography, magnetic resonance imaging, computed tomography, myelography, and scintigraphy. The radiography is used to evaluate bone anatomy and structure. In cases of trauma, and concern for alignment changes, an anterior-posterior view is taken. A lateral view, with flexion and extension views can determine instability or movement of vertebrae. The computed tomography and MRI can be used for more detailed views, and provide axial and sagittal views. The MRI is helpful for visualizing soft tissue, disk structure. With the addition of contrast, evaluation of the spine in post-surgical patients can be done as well. The CT scan is also an option for lumbar spine evaluation, and may be an alternative to MRI in those patients with hardware, which may obstruct MRI use.[4]

The MRI and CT scan are helpful to determine degenerative changes in the facets, the disks, as well as looking at the neuroforamina and the central spinal canal. The CT can provide good bony anatomy and detail. While, MRI is helpful to identify disk, ligament, and nerve pathologies.[17]

The scintigraphy is a scan which uses a radionucletide that can be used to look for inflammation, fractures, infections, and metastatic disease. Many a times, it can be combined with single-photon emission computed tomography for better anatomic detail, and determine location of picks up. The milligram, often ordered to evaluate the dura and nerve roots in the lumbar spine. This involves a spinal tap with the introduction of contrast media and then followed with CT scan. Since the development of MRI, milligram is not utilized as often.

The nerve conduction and electromyography may also be used in the diagnostic phase of lower lumbar pain. This test allows for the evaluation of peripheral nerves and muscles. It can help diagnosis location of lesion in nerves, and the degree in which damage, if any, is occurring to the nerve or muscles.[18]

Finally, the laboratory studies can be done to evaluate for inflammatory markers. Some of these include such markers as the C-reactive proteins, and erythrocyte sedimentation rate.

DIFFERENTIAL DIAGNOSIS

Depending upon the physical examination finding and history, a differential diagnosis can be generated. More common diagnosis may include mechanical low back pain, muscle imbalance/overuse/spasm, lumbar spondylosis, disk-mediated pain from a herniation or bulge, spinal central/ neuroforaminal stenosis, lumbar radiculopathy, lumbar facet arthropathy, sacroiliac joint dysfunction, hip mediated pain, and/or spondylolisthesis. These diagnoses may present in isolation or combination. Therefore, it is important to take a detailed history, correlate the symptoms to the physical examination, and determine concordant pain patterns. In more refractory cases, or abnormal presentations, examiners should always have a high index of suspicion for more life threatening conditions, such as tumors, fracture, or other less common pathologies.

TREATMENT PROTOCOL

The treatment plans should be tailored in case-by-case basis. Most cases will respond to conservative treatments. However, a combination of treatments have been shown to improve outcomes. This should include medications, education, counseling, interventions, physical therapy, manipulation, and development of long-term exercise programs for patients. The treatments should be discussed with patients and developed to accommodate their lifestyle, social situations, and personal goals.

CONCLUSION

The clinical examination of lumbar spine is the key to the success of assessment and pain relief in chronic lumbar radiculopathy pain.

REFERENCES

1. Frymoyer JW, Cats-Baril WL. An overview of the incidence and cost of low back pain. Orthop Clin N Am. 1991;22: 263-71.
2. Martin BI, et al. Expenditures and health status aming adults with Low Back Pain. JAMA. 2008;299:656-64.
3. NASS Task Force on Clinical Guidelines. Phase III clinical guidelines for multidisciplinary spine care specialist. Unremitting Low Back Pain, 1st ed. Burr Ridge, IL: North Am Spine Soc; 2000.
4. Bigos S, et al. Acute low back problems in adults. In: Clinical practice guideline, Quick reference guide number 14. AHCOR Pub. No. 95-0643, December 1994.
5. Bhangle SD, et al. Back pain made simple: An aprroach based on principles and evidence. Cleveland Clin J of Med. 2009;76:393-99.
6. Reuler JB. Low Back Pain. West J Med. 1985;143:259-65.
7. Nadler SF, et al. Hip muscle imbalance and low back pain in athletes: influence of core strengthening. Med Sci Sports Med Rep. 2005;4:179-83.
8. Nadler SF, et al. The relationship between lower extremity injury, low back pain, and hip muscle strength in male and female college athletes. Clin J Sport Med. 2000; 80:89-97.

9. Deyo RA, et al. What can the history and physical examination tell us about back pain? JAMA. 1992; 268:760-65.
10. Magee DJ. Lumbar spine. In: Magee DJ (Ed). Orthopedic Physical Exam, 4th ed. Philadelphia: Elsevier; 2002. pp. 467-566.
11. Nader SF. Visual vignette: injury in a throwing athlete: understanding the kinetic chain. Am J Phys Med Rehabil. 2004;83:79.
12. Parks KA, et al. A comparison of lumbar range of motion and functional ability scores in patients with low back pain: assessment for range of motion validity. Spine. 2003;28:380-4.
13. Barr KP. Low back pain. In: Braddom RL Physical medicine and Rehabilitation, 3rd ed. Saunders; 2007.
14. Malik M, Benzon HT. Low back pain. In: Raj's Practical Management of Pain. 4th ed. Philadelphia: Mosby; 2008.
15. Dreyfuss P, et al. The value of medical history and physical examination in diagnosis of sacroiliac joint syndrome. Spine. 1996;21:2594-602.
16. Scavone JG, et al. Use of lumbar spine films: Statistical evaluation of a university teaching hospital. JAMA. 1981; 246:1105.
17. Deen HG. Diagnosis and management of lumbar disc disease. Mayo Clin Proc. 1996;71:283-7.
18. Robinson LR. Electromyography, magnetic resonance imaging and radiculopathy: it's time to focus of specificity. Muscle Nerve. 1999;22:149-50.

SECTION 3

Understanding Imaging Modalities for Pain Patient

CHAPTER 8

Interpretation of X-ray Spine

Muthusamy Chandramohan

AIMS

- To understand the role of plain X-ray in pain medicine
- To review the key radiological anatomy of spine
- To recognize common variations in spine anatomy
- To familiarize with common pathologies that one can encounter in day-to-day practice.

ROLE OF X-RAY IN PAIN MEDICINE

- There is no specific role for plain X-ray in pain medicine
- X-ray is indicated only if the back pain persists despite 6 weeks of conservative management in the absence of trauma (Royal College of Radiologists Guidelines)
- Can be useful to confirm the presence of degenerative disease
- Can be useful to exclude other causes of back pain such as osteoporotic spinal fractures, inflammatory spondyloarthropathy, infection, and malignancy.

RADIOLOGICAL ANATOMY OF SPINE

Cervical Spine

- Lateral view: Normal cervical spine has gentle lordosis with anterior convexity (Fig. 1). The odontoid process (dens) of

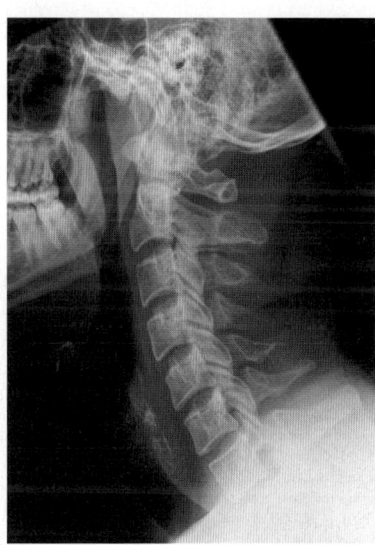

FIG. 1: Normal X-ray cervical spine lateral projection

C2 protrudes in to the C1 arch. The joint between anterior arch of C1 and odontoid process of C2 is called atlantoaxial joint (Fig. 2), which normally measures 2 mm in distance. The atlantoaxial joint space can be widened in rheumatoid arthritis due to ligament laxity resulting in atlantoaxial instability (can be radiologically assessed with flexion and extension lateral views) (Fig. 3).

- Anteroposterior view: The C1 and superior half C2 is obscured in the AP view due to superimposition of jaw bone (Fig. 4).

> **Key Points**
> - How to differentiate C7 from T1 in AP view?
> - The transverse process of C7 point downwards whereas the transverse process of T1 point upwards (Fig. 4).

- Oblique view: It is commonly used position during fluoroscopy guided spine intervention to demonstrate the neural foramina adequately (Fig. 5). Always look for signs of nerve root/neural foramina compromise such as disk osteophyte bar or bony spur (Fig. 5). Uncovertebral joint/ neurocentral joint (Fig. 6). Arthrosis is common in cervical spine, which can impinge on the nerve in the lateral recess.

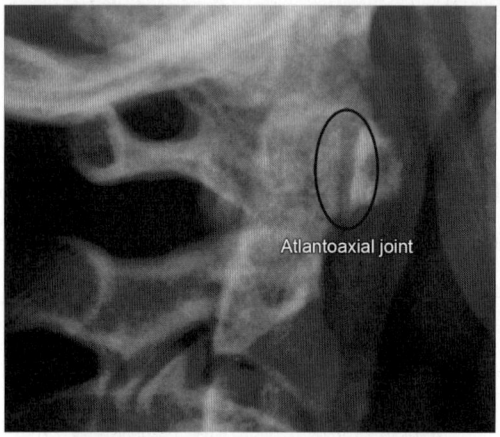

FIG. 2: Cervical spine (coned view) lateral view showing normal atlantoaxial joint space (C1-C2 articulation)

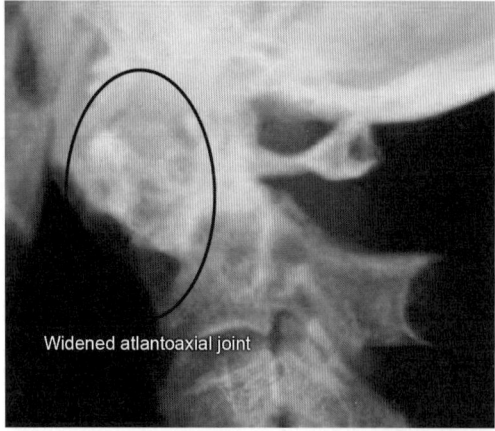

FIG. 3: X-ray cervical spine lateral projection (coned view) of a patient with rheumatoid arthritis showing gross widening of the atlantoaxial joint due to ligament laxity

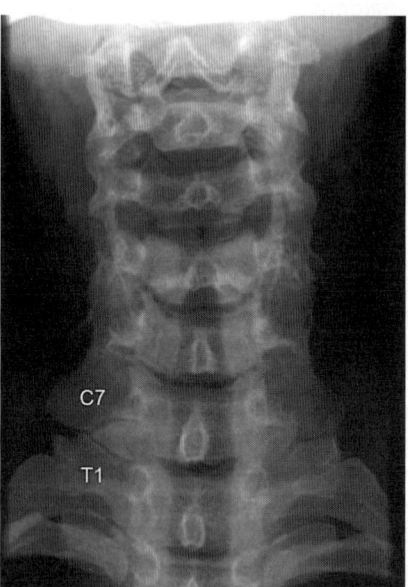

FIG. 4: Normal X-ray cervical spine (anteroposterior projection). Note the transverse process of C7 points downwards whereas the transverse process of T1 points upwards

Chapter 8: Interpretation of X-ray Spine

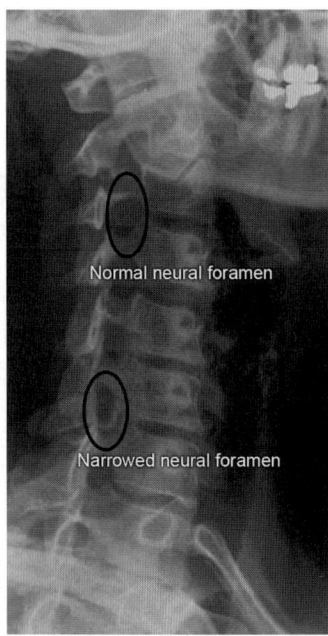

FIG. 5: X-ray cervical spine oblique view demonstrating the neural foramina adequately. There is narrowing of the C6-C7 neural foramina due to osteophytic disease

Thoracic Spine

- Lateral view: Normal thoracic spine has gentle kyphosis with posterior convexity (Fig. 7). Weight bearing thoracic vertebral bodies is slightly wedge shaped anteroposteriorly
- Thoracic intervertebral disk spaces are relatively shorter than cervical and lumbar disks and are less frequently involved in degeneration
- Osteoporotic collapse: It typically occurs in the thoracolumbar region (D11-L1) (Fig. 8)
- Costovertebral joints and costotransverse joints are difficult to assess on the X-ray, which are not infrequently involved in inflammatory, spondyloarthropathy, and crystal deposition disease.

Key Point

- Thoracic spine is relatively fixed by the rib cage and therefore degenerative disk disease is less common when compared with cervical and lumbar spine

Lumbar Spine

- Lateral view: Normal lumbar spine has gentle lordosis with anterior convexity (Fig. 9)
- Anteroposterior view: The interpedicular distance gradually widens from L1 down to L5 (Fig. 10). Failure of divergence of interpedicular distance from L1 down to L5 indicates spinal canal stenosis on AP view (Fig. 11)

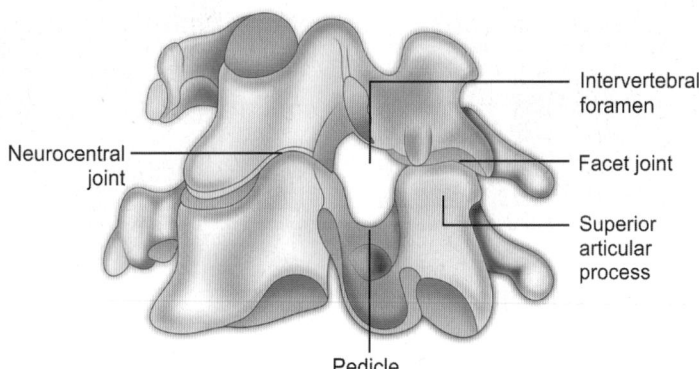

FIG. 6A: Line diagram showing the anatomy of the neurocentral joint (uncovertebral joint)

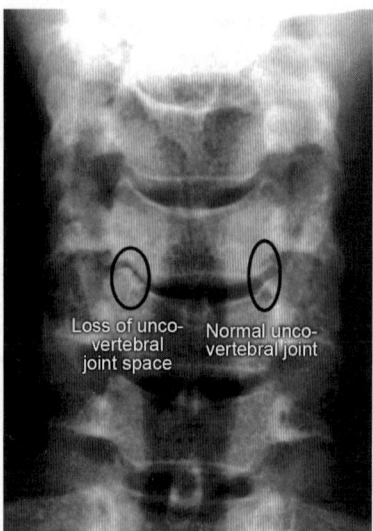

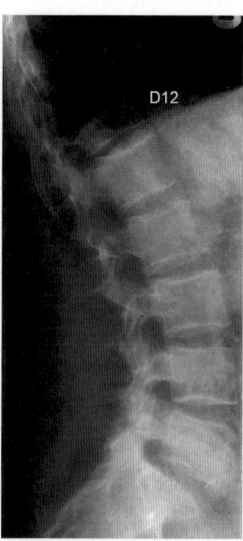

FIG. 6B: X-ray cervical spine anteroposterior view showing the normal C4/C5 uncovertebral joint on the left and early arthritis (loss of joint space) of the C4/C5 uncovertebral joint on the right

FIG. 8: X-ray thoracolumbar spine lateral spine— lateral view showing moderate wedge fracture of the D12 vertebral body due to osteoporosis

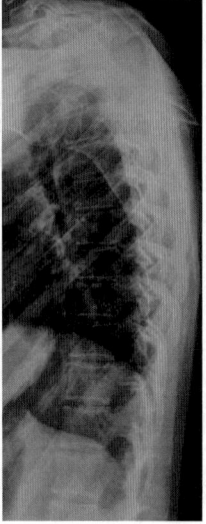

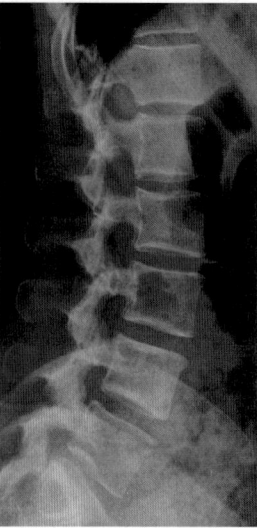

FIG. 7: Normal X-ray thoracic

Fig. 9: Normal X-ray lumbar

- Oblique view: "Scottish Terrier dog" appearance. Look for a break in the neck of the "Scottish Terrier dog" to diagnose spondylolysis/pars inter articularis fracture (Fig. 12).

Key Points
- Lumbosacral transitional vertebra is common
- Provocative diskogram/diagnostic injections indicated to identify the symptomatic level

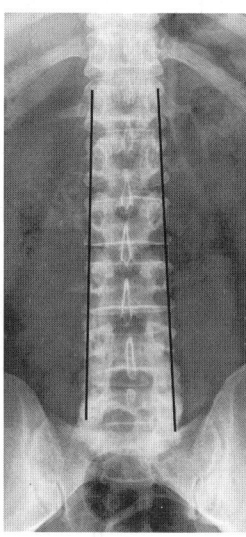

Fig. 10: Normal X-ray lumbar spine—anteroposterior, spine lateral projection. Note the gradual widening of the interpedicular distance from L1 down to L5

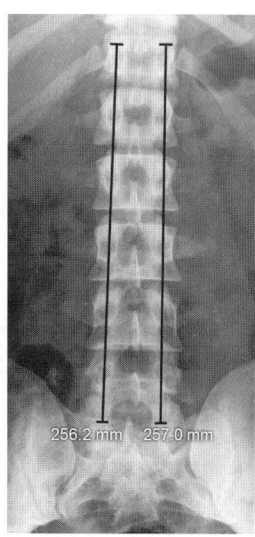

FIG. 11: Non-divergence of interpedicular distance from L1 down to L5 on anteroposterior view indicates spinal canal stenosis

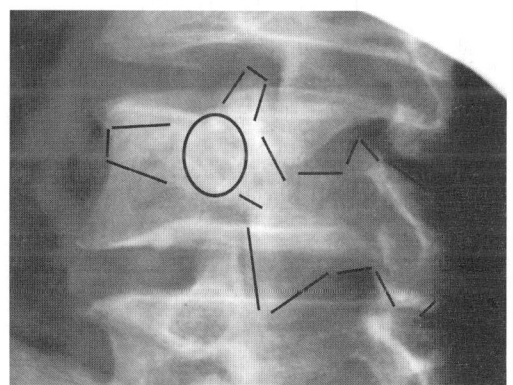

FIG. 12A: Lumbar spine oblique view demonstrates 'Scottish Terrier' dog appearance of the vertebral body (transverse process–nose, pedicle–eye, superior articular process–ear, inferior articular process–forelimb, pars interarticularis–neck)

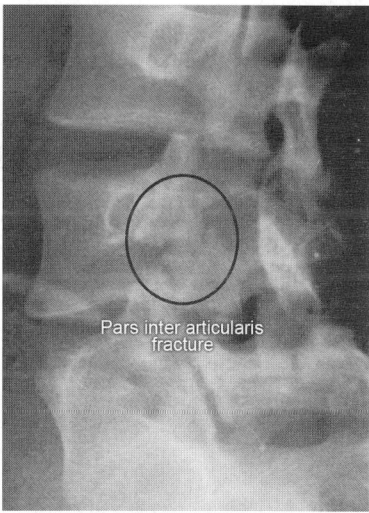

FIG. 12B: Lumbar spine oblique view of another patient showing discontinuity of the pars interarticularis (defect in the neck of 'Scottish Terrier' dog) of L4 consistent with spondylolysis (pars defect)

Sacroiliac Joints

- Radiological evaluation of spine is incomplete without assessing the sacroiliac joints sacroiliac joints
- The superior two-thirds of the sacroiliac joints is fibrous joint and the inferior one-third of the joint is synovial

- Degenerative changes are common in sacroiliac joints and can resemble sacroiliitis
- Bilateral symmetrical triangular sclerosis of the sacroiliac joints on the iliac side are not infrequent (osteitis condensans ilii) and can be mistaken as sacroiliitis (Fig. 13).

Key Point
• The anteroinferior portion of the sacroiliac joint is synovial and therefore commonly involved in inflammatory sacroiliitis (Fig. 14)

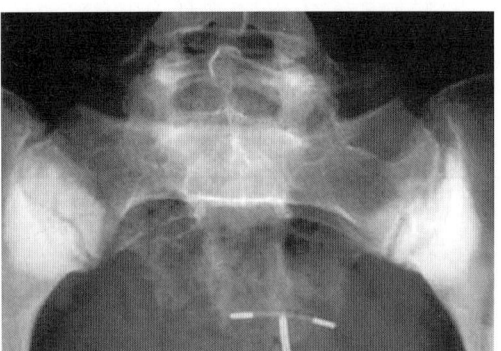

FIG. 13: X-ray sacroiliac joints of a multiparous female patient demonstrating a well-defined sclerosis on the iliac side of the sacroiliac joints bilaterally, typical of osteitis condensans ilii

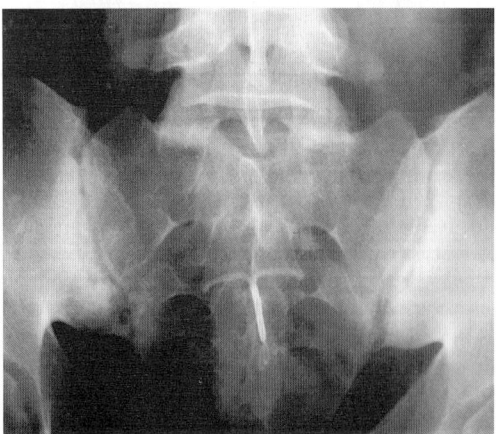

FIG. 14: Bilateral sacroiliitis. X-ray showing irregular articular surfaces and subchondral sclerosis of the sacroiliac joints bilaterally

HOW TO INTERPRET A SPINE X-RAY?

- Remember ABCDEF.

A: Alignment

In the absence of trauma, malalignment is usually secondary to degenerative disk or facet joints (Fig. 15). The other cause of malalignment is spondylolisthesis (slip of one vertebra over another) secondary to spondylolysis (pars interarticularis fracture or defect) in the lower lumbar spine (Fig. 16).

B: Bone Morphology

Height/size of the vertebral body—reduced height of a vertebral body is either due to osteoporotic collapse or due to metastatic collapse (Fig. 17). Bone expansion is a feature of Paget's disease (Fig. 18) and vertebral hemangioma.

Contour—irregular/shiny vertebral corners suggest enthesitis/inflammatory spondyloarthropathy (Fig. 19).

Cortical thickening is a feature of Paget's disease (Fig. 18).

Coarsened trabeculations can be due to vertebral Paget's (Fig. 18) or hemangioma.

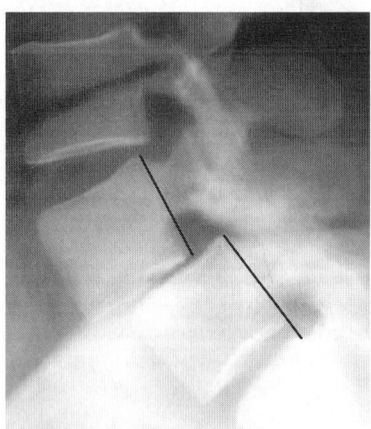

FIG. 15: X-ray lumbar spine lateral projection (coned view) showing anterior slip (spondylolisthesis) of L5 on S1 due to degeneration. Note narrowing of the L5/S1 disk space and L5/S1 facet joint arthrosis

Focal lesions can be either lytic or sclerotic, which can occur in infection, benign, and malignant bone lesions (Fig. 20).

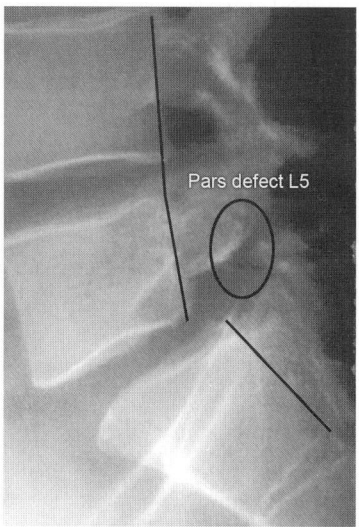

FIG. 16: Spondyolisthesis (slip) of L5 on S1 due to pars fracture of L5

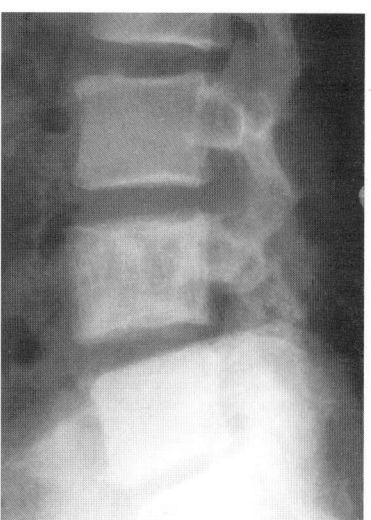

FIG. 18: Ivory vertebra (solitary sclerotic vertebra) of L4 due to Paget's disease. The L4 vertebral body is expanded with cortical thickening and coarsened trabeculations

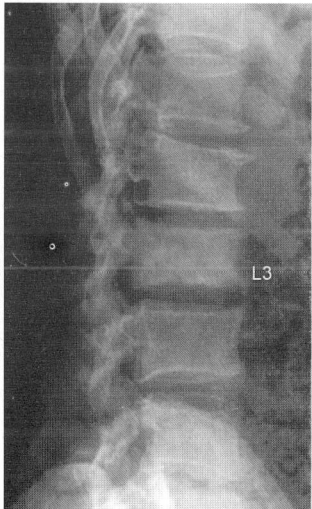

FIG. 17: There is collapse of the L3 vertebral body due to metastasis from known breast carcinoma. The L3 vertebral body appear dense when compared with the rest of the spine

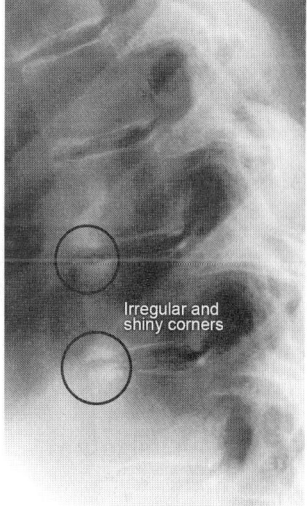

FIG. 19: X-ray lower thoracic spine of an adult male with back pain shows irregular and sclerosed anterior corners of multiple vertebral bodies consistent with inflammatory spondyloarthropathy (ankylosing spondylitis)

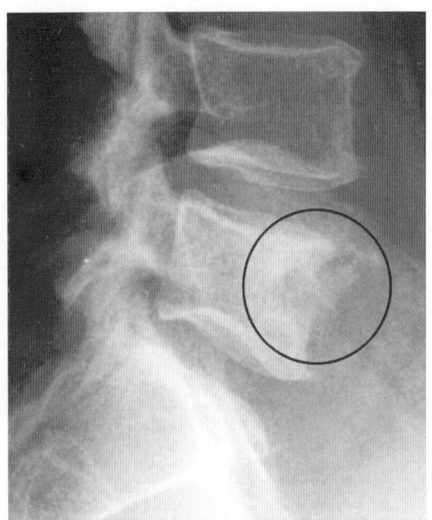

Fig. 20: Focal bone destruction of L5 due to infection (TB). The other common causes of focal bone lesion is metastasis and myeloma

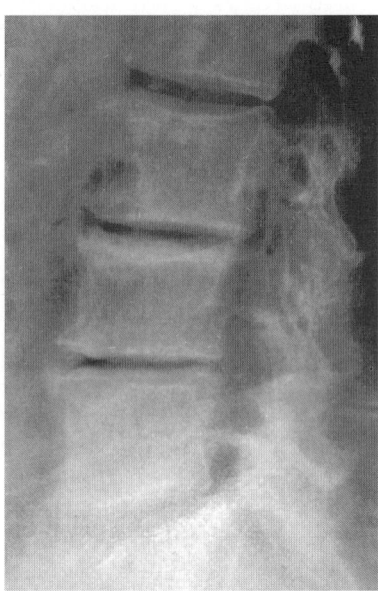

FIG. 21: Severe degeneration of the lumbar spine. Note complete loss of disk height at multiple levels. The presence of intradiskal gas, vertebral end-plate sclerosis and facet joint arthritis indicates degeneration

C: Cartilage

Loss of joint space equals cartilage loss—a feature of degeneration typically seen in atlantoaxial joint and uncovertebral joints in cervical spine. The other findings of degeneration are intra-articular gas, subchondral sclerosis, and osteophytosis.

D: Disk Height

Reduced disk height is a feature of degenerative disk disease. Additional findings are end-plate sclerosis, osteophytes and facet joint arthrosis (Fig. 21).

Reduced disk space with destruction of the adjacent vertebral end-plate equals diskitis.

E: End-plate of the Vertebral Body

End-plate sclerosis usually indicates degenerative Modic changes.

End-plate destruction with or without reduction in the height of the disk suggests diskitis/infection (Fig. 22).

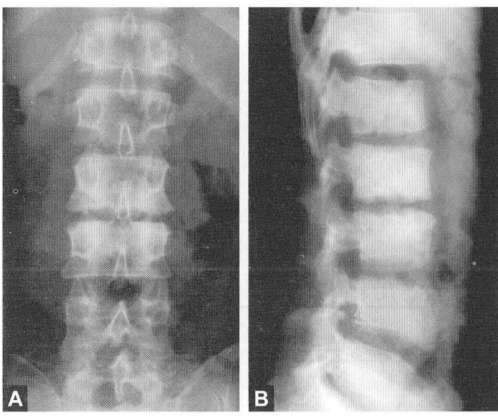

Fig. 22: X-ray lumbar spine AP and lateral view showing L2/L3 diskitis. There is loss of L2/L3 disk space with irregularity and sclerosis of the adjacent vertebral end-plates

F: Facet Joints

Loss of facet joint space with or without osteophyte and subchondral sclerosis indicates degeneration.

Chapter 8: Interpretation of X-ray Spine

S: Soft Tissue and Structures Around

Suspect spinal infection or tumor if prevertebral or paravertebral soft tissue mass is present in the absence of trauma (Fig. 23).

Do not forget to assess the review areas, i.e. SI joints in a lumbar spine X-ray (Fig. 24) and Pancoast tumor in a thoracic spine X-ray (Fig. 25).

- Remember FACE. You should see two eyes (end on view of pedicles), two ears (transverse processes), and a nose (spinous process). That is how an individual thoracic and lumbar vertebral body's look like in an AP view. In contrast the cervical vertebral body looks like an "alien" face (Fig. 26).

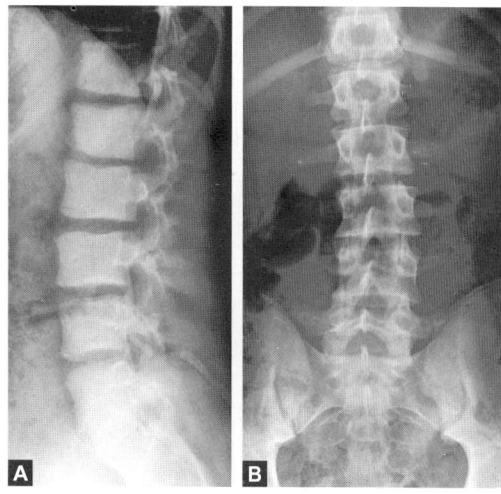

FIG. 24: Male aged 22 presented with low back pain following injury in rugby sport. X-ray lumbar spine lateral view demonstrates irregular erosion of the anteroinferior corner of L1 vertebral body. Note the presence of bilateral sacroiliitis in the AP view. Based on the X-ray findings a diagnosis of early ankylosing spondylitis was made

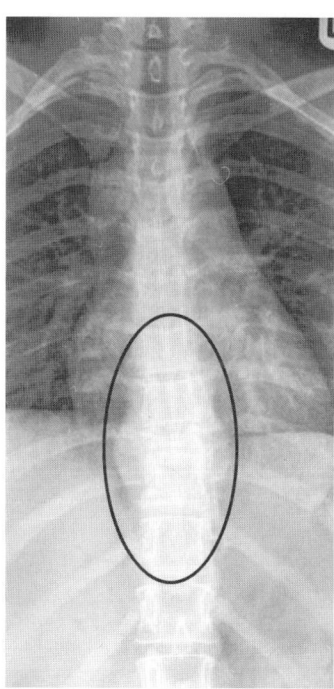

FIG. 23: TB spine in a 25 year old female patient who presented with mid thoracic pain. X-ray showing collapse of T9 vertebra with large paraspinal soft tissue mass

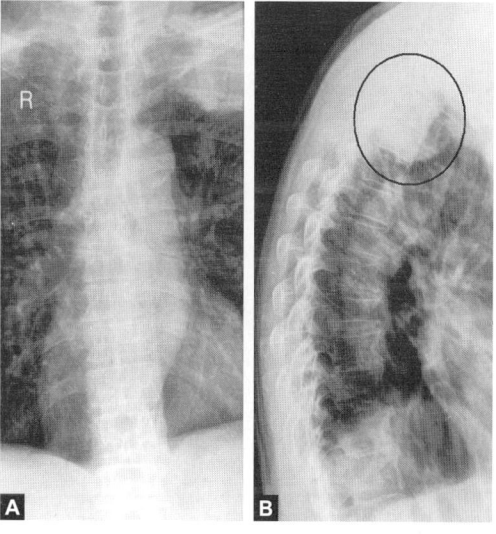

FIG. 25: Adult male with interscapular pain. The left apical lung cancer was missed in the initial radiograph of the thoracic spine

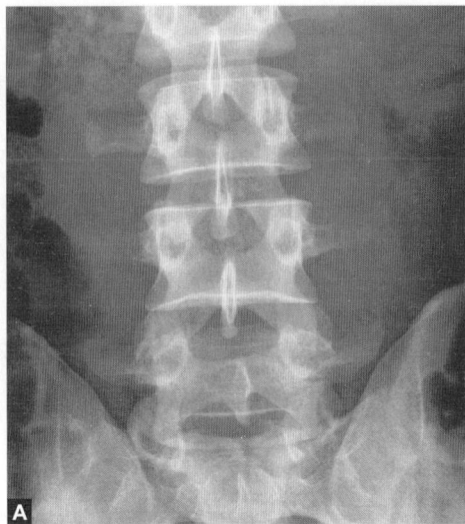 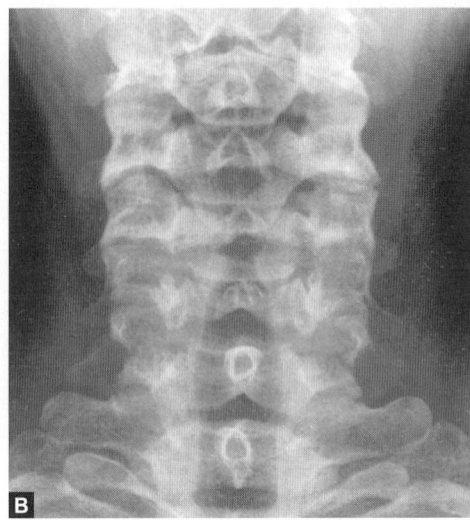

FIG. 26: Anteroposterior view of the lumbar spine and cervical spine, respectively. Each lumbar vertebra resembles a human face and each cervical vertebra resembles an "alien" face

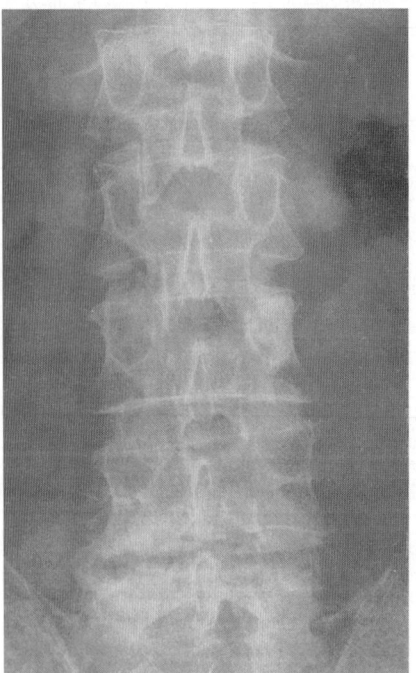

FIG. 27: Winking eye—sclerosed/dense left pedicle of L3, typical appearance of metastasis

Winking eye (sclerosed/destroyed pedicle) indicates metastasis (Fig. 27).

CONCLUSION

X-ray is indicated only if the back pain persists despite six weeks of conservative management in the absence of trauma. Remember ABCDEF when interpreting spine X-ray. Radiological evaluation of spine is incomplete without assessing the sacroiliac joints.

CHAPTER 9

Interpretation of Computer Tomography Scans for Interventional Pain Treatment Procedures

Sunil A Waghmare

INTRODUCTION

Pain management specialists pose a challenge in the 21st century as spinal and perispinal pain has emerged to be the cause of loss of man hours and increasing disability with respect to physical and emotional drain.

Computed tomography (CT) scan today is already being used as a powerful tool to aid interventional pain physician in performing various intervention, basic and advanced.

While basic interventions involving infiltrations are easy to perform, advanced infiltrations require proper training and experience. Radiologist should be available for difficult interventions.

Computed tomography fluoroscopy is a tool which is indispensable for pain interventions as it decreases the procedure time as well as makes the procedure more precise.

Sometimes CT fluoroscopy-guided interventions can avoid a major surgery and thus less burden to the patient and his family in monetary as well as risk avoidance.

The materials and techniques used in CT guidance although remain the same, it gives an interventional pain physician additional advantage of three-dimensional comprehension of the anatomy with regards to final needle positions and very high accuracy too (Table 1).

TABLE 1: Types of procedures

Basic interventions	Advanced interventions
• Cervical spine	• Neurolysis/radio frequency (RF)
○ Greater occipital nerve	○ Trigeminal nerve
○ Periradicular infiltration	○ Sphenopalatine ganglia
• Thoracic spine	• Neurolysis
○ Costovertebral joints	○ Stellate ganglia
○ Facet joints	○ Thoracic sympathetic
• Lumbar spine	○ Splanchnic nerves
○ Epidural	○ Celiac ganglia
○ Periradicular	○ Lumbar plexus
○ Facet joints	• Nucleoplasty
○ Spondylolysis	• Vertebroplasty
○ Synovial cyst	–
• Sacroiliac joint or SI joint	–

BASIC PROCEDURES

Arnold Nerve Infiltration

It is useful to diagnose as well as treat greater occipital neuralgia (GON).

Patient is placed in a prone position on the CT scan table. Scanning is performed from C0 to

C3 vertebral bodies. This confirms the anatomy of muscles, bones, foramen and the anteriorly placed vertebral artery. GON originates between the posterior arches of C1 and C2, immediately next to the atlas-axis facet joint. Hence, a dorsal paramedian approach is planned. A 25-Gauge (G) needle is passed under CT-fluoroscopy guidance for faster procedure and the target is the C2 bony facet where the needle upon landing should produce neuralgic symptoms and if the symptoms produced are different than the patient's initial complaints, the most likely cause is that the needle is stimulating a facet joint (C1–C2), which is known as pseudo Arnold's neuralgia. Repositioning the needle towards C2 facet is required.

The same protocol should be followed while performing rhizotomy with radio frequency (Fig. 1).

Cervical Root Injections

It is indicated for patients with radicular hand pain due to disk herniation.

Patient is placed in supine position and scanning performed from C4 to T1 vertebral bodies. Target the neural foramina with a lateral approach just lateral to sternocleidomastoid muscle using a 25-G spinal needle carefully avoiding the anteriorly placed vertebral artery. Stop at the anterior aspect of facet joint. Carefully install the steroid and local anesthetic (LA) cocktail up to 0.3–0.5 mL. If the radicular pain increases upon start of injection (severe inflammation), then withdraw the needle and reposition it little outside the facet ventral margin till pain is elicited, then reinject the cocktail (Fig. 2).

Thoracic Costovertebral and Facet Injection

It is indicated in patients with intercostal neuralgia and localized paraspinal pain.

Patient is place in prone position, painful level marked on the skin and limited scan performed. 22-G needle in a paraspinal and oblique approach towards the desired costovertebral or facet joint. CT fluoroscopy aids in the faster placement of the needle (Fig. 3).

Lumbar Epidural Injections

It is used for sciatic pain. Patient is placed in prone position and the target area is based on diagnostic tests and clinical findings. Target is the epidural space posteriorly between ligamentum flavum, facet joint, dura and the affected nerve root. Target slice is selected and under CT fluoroscopy a 22G needle is passed paramedially till it reaches the dorsal margin of ligamentum flavum. Further advancement should be carefully done till a give way is encountered. Push 0.3 mL of air to confirm epidural positioning. On CT image, it

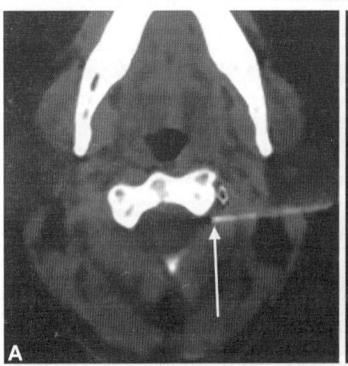
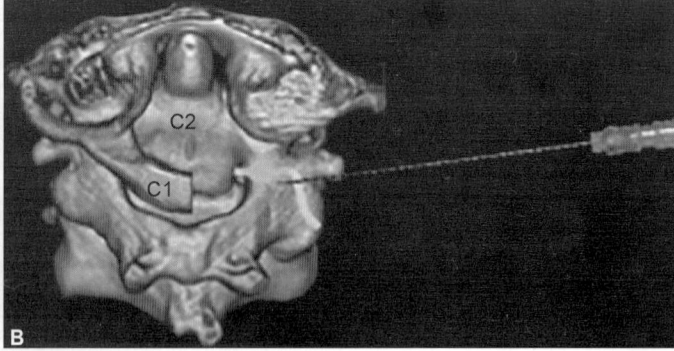

FIGS 2A and B: (A) Final position of needle at the level of C2 facet; (B) 3D scan depicting the needle position before infiltration *(For color version, see Plate 2)*

Chapter 9: Interpretation of Computer Tomography Scans for Interventional Pain Treatment...

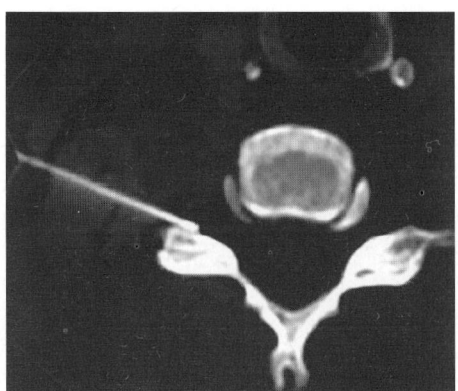

FIG. 2: Needle position anterior to the facet joint for cervical root injections

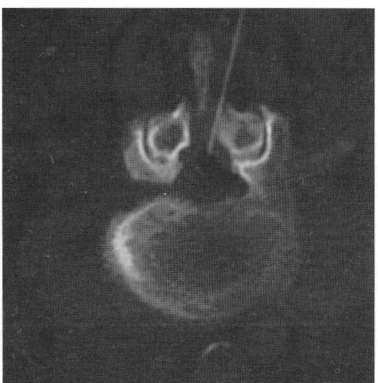

FIG. 4: Lumbar epidural injection of air in epidural space to confirm the spread

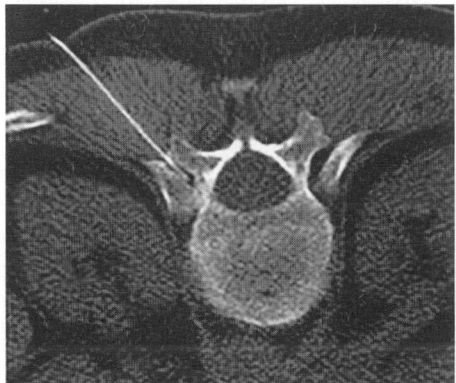

FIG. 3: Facet injection with posterolateral approach

scan begins with scanning of the desired level. Tilt the gantry according to lordosis so that it is parallel with targeted intervertebral disk space. Target is to reach the level of spinal dorsal root ganglion (DRG) anteriorly. Generally, target slice of region of interest (ROI) is selected and needle is aligned with the gantry tilt and entered postern-laterally about 5–6 cm from midline. Needle passing through the muscular plane should stop at the level of facet joint anteriorly near the exit of foramina and spinal ganglion in the vicinity. The risk of procedure is low when performed under continuous CT fluoroscopy (Figs 5A and B).

Lumbar Facet Joint Injections

It is indicated for lumbar facet joint injections. Target of injection is the inferior recess part of the degenerated facet join and the cartilage being still intact. Under continuous CT fluoroscopy the needle is introduced posterolaterally and the facet joint entered with the 22-G needle as explained above. Steroid and LA is injected (Fig. 6).

Lumbar Spondylolysis Test Infiltration

It is low back pain attributable to degenerative disk disease. Test infiltration aims to guide further strategies of management.

will remain there thus creating space between dura and flavum for further injection of steroid and LA. Chances of dural perforation must be kept in mind. First sign is cerebrospinal fluid (CSF) aspiration through needle and second sign being washout of injected air. Hence, needle needs to be retracted till no CSF is aspirated or the injected air stays in place. Considered blood patch for dural tear, which is about 1 mL of blood through the same needle (Fig. 4).

Lumbar Periradicular Injection

It is indicated for foraminal or postforaminal symptoms correlating with imaging. Generally,

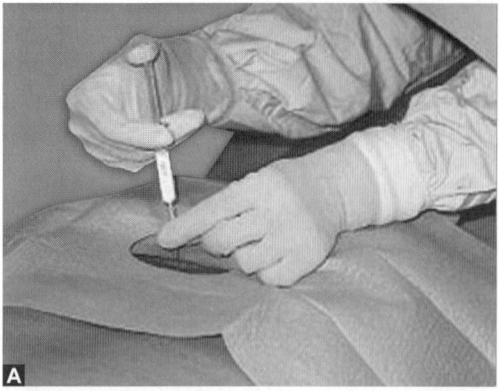
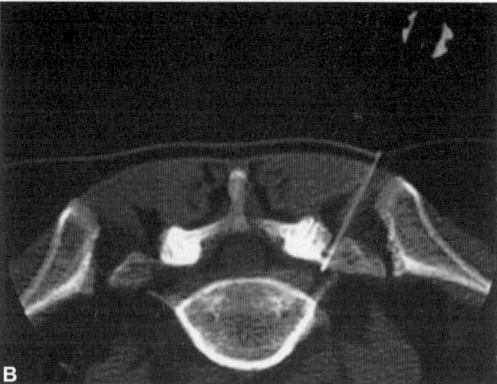

FIGS 5A and B: (A) Injection of steroid in the foramen; (B) Final position of needle tip in the foramen prior to the injection

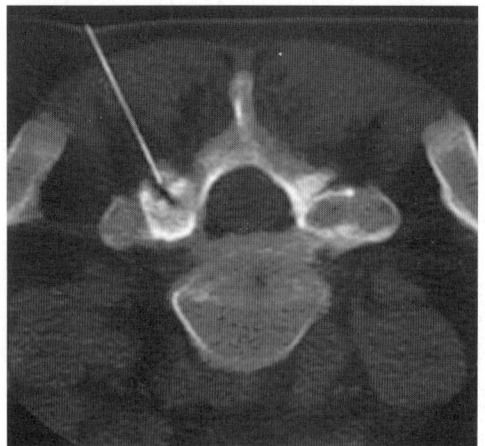

FIG. 6: Injection into facet joint

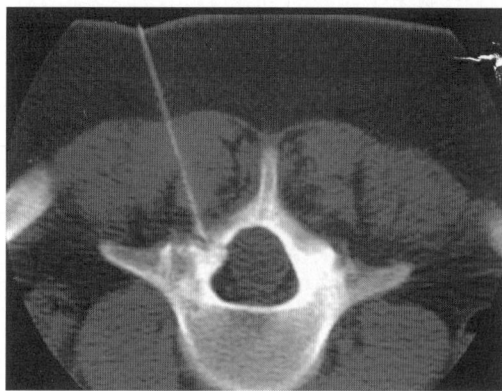

FIG. 7: Injection into spondylolytic defect

Patient is placed in prone position and the desired CT slice with spondylolysis in view is selected and injection is performed with a 22-G needled through postern-lateral approach. Then once inside the spondylolytic site, 1 mL of lignocaine is injected. Within 5 minutes the patient's pain should reduce significantly in extension, this implies that the test is positive and the back pain is due to spondylolysis only (Fig. 7).

Lumbar Synovial Cyst Infiltration

It is indicated for synovial facet cyst causing nerve compression or radicular symptoms. Patient is placed prone on CT table and rest of the procedure is performed similar to lumbar facet injection using a 20-G needle. Then air is injected to opacify the facet joint and the cyst. Saline is injected in order to rupture the cyst. If unbearable pain occurs then the technique of lumbar epidural injection is performed with direct puncture of the cyst and then saline is injected to rupture the cyst wall, and finally LA alone with steroid is injected to finish the procedure (Fig. 8A and B).

Sacroiliac Joint Injection

It is indicated in patients with acute or chronic sacroiliac (SI)-joint pain not controlled

Chapter 9: Interpretation of Computer Tomography Scans for Interventional Pain Treatment...

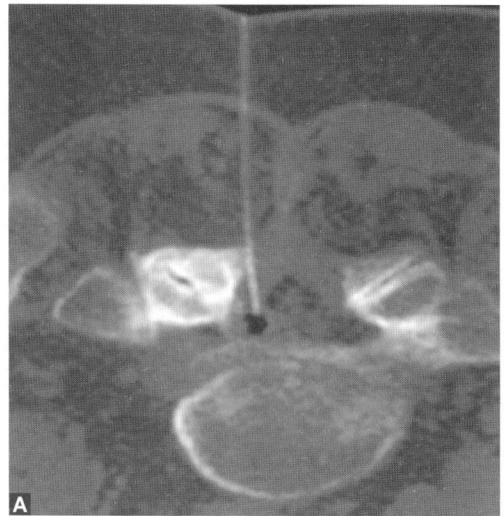
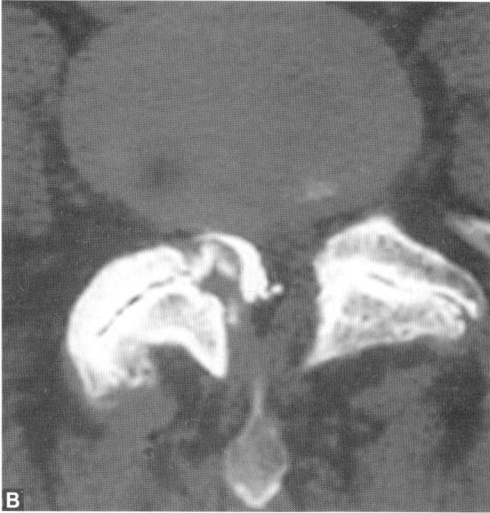

FIGS 8A and B: (A) Puncture of facet cyst under CT guidance; (B) Contrast injection into facet cyst

with nonsteroidal anti-inflammatory drug (NSAIDs) or conservative management. Not infrequently the procedure is performed in patients with seronegative inflammatory sacroiliitis. With patient in prone position, needle is advanced under continuous fluoroscopy in an angulated trajectory in line with the SI-joint. Target is to reach the center of the SI-joint, this is felt like a sudden decrease in needle advancement upon crossing the dorsal margin of the joint, which is covered by strong posterior longitudinal ligaments. Avoid entering the anterior joint space or presacral space. Nonionic contrast is injected to watch for diffusion and correct needle placement.

Steroid mixed with local anesthetic is followed after (Fig. 9).

ADVANCED PROCEDURES

Trigeminal Ganglia Neurolysis or Radiofrequency

The procedure is carried out under hypnotic anesthesia so as to keep the patient calm and responding to verbal command. Patient is placed in supine position with neck extended.

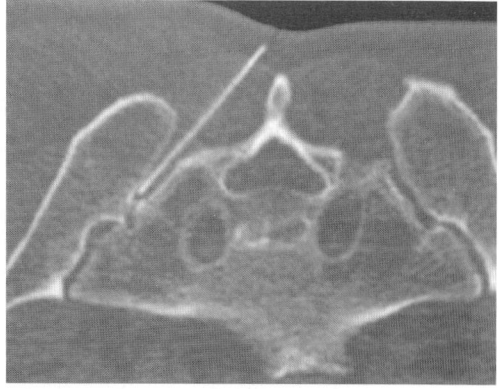

FIG. 9: Injection into sacroiliac joint

A skin wheal is raised 2.5–3 cm lateral to the angle of the mouth, with CT guidance the needle is inserted in frontal-mentonian plane and along the homo-lateral pupil, 45^0 to the sagittal plane. The needle is advanced in the foramen ovale (Fig. 10A). Noting the absence of CSF, contrast is injected to depict the spread in Meckel's cave along with demonstration of all the three branches (Fig. 11B). Neurolysis is performed at this juncture using glycerol. For the purpose of radiofrequency (RF) the 20-G RF needle with 8–10 mm exposed is advanced

5 mm anterior to the clival plane for third division and at the clival plane for second division. RF is performed at 70° C for 60 seconds after sensory and motor stimulation. During RF procedure, patient should be administered adequate hypnotic analgesia for pain relief (Figs 10A to D).

Sphenopalatine Ganglia Neurolysis or Radiofrequency

Neurolysis or RF of sphenopalatine ganglia is contemplated in patients with cluster headaches, pterygopalatine ganglion (PPG) neuritis, postherpetic neuralgia and severe intractable cancer pains.

Computed tomography gives the correct position of sphenopalatine ganglion (SPG) in the pterygopalatine fossa. The important contents of the PPG fossa are the SPG, internal maxillary artery and the maxillary nerve.

Approach to the PPG should be by placing the patient supine on the CT table with the head turned towards the opposite side. Scanning is performed from the anterior zygomatic process till the maxillary bone. The SPG lies posteriorly within the PPG fossa and the artery is anterior. Hence, under continuous CT fluoroscopy the needle is advanced from above the zygomatic arch (lateral approach) and advanced till the tip lies anterior to the lateral pterygopalatine plane posterior to the maxillary sinus. A test injection (20:80—contrast; local anesthetic 1%) to confirm the needle tip as well as to perform a block. For neurolysis 1 mL of alcohol is instilled and the effects are noticed on CT scan with washing of the contrast and it becoming hypodense.

Radiofrequency is carried out in continuous mode 70° C for 90 seconds and is performed three times. Post-RF small amount

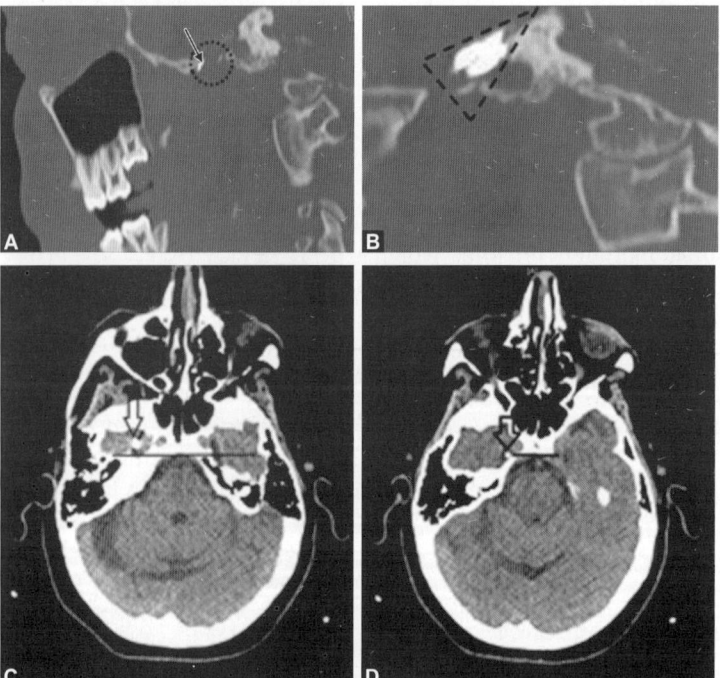

FIGS 10A to D: (A) Final position of needle tip in the foramen ovale behind clivus; (B) Contrast injection to depict the nerve roots of trigeminal nerve; (C) Needle position 5 mm anterior to clival plane, horizontal line represents clival plane; (D) Needle tip at the level of clival plane, horizontal line represents clival plane of local anesthetic mixed with steroid is instilled for preventing postprocedure pain and inflammation.

Some patients experience epistaxis following the procedure. It should be satisfactorily corrected before discharge (Fig. 11).

Stellate Ganglion Neurolysis or Radiofrequency

Neurolysis or RF is an accepted method of treating acute and chronic sympathetic upper limbs, causalgia of head and neck, postherpetic neuralgia, reflex sympathetic dystrophy, cancer pain involving stellate ganglia from lower neck and thoracic apex (along with thoracic sympathetic procedure).

Stellate ganglia is located anterior to C7 and the neck of first thoracic vertebra, it measures 2.5 cm in long axis, 1 cm wide and 0.5 cm in thickness.

Patient is placed supine with head turned towards the opposite side. Anterolateral approach is chosen and the entry point is chosen anterior to C7 vertebra and anterior to T1 thoracic rib for RF. For neurolysis the target is anterior to C7 vertebral body. Scanning is performed for C6 vertebral body (superior level) till T2 vertebral body (superior level). Entry point is anterolateral and is selected in line with the target avoiding the carotid artery and the jugular vein anteriorly and the vertebral artery posteriorly (where it emerges from the subclavian artery).

Upon reaching the target, small volume is contrast is injected in order to confirm the position and to also look for vascular injection. RF or neurolysis is performed at above-mentioned targets. Usually 1 mL of alcohol should suffice. Advantage of RF over neurolysis is that it gives good pain relief without producing Horner's syndrome (Figs 12A to C).

Splanchnic Nerve Neurolysis

It is indicated and is efficient in management of pain due to celiac ganglia encasement due to neoplastic infiltrations (pancreatic and

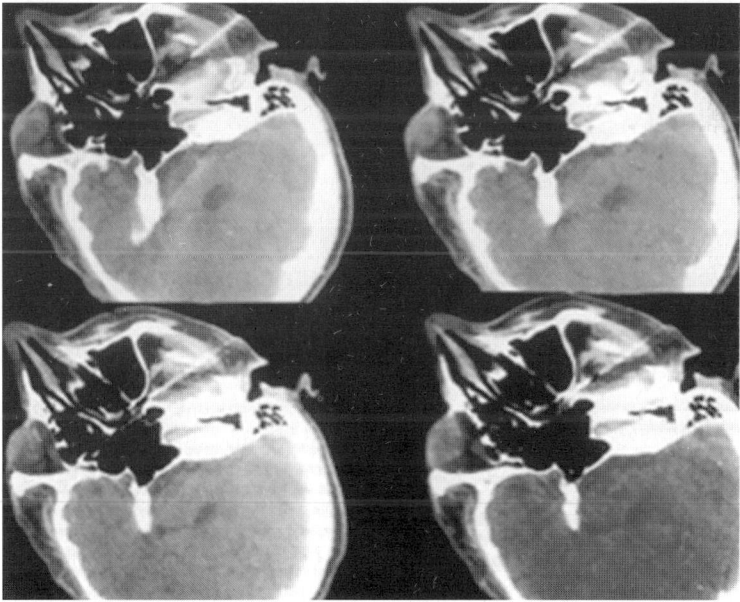

FIG. 11: Sequential images depicting advancement of needle to the final position posterior to maxillary sinus and anterior to the lateral pterygoid plate

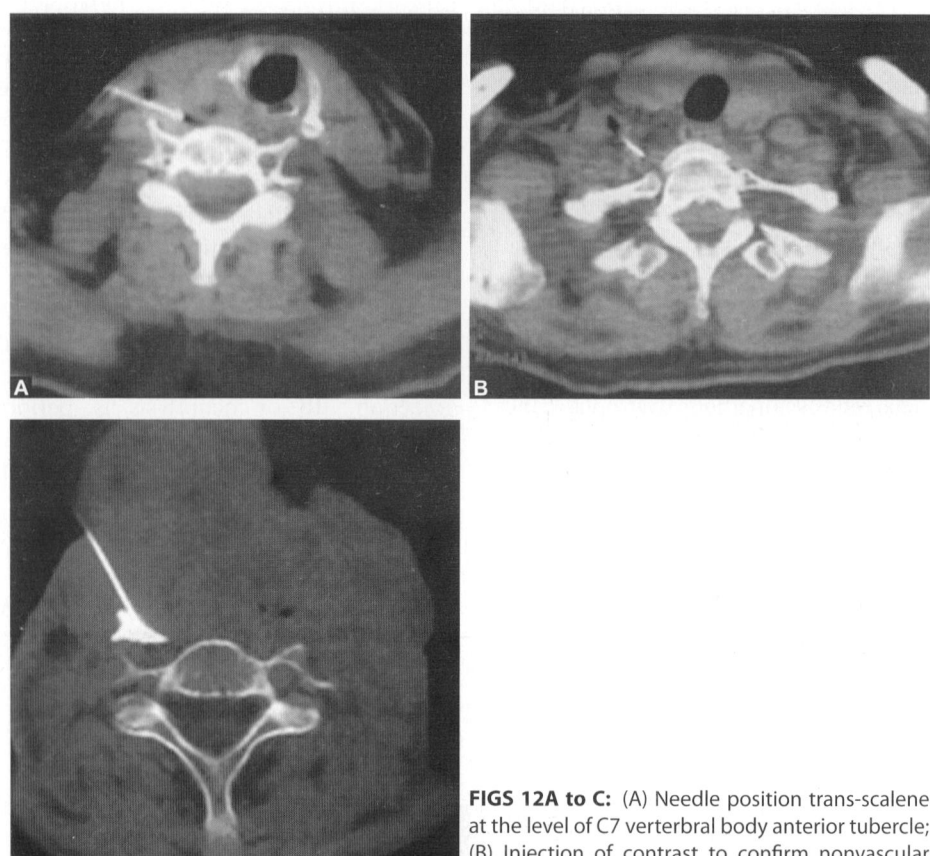

FIGS 12A to C: (A) Needle position trans-scalene at the level of C7 verterbral body anterior tubercle; (B) Injection of contrast to confirm nonvascular dye spread

gastric tumors), neoplastic infiltrations of retroperitoneal tissues and pain of chronic pancreatitis.

Target is to perform neurolysis at anterior third of paravertebral space at the level of T12 vertebral body where lies the splanchnic nerves.

Patient lies in prone position, scans performed from T11 till L2 vertebral body after I.V contrast. Target as explained above is approached bilaterally with a 22-G needle posterior paramedian approach under continuous CT-fluoroscopic guidance. Upon reaching the target, lignocaine mixed with contrast is injected and nonvascular spread is confirmed using CT fluoroscopy. Also diffusion of contrast is noted behind the crux of the diaphragm and paravertebral space.

Neurolysis is performed with 5 mL of 8% phenol bilaterally. Infuse 1 mL of lignocaine before withdrawal of needle (Figs 13A and B).

Coeliac Ganglia Neurolysis

Its indications are the same as splanchnic nerve neurolysis.

Approach using prone position is paramedian with needle passing through the paravertebral space to reach the celiac ganglia, either by the side of aorta or through the aorta below the celiac trunk. It is advisable to perform this procedure under CT fluoroscopy. A total of 3 mL nonionic contrast mixed with lignocaine (25–75%) is injected to demonstrate the extravascular spread and diffusion. Neurolysis is performed using 15 mL of 8% phenol or 15 mL

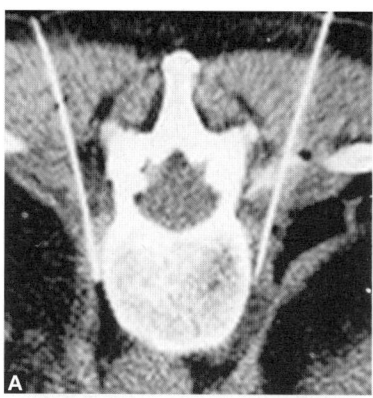 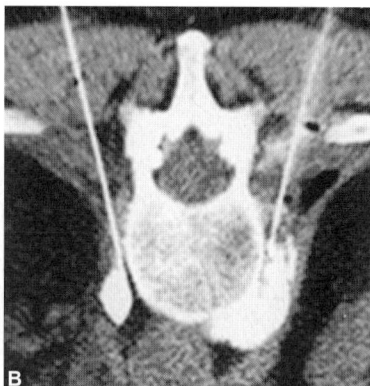

FIGS 13A and B: (A) Correct needle placement for splanchnic neurolysis; (B) Local and dye injection to observe the spread before neurolysis

of pure ethanol. Postprocedure the needle is flushed with 1 mL of lignocaine (Figs 14A to C).

Anterior Approach

The patient in prone position with scanning from Th11 to L2.

Needle passes transhepatically, eventually transgastric, transintestinal and tip being position anterior to the aorta and celiac trunk. A total of 3 mL of nonionic contrast is injected to demonstrate nonvascular and preaortic spread. Eventually, 15 mL 8% phenol or pure ethanol is injected. Needle is flushed with 1 mL of lignocaine before withdrawal (Figs 14D to G).

Lumbar Plexus Neurolysis

It is indicated in patients with significant peripheral arterial disease and complex regional pain syndrome with sympathetic component.

Target area paravertebral space at l2 and l4 vertebral body between aorta (left) or inferior vena cava (IVC) and IVC (right) and psoas muscle.

With the patient lying prone, scan is performed for Th12 to L5 vertebral body level with IV contrast to delineate the position of ureters. A 15-cm-long 22-G needle being inserted paracentrally to reach the target as described above and contrast is injected along with lignocaine to observe the diffusion and to rule out intravascular, intraureteric and posterior paravertebral spread. A total of 10 mL of 8% phenol mixed with glycerol is injected to perform neurolysis. Postprocedure pain and orthostatic hypotension could be expected (Figs 15A to C).

Nucleoplasty—Disc Decompression with Laser/RF

This technique is indicated for sciatica pain beyond 6 weeks and postfailure of conservative management in a contained disk herniation. The patient is placed in prone position and axial scans are obtained at the desired disk level.

Local anesthesia administered from skin to the facet joint under CT fluoroscopy. An 18-G needle is passed under fluoroscopy anterior to facet joint from a posterolateral approach. Disk is punctured and needle placed in the center of the disk in anteroposterior (AP) and lateral position. Laser fiber is passed through the needle projecting 3 mm beyond the needle tip and the laser fiber and needle combination readjusted in the disk center. The same procedure can be performed using a combination of RF needle and thermocouple. The idea is to deliver enough energy so as to desiccate the nucleus thereby causing decompression enough to reduce the protrusion.

Complications like diskitis, infectious or thermal could be avoided by adequate anti-

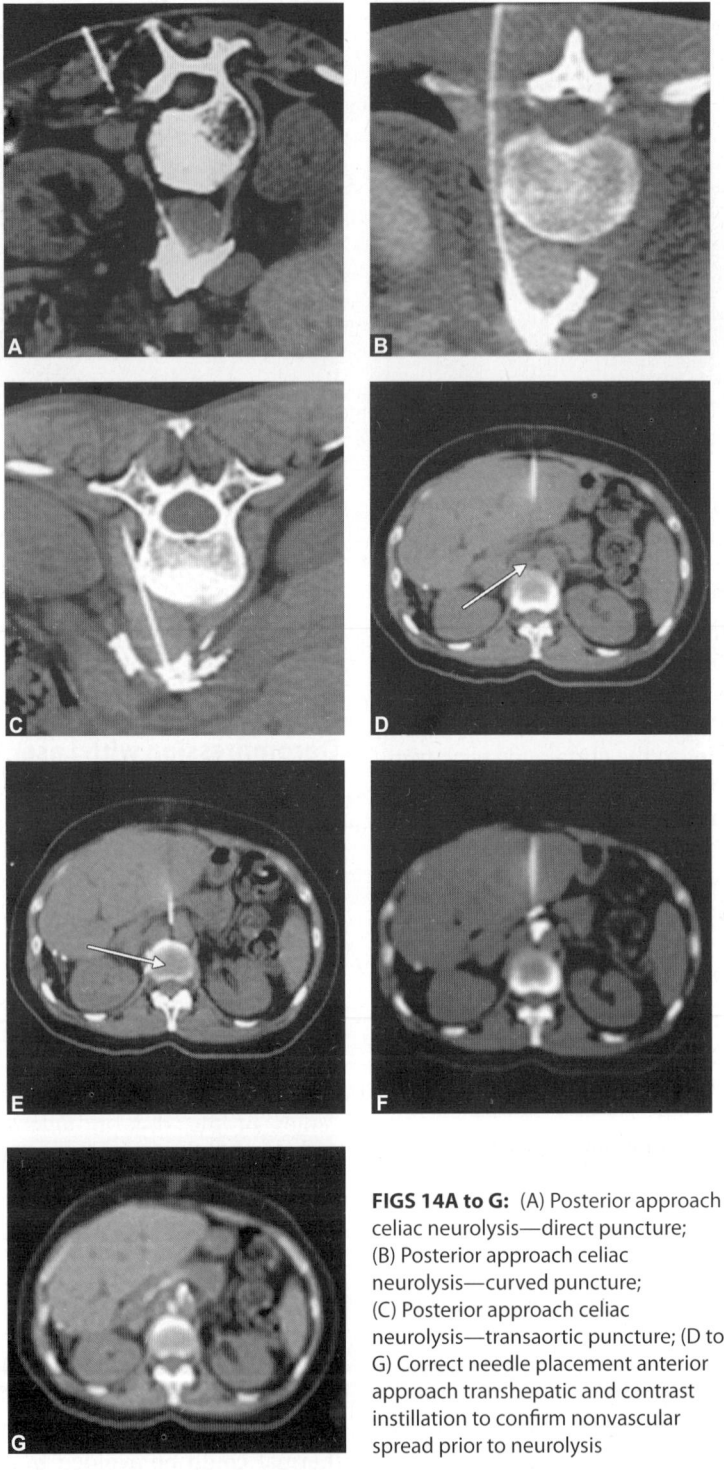

FIGS 14A to G: (A) Posterior approach celiac neurolysis—direct puncture; (B) Posterior approach celiac neurolysis—curved puncture; (C) Posterior approach celiac neurolysis—transaortic puncture; (D to G) Correct needle placement anterior approach transhepatic and contrast instillation to confirm nonvascular spread prior to neurolysis

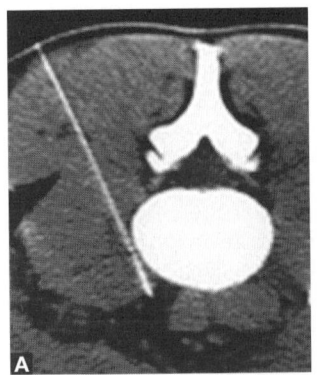 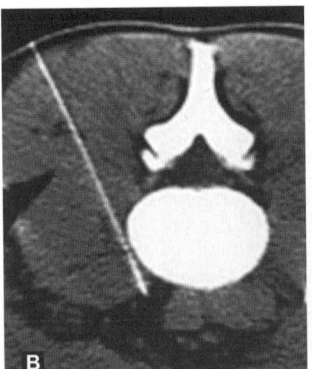 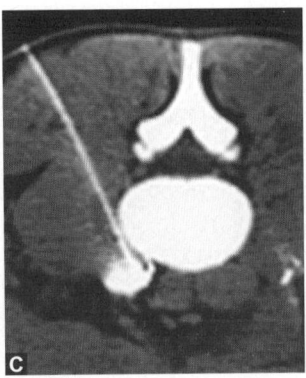

FIGS 15A to C: (A) Lumbar plexus target slice; (B) Correct needle positioning; (C) Opacification and neurolysis

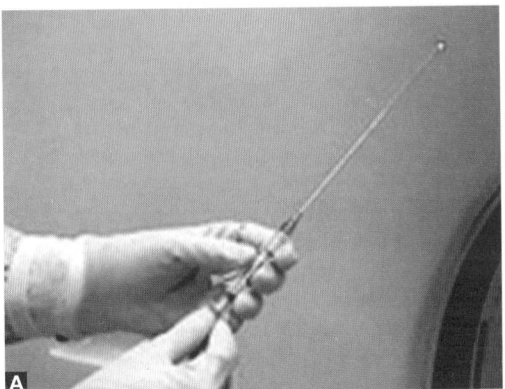 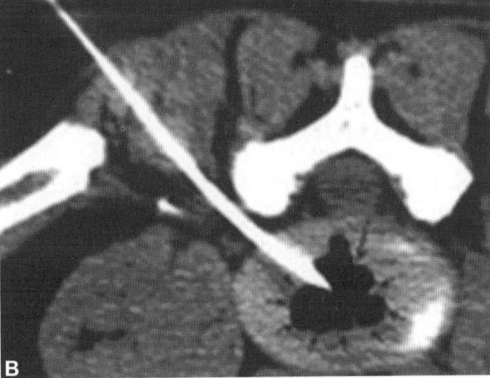

FIGS 16A and B: (A) Needle and laser fiber assembly for percutaneous laser disc decompression (PLDD); (B) Vaporization of nucleus allowing disc decompression

biotics (intradiscal postprocedure and IV at the start of the procedure. Postprocedure 5 days course should follow) (Figs 16A and B).

Vertebroplasty

Indicated in (1) fractured endplates due to trauma, neoplasm or osteoporosis, (2) lytic neoplasm and (3) painful hemangiomas.

With the patient lying prone, axial scan is obtained at the level of the affected vertebral body including adjacent vertebral bodies' end plates.

Approach is transpedicular mostly and could be posterolateral at lumbar levels and intercostovertebral at thoracic levels.

Transpedicular Approach

Under CT fluoroscopy the trajectory is marked and adequate anesthesia is delivered from skin to the bone (pedicle). 11 or 13-G vertebroplasty needle is advanced with small jolts of hammer avoiding the medical cortex of the pedicle thus entering the vertebral body, preferably short of anterior third of the cortex and in the center of vertebral body.

Approximately 3-6 mL of cement is injected under CT-fluoroscopy guidance avoiding leak in the epidural space and venous leak. Stop procedure if the cement is advancing towards posterior cortex.

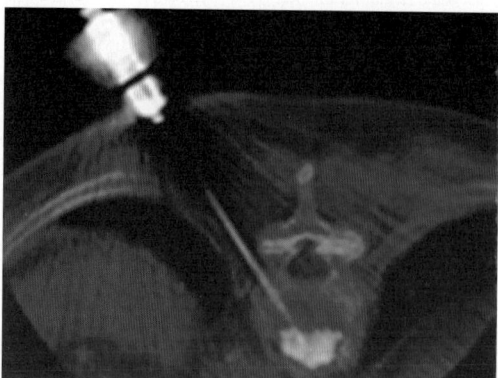

FIG. 17: Cement injection under CT-fluoroscopic guidance during vertebroplasty

Posterolateral Approach

Avoid hitting the exiting nerve root (Fig. 17).

CONCLUSION

Computed tomography-guided procedures are much safer and performed at an out-patient basis. It allows step-by-step control over the procedure with 2D and 3D perspective of the anatomic location of the target as compared to fluoroscopy guidance. It can be used as an alternative modality or in conjugation with other modalities of image guidance during pain interventions. However, the pain interventionist has to be skilled in the interpretation of axial, coronal and 3D anatomy from CT perspective and is a laborious but fruitful task.

BIBLIOGRAPHY

1. Begemann PGC. CT-guided interventions–indications, technique and pitfalls. In: Mahnken AH, Ricke J (Eds). CT- and MR-guided interventions in radiology. Berlin Heidelberg: Springer Berlin Heidelberg; 2009. pp. 11-20.
2. Bhaskar AK. Interventional management of cancer pain. Curr Opin Support Palliat Care. 2012;6(1):1-9.
3. Brat H. (2007). CT fluoroscopy-guided spine interventions. [online] Available from *www.diagnosticimaging.com/articles/ct-fluoroscopy-guides-spinal-interventions* [Accessed December, 2016].
4. Gangi A, Dietemann JL, Mortazavi R, Pfleger D, Kauff C, Roy C. CT guided interventional procedures for pain management in lumbo-sacral spine. Radiographics. 1998;18(3):621-33.
5. Jain P, Dutta A, Sood J. Coeliac plexus blockade and neurolysis: an overview. Indian J Anaesth. 2006;50(3):169-77.
6. Kastler A, Aubry S, Sailley N, Michalakis D, Siliman G, Gory G, et al. CT-guided stellate ganglion blockade vs. radiofrequency neurolysis in the management of refractory type I complex regional pain syndrome of the upper limb. Eur Radiol. 2013;23(5):1316-22.
7. Lim SM, Lee C-S, Seo N, Chae E-Y, Suh DC. CT guided epidural steroid injection. Neurointervention. 2010;5:8-12.
8. Lai GH, Tang YZ, Wang XP, Qin HJ, Ni JX. CT-guided percutaneous radiofrequency thermocoagulation for recurrent trigeminal neuralgia after microvascular decompression. Medicine (Baltimore). 2015;94(32):e1176.
9. McArthur TA, Millsap JL, Clayton NG, Lambertsen Z, Narducci CA. CT-guided lumbar facet synovial cyst intervention: what the radiologist needs to know. Birmingham: University of Alabama; 2016.
10. Piagkou M, Demesticha T, Troupis T, Vlasis K, Skandalakis P, Makri A, et al. The pterygopalatine ganglion and its role in various pain syndromes: from anatomy to clinical practice Pain. Pract. 2012;12(5):399-412.
11. Quek LH, Pua U, Chua GC, Tsou IY. Computed tomography fluoroscopic-guided percutaneous spinal interventions in the management of spinal pain. Ann Acad Med Singapore. 2009;38(11):980-8.
12. Rizzo CC, Ventura LM, Antônio de Castro L. CT-guided anterior celiac plexus neurolysis: case report. Rev Dor. 2011;12.
13. Ruiz Lopez R (2016). Treatment of craniofacial pain with radiofrequency procedures. [online] Available from *docslide.us/documents/treatment-of-cranio-facial-pain-with-radiofrequency-procedures.html* [Accessed December, 2016].
14. Sahin O, Harman A, Akgün RC, Tuncay IC. An Intra-articular sacroiliac steroid injection under the guidance of computed tomography for relieving sacroiliac joint pain: A clinical outcome study with two years of follow-up. Arch Rheumatol. 2012;27(3):165-73.
15. Timpone VM, Hirsch JA, Gilligan CJ, Chandra RV. computed tomography guidance for spinal intervention: basics of technique, Pearls, and avoiding pitfalls. Pain Physician. 2013;16(4):369-77.
16. Yang JT, Lin M, Lee MH, Weng HH, Liao HH. Percutaneous trigeminal nerve radiofrequency rhizotomy guided by computerized tomography with three-dimensional image reconstruction. Chang Gung Med J. 2010;33(6):679-83.

CHAPTER 10

Magnetic Resonance Imaging in Pain Management

Makarand M Kulkarni

INTRODUCTION

There are various imaging modalities for the investigation of pain. In the present era, pain management is incomplete without radiological investigation. The various radiological investigations including X-ray, computerized axial tomography (CAT) scan, ultrasonography, magnetic resonance imaging (MRI) and bone scan. With newer sequences and increase in magnetic field strength, the role of MRI has increased in imaging of spinal, abdominal, musculoskeletal, neurological causes of pain. The most common pain in the clinical practice is back pain and hence the spinal MR imaging is important investigation in the work-up of back pain.

MRI IN BACK PAIN

The Degenerative Spinal Disease

Lumbar Spine

The commonest cause of back pain and neck pain in the clinical practice is the degenerative spinal disorders which include the diskogenic pain, pain due to facet degeneration, spinal canal stenosis, and spinal instability. MR imaging is the choice of investigation in cases of back pain.

MR Imaging of Normal Disk and Disk Pathologies

The normal intervertebral disk has peripheral annulus fibrosus and central nucleus pulposus. The nucleus pulposus consist of collagen and hydrophilic proteoglycanes.[1,2] The normal hydrated disk has high-signal intensity on T2-weighted images in the center with low signal intensity in the periphery of annulus fibrosus (Figs 1A and B). While on T1-weighted sequence the distinction between the 2 zones of the disk is difficult. A low signal intensity band within the central nucleus region is attributed to internuclear cleft is commonly seen in patients older than 30 years[3] (Fig. 1B).

Degeneration of central nucleus may lead to instability and may be a cause low back pain. The desiccated disk shows hypointense signal on T2-weighted images with loss of internuclear cleft (Fig. 2A).[1] The outer annular fibers of the disk are innervated by free nerve endings. The disruption of the fibers known as annular tear can be a source of the back pain. The annular tear is seen as high-signal intensity zone on T2-weighted images in the posterior annulus of the bulging disk (Fig. 2B).

The lumbar disk herniation is a focal extension of the nucleus pulposus beyond

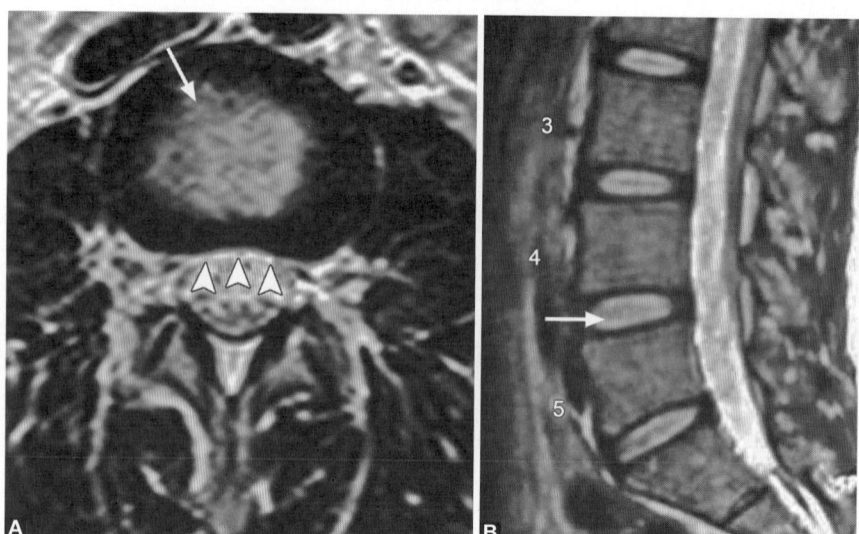

FIGS 1A and B: (A); T2-weighted axial images through the intervertebral disk showing central bright signals of hydrated nucleus pulposus (white arrow) and peripheral rim of hypointense signals of annulus fibrosus; (B) Sagittal T2-sections of spine showing normal appearance of disk with central nuclear cleft of low signals

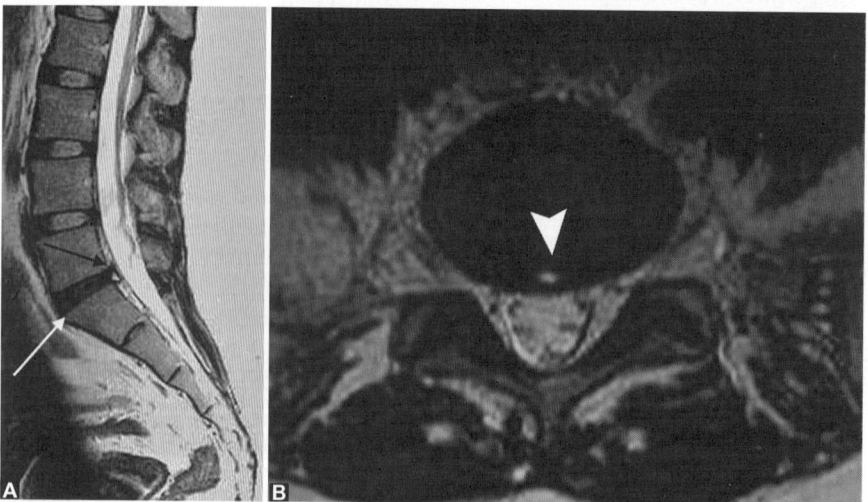

FIGS 2A and B: T2W sagittal and axial sequence showing diffuse dark signals in a desiccated disk (white arrow) with focal T2W bright signals in the posterior annulus of the disk (black arrow in Figure A and white arrowhead in Figure B) suggestive of annular tear

the margins of the disk. Posterior disk herniation can cause compression of the nerve roots and severe radicular pain. There are various terminologies of the disk herniations including disk bulge, protrusion, and extrusion. The disk bulge is symmetrical, circumferential disk extension beyond the interspace. Protrusion indicates focal or asymmetrical disk extension beyond the interspace with broad base against the parent

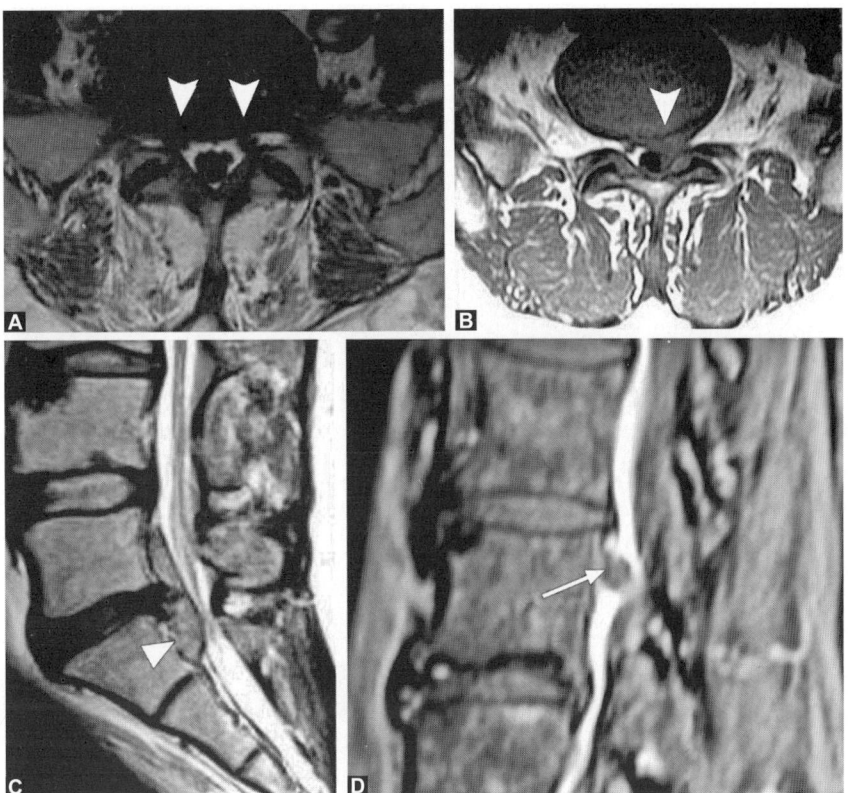

FIGS 3A to D: Disk bulge, protrusion, extrusion, and sequestration

disk. Extrusion refers to focal extension beyond the interspace with a narrow neck against parent disk (Figs 3A to D). The location of the disk herniation is also important which can be well assessed on MRI. On the axial images the location of disk herniation can be characterized by posterocentral, paracentral, foramina and extraforaminal (Figs 4A to D).[4]

Degenerative Pathologies other than Disk

The Facet Joints and Pathologies

Low back pain can be associated with degenerative changes in the posterior vertebral elements. The osteoarthritis of the apophyseal joint is one of the frequent causes of low back pain. MR imaging is inferior to CT scan for detecting the bony changes in the facet joint however, the effect of facet arthritis over the spinal canal and the lateral recess is better assessed on MR imaging. Similarly the soft tissue changes associated with degenerative changes in the facet joints like ligamentum flavum bulging, facet joint synovial cyst are better assessed on MR imaging.

The normal facet joint space shows bright signals on T2-weighted images due to hyaline articular cartilage. In case of osteoarthritis of facet joints, there is loss of this bright signals with loss of joint space and surface irregularity with subchondral cystic changes (Figs 5A and B). Facet joint subluxation can cause degenerative spondylolisthesis which cause significant

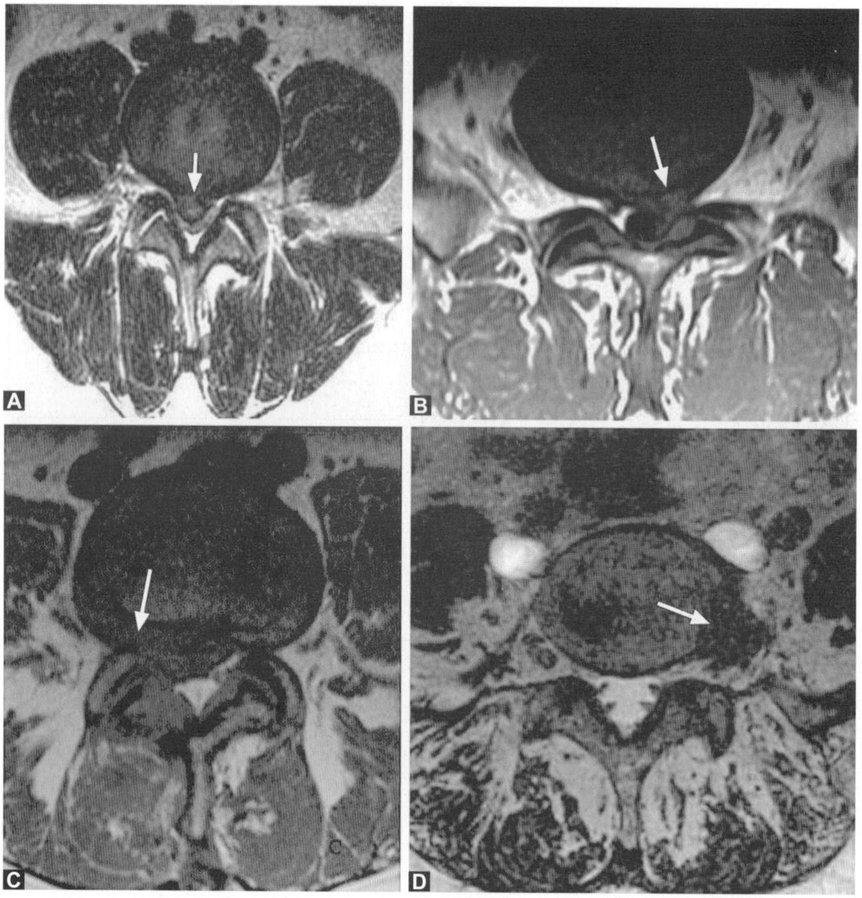

FIGS 4A to D: Location of disk herniation (A) Posterocentral; (B) Paracentral; (C) Foraminal; (D) Extraforaminal

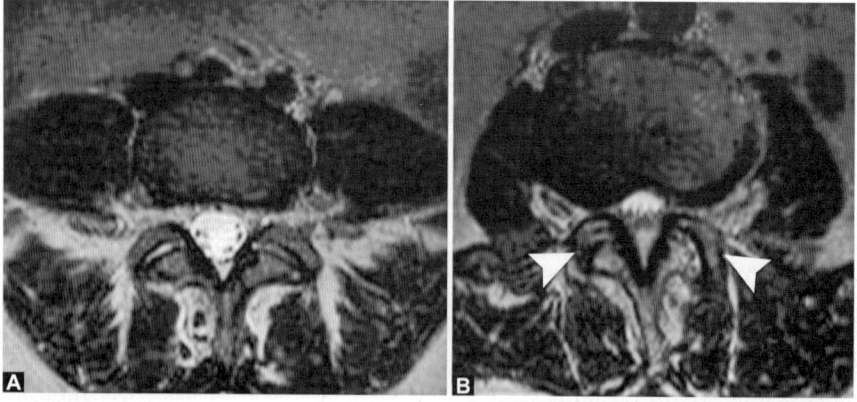

FIGS 5A and B: (A) Normal facet joint on T2W images with bright signals of facet joint fluid; (B) Reduced signals from the facet joint in a degenerated facet joint

narrowing of the spinal canal and leading to compression of neural structures and severe radiculopathy.[6] In a normal individual, unlike thoracic facet joints which are more coronal, the lumbar facet joints are oriented in Sagittal plane. However, there is a variation in the angulation of the facet joint with mean angulation between 39.1° on left and 42.9° on right.[5] In case of facet joint subluxation, the joint space is oriented more in the sagittal plane on axial CT images (Fig. 6). Degenerative changes in facet joint may lead to formation of facet joint synovial cyst which can be better appreciated on MR images[7] (Figs 7A and B). The facet joint synovial cyst can cause compression of the traversing nerve roots and may contribute to spinal canal stenosis, leading to severe radiculopathy.

Bulging/thickening of the ligamentum flavum can be associated with facet joint subluxation and may lead to severe spinal canal stenosis and radiculopathy (Fig. 8). The normal thickness of the ligamentum flavum on axial CT/MR images is about 4 mm.

The osteophytes associated with arthritis of the facet joints can cause severe neural foraminal stenosis. These osteophytes are better appreciated on CT scans. The other degenerative changes of the facet joints like hyperostosis on either sides of the joint space, subarticular cyst, osteophytes are better appreciated on CT scan.[7]

Imaging in spinal instability: There is no accepted definition of spinal instability, however, the most precise definition is given by Pope and Punjabi. According to them, instability is defined as abnormal response to applied loads characterized kinematically by abnormal movement in motion segment beyond normal constrains.[8] The instability

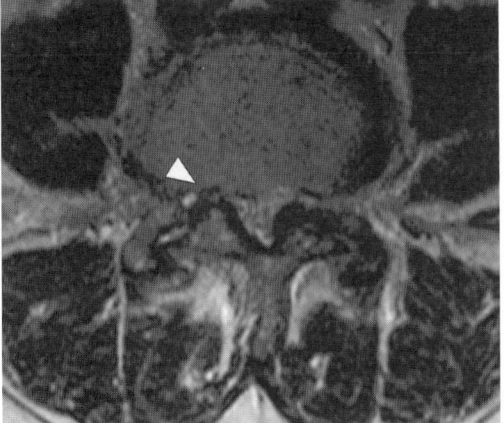

FIG. 6: Subluxation of the facet joint causing right lateral recess stenosis. Note the sagittal orientation of joint space (arrowhead)

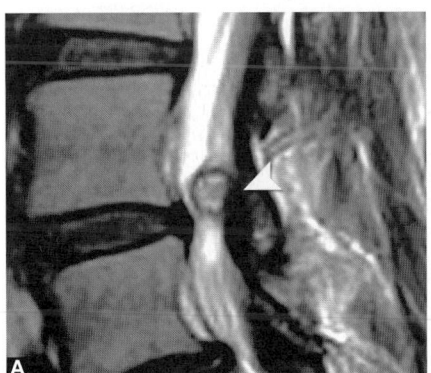 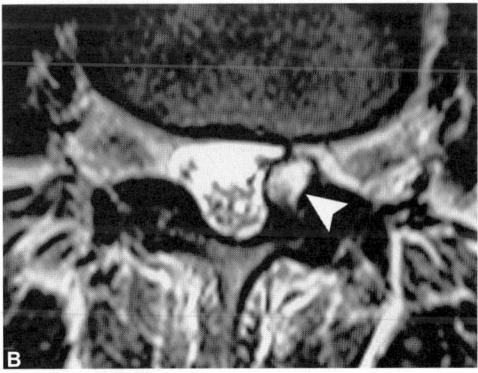

FIGS 7A and B: (A) Sagittal and (B) Axial T2-weighted images of facet joint synovial cyst causing severe compromise of left lateral recess

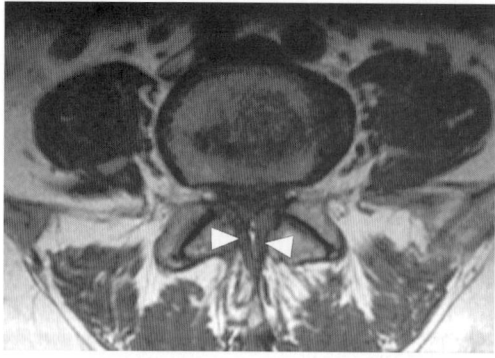

FIG. 8: T1W axial image showing hypertrophy of the ligamentum flavum (arrowheads)

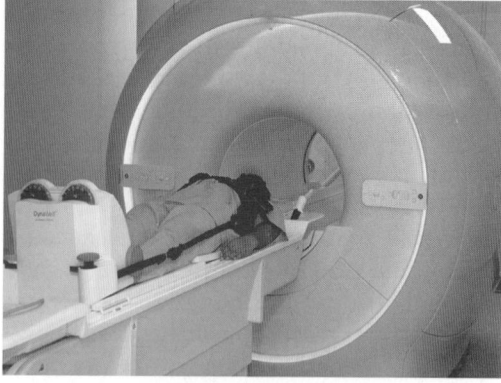

FIG. 9: Photograph of axial loading device in stress MRI

occur due to damage to restraining structures like facet joints, disks, ligaments and muscles, which leads to altered equilibrium.[9] Vertebral instability is one of the major causes of spinal pain and is often an important factor in determining the surgical indication for spinal fusion and with decompression. Vertebral instability can be imaged by flexion and extension lateral radiograph of spine. Axial loading of spine during MRI in supine position may mimic the standing position MRI and thus helps in evaluation of spinal instability[10,11] (Fig. 9).

THE CERVICAL SPINE

The mechanism of disk degeneration and herniation in cervical region is similar to that of the lumbar spine. However, unlike lumbar region, because of circumferential diameter of the spinal cord and anatomical conflagration of the vertebral bodies, a small disk herniation can produce severe radicular pain. A central disk herniation can cause cord compression leading to paraparesis or paraplegia while foraminal disk herniations can cause compression of the nerve roots and radicular pain[12] (Figs 10A and B).

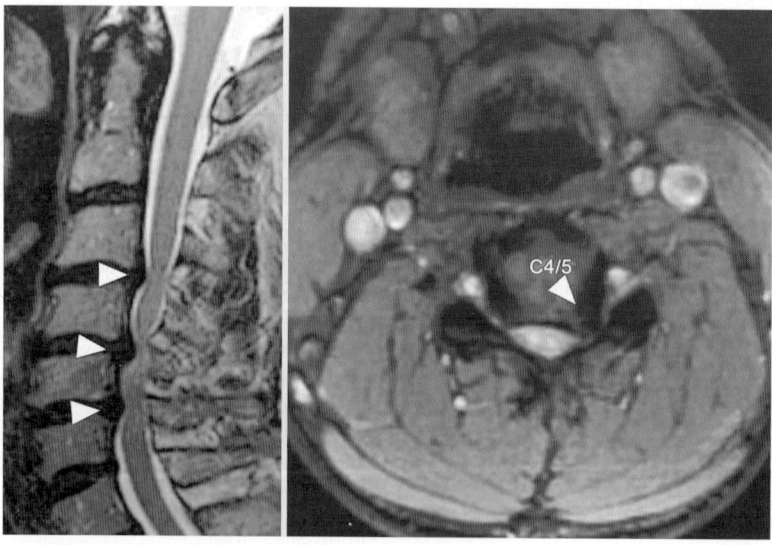

FIGS 10A and B: Disk herniation (A) Central; (B) Lateral

Chapter 10: Magnetic Resonance Imaging in Pain Management

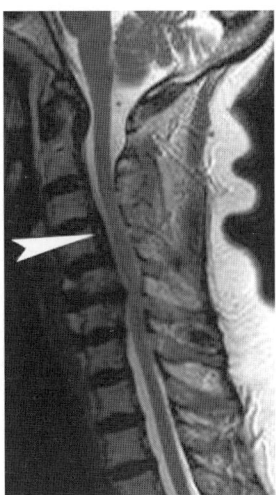

FIG. 11: Ossified posterior longitudinal ligament (arrowhead)

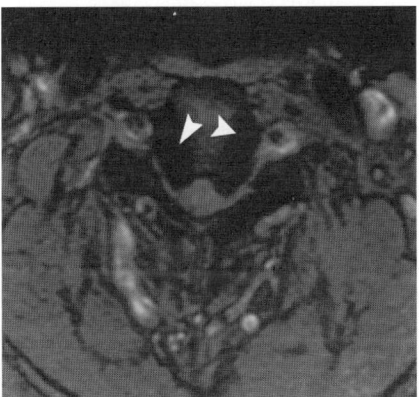

FIG. 12: Hypertrophy of uncinate process

Apart from disk herniation/disk degeneration, the degenerative changes in the diskovertebral complex and apophyseal joint can also cause severe pain and radiculopathy. Ossified posterior longitudinal ligament is seen as low signal intensity band on T2W sequence along the posterior border of vertebral bodies extending to several vertebral levels (Fig. 11). On T1 images, the signals may be variable depending on marrow formation signals within the ossified ligament. The hypertrophy of the uncinate process can cause spinal canal and neural foraminal compromise[13] (Fig. 12).

VERTEBRAL BODY COLLAPSE

There are various causes of solitary vertebral collapse including trauma, tumor and infection. In old patient, it is often a diagnostic problem between ostoporotic and malignant compression on plain X-ray. MR imaging can help in differentiating between the various causes of vertebral body collapse[14,15] (Table 1).

IMAGING IN INFLAMMATORY SPONDYLOARTHROPATHY

With development of more promising treatment like TNF-α, there is increasing need for the development of low back pain protocol with complete evaluation of whole spine, sacroiliac joint and hip joints. Spinal changes associated with inflammatory spondyloarthritis are florid anterior spondylitis (Romanus lesions), diskitis (Anderson's lesion), ankylosis, insufficiency fracture of ankylosed spine, syndesmophytes, arthritis of apophyseal and costovertebral joint, enthesitis of interspinous ligament. Syndesmophytes are well depicted on plain radiograph while all other radiological manifestations are better seen on MRI[16] (Figs 24A and B).

THE SPINAL TUMORS

The spinal tumors can be divided into intramedullary spinal tumors, extramedullary-intradural spinal tumors and extradural tumors. Most of the extradural spinal tumors are vertebral origin. The location of the tumor in the spinal canal is most important as both, the differential diagnosis and the management differs. MRI is the best imaging investigation which can differentiate the location of tumor in the spinal canal. The intramedullary tumors are usually associated with widening of the spinal cord and narrowing of the adjacent CSF spaces (Figs 25A and B). The extramedullary and intradural tumors are located between the spinal cord and dura and result in widening

TABLE 1: Causes of vertebral body collapse

Osteoporotic	Malignant	Infective
Concave posterior border with retropulsion or angulated posterior superior or inferior corner in the spinal canal—a very uncommon finding in malignant collapse. 2–19% of benign osteoporotic compression may show posterior bulging-convex border (an important sign of malignant collapse)	Posterior border convexity seen in 33–70% of malignant vertebral collapse (Fig. 13)	Posterior border convexity can be seen in infective spondylitis (Fig. 14)
Preservation of some normal fatt marrow on T1W images (Fig. 15)	The marrow infiltration by the tumor is usually complete. Vast majority of vertebral metastasis will not cause fracture unless there is complete replacement. In one-third cases there may be incomplete marrow replacement as seen in osteoporotic collapse however the configuration of marrow replacement (round/focal) may help in differentiating (Fig. 16)	
A band like hypointensity on T1W images along the fracture end plate—one of the specific signs of benign osteoporotic compression. It represents the compact bone or marrow replacement by fibrosis and is seen after restoration of normal fatty marrow in 2–3 months time which is specific sign of benign compression (Fig. 17)	Restoration of normal fatty marrow almost never occurs in malignant collapse	
An intraveretebral fluid cleft along the fractured end-plate seen in 12–50%. It can be due to intravertebral vacuum or due to ischemia of the vertebral body (Fig. 18)	Fluid cleft sign is seen in only 5–6% of the malignant vertebral collapse	
Usually, there is single vertebral involvement. In 19% cases, there may be focal areas of signal alteration in other vertebrae, most of these are benign (Schmorl's node, fracture line) (Fig. 19)	Multiple lesions are seen in more than 63–88% cases. The lesions in the other vertebrae are usually rounded and focal (Fig. 20)	Multiple vertebral involvements with skip lesions common in tubercular infection (Fig. 21)
Fragmentation seen in 10% of benign osteoporotic collapse	Fragmentation is caused due to higher force required to fracture a normal or osteoporotic vertebra than a malignant vertebra; hence, in malignant lesion fragmentation is less often seen	

Contd...

Contd...

Osteoporotic	Malignant	Infective
Hypointense on diffusion and high ADC	*Hyperintense on diffusion with low ADC*	*Hyperintense on DWI with low ADC*
Intense enhancement can be seen in acute collapse while the subacute and chronic collapse may show mild or no enhancement. The fracture line may be seen as hypointense line in enhanced vertebral body (Fig. 22)	Intense heterogeneous enhancement with diffuse or patchy distribution and without any linear hypointensity	Intense enhancement of the end-plate and adjacent marrow
No epidural soft tissue	*Presence of anterior epidural or paraspinal soft tissue*	*Anterior epidural and paraspinal soft tissue present*
No disk involvement	Since metastasis occurs through hematogeneous route hence, there is absence of involvement of avascular structures like end-plates and disks. In the primary malignant lesion, however, there may be disk involvement as is seen in infection	Destruction of the adjacent end-plate with involvement of the disk (Fig. 23)

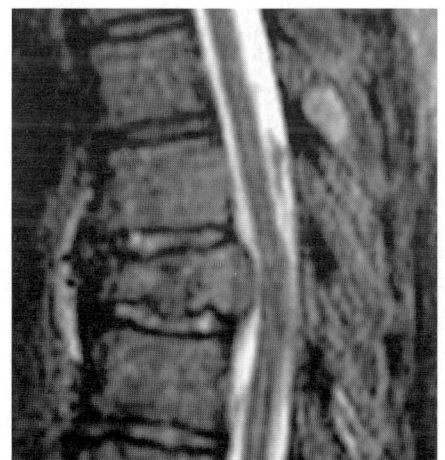

FIG. 13: Sagittal T2W image showing posterior border convexity

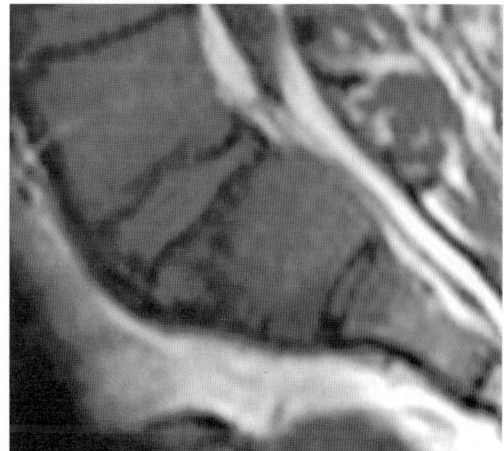

FIG. 14: T2W MRI showed a soft tissue mass in S1 vertebral segment with posterior border convexity. On biopsy it was tubercular spondylitis

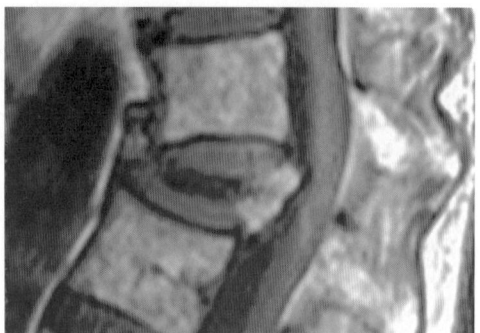

FIG. 15: Posterior border concavity and preservation of normal fatty marrow in the posterior part of vertebral body

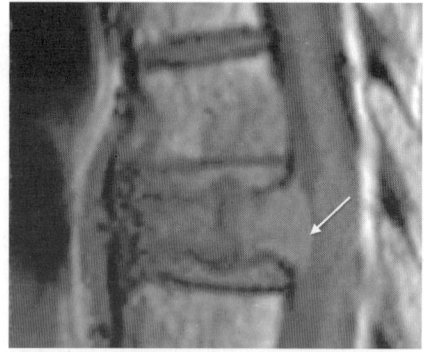

FIG. 16: Incomplete marrow replacement

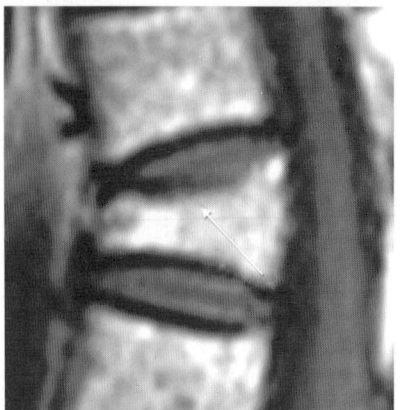

FIG. 17: Benign osteoporotic compression

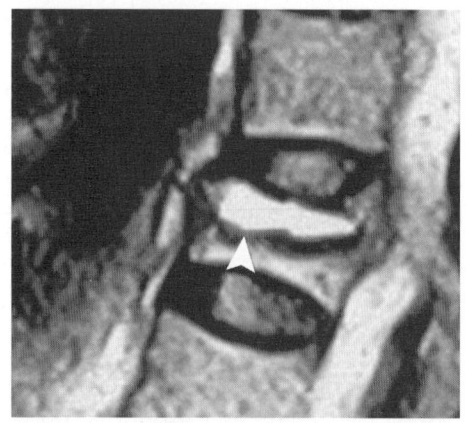

FIG. 18: Fluid cleft (arrowhead)

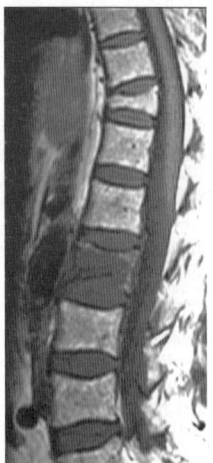

FIG. 19 Acute compression of L2 with marrow signal changes while chronic compression of D11 without marrow signals changes

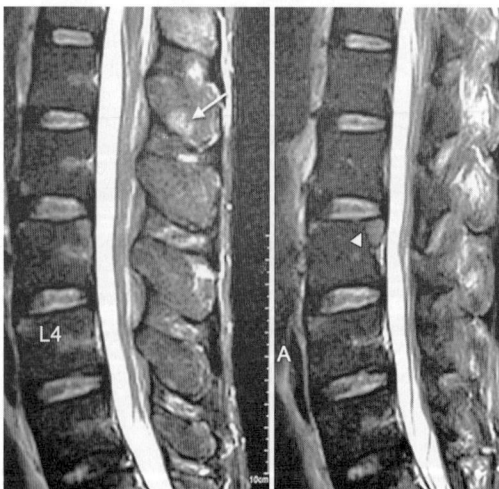

FIG. 20 Multiple lesions usually are rounded and focal

of the adjacent subarachnoid spaces. Most of these tumors are either neurofibroma or meningiomas. Extradural tumors are mostly vertebral origin and the most common are metastasis and myeloma.[17]

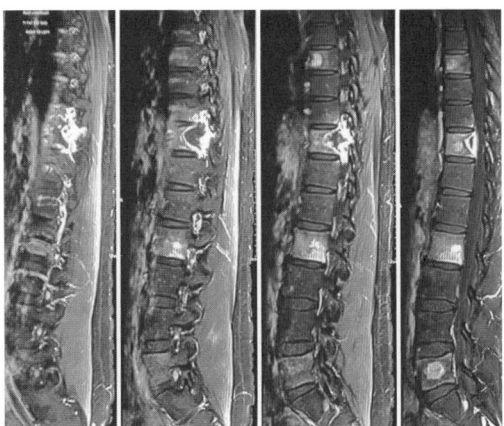

FIG. 21 Multiple lesions in tubercular infection

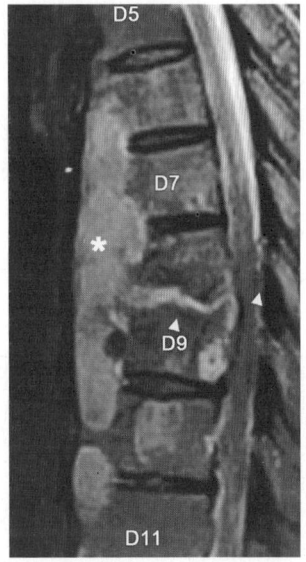

FIG. 23 Spinal infection. T2W sagittal MRI showing erosion of the adjacent end-plates causing partial collapse of the vertebrae with involvement of the adjacent disk space (arrow heads), anterior epidural abscess and a large prespinal abscess (asterisk)

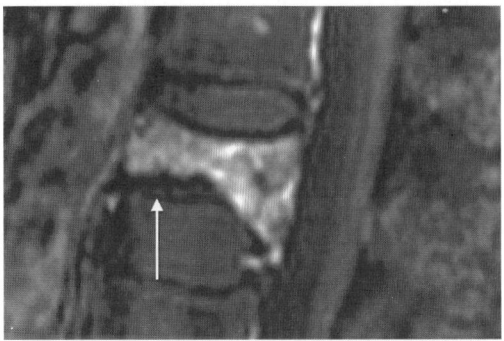

FIG. 22 Hypointense line

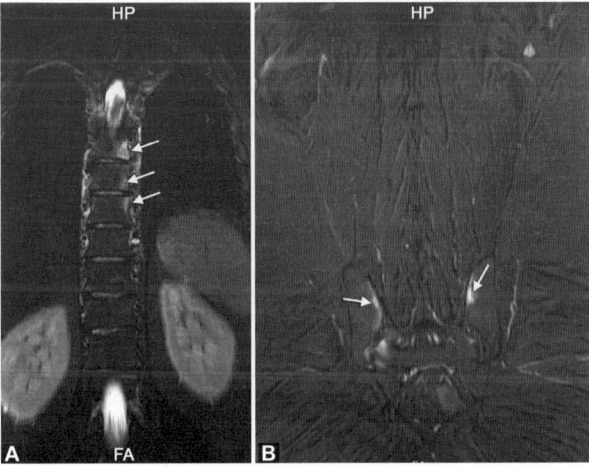

FIGS 24A and B: STIR coronal images of dorsal spine and SI joints in 43-year-old, male patient with nonspecific back pain showing foci of bright signals on sacral and iliac sides of bilateral SI joints suggestive of sacroiliitis and at costovertebral junctions in dorsal spine suggestive of inflammatory arthritis

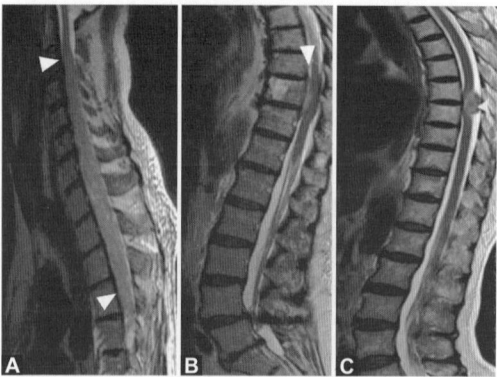

FIGS 25A to C: T2W sagittal images showing intramedullary, extradural, intradural-extramedullary lesions revealing changes of subdural CSF spaces in all three conditions

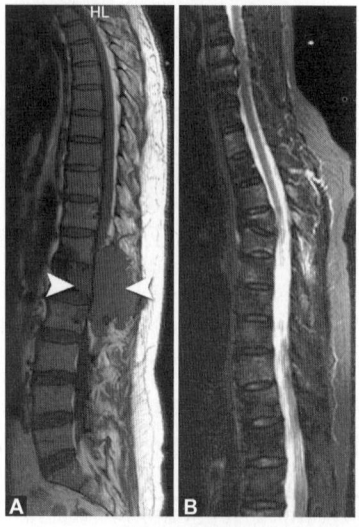

FIGS 26A and B: (A) T2W image of the spine showing a large vertebral tumor in a case of plasmacytoma; (B) Metastatic lesions in multiple vertebral bodies

THE BONE MARROW PATHOLOGIES

The composition of the bone marrow of the spine changes as the age advances and hence MR signals on T1 and T2. The hematopoietically active marrow or red marrow contain approximately 40% water, 40% fat and 20% proteins while hematopoietically inactive marrow contain 80% fat, 15% water and 5% protein. As the age advances the red marrow is converted to yellow marrow, with older individuals commonly having spine and pelvis dominated by yellow marrow. The signal intensity changes of yellow and red marrow can be well appreciated on T1W images. The fatty marrow being rich in fat is brighter on T1W images (Fig. 27A) while the red marrow or any marrow infiltrative disorder which leads to increased water containing lesion becomes darker (hypointense) on T1W images[18] (Fig. 27B).

SPINAL INFECTIONS

The spinal infections are an important cause of back pain and may involve the vertebra and the adjacent disk. The vertebral osteomyelitis and involvement of the adjacent intervertebral disk are together called as infective spondylodiskitis. The spread

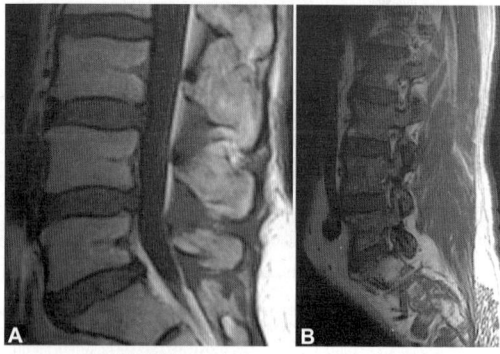

FIGS 27A and B: (A) T1W image of an adult spine showing bright marrow signals compared to adjacent intervertebral disk; (B) Diffuse marrow hypointensity of the vertebral bodies in a known case of multiple myeloma. Note the signal intensity is less than adjacent intervertebral disk

The vertebral tumor can be seen as focal marrow replacement by a soft tissue tumor with paraspinal soft tissue or intraspinal (extradural) mass with or without compression of the spinal cord (Fig. 26A). Vertebral metastasis is characterized by multiple vertebral lesions showing focal marrow signal alteration (Fig. 26B).

of infection to spine is mostly through hematogenous route. The spinal infections can be tubercular/fungal or pyogenic.

On MRI the infectious spondylodiskitis shows altered marrow signals of one or more vertebra with low signals on T1-and bright on T2-weighted images suggestive of marrow edema. Marrow edema is the earliest sign of any bone pathology and is nonspecific. This is followed by erosions or destructions of the vertebral end plates with involvement of adjacent disk space causing diskitis, which shows abnormal bright signals in the disk on T2-weighted images. There may be associated paraspinal soft tissue edema or abscess formation which shows bright signals on T2W images and peripheral enhancement on post-contrast MRI[19] (Fig. 28).

Differentiating between the various organisms as the cause of spinal infections is difficult on imaging alone. However, few general features like large paraspinal and epidural abscess and thick rim enhancement of abscess favors possibility of tuberculosis.[15] Unlike pyogenic osteomyelitis, disk space is sometimes preserved. Subligamentous spread (usually anterior longitudinal ligament), paraspinal and epidural extension and development of paraspinal abscess below the level of spondylitis, mainly in Psoas muscle is common in tubercular infections.[15]

MRI IN POSTOPERATIVE SPINAL PAIN

There is a high incidence of unsuccessful spinal surgery with persistent symptoms and known as failed back surgery syndrome. There are many causes of failed back surgery which are divided into early postoperative and late postoperative.

The early postoperative causes are those with persistent/recurrent pain in first few hours or days after the surgery and include bleeding, infection, dural tear leading to pseudo-meningocele, nerve root lesion, residual disk.

Late postoperative causes of failed back surgery lead to back pain, months to years after the surgery. These include textiloma, arachnoiditis, recurrent disk and scar, stenosis, instability.[20]

The most important role of MRI in post-operative spine is to differentiate recurrent/residual disk from postoperative scar. The MRI is about 95–100% accurate in differentiating the two entities. On post-contrast study the epidural scar will enhance homogeneously while the disk will show peripheral enhancement. There is no central enhancement as the disk material lacks the blood vessels.[21] The accuracy of contrast enhanced MRI in differentiating recurrent disk from postoperative scar is about 95–100%[22] (Figs 29A and B).

Postoperative spinal infection is one of the important causes of failed back surgery. The diagnosis of postoperative

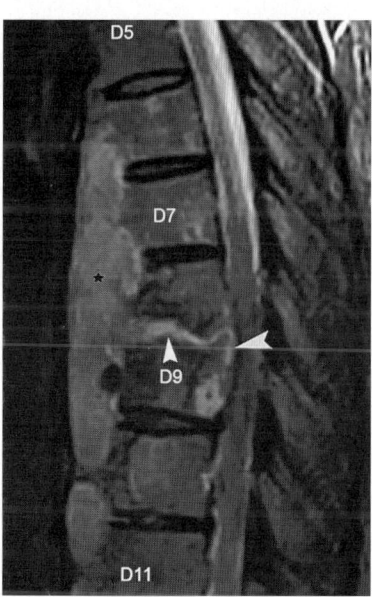

FIG. 28: Spinal infection. T2W sagittal MRI showing erosion of the adjacent end plates causing partial collapse of the vertebrae with involvement of the adjacent disk space (arrowheads), anterior epidural abscess and a large prespinal abscess (black asterisk)

spinal infection depends on clinical data, laboratory findings and imaging. The clinical data of postoperative spinal pain, fever, and muscle spasm should give a suspicion of post-operative spinal infection. The elevated WBC counts, ESR, C-reactive protein are the laboratory findings which further support to diagnosis. The imaging findings of marrow signal changes in the vertebral bodies adjacent to end plates along with end plate changes and involvement of the intervertebral disk should suggest possibility of infection and needs to be correlated with laboratory and clinical findings. At times a large abscess may be formed at the site of surgery[21] (Figs 30A and B).

Chronic sterile arachnoiditis is one of the important conditions causing persistent pain in postoperative period in 6–16% of the patient's. The various MRI findings in chronic sterile arachnoiditis are clumped and matted nerve roots, adhered to walls of the thecal sac giving empty thecal sac appearance. There may be enhancement of the nerve roots on postcontrast study[21] (Fig. 31).

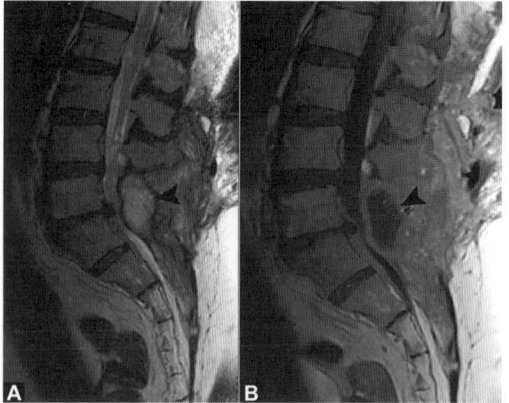

FIGS 30A and B: (A) T2W and (B) Postcontrast T1W images showing postoperative spinal abscess (black arrow-head) at the site of surgery showing peripheral enhancement on postcontrast

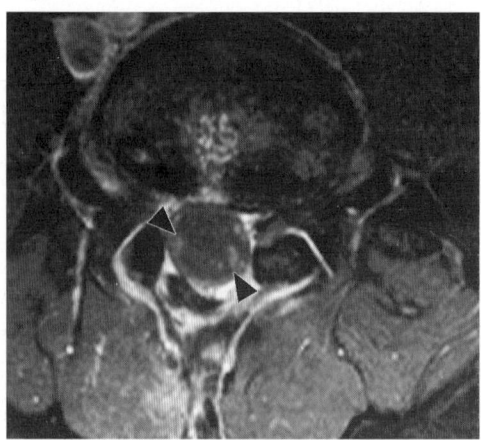

FIG. 31: Post contrast MRI, 2 years after laminectomy with persistent pain showing clumping and enhancement of the nerve roots of cauda equine (black arrowheads)

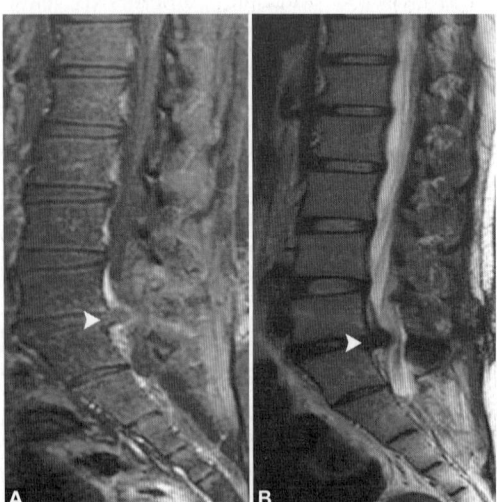

FIGS 29A and B: Postoperative recurrent disk (A) Postcontrast scan showing peripheral enhancement of the disk. There is no enhancement in the center of the disk; (B) T2-weighted image of the same patient

MRI IN CHRONIC ABDOMINAL PAIN

The role of MRI in the abdominal imaging is increasing after the development of fast imaging techniques and development of new liver specific contrast agents. The advantages of MRI over all the other imaging modalities are better soft tissue contrast, lack of ionizing radiations, no nephrotoxicity and less allergic reaction of gadolinium as compared to iodinated contrast agents. MRI is now the investigation of choice in imaging the lesions of liver, spleen, pancreas, biliary system, adrenals, kidneys, gynecological and pelvic masses. MRI with magnetic resonance cholangiopancreatography (MRCP) is one stop solution in work-up of the patients with hepatobiliary pathologies and in cases of chronic pancreatitis.

MR imaging is more accurate for detection and characterization of liver masses than CT scan[23] (Fig. 32). The MR imaging features of different neoplastic lesions is beyond the scope of this chapter.

There is an increasing role of MRI in imaging the pancreatic pathologies like pancreatitis, pancreatic tumors. High field strength (1.5 and 3 Tesla) MRI has increased the role of MRI in imaging of pancreatic diseases. MRI has better sensitivity and better tissue characterization than CT scan in diagnosing pancreatic diseases. The normal pancreas is the brightest abdominal organ on fat saturated T1 sequence (Fig. 33A). Pancreatic tumor/chronic focal pancreatitis can be seen as focal area of abnormal signals (Fig. 33B). The status of pancreatic duct can be simultaneously evaluated on MRCP[24] (Fig. 33C).

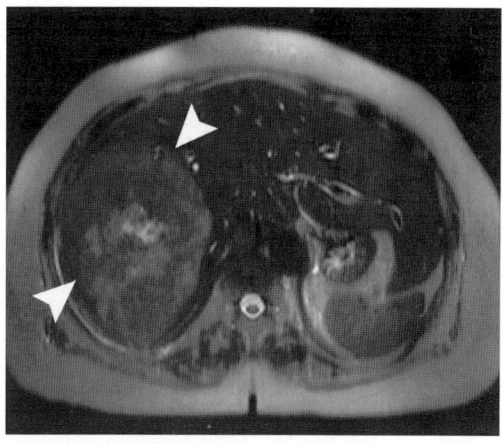

FIG. 32: T2W MRI section of liver showing a large mass lesion (hepatocellular carcinoma) in the posterior segment of liver

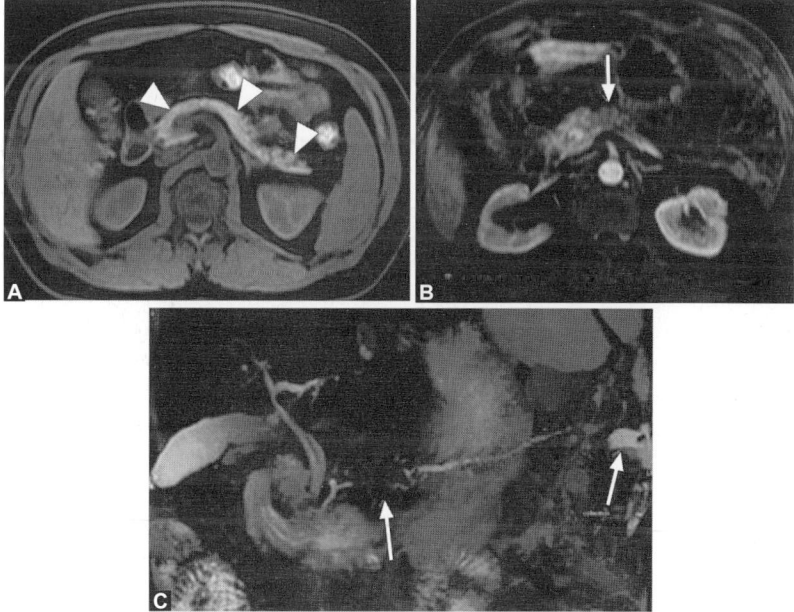

FIGS 33A to C: (A) Normal pancreas is the brightest abdominal organ on fat saturated T1 images; (B) Small tumor showing focal area of low signals in the region of body of pancreas; (C) MRCP of the same patient showing cutoff of the pancreatic duct at the site of tumor, resulting into distal duct dilatation

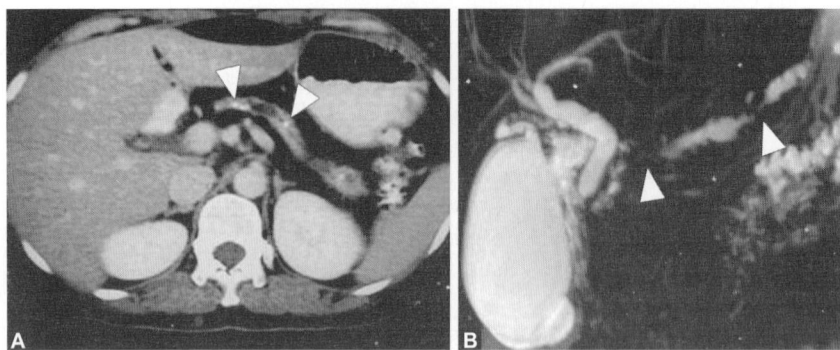

FIGS 34A and B: Case of chronic pancreatitis with (A) CT scan showing intraductal calcifications (white arrowheads) and (B) MRCP images of the same patient showing ductal obstruction (white arrowheads)

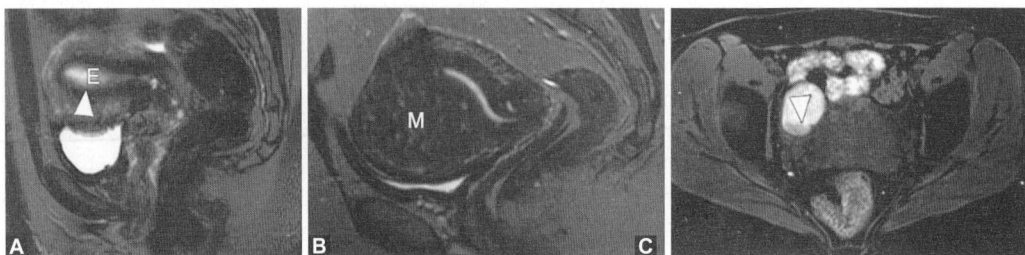

FIGS 35A to C: (A) Normal uterus with endometrium (E), junctional zone (arrowhead); (B) Focal adenomyosis M along the anterior uterine wall, indistinct from the junctional zone; (C) Endometriosis in right ovary with fluid level (arrowhead)

Chronic pancreatitis is one of the frequent causes of abdominal pain. Calcifications in cases of chronic pancreatitis either intraductal or parenchymal are better seen on CT scan however, the ductal anatomy is better seen on MRCP (Figs 34A and B).

MRI is now the most important diagnostic modality in pelvic pathologies. Endometriosis, adenomyosis are frequent causes of chronic lower abdominal pain and sometimes referred back pain. MRI due to its higher soft tissue resolution is the best modality of investigation in gynecological diseases including endometriosis, endometrial malignancies, ovarian pathologies, cervical malignancies, etc.[25] (Figs 35A to C).

CONCLUSION

MRI is one of the most important investigations in the workup of pain mainly the back pain, musculoskeletal pain. For evaluation of spinal and musculoskeletal pathologies, MRI is the imaging modality of choice. There is increasing role of MRI in the abdominal imaging.

The advantages of MRI is noninvasive, better soft tissue resolution, no ionizing radiations, gadolinium is less allergic as compared to iodinated contrast used in other radiological investigations. MRI gives better characterization of the lesions than any other imaging modality. The disadvantages of MRI are less availability, claustrophobia, more time consuming. The cortical bone and calcifications are better assessed by CT scan while the marrow pathologies are better evaluated by MRI. The MRI is contraindicated in patients with aneurismal clips, cochlear implants and pacemaker.

REFERENCES

1. Jeffrey G and Richard A Deyo. Imaging of lumbar intervertebral disk degeneration and aging, excluding disc herniation. Radiology clinics of North America. 2000;38(6):1255-566.
2. Czervionke LF. Lumbar intervertebral disc disease. Neuroimaging Clinics of North America. 1993;3:465-85.
3. Aguila LA, Piraino DW. Modiac MT, et al. The intranuclear cleft of intervertebral disc: Magnetic resonance imaging. Radiology. 1985;155:155-8.
4. Pierre C. Milette Classification, diagnostic imaging and imaging characterization of a herniated lumbar disc. Imaging of low back pain 1. Radiologic Clinics of North America. 2000;38(6):1267-91.
5. Dieter Schellinger, Louis Wener, Bruce Ragsdale, Nicolas Patronas. Facet Joint disorder and their role in production of back pain and sciatica. Radiographics. 1987;7(5):923-44.
6. Remy S Nizard, Marc Wybier and Jean-Denis Laredo- Radiological assessment of Lumbar intervertebral instability and degenerative spondylolisthesis. Imaging of low back pain II. Radiologic Clinics of North America. 2001;39(1):55-72.
7. Marc Wybier. Imaging of lumbar degenerative changes involving structures other than disc space. imaging in low back pain II. Radiologic Clinics of North America. 2001;39(1):101-14.
8. Bidhya Bhushan Tamarkar, Nitin Tandra, Huang Yonghui, Li Dapeng, Sun Jifu. Radiological evaluation of lumbar instability. 2014;13(4):83-7.
9. Antonio Leone, Giuseppe Guglielmi, Victor N Cassar-Pullicino, Lorenzo Bonomo. Lumbar Intervertebral instability: A review. Radiology. 2007;245(1):62-77.
10. Barbro Danielson, J Willen, A. Gaulitz, T Niklason and TH Hansson. Axial loading of spine during CT and MRI in patients with suspected spinal canal stenosis. Acta Radiologica. 1998;39:604-11.
11. Nils Schonstrom, Jan Willen. Imaging of lumbar spinal stenosis. Imaging of low back pain II. Radiologic Clinics of North America. 2001;39(1):31-53.
12. KCVG Rao/JP Williams. Degenerative disc and vertebral diseases. MRI and CT of the spine. Williams and Wilkins. pp. 129-210.
13. Shoichiro Otake, Michimasa Matsuo, Sadahiko Nishizawa, Akira Sano and Yasumasa Kuroda. Ossification of posterior longitudinal ligament: MR evaluation. AJNR. 1992;13:1059-067.
14. Hee-Sun Jung, Won-Hee Jee, Thomas R Mc Cauley, Kee-Yong Ha, Kyu-Ho Choi. Discrimination of metastasis from osteoporotic compression spinal fractures with MR imaging. Radiographics. 2003;23:179-87.
15. Jamshid Tehranzadeh and Cliff Tao. Advances in MR imaging of vertebral collapse. Seminars in Ultrasound, CT scan and MRI. 2004;25:440-60.
16. Kay-Geert A Hermann, Christian E Althoff, et al. Spinal changes in patients with spondyloarthritis: Comparision of MR imaging and radiographic appearances. Radiographics 2005;25:559-70.
17. RS Williams, JP Williams Tumors. MRI and CT of the spine. Williams and Wilkins. pp. 347-428.
18. Lia A Moulopoulos and Meletious A. Dimopoulos. Magnetic Resonance Imaging of Bone Marrow in Hematological Malignancies Blood. 1997;90:2127-47.
19. Axel Stabler and Maximillann F. Reiser-Imaging of spinal infection. Low back pain II. Radiologic clinics of North America. 2001;39(1):115-35.
20. KCVG. Rao and JP Williams. Post operative spine. MRI and CT of the spine. Williams and Wilkins: pp. 211-249.
21. J Randy Jinkins and Johan WM Van Goethem. The post surgical lumbosacral spine. Imaging of low back pain II. Radiologic Clinics of North America. 2001;39(1):1-29.
22. Shafaie FF, Bundeschuh C, Jinkins JR. The post therapeutic lumbosacral spine. In: Jinkins JR (Ed). Post therapeutic Neurodiagnostic Imaging. Philadelphia, Lippincott-Raven. 1997. pp. 223-43.
23. Ihab R Kamel, David A Bluemake. MR imaging of liver tumors. Radiologic Clinc of North America. 2003;41:51-6.
24. John N Ly, Frank H Miller. MR imaging of Pancreas-A practical approach. Radiologic Clinics of North America. 2002;40:1289-309.
25. Julia R Fielding. MR Imaging of female pelvis. Radiologic Clinics of North America. 2003;41:179-92.

Role of Electrodiagnosis in the Management of Neck and Back Pain

Mansukhani A Khushnuma

INTRODUCTION

Electrodiagnosis (EDX), more correctly called electroneuromyography (ENMG)[1] is an assessment of a patient by a physician using a series of tests to establish an accurate diagnosis of the presenting clinical problem that suggests a neuromuscular disorder and is localized to peripheral nerves, plexuses, motor and sensory roots, anterior horn cells, neuromuscular junction or muscles.[2] In subjects who present with neck or arm pain and back or leg pain, there is always a clinical suspicion of a radiculopathy and ENMG studies would help detect this. This chapter gives a very basic outline of electrodiagnosis and its utility. For more detailed description of techniques, other books and articles should be referred to.[3-8]

HOW DOES ELECTRONEURO-MYOGRAPHY HELP?

- Objective record documentation and later comparison
- Predominant pathology determined: axonal/demyelinating/combined
- Extent of lesion
- Distribution of abnormalities
- Predominant fibers involved sensory, motor
- *Temporal profile*: Acute, chronic, old, and progressive
- Severity of lesion
- Other disorders
- Assess progress.

WHY ELECTRONEUROMYOGRAPHY IN BACK AND NECK PAIN?

- To know whether there is a neural deficit responsible for the pain
- If there is a deficit, to objectively document it
- To know, which nerve root function is affected
- To know whether the deficit is solely sensory or is there subclinical motor axon loss
- How severe is the damage?
- Is it due to focal demyelination, axon loss or a combination of the two?
- Is it unilateral or bilateral?
- Is the involvement acute, chronic or acute or chronic?
- Is the finding on the MRI correlating with the deficit?
- Is the presenting neurodeficit a manifestation of noncompressive radiculitis?
- For assessing the progress of the deficit
- For diagnosing the presence of other conditions (MND, entrapment and generalized neuropathies, noncompressive radiculopathy, cervical myelopathy)
- Postoperative follow-up.

Chapter 11: Role of Electrodiagnosis in the Management of Neck and Back Pain

PROTOCOL

- History is a must
- Clinical examination
- Plan the ENMG study
- Interpret the report
- Correlate with presenting symptoms. It must be borne in mind that ENMG is an extension of the clinical examination and not a replacement and hence, a good history and clinical examination are prerequisites to the test. A good referral letter from the referring physician is useful to customize the procedure for each patient. A sound technique, knowledge of neuromuscular disorders and interpretation of results with the presenting problem provide a good ENMG study.

EQUIPMENT

An electromyograph is the machine used for the study. It picks up undistorted biological signals evoked from nerves and muscles with minimal noise disturbance. It is basically a computer with facilities of a head box, stimulator, display screen, amplifiers and filters. Since needle electromyography is an audiovisual test a loudspeaker is also fitted (Fig.1).

ELECTRONEUROMYOGRAPHY TESTS

- Nerve conduction studies
- Needle electromyography
- *Late responses*: F-waves and H reflex
- *Somatosensory evoked potential study*: For conduction along the spinal cord (posterior columns).

Nerve Conduction Studies

A method of measuring changes in a peripheral nerve by stimulating it electrically and recording the action potential generated. There are two types of studies done: sensory nerve conduction and motor nerve conduction studies.

Sensory Nerve Action Potential SAP/SNAP

The potential obtained from recording electrodes placed over a sensory nerve, while stimulating it at a point some distance away is called a sensory nerve action potential (SAP/SNAP) (Figs 2 and 3). The SAP assesses integrity of the postganglionic sensory fibers and is a sensitive and specific test to localize the site of the lesion to the peripheral nerve. A lesion proximal to the dorsal root ganglion, i.e. at the roots level will cause clinical sensory loss but on nerve conduction study the relevant SAP will be normal. Hence, the relevant SAP will be normal in root lesions in spite of clinical sensory affection, e.g. in a L5 radiculopathy there will be sensory affection over the dorsum of the foot, but the superficial peroneal SAP recorded will be normal. Rarely, when there is a far lateral/foraminal

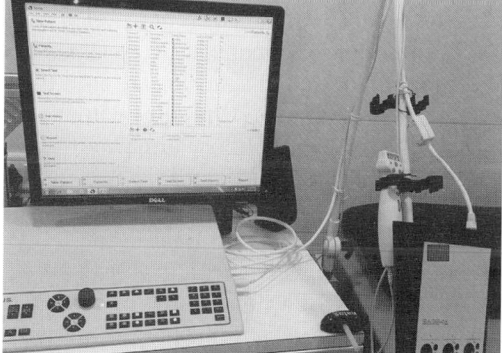

FIG.1: Electromyograph

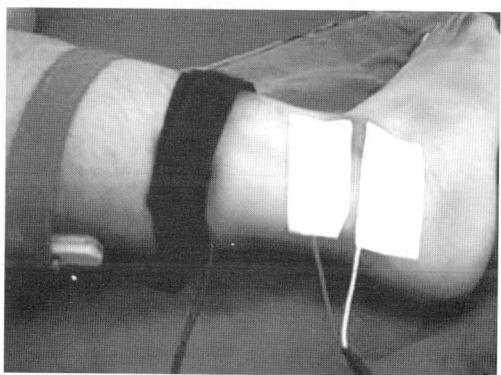

FIG. 2: Sural sensory conduction technique

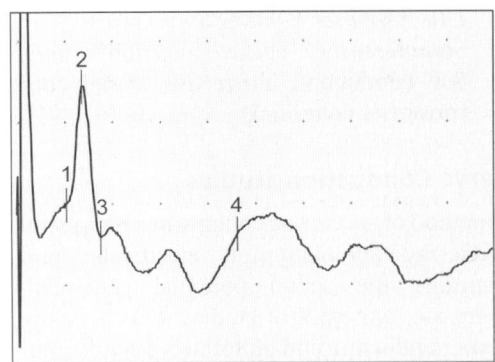

FIG. 3: Sural sensory nerve action potential

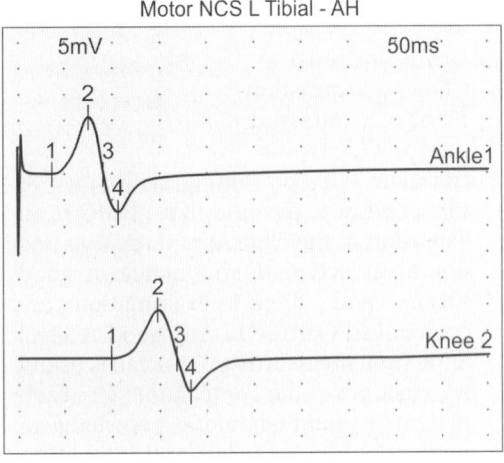

FIG. 5: Tibial compound muscle action potentials

disk prolapse the SNAP may be, affected due to involvement of the dorsal root ganglion especially the L5 dorsal root ganglion.[9-11]

Motor Nerve Conduction

Motor nerve conduction study is a technique of stimulating a motor nerve at two sites serially and picking up the muscle action potential using surface electrodes from the relevant muscle (Figs 4 and 5). The amplitude of the compound muscle action potential (CMAP) indicates the number of functioning axons and muscle fibers and reflects the amount of axon loss; hence, is absent or low amplitude in severe lesions. However, the CMAP in most root lesions is not affected, as 50% of the motor fibers need to be lost to show a significant drop in the amplitude and this is not often the case and also there is an overlap in the myotomes.[12]

Needle Electromyography Examination or Electromyography

A method of studying the electrical activity of a muscle, by placing a needle electrode within it and observing (Fig. 6):
  i. The spontaneous activity in the muscle at rest.
  ii. The motor unit action potentials (MUAPs) generated by voluntary contraction of the muscle by the patient.

This is an audiovisual diagnosis and both the configuration and sound of the potentials is used. This test is the most important one for the diagnosis of root lesions, as it is most sensitive and specific for identification of axon loss motor radiculopathy. It detects the level and extent of root involvement, degree of axon loss and whether the lesion is active or chronic. Paraspinal muscle electromyography (EMG) in root lesions adds support, if abnormal, but does not rule root lesion, if normal.

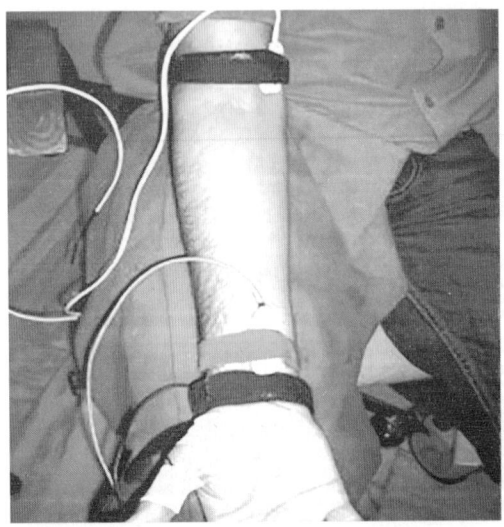

FIG. 4: Median motor conduction technique

Spontaneous activity on EMG in the form of fibrillation potentials is detected with the muscle at rest. It is a sign of acute/ongoing axon loss especially when detected in proximal muscles or in distal muscles with recent onset symptoms. In acute root lesions, spontaneous activity is seen in the paraspinal muscles after 7 days and limb muscles after 14–21 days (Fig. 7).

The motor unit action potential (MUAP) is the activity seen with mild to moderate voluntary effort and the configuration, size and duration of the MUAP localizes the site of the lesion and its chronicity. The small jagged polyphasics MUAPs (Fig. 8) suggest ongoing involvement and large and wide triphasic motor unit action potentials suggest that the lesion is chronic (Fig. 9). Once the MUAPs become abnormal they do not return to normal configuration and the abnormalities would be evident even when the patient becomes asymptomatic. The abnormalities should be present in at least two muscles of the same myotome and innervated by different peripheral nerves. The muscles of one myotome above and below the lesion should also be examined.[13]

To summarize the abnormalities on needle EMG, which predict a root lesion are:
- Spontaneous activity—fibrillations

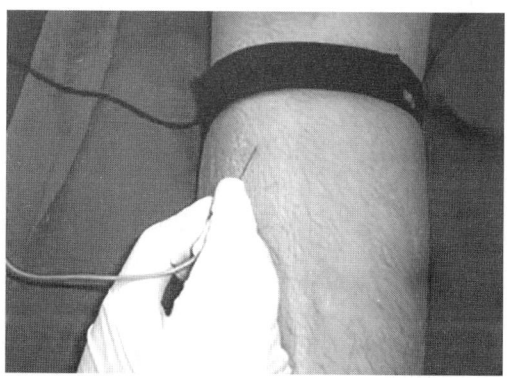

FIG. 6: Needle electromyography

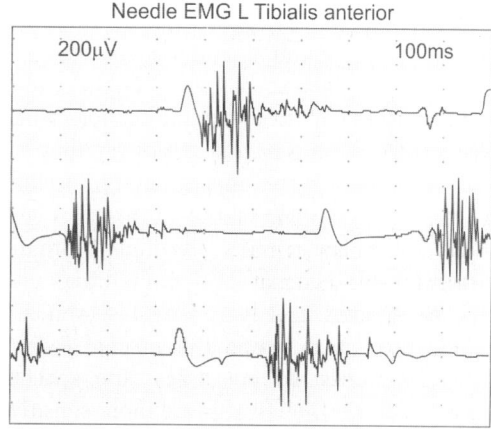

FIG. 8: Polyphasic units

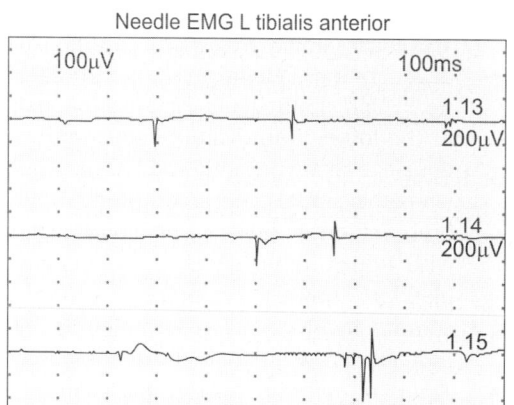

FIG. 7: Fibrillation potentials

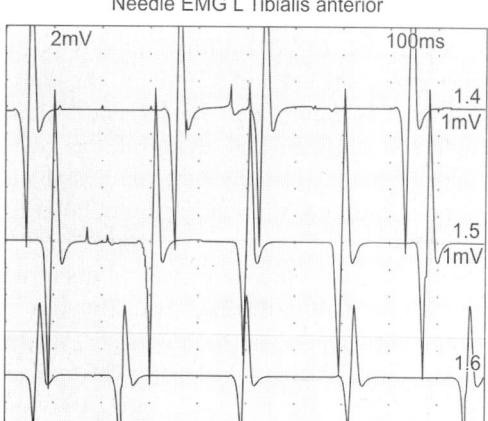

FIG. 9: Large wide triphasic units

- Reduced recruitment of motor units
- Increased duration and amplitude of motor units
- Increase in polyphasics.

Late Responses

F-Waves

These are waves that occur after the direct motor response and were first described by McDougal and Magladery in 1950. They were first evoked from the small muscles of the foot and hence the name. They arise from the motor neurons, which fire impulses when activated by an antidromic volley from the nerve being examined and hence represent proximal conduction in motor fibers, which are not accessible to direct stimulation, when distal conduction is normal. However, they are not sensitive for demonstrating root lesions as the segment being examined (roots) is very short and the abnormality gets diluted with the normal distal segment. Also all the fibers may not be affected and even few-preserved fast conducting fibers would give normal F-wave latencies.[14] They do not assess the sensory pathway at all. The F-waves are more sensitive to abnormalities in the peripheral nerve conduction.[15]

H Reflex Study

H reflex also called Hoffmann reflex is the electrically elicited ankle jerk in the lower limbs and is abnormal in S1 radicular lesions. Unilateral absence and delay of the reflex elicited from the rested gastrocnemius-soleus group of muscles, stimulating the tibial nerve at the knee is an important finding to localize the root lesion to the sensory S1 fibers in the absence of motor involvement. The use of nomograms increases the diagnostic yield.[16] In the upper limbs, the flexor carpi radialis H reflex is useful to localize the lesion to the sensory C6 or C7 root when needle electromyography is normal.[17]

Somatosensory Evoked Potential Study

This is a study to assess the conduction along the posterior columns of the spinal cord and is indicated when a cord compression is suspected. It is not useful for detecting root lesions. Electrical stimulus is given to mixed nerves distally and the responses are picked up from the lumbar spine and the cortex in lower limbs and from the neck, cervical spine, and opposite cortex in the upper limbs.[18] Dermatomal somatosensory evoked potentials (SSEPs) were used initially where instead of stimulating a cutaneous or mixed nerve as in routine SSEPs a dermatome was stimulated and the evoked response was recorded from the opposite cortex.[19] However, their usefulness over the routine tests has not been established and they are no longer used for the diagnosis of radiculopathies.[20]

Neural Deficits Associated with Back or Neck Pain

- *Acute nerve root compression* due to an acutely prolapsed disk. This causes initially a conduction block in the fibers, which are compressed and later acute axon loss. Presents with back/neck and radicular pain in the limb with or without sensory +/− motor loss.
- *Chronic nerve root compression* due to degenerative changes, which reduce the dimensions of the central or lateral canal. This causes slowly progressive chronic axon degeneration. Patient presents with back/neck pain, neurogenic claudication pain in the lower limbs. Clinical sensorimotor deficits may be present. In the upper limb when the central canal is compromised the presentation would be of cord compression with upper motor signs in lower limbs, bladder bowel symptoms, posterior column involvement in lower limbs and radicular involvement in the upper limbs.
- *Acute or chronic compression* shows a combination of lesions—chronic axon loss + conduction block initially and acute

axon loss as well. Presents with acute recent onset pain + sensory-motor deficit and previous history of such attacks or chronic pain.
- *Predominantly sensory* or only sensory nerve root compression—involvement of only sensory fibers. Presents with pain +/− sensory loss.
- *Multiple root lesions* commonly seen with central disc lesions and lumbar canal stenosis and are usually bilateral even if symptoms are unilateral.

Electroneuromyography in Root Lesions Correlated with Pathophysiology

- Recent acute involvement is detected by noting fibrillations in proximal muscles of the same myotome.
- Chronic root compression is detected by noting large and wide triphasic or polyphasic units in muscles of the same myotome.
- Acute or chronic radicular lesions are detected by noting fibrillations and small wide polyphasic units in the proximal muscles of the myotome.
- Conduction block is detected by noting a good amplitude motor response from a clinically weak muscle (on NCS) and fast firing but normal configuration MUPs with a reduced interference pattern on NEE.
- When there is cord compression the somatosensory evoked potential shows delayed cortical responses.

CONCLUSION

ENMG in root lesions would show active or chronic motor axon degeneration in a myotomal distribution with/without proximal muscle involvement and normal relevant SNAPs with clinical e/o sensory involvement.

The findings depend on the exact root involved, whether compression involves motor/sensory fibers, percentage of fibers compressed, type of pathophysiology, and duration of lesion, completeness of study and skill of the examiner.

Limitations of Electroneuromyography

- It identifies the root involved and not the vertebral level.
- Timing of study is important as defined by appearance of fibrillation potentials.
- All meaningful postoperative studies require preoperative evaluation.
- Can be normal even with a prolapsed intervertebral disk, which causes no neural compression (false-negative).
- ENMG findings do not *Always* correlate with the symptoms.
- Severity of "sensory involvement" cannot be assessed.
- Etiology is not determined.

It can be *false positive*, if:
- The examiner is not experienced.
- Diagnosis criteria are not followed.
- Inadequate study without clinical correlation
- Biased examiner.

Electroneuromyography in Postoperative Care

- Postoperative evaluation has value, if a preoperative study has been done
- EMG cannot answer the question, "Whether adequate decompression has been achieved?"

Electroneuromyography Versus Imaging

Over the years, MRI localization had reduced the importance of ENMG; however, it is the *ONLY* test for the function of the nervous tissue and is abnormal in non-compressive lesions, where an MRI without contrast would be normal. It detects additional lesions which may be contributing to the symptoms. Since ENMG tests the functional integrity and MRI the anatomical lesion, both tests must be done as they complement each other.

What Should Your Patient Expect?
Nerve Conduction Studies

- Nerve conduction studies (NCS) are done with surface electrodes

- The 'shocks' given are in mille amperes and are quite bearable
- The stimulus is local and does not travel all over the body
- NCS are ALWAYS required
- Can be done very safely even in the new born
- The motor conduction stimulus feels like a tap and moves the muscle
- The NCS may be contraindicated in patients with pacemakers.

Electromyography

- The needle EMG examination is done using fine disposable electrodes, which are solid pins but thin and very sharp
- No shocks are given
- The needle is inserted just into the muscle for few seconds
- The patient is asked to contract the muscle and the activity is picked up by the electrode and displayed on the monitor and through a loud speaker–audiovisual diagnosis is made online
- The number of muscles examined depend upon the working diagnosis
- Needle EMG should be avoided in patients with bleeding disorders, on anticoagulants and in local infection.

How can the Referring Doctor Help?

- The working diagnosis or differential diagnosis should be stated in the referral note.
    - It does not introduce a bias; in fact it helps to customize the procedure.
- Relevant reports and supportive radiography should be sent with the patient
- If the patient is HbsAg or HIV positive/has a pacemaker or is on anticoagulants the electromyographer must be alerted
- Remember the limitations of the test before asking for it.

What if the Working Diagnosis is Inaccurate?

ENMG is an objective test and an experienced examiner will definitely be able to localize the lesion.

What to Look for in an ENMG Report?

Besides the final impression:
1. Check whether clinically relevant sites have been examined, e.g. if there is foot drop? Superficial peroneal SNAP should be done.
2. Does the report correlate with the symptoms? A foot drop can be due to: Peroneal neuropathy, L5 radiculopathy, presentation of MND or a lesion in the opposite frontal cortex.

A restricted anterior horn cell lesion and a radiculopathy show identical findings on EMG. Here the history and clinical examination are important and extensive NEE is required.

The following case illustrates the use of ENMG:

A 63-old-lady, not diabetic, was referred to the ENMG department with c/o painless, bilateral, non-healing, heel ulcers since 9 months, to confirm a Hansen's neuropathy (Fig. 10).

ENMG showed normal sensory nerve action potentials from all nerves including the medial plantar nerves (Fig. 11).

Needle electromyography showed severe, active, ongoing and chronic motor axon degeneration in bilateral distal + proximal S1>L5 innervated muscles, likely to be a root lesion.

On inquiry she had weakness in the feet since 15 years and backache more than 25 years back, for which she had taken no treatment. Denied bladder bowl-related symptoms (but had smell of urine).

On examination there were no thickened nerves/patches.

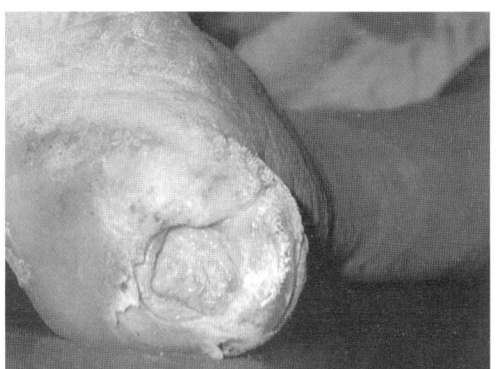

FIG. 10: Heel ulcer *(For color version, see Plate 2)*

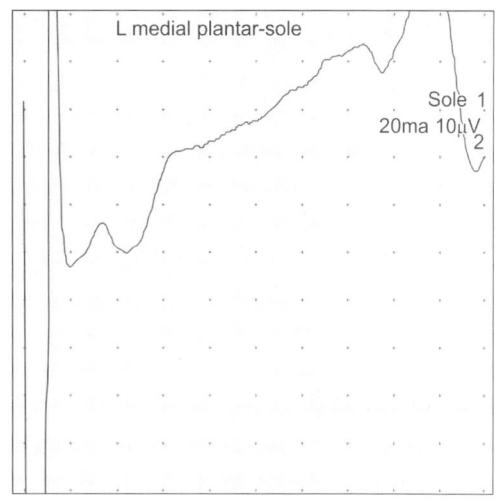

FIG. 11: Medial plantar sensory nerve action potential

Ankle jerks were absent, knee jerks were normal. Sensations were lost over soles. Feet were wasted and she could not stand on her toes. Imaging of the lumbosacral spine showed a large disk completely obliterating the thecal sac.

To conclude, electroneuromyography is a useful test for diagnosis and prognosis of root lesions as it is the only test to assess the function of the nervous tissue being examined. It should be used along with imaging as the two tests complement each other.[21] Its best use is when the clinician can tell the electromyographer what questions he/she wants answered regarding his/her patient.

REVIEW OF RECENT LITERATURE

A recent study stressed the usefulness of electrodiagnosis in detecting functional abnormalities at the root level which proved to be important for surgical out comes in patients of lumbar canal stenosis or lumbar disc herniation.[22] Mulford and Cohen in their paper stressed the need of a well directed electrodiagnostic test as an extension of clinical examination for evaluation of low back pain.[23] A study in Muscle and Nerve stressed the importance of correlating MRI findings with electrodiagnosis to avoid confounding age-related changes with actual nerve root compressions.[24] Another study confirmed the utility of sensory conduction studies in the differentiation of plexus lesion from lumbar radiculopathies.[25] A study done in 51 patients of cervical or lumbar radiculopathy for comparison between clinical inference and electrodiagnosis concluded that neurological examination and electrodiagnosis should be used and interpreted together.[26] A review article states that there is strong support of electrodiagnosis as a predictor for outcomes after epidural steroid injections in lumbosacral radiculopathies, though not yet or cervical radiculopathies.[27] Another excellent paper discusses the utility of the electrodiagnostic study with reference to lumbar radiculopathies and concludes that the utility of electrodiagnosis depends on the expertise of the physician who conducts the test and when adequate helps to rule out competing diagnoses, gives information about the function and is useful because it is specific for lumbar root lesions. It complements the MRI test.[28]

A study done on 200 patients suspected to have cervical or lumbar radiculopathy showed that the sensitivity of the electrodiagnostic test was most when there was dermatomal pain or numbness with l reflex loss and myotomal weakness. The specificities were 78% for lumbosacral disease and 99% for cervical disease. They concluded that all tests should be clinically directed.[29] Tsao reviewed the usefulness of the electrodiagnostic study in determining the functional level of involvement, it's severity and providing a correlate to the MRI findings.[30] Hakimi et al concluded that electrodiagnosis is useful in patients suspected to have cervical radiculopathy when they have atypical symptoms, pain-related weakness and non-localizing MRI findings.[31] A report supports the value of multiparameter clinical neurophysiological evaluations in patients with lumbar radiculopathy including CMAPs and F-waves.[32]

REFERENCES

1. Katirji B. The clinical electromyography examination: an overview. Neurolo Clin N Am. 2002;20:291-303.
2. Wilbourn AJ, et al. Clinical electromyography. Baker's clinical neurology. WB. Saunders; 2000.
3. Wilbourn AJ, et al. Radiculopathies. Clinical Electromyography. Butterworth-Heinemann; 1993. pp.177-209.
4. Wilbourn AJ, Aminoff MJ. AAEE minimonograph #32. The electrophysiologic examination in patients with radiculopathies. Muscle Nerve. 1988;11:1099-114.
5. Levin KH. Electrodiagnostic approach to the patient with suspected radiculopathy. Neurolo Clin N Am. 2002; 20:397-421.
6. Clairmont AC, et al. Evaluation of the patient with possible radiculopathy. Practical Electromyography. Williams and Wilkins; 1997. pp.115-30.
7. Stewart JD. Lower cervical nerve roots and spinal nerves. Focal peripheral neuropathies. Lippincott Williams and Wilkins; 2000. pp. 97-116.
8. Stewart JD, Cauda Equina. Lumbar and sacral nerve roots and spinal nerves. Focal peripheral neuropathies. Lippincott Williams and Wilkins; 2000. pp. 315-54.
9. Levin KH. Neurological manifestation of compressive radiculopathy of the first thoracic root. Neurology. 1999; 53:1149-51.
10. Wiltse LL, Guyer RD, et al. Alar transverse process impingement of the L5 spinal nerve: the far-out syndrome. Spine. 1984;9:31-41.
11. Levin KH. L5 radiculopathy with reduced superficial peroneal sensory responses: intraspinal and extraspinal causes. Muscle Nerve. 1998;21:3-7.
12. Bromberg AR, Sharma K, et al. Comparison of motor conduction abnormalities in lumbosacral radiculopathy and axonal polyneuropathy. Muscle Nerve. 1999; 22:1053-7.
13. Levin KH, et al. Cervical radiculopathies: comparison of surgical and EMG localization of single root lesions. Neurology. 1996;7:673-83.
14. Aminoff MJ, et al. Electrophysiological evaluation of lumbosacral radiculopathy: electromyography, late responses and somatosensory evoked potentials. Neurology (NY). 1985;35:1514-8.
15. Berger AR, et al. Comparison of motor conduction abnormalities in lumbosacral radiculopathies. Electromyogr Clin Neurophysiol. 1997;37:19-26.
16. Braddom RI, et al. Standardization of H–reflex and diagnostic use in S1 radiculopathy. Arch Phys Med Rehabil. 1974;55:161-6.
17. Schimsheimer RJ, et al. The flexor carpi radialis H-reflex in lesions of the sixth and seventh cervical nerve roots. J Neurol Neuro Surg Psychiatry. 1985;48:445-9.
18. Aminoff MJ, et al. Electrophysiological evaluation of lumbosacral radiculopathy: electromyography, late responses and somatosensory evoked potentials. Neurology. 1985;35:1514-8.
19. Aminoff MJ, et al. Dermatomal somatosensory evoked potentials in unilateral lumbosacral radiculopathy. Ann Neurol. 1985;17:171-6.
20. Aminoff M.J., Douglas S., et all Dermatomal Somatosensory Evoked Potentials in Unilateral Lumbosacral Radiculopathy Ann Neurol. 1985;17:171-76.
21. Nardin RA, et al. Electromyography and magnetic resonance imaging in the evaluation of radiculopathy. Muscle Nerve. 1999;22:151-5.
22. Lee JH, Lee SH. Clinical usefulness of electrodiagnostic study to predict surgical outcomes in lumbosacral disc herniation or spinal stenosis. Eur. Spine J. 2015;24 (10): 2276-80.
23. Mulford GJ, Cohen SJ. The role of electrodiagnosis in the evaluation of low back pain. Clin Occup. Environ Med. 2006;5(3):591-613.
24. Botez SA, Zynda-Weiss AM, Logigian EL. Diffuse age-related lumbar MRI changes confound diagnosis of single (L5) root lesions. Muscle Nerve. 2014;50 (1):135-7.
25. Mondelli M, Aretini A, et al. Clinical findings and electrodiagnostic testing in 108 consecutive cases of lumbosacral radiculopathy due to herniated disc. Neurophysiol Clin. 2013;43(4):205-15.
26. Inal EE, Eser F, Aktekin LA, Oksüz A, Bodur H. Comparison of clinical and electrophysiological findings in patients with suspected radiculopathies. J Back Musculoskelet Rehabil. 2013;26(2):169-73.
27. Annaswamy TM, Bierner SM, Avraham R. Role of electrodiagnosis in patients being considered for epidural steroid injections. PMR. 2013; 5(5 Suppl):S96-9.
28. Barr K. Electrodiagnosis of lumbar radiculopathy. Phys Med Rehabil Clin N Am. 2013;24(1):79-91.
29. Hassan A, Hameed B, Islam M, Khealani B, Khan M, Shafqat S. Clinical predictors of EMG-confirmed cervical and lumbosacral radiculopathy. Can J Neurol Sci. 2013; 40(2): 219-24.
30. Tsao B. The electrodiagnosis of cervical and lumbosacral radiculopathy. Neurol Clin. 2007;25(2):473-94.
31. Hakimi K, Spanier D. Electrodiagnosis of cervical radiculopathy. Phys. Med. Rehabil Clin N Am. 2013; 24(1):1.
32. Fischer MA, Bajwa R, Somashekar KN. Routine electrodiagnosis and a multiparameter technique in lumbosacral radiculopathies. Acta Neurol Scand. 2008;118(2):99-105.

CHAPTER 12

Bone Mineral Density: Interpretation, Treatment, and Prevention

Shirish Kataria

INTRODUCTION

Originating from the Greek words *osteon* (bone) and *poros* (passage, pore); osteoporosis literally translates to porous bones.

It is defined by the World Health Organization as a generalized skeletal disorder characterized by low bone mass and deteriorating bone architecture, causing increased susceptibility to fracture. While the chances of developing osteoporosis are greater with increasing age, it has a wide reach that affects all populations irrespective of sex or race. It falls under the realm of public health issues, acting as a silent disease until it manifests as a fracture. Contrary to popular belief, it can be both treated and prevented.[1]

PATHOPHYSIOLOGY

To understand the pathophysiology that surrounds osteoporosis, it is important to know the structural composition of bones in our bodies. This includes cells and tissues, each with their own functions, that repair bones and help them grow. The *cortical bone* or compact bone is the tissue, which forms the hard outer layer in a bone. Whereas, the trabecular or cancellous bone is the lighter, less compact tissue that makes up the inner spongy layer.[2]

Bones consists of a number of cells of which are: *Osteoblasts* that keep bone mineralization in check and form the organic bone matrix by generating proteins; *Osteocytes* that assist in bone remodeling; and *Osteoclasts* that are responsible for resorption of the bone. These processes are controlled by various hormones such as parathyroid hormone (PTH), calcitonin, vitamin D and estrogen.[3]

The remodeling of bone tissue through the functioning of these cells, takes place under local and systemic factors that are responsible for maintaining the balance between formation and resorption, i.e. bone homeostasis. When this balance is disturbed, it could result in osteoporosis.[4-6]

In osteoporosis there is decreased cortical and trabecular bone which increases porosity. This in turn leads to a fragility fracture.

RISK FACTORS

The International Osteoporosis Foundation characterizes a risk factor as something that increases ones probability of contracting a particular disease. They categorized the risk factors for osteoporosis into two groups: Fixed risks and modifiable risks. The presence of a risk factor/s does not, however, presuppose the presence of osteoporosis.

Fixed Risks

Fixed risks (those we cannot change) include the following:
- Age
- Female gender
- Family history of osteoporosis
- Previous fracture
- Ethnicity
- Menopause or hysterectomy
- Long-term glucocorticoid therapy
- Rheumatoid arthritis
- Primary or secondary hypogonadism in men.

Modifiable Risks

Modifiable risks (those that we have control over) include the following:
- Alcohol
- Smoking
- Low body mass index
- Poor nutrition
- Vitamin D deficiency
- Eating disorders
- Insufficient exercise
- Low dietary calcium intake
- Frequent falls.[7-11]

DIAGNOSIS

Diagnosis of osteoporosis by conventional radiography is not as accurate as bone mineral density (BMD) testing. An appreciable amount (usually 30–80%) of bone mineral loss has to be present for it to become noticeable on radiographs.[12,13] Radiographs display an increase in radiolucency and cortical thinning while detecting generalized osteoporosis. The trabecular bone tissue could be subject to thinning and loss, which along with resorption results in increased radiolucency. Radiographs also detect fragility fractures. However, there are technical limitations that impede a perfect diagnosis, caused by inconsistencies in factors like film development, soft-tissue thickness in patients and radiographic exposure.[14]

Radiographs showing osteoporosis are given in Figures 1 and 2.

Bone densitometry is considered an invaluable test to diagnose osteoporosis.
Following are the several methods used for measuring bone mineral density:

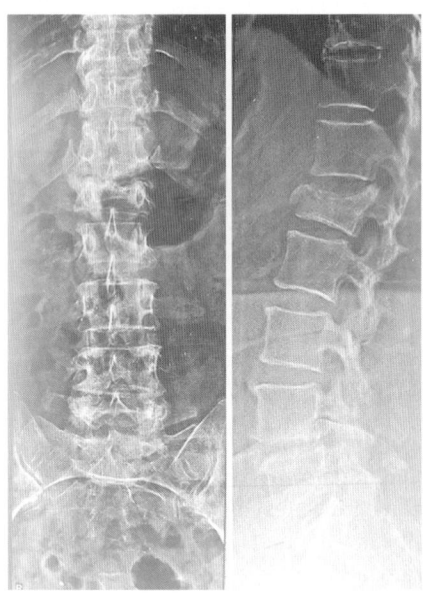

FIG. 1: X-ray of lumbosacral spine showing osteoporosis with compression fracture of L1 vertebra

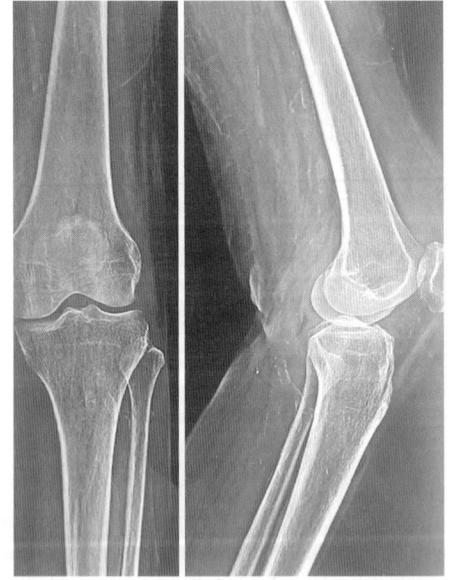

FIG. 2: X-ray of knee joint showing osteoporosis

- Dual energy X-ray absorptiometry (DXA SCAN)
- Peripheral dual energy X-ray absorptiometry (p-DXA)
- Quantitative computed tomography
- Dual photon absorptiometry
- Quantitative ultrasound.

Dual energy X-ray scan is the most accurate and standardized test for measuring BMD. It is quick, easy and noninvasive. It is used to calculate BMD at the lumbar spine, hip and forearm. Whole body BMD also can be measured.

INDICATIONS

- All women aged 65 years or more and men above 70 years of age.
- Postmenopausal women under age of 65 years, and men between 50 years and 70 years, having one or more risk factors
- Adults who have fracture at or after age of 50 years
- Patients who are on long-term steroids.

CONTRAINDICATIONS

- Pregnancy
- Recent contrast studies
- Body weight more than 120 kg.

Dual energy X-ray test results are reported as T-score and Z-score:

- T-score compares bone density with that of healthy young adult
- Z-score compares bone density with that of other people of same age and gender
- T-score is generally considered for diagnosis of osteoporosis.

Z-score should be used in the following patients:

- Premenopausal women
- Men younger than 50 years
- Children.

World Health Organization T-score and Z-score criteria:

World Health Organization (WHO) criteria define a normal T-score within one standard deviation of the mean BMD value in young healthy adult (Table 1).

TABLE 1: World Health Organization criteria for T-score

	T- Score
Normal	At or above −1 SD
Osteopenia	Between −1 to−2.5 SD
Osteoporosis	At or below −2.5 SD
Severe osteoporosis	Less than −2.5 SD with fragility fracture

Z-score value of −2 SD or lower defined as below the expected range for age and those above −2 SD as within expected range for age.

Patients with low Z-score should be investigated for secondary causes of osteoporosis.

Monitoring of osteoporosis: Repeat DXA scans are usually done every 2 years. Testing more frequently than 2 years can be done for patients having hyperparathyroidism or patients who are receiving steroids.[15,16]

The interpretation formats for DXA scans are given in Figures 3 to 9.

TREATMENT

Prevention of fractures, maintenance or increasing BMD, improving physical functions are major objectives in management of osteoporosis.

Following patients should be considered for treatment:

- Hip or vertebral fracture
- T-score −2.5 or less at femoral neck or lumbar spine by DXA
- In postmenopausal women and men age 50 years or older, whose T-score is between −1 SD and −2.5 SD.

Following pharmacologic options are considered for prevention or treatment of osteoporosis:

- Bisphosphonates
- Calcitonin
- Estrogens
- Estrogen agonist or antagonist
- Parathyroid hormone.[17,18]

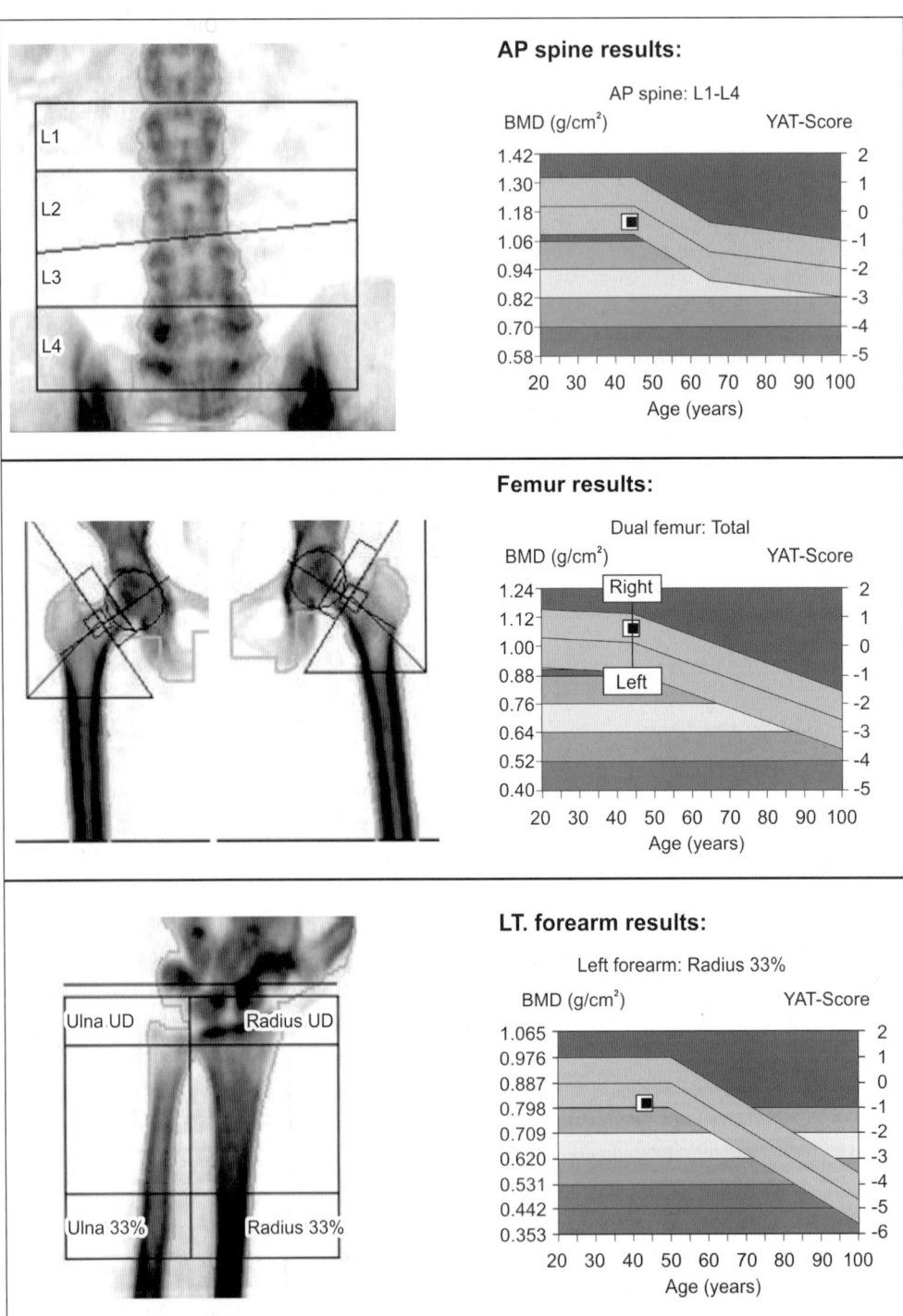

FIG. 3: Anterior-posterior spine, neck of femur and radius showing normal bone mineral density *(For color version, see Plate 3)*

Chapter 12: Bone Mineral Density: Interpretation, Treatment, and Prevention

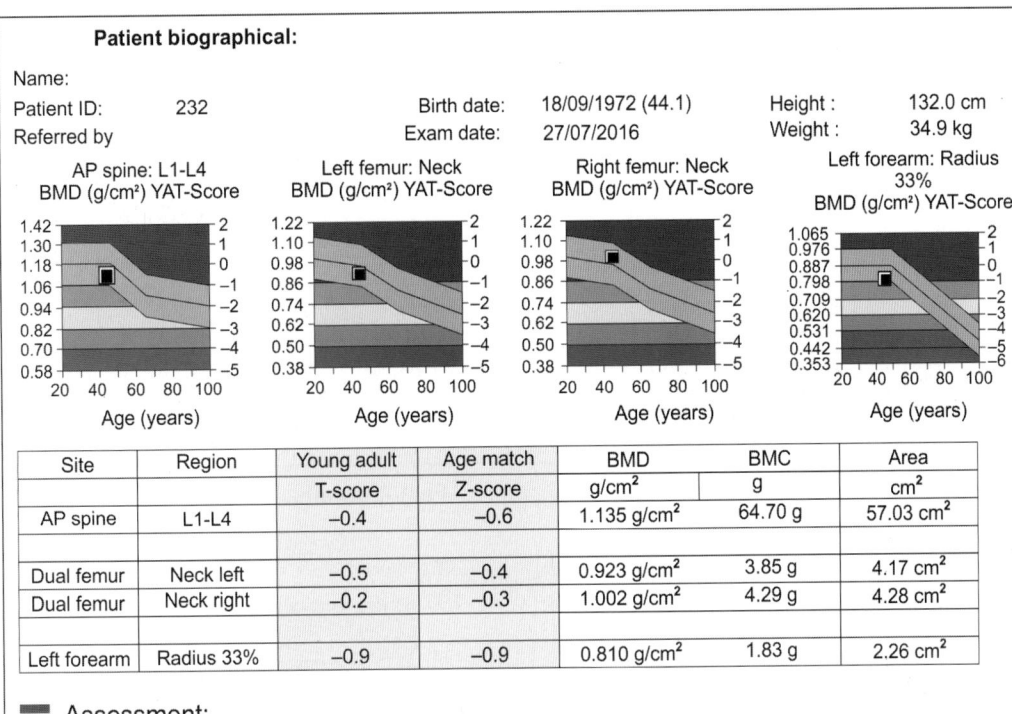

FIG. 4: Normal bone mineral density *(For color version, see Plate 4)*

PREVENTION

As mentioned above, people can be informed and made aware of the ways in which they can help to prevent osteoporosis and related fractures. A good diet and physical activity influence bone development in adolescents. Bone mass acquired during youth is an important factor which determines the risk of fragility fracture later in life. Hence, nutritional and lifestyle modifications are essential factors to prevent osteoporosis.

The Clinician's guide to Prevention and Treatment of Osteoporosis suggests adequate dietary calcium requirement. Suggested intake is as follows:
- 1,000 mg/day for men between 50 years and 70 years
- 1,200 mg/day for women 51 years and older and men 71 years and older.

Additionally, vitamin D intake 800–1,000 IU/day is to be included, regular physical exercise should be performed and excessive alcohol consumption or smoking should be avoided. All risk factors should be assessed and modified accordingly.[17]

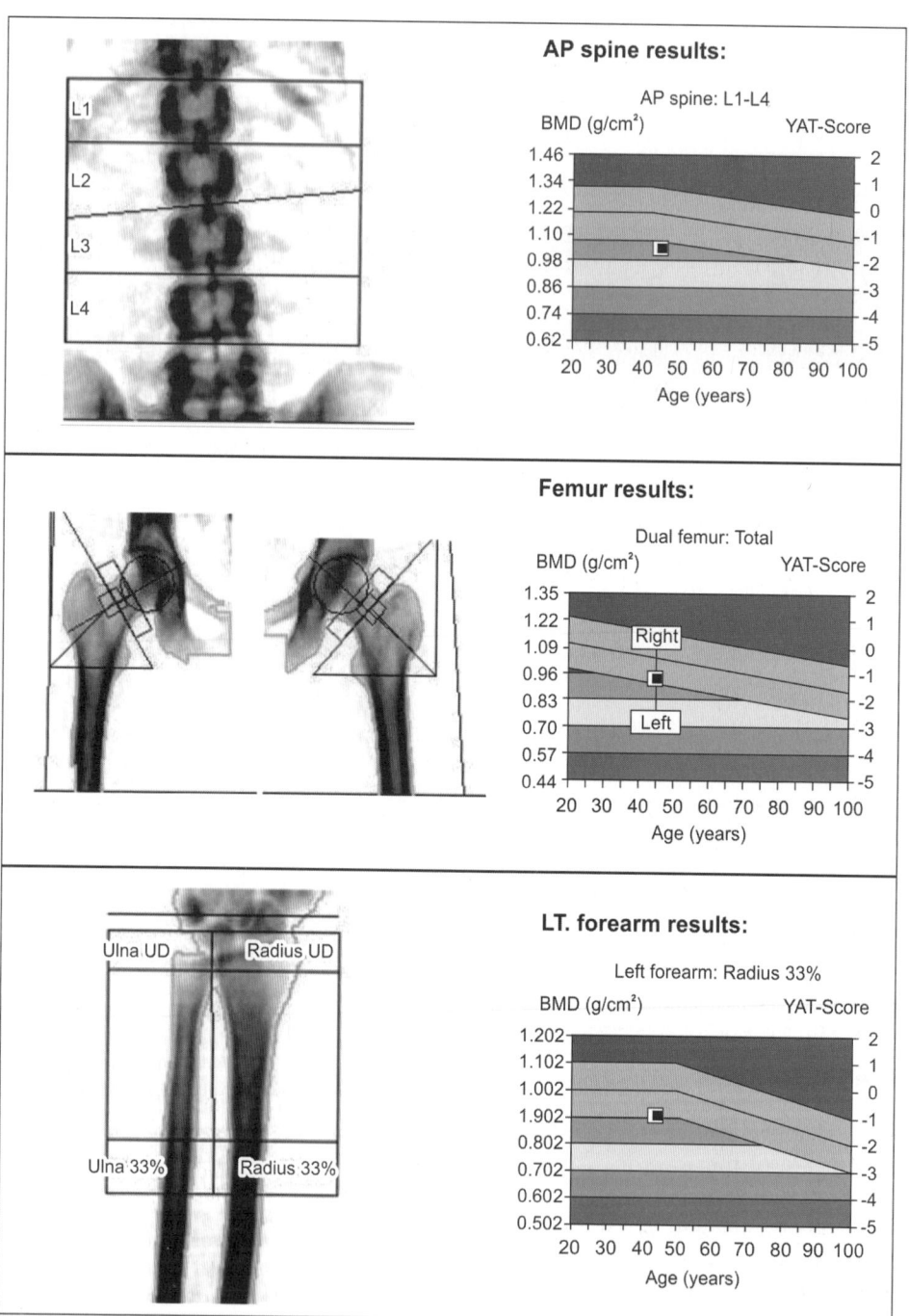

FIG. 5: Anterior-posterior spine, neck of femur, and radius showing osteopenia *(For color version, see Plate 5)*

Chapter 12: Bone Mineral Density: Interpretation, Treatment, and Prevention

Patient biographical:

Name:
Patient ID: 203 Birth date: 13/11/1971 (44.1) Height: 177.0 cm
Referred by Exam date: 27/07/2016 Weight: 72.5 kg

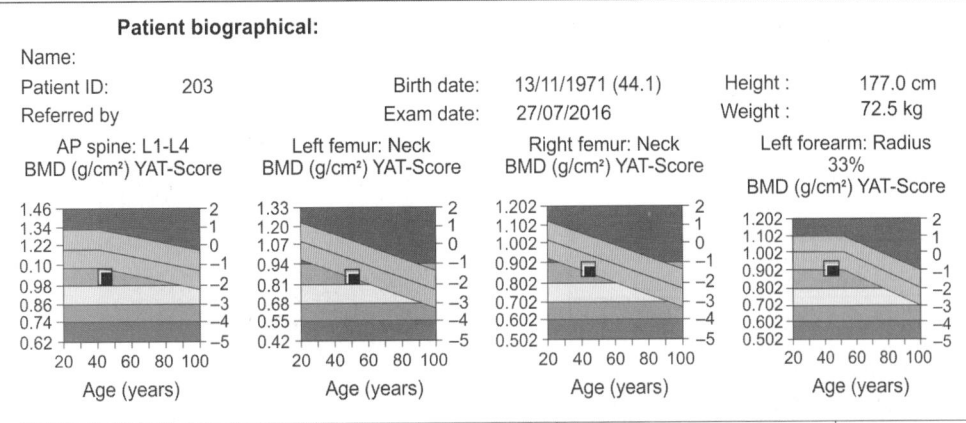

Site	Region	Young adult T-score	Age match Z-score	BMD g/cm^2	BMC g	Area cm^2
AP spine	L1-L4	–1.5	–1.3	1.035 g/cm^2	52.51 g	50.72 cm^2
Dual femur	Neck left	–1.7	–1.1	0.853 g/cm^2	4.25 g	4.98 cm^2
Dual femur	Neck right	–1.4	–0.8	0.887 g/cm^2	4.31 g	4.86 cm^2
Left forearm	Radius 33%	–1.0	–1.0	0.904 g/cm^2	2.35 g	2.60 cm^2

Assessment:

The BMD measured at AP spine L1-L4 is 1.035 g/cm^2 with a T-score of –1.5 is considered moderately low. Fracture risk is moderate. Treatment is advised if there are other risk factors.

The BMD measured at AP spine L1-L4 is 0.853 g/cm^2 with a T-score of –1.7 is considered moderately low. Fracture risk is moderate. Treatment is advised if there are other risk factors.

The BMD measured at AP spine L1-L4 is 0.887 g/cm^2 with a T-score of –1.4 is considered moderately low. Fracture risk is moderate. Treatment is advised if there are other risk factors.

The BMD measured at forearm radius is 0.904 g/cm^2 with a T-score of –1.0 is considered moderately low. Fracture risk is moderate. Treatment is advised if there are other risk factors.

World Health Organization (WHO) criteria for osteoporosis
Normal: T-score at or above –1 SD
Osteopenia: T-score between –1 and –2.5 SD
Osteoporosis: T-score at or below –2.5 SD

FIG. 6: Osteopenia *(For color version, see Plate 6)*

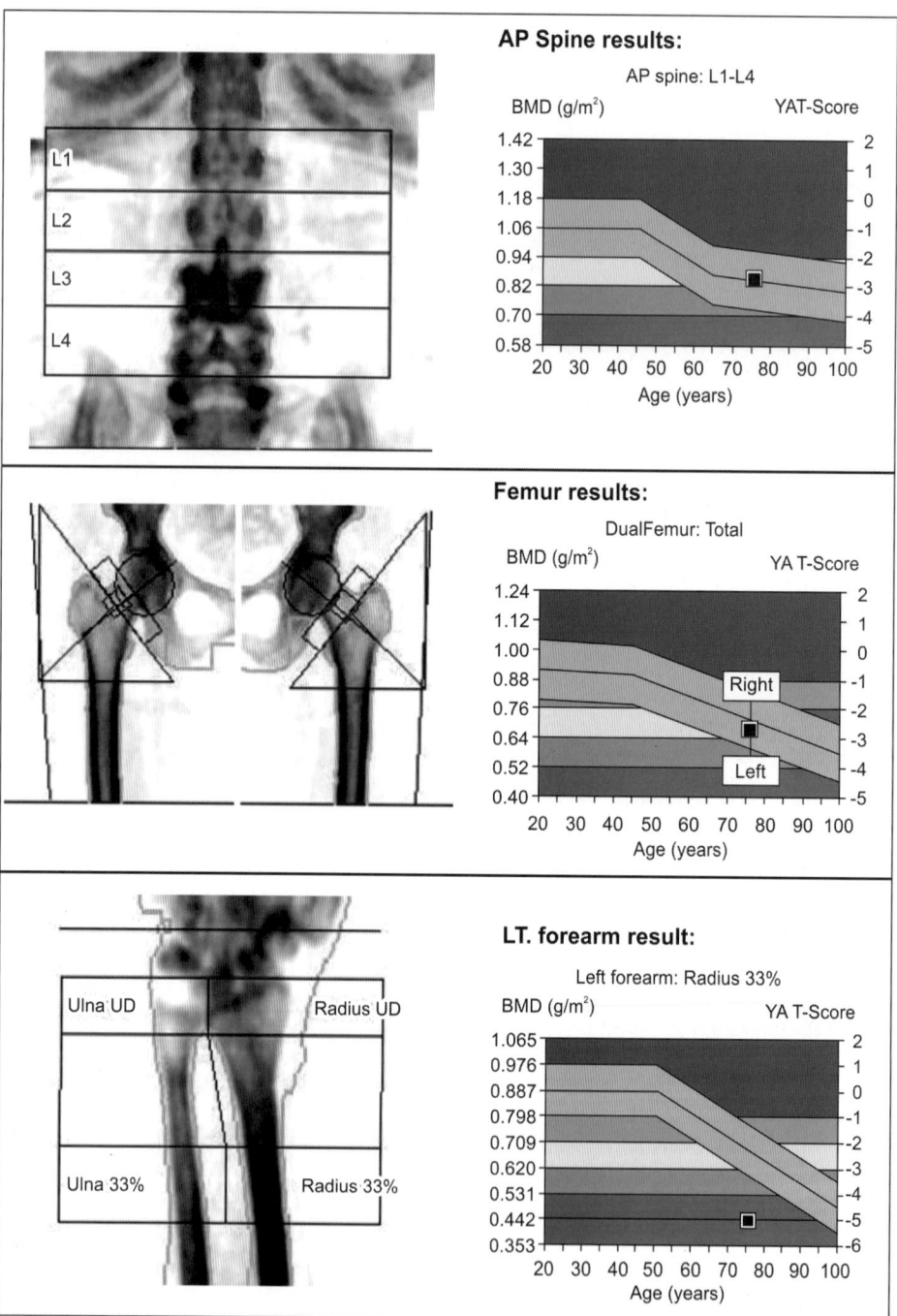

FIG. 7: Anterior-posterior spine, neck of femur and radius showing osteoporosis *(For color version, see Plate 7)*

Chapter 12: Bone Mineral Density: Interpretation, Treatment, and Prevention

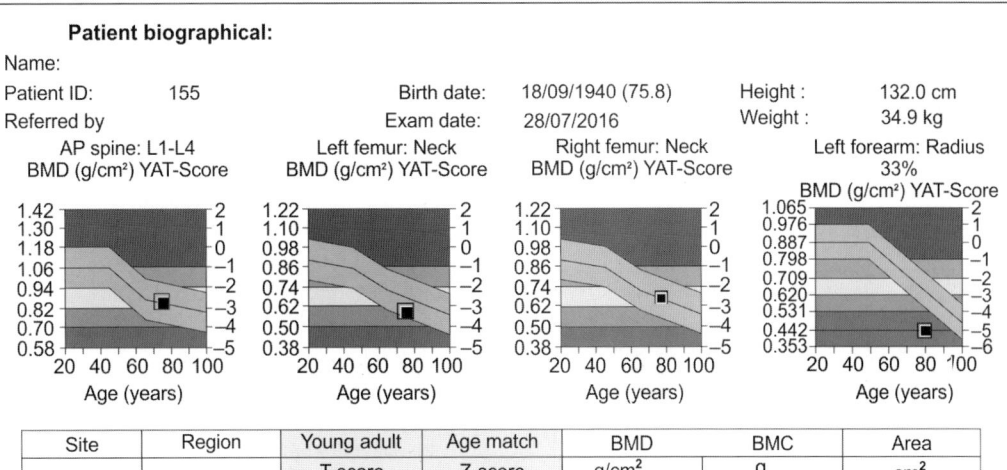

Patient biographical:
Name:
Patient ID: 155
Referred by

Birth date: 18/09/1940 (75.8)
Exam date: 28/07/2016

Height: 132.0 cm
Weight: 34.9 kg

Site	Region	Young adult T-score	Age match Z-score	BMD g/cm²	BMC g	Area cm²
AP spine	L1-L4	–2.7	0.0	0.850 g/cm²	27.00 g	31.76 cm²
Dual femur	Neck left	–3.3	–0.8	0.586 g/cm²	2.67 g	4.56 cm²
Dual femur	Neck right	–2.6	–0.1	0.664 g/cm²	2.74 g	4.13 cm²
Left forearm	Radius 33%	–5.1	–2.7	0.438 g/cm²	2.94 g	2.14 cm²

Assessment:

The BMD measured at AP spine L1-L4 is 0.850 g/cm² with a T-score of –2.7 is low. Fracture risk is high. A follow-up DXA test is recommended in one year to monitor response to therapy.

The BMD measured at femur neck left is 0.586 g/cm² with T-score of –3.3 is markedly low. Fracture risk is high. Treatment, if not already being done, should be started. A follow-up DXA test is recommended in one year to monitor response to therapy.

The BMD measured at femur neck right is 0.664 g/cm² with a T-score of –2.6 is low. Fracture risk is high. A follow-up DXA test is recommended in one year to monitor response to therapy.

The BMD measured at forearm radius 33% is 0.438 g/cm² with a T-score of –5.1 is severely low. Fracture risk is high. Treatment, if not already being done, should be started. A follow-up DXA test is recommended in one year to monitor response to therapy.

World Health Organization (WHO) criteria for osteoporosis
Normal: T-score at or above –1 SD
Osteopenia: T-score between –1 and –2.5 SD
Osteoporosis: T-score at or below –2.5 SD

Fig. 8: Osteoporosis *(For color version, see Plate 8)*

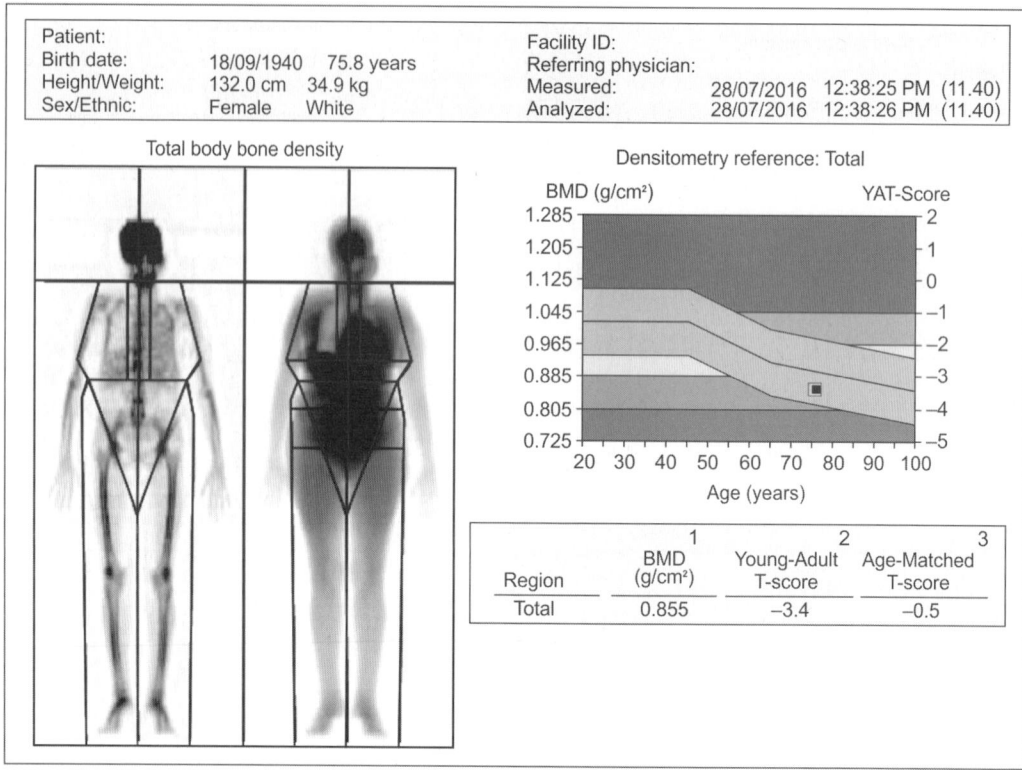

FIG. 9: Whole body scan showing osteoporosis *(For color version, see Plate 9)*

CONCLUSION

Concerning the management of osteoporosis, the main objective is preventing fractures and preserving bone mass.

Proper risk modification, adequate nutrition, and physical activity- all help in preventing osteoporosis. There are effective medications available for its treatment also. Lastly, DXA scan remains to be the most important tool in diagnosing bone mineral density.

REFERENCES

1. National Institute of Arthritis, Musculoskeletal and Skin Diseases. (2016). Osteoporosis handout on health. [online] Niams.nih.gov. Available from www.niams.nih.gov/health_info/Osteoporosis/default.asp [Accessed December, 2016].
2. International Osteoporosis Foundation. (2015). Introduction to bone biology: all about our bones [Internet]. [online]. Available from: https://www.iofbonehealth.org/introduction-bone-biology-all-about-our-bones [Accessed December, 2016].
3. Oursler M, Bellido T. American Society for Bone and Mineral Research. (2003). Bone cells. [online] Available from: https://depts.washington.edu/bonebio/ASBMRed/cells.html#oblasts [Accessed December, 2016].
4. Dallas SL, Prideaux M, Bonewald LF. The osteocyte: an endocrine cell and more. Endocr Rev. 2013;34(5):658-90.
5. Sobacchi C, Schulz A, Coxon FP, Villa A, Helfrich MH. Osteopetrosis: genetics, treatment and new insights into osteoclast function. Nat Rev Endocrinol. 2013;9(9):522-36.
6. Florencio-Silva R, Sasso G, Sasso-Cerri E, Simões M, Cerri P. Biology of bone tissue: structure, function, and factors that influence bone cells. Biomed Res Int. 2015;2015: 421746.
7. Kanis JA, Johnell O, Odén A, Dawson A, De Laet C, Jonsson B. Ten year probabilities of osteoporotic fractures according to BMD and diagnosis thresholds. Osteoporosis Int. 2001;12(12):989-95.
8. Kanis JA, Johansson H, Odén A, Johnell O, De Laet C, Eisman JA, et al. A familiy history of fracture and fracture risk: a meta-analysis. Bone. 2004;35:1029-37.

9. Kanis JA, Johnell O, De Laet C, Johansson H, Oden A, Delmas P, et al. A meta-analysis of previous fracture and subsequent fracture risk. Bone. 2004;35(2);375-82.
10. Kanis JA, Johansson H, Odén A, Johnell O, De Laet C, Melton LJ III, et al. A meta-analysis of prior corticosteroid use and fracture risk. J Bone Miner Res. 2004;19(6). 893-9.
11. International Osteoporosis Foundation. (2015). Who's at risk? [online] Available from https://www.iofbonehealth.org/whos-risk [Accessed December, 2016].
12. Harris WH, Heaney RP. Skeletal renewal and metabolic bone disease. N Engl J Med. 1969;280(6): 303-11.
13. Guglielmi G, Muscarella S, Bazzocchi A. Integrated Imaging approach to osteoporosis: state-of-the-art review and update. Radiographics. 2011;31(5):1343-64.
14. Guglielmi G, Muscarella S, Leone A, Peh WC. Imaging of metabolic bone diseases. Radiol Clin North Am. 2008;46(4):735-54, VI.
15. World Health Organisation. Assessment of fracture risk and its implication to screening for postmenopausal osteoporosis: Technical report series 843. Geneva: WHO; 1994.
16. Kanis J. Diagnosis of osteoporosis and assessment of fracture risk. Lancet. 2002;359:1929-36.
17. Cosman F, de Beur SJ, LeBoff MS, Lewiecki EM, Tanner B, Randall S, et al. Clinician's guide to prevention and treatment of osteoporosis. Osteoporos Int. 2014;25(10):2359-81.
18. Gallagher JC, Tella SH. Prevention and treatment of postmenopausal osteoporosis. J Steroid Biochem Mol Biol. 2013;142:155-70.

SECTION 4

Cervical/Neck Pain

CHAPTER 13

Headache: Causes and Treatment Modalities

K Ravishankar

INTRODUCTION

Headache is the most common of medical complaints and the differential diagnosis of headache is probably one of the longest in all of medicine. In spite, only a small proportion of headache patients consult physicians, most continue to self-medicate and when they do consult, they are often misdiagnosed or treated suboptimally.

Headache is a symptom with numerous causes that could range from a mild head injury to a serious brain tumor or as happens more often, it could be a disorder unto itself, such as migraine. Different headaches have different treatments, and the final outcome in treating a patient with headache will therefore depend on getting the diagnosis right. The aim of this chapter will be to discuss the right approach to the diagnosis of this common complaint and detail the management strategies for some of the more important headache entities.

CAUSES

All headaches can be grouped under two broad categories—primary and secondary. Primary headaches are those benign headaches where clinical examination and investigation including imaging are normal and not suggestive of any underlying etiology, but yet the patient continues to suffer.

Secondary headaches are those headaches where there is an underlying structural or vascular or metabolic or infective cause that can be detected on clinical examination or by appropriate investigation. Approximately 90% of headaches seen in practice are primary headaches. Less than 10% of headaches are secondary headaches due to an underlying identifiable problem. All these headaches have been listed in table 1 using the same rubrics as in the revised International Headache Society Classification (ICHD-3 beta 2013).

TABLE 1: The International Classification of Headache Disorders, 3rd edition (beta version; 2013)

Primary headache disorders

1. Migraine
    1.1 Migraine without aura
    1.2 Migraine with aura
        1.2.1 Migraine with typical aura
            1.2.1.1 Typical aura with headache
            1.2.1.2 Typical aura without headache
        1.2.2 Migraine with brainstem aura
        1.2.3 Hemiplegic migraine
            1.2.3.1 Familial hemiplegic migraine
                1.2.3.1.1 Familial hemiplegic migraine type 1
                1.2.3.1.2 Familial hemiplegic migraine type 2
                1.2.3.1.3 Familial hemiplegic migraine type 3
                1.2.3.1.4 Familial hemiplegic migraine, other loci
            1.2.3.2 Sporadic hemiplegic migraine
        1.2.4 Retinal migraine
    1.3 Chronic migraine
    1.4 Complications of migraine
        1.4.1 Status migrainosus
        1.4.2 Persistent aura without infarction
        1.4.3 Migrainous infarction
        1.4.4 Migraine aura-triggered seizure
    1.5 Probable migraine
        1.5.1 Probable migraine without aura
        1.5.2 Probable migraine with aura
    1.6 Episodic syndromes that may be associated with migraine
        1.6.1 Recurrent gastrointestinal disturbance
            1.6.1.1 Cyclical vomiting syndrome
            1.6.1.2 Abdominal migraine
        1.6.2 Benign paroxysmal vertigo
        1.6.3 Benign paroxysmal torticollis
2. Tension-type headache
    2.1 Infrequent episodic tension-type headache
        2.1.1 Infrequent episodic tension-type headache associated with pericranial tenderness

Continued

        2.1.2 Infrequent episodic tension-type headache not associated with pericranial tenderness
    2.2 Frequent episodic tension-type headache
        2.2.1 Frequent episodic tension-type headache associated with pericranial tenderness
        2.2.2 Frequent episodic tension-type headache not associated with pericranial tenderness
    2.3 Chronic tension-type headache
        2.3.1 Chronic tension-type headache associated with pericranial tenderness
        2.3.2 Chronic tension-type headache not associated with pericranial tenderness
    2.4 Probable tension-type headache
        2.4.1 Probable infrequent episodic tension-type headache
        2.4.2 Probable frequent episodic tension-type headache
        2.4.3 Probable chronic tension-type headache
3. Trigeminal autonomic cephalalgias
    3.1 Cluster headache
        3.1.1 Episodic cluster headache
        3.1.2 Chronic cluster headache
    3.2 Paroxysmal hemicrania
        3.2.1 Episodic paroxysmal hemicrania
        3.2.2 Chronic paroxysmal hemicrania
    3.3 Short-lasting unilateral neuralgiform headache attacks
        3.3.1 Short-lasting unilateral neuralgiform headache attacks with conjunctival injection and tearing (SUNCT)
            3.3.1.1 Episodic SUNCT
            3.3.1.2 Chronic SUNCT
        3.3.2 Short-lasting unilateral neuralgiform headache attacks with cranial autonomic symptoms (SUNA)
            3.3.2.1 Episodic SUNA
            3.3.2.2 Chronic SUNA

Continued

Continued

- 3.4 Hemicrania continua
- 3.5 Probable trigeminal autonomic cephalalgia
  - 3.5.1 Probable cluster headache
  - 3.5.2 Probable paroxysmal hemicrania
  - 3.5.3 Probable short-lasting unilateral neuralgiform headache attacks
  - 3.5.4 Probable hemicrania continua
4. Other primary headache disorders
  - 4.1 Primary cough headache
    - 4.1.1 Probable primary cough headache
  - 4.2 Primary exercise headache
    - 4.2.1 Probable primary exercise headache
  - 4.3 Primary headache associated with sexual activity
    - 4.3.1 Probable primary headache associated with sexual activity
  - 4.4 Primary thunderclap headache
  - 4.5 Cold-stimulus headache
    - 4.5.1 Headache attributed to external application of a cold stimulus
    - 4.5.2 Headache attributed to ingestion or inhalation of a cold stimulus
    - 4.5.3 Probable cold-stimulus headache
      - 4.5.3.1 Headache probably attributed to external application of a cold stimulus
      - 4.5.3.2 Headache probably attributed to ingestion or inhalation of a cold stimulus
  - 4.6 External-pressure headache
    - 4.6.1 External-compression headache
    - 4.6.2 External-traction headache
    - 4.6.3 Probable external-pressure headache
      - 4.6.3.1 Probable external-compression headache
      - 4.6.3.2 Probable external-traction headache
  - 4.7 Primary stabbing headache
    - 4.7.1 Probable primary stabbing headache
  - 4.8 Nummular headache

Continued

Continued

- 4.8.1 Probable nummular headache
- 4.9 Hypnic headache
- 4.9.1 Probable hypnic headache
- 4.10 New daily persistent headache
- 4.10.1 Probable new daily persistent headache

Secondary headache disorders

5. Headache attributed to head and/or neck trauma
6. Headache attributed to cranial or cervical vascular disorder
7. Headache attributed to nonvascular intracranial disorder
8. Headache attributed to a substance or its withdrawal
9. Headache attributed to infection
10. Headache attributed to disorder of homeostasis
11. Headache or facial pain attributed to disorder of cranium, neck, eyes, ears, nose, sinuses, teeth, mouth or other facial or cranial structures
12. Headache attributed to psychiatric disorder
13. Cranial neuralgias and central causes of facial pain
14. Other headache, cranial neuralgia central or primary facial pain

CLINICAL EXAMINATION

History

Establishing a diagnosis when a patient presents with headache depends almost entirely on taking an accurate history. Pattern recognition is most important for headache diagnosis. It is a better practice to generate a routine set of questions under preset headings. At the end of the history, keeping in mind a checklist of the various causes of headache, we can arrive at a conclusion as to the diagnosis of the underlying cause. The same patient can have more than one type of headache.[1]

Temporal Profile

The mode of onset and progress over time are critical issues in deciding whether one is dealing with a benign or a serious headache. A chronic recurrent headache or a chronic nonprogressive daily headache most likely represents a primary headache. Sudden onset of a severe headache suggests possible vascular involvement such as a subarachnoid bleed or an acute infective cause like meningitis. Progressively worsening headache suggests increasing intracranial pressure or uncontrolled systemic disease. The presence of focal or lateralizing features makes the diagnosis easier. One must, therefore, specifically obtain information regarding progressive worsening.

Age

The age of onset of the headache is also important. Migraine generally begins at a younger age and is more common in females between 25 and 40 years of age whereas tension-type headache is more common around middle age.

Headaches that begin after 50 years of age should always be investigated to rule out potential secondary causes such as temporal arteritis.

Location and Type

The type of pain, the severity, and the location of the head pain are important parameters for diagnosis. Unilateral pulsating or throbbing headaches most likely indicate an underlying vascular involvement as with migraine but it is important to note that migraine headaches need not always be unilateral; it can often be bilateral and can involve any part of the head and can also radiate to the neck and shoulder. Cluster headaches are almost always unilateral in the same location during a cluster period, and rarely shift sides.

Tension-type Headache

It is diffuse, dull and generally bilateral. With secondary headaches, the location of the headache, the nature and severity would vary depending on the anatomical location of the lesion and the mechanism involved in pain production.

Accompaniments

In all headache patients, one must ask for the presence or absence of nausea, vomiting, hypersensitivity to light and noise and associated neurological involvement. Associated features like fever, arthralgias, and malaise should suggest a systemic problem. It is essential to get a detailed history of associated neurological deficits or auras, such as transient visual symptoms or hemisensory deficits which would support the diagnosis of migraine with aura.

Sometimes, it helps in the diagnosis of a headache to ask about behavior during the acute headache attack. The typical behavior of a migraine patient who tries to sleep undisturbed in a darkroom is quite in contrast to that of the patient with a cluster headache who cannot stay still and keeps pacing around.

Headache that occurs regularly just before or during the menstrual periods is more likely to be due to menstrual migraine. Hypertensive headache is more common in the morning whereas sinusitis induced headache is worse on bending.

Provoking and Relieving Factors

Primary headaches such as migraine can frequently be provoked by missing meals or going out in the hot sun. Trigger factors vary in different regions. Trigger factors in the Indian setting are listed in table 2.

Past Medical History

Careful questioning for systemic illnesses are essential for the complete evaluation of a headache patient, e.g., malignancy anywhere in the body should raise the possibility of metastases. Always enquire about other coexisting medical illnesses. The presence of a particular systemic problem

TABLE 2: Migraine triggers

Food items: Cheese, dairy products, paneer (cottage cheese), citrus fruits, chocolates, onions, sea food
Food additives: Monosodium glutamate, aspartame, nitrates, caffeine
Alcohol: Red wine, beer
Hormonal changes: Menstruation, ovulation
Physical exertion: Excessive exercise, fatigue
Visual stimuli: Bright lights, glare
Auditory stimuli: Loud noise or music
Olfactory stimuli: Perfumes and certain odors
Sleep: Too much or too little
Weather changes
Head or neck trauma
Hunger
Stress and anxiety

may be a contraindication for the use of certain headache drugs, e.g., β-blockers would be contraindicated in a diabetic or asthmatic patient.

Physical Examination

Physical examination helps to confirm the information obtained from the history. Routine examination in patients with headache can help exclude causes like hypertension, meningitis, or systemic febrile illnesses. It may be necessary to palpate over the head and neck for detection of tender trigger points, to auscultate over the skull, over the carotid and vertebral vessels for bruits, to evaluate the temporomandibular joint for tenderness and movement limitations, to palpate the cervical spine for tenderness and to palpate the temporal artery to rule out temporal arteritis. The neurological examination in headache patients is most often normal, but this should in no way reduce the level of alertness of the physician.[2]

DIAGNOSTIC CRITERIA

Criteria for each type of headache is beyond the scope of this chapter but listed in table 3 are the criteria for the most common headache seen in practice, viz., migraine. This will give you an idea of how the ICHD2 has laid down diagnostic criteria for every type of headache.

INVESTIGATIONS

Headaches are more often due to benign causes, but because headache may be a symptom of a wide variety of diseases, recognizing those headaches that warrant further investigation continues to be a challenge for any physician. A range of different investigational techniques are now at the disposal of the clinician. One or more of the tests outlined below may be appropriate for a particular situation.[3]

Laboratory Testing

The complete blood count (CBC) erythrocyte sedimentation rate (ESR), and relevant blood chemistry should be obtained in all headache patients whom you decide to investigate. It helps rule out unsuspected systemic diseases such as temporal arteritis. Further specific laboratory tests should be done when necessary, depending on the etiology you are suspecting.

Cerebrospinal Fluid Examination

Cerebrospinal fluid (CSF) examination must be considered in headache patients when there is fever or when the onset is sudden or when there are associated cranial nerve deficits. The spinal tap should preferably be performed after a computed tomography (CT) or magnetic resonance imaging (MRI) scan has ruled out the presence of raised pressure due to intracranial structural disease.

Neuroimaging

Imaging must be done in a headache patient whenever there are danger signals. Magnetic resonance imaging is now rapidly becoming the standard diagnostic test for head and face pain, particularly in view of the advantage of noninvasive evaluation of the vasculature

TABLE 3: Criteria for migraine with and without aura

S. No.	Migraine without aura		Migraine with aura
1.	At least five attacks fulfilling criteria 2–4	1.	At least two attacks fulfilling criterion 2
2.	Headache lasting 4–72 h (untreated or unsuccessfully treated)	2.	At least three of the following four characteristics: a. One or more fully reversible aura symptoms indicating brain dysfunction
3.	Headache has at least two of the following characteristics: a. Unilateral location b. Pulsating quality c. Moderate or severe intensity (inhibits, or prohibits daily activities) d. Aggravation by walking stairs or similar routine physical activity		b. At least one aura symptom develops gradually over more than 4 min or 2 or more symptoms occur in succession c. No single aura symptom lasts more than 60 min d. Headache follows aura with a free interval of less than 60 min (it may also begin before or with the aura)
		3.	History, physical examination and, when appropriate, diagnostic tests exclude a secondary cause
4.	During headache at least one of the following: a. Nausea and/or vomiting b. Photophobia and phonophobia		
5.	History, physical, and neurologic examinations do not suggest another disorder		

by magnetic resonance angiography and magnetic resonance venography. As and when necessary and in the appropriate situation, one must investigate further with digital subtraction angiography (DSA).

DIFFERENTIAL DIAGNOSIS

Primary Headaches

Migraine

Migraine is a complex neurological brain disorder that manifests with recurrent headaches and is associated with nausea, vomiting, photophobia, or photophobias. There may or may not be a neurological accompaniment in the form of an aura. It is more common in women than in men (2 to 3:1) and a family history is present in more than 60% of cases. Attacks often begin in late childhood, adolescence and early twenties. Migraine should always be thought of as a complex neurological disorder with headache being one of the most common presenting features. There may be other accompanying neurological, gastrointestinal or autonomic features as shown in the typical attack of migraine consists of a sequence of events with four different phases: the prodrome, the aura, the headache and the postdrome and these phases blend imperceptibly with one another during the course of an attack.[4]

Treatment

Once trigger factors are identified and controlled, drug treatment needs to be selected depending on the severity and the level of disability. Ideal management of migraine should concentrate on four major areas (Table 4):

1. Control of trigger factors
2. Treatment of the acute attack
3. Long-term prophylactic medication[5]
4. Nonpharmacologic management.

TABLE 4: Pharmacotherapy of migraine

Abortive therapy	Prophylactic therapy
Simple analgesics	Beta blockers
Combination analgesics	Calcium channel antagonists
Nonsteroidal anti-inflammatory drugs	Antidepressants
Erogtamine tartrate	Serotonin antagonists
Dihydroergotmine	Nonsteroidal anti-inflammatory drugs
Sumatriptan and other triptans	Anticonvulsants—divalproex sodium, topiramate
Corticosteroids	OnabotulinumtoxinA

Tension-type Headache

Tension-type headache occurs more commonly in patients subjected to stress, anxiety, and depression. Tension type headache usually begins in an episodic form and progresses to a chronic form where headaches occur almost daily and do not appear to be associated with any overt psychological factors.

The head pain in tension-type headache is usually generalized and of long duration. The patient experiences a constant pain and obtains temporary relief with analgesics and sleep. Nevertheless, there are no associated accompaniments such as vomiting and photophobia, and the diagnosis can be established by a good history.[6]

Treatment

Attempt to identify the stress or emotional problem underlying the headache. The mechanism of the head pain should be explained to the patient. The patient should be reassured that there is no underlying disease. When tension-type headaches are due to a severe emotional problem, the patient should be referred for psychiatric for evaluation and treatment.

Cluster Headache

It is a devastating painful headache, mostly affecting men. It is the most easily diagnosable headache. The term "cluster headache" reflects the clustering of headache attacks in time. There is a periodicity to the attacks with seasonal clustering. Typically, the pain peaks in 10–15 minutes and lasts 45–180 minutes and may occur 1–3 times per day. The pain is usually spontaneous, but can be provoked by alcohol. Patients describe the pain as excruciating or penetrating and on the same side during each cluster. The pain is accompanied by lacrimation, rhinorrhea or ptosis.[7]

Treatment

Symptomatic treatment includes oxygen inhalation at about 7 L/min, parenteral dihydroergotamine, or parenteral sumatriptan 6 mg. The following drugs have been shown to be beneficial in the prophylactic therapy of cluster headache:[8]

- Verapamil (120–240 mg daily)
- Lithium carbonate (300 mg daily)
- Methysergide (2 mg)
- Steroids are very effective in preventing attacks.

When cluster headache is intractable, one may need to resort to other invasive measures such as occipital nerve blocks or neurostimulation procedures such as sphenopalatine ganglion stimulation or vagal nerve stimulation, or occipital nerve stimulation.

Other Trigeminoautonomic Cephalgias and Short-lasting Headaches

There are some head pains which are considered variants of cluster headache, but there are a number of differences between cluster headache and these pains—the most important of them being the fact that many of them are characterized by a prompt response to indomethacin. They should not be confused with cluster headache and can be easily distinguished by their short duration and high frequency of attacks. The best example of this type of indomethacin responsive cluster variant is chronic paroxysmal hemicrania. There are some other rare short-lasting headaches such as SUNCT syndrome (short lasting neuralgiform attacks with conjunctional tearing) that are responsive to lamotrigene.

Secondary Headaches
Raised Intracranial Pressure
Any lesion that increases intracranial pressure is likely to cause a progressively increasing headache. Headache as a presenting feature will depend on the nature and location of the mass. The headache is usually generalized, may not fit into any particular pattern, slowly increases in intensity and leads to drowsiness and confusion.

Intracranial Hemorrhage
Collection of blood in different areas of the brain can produce headache. Intracerebral hemorrhage is usually sudden in onset and can produce incapacitating headache with focal neurological symptoms and decreased levels of consciousness.

Meningitis
It is an inflammation of the meninges and spinal fluid caused by any type of infection or toxic reaction. It may be aseptic (viral), chemical or infectious. The headache is usually accompanied by fever, stiff neck, vomiting, and the diagnosis is confirmed by CSF examination.

Idiopathic Intracranial Hypertension
Idiopathic intracranial hypertension or pseudotumor cerebri has a variety of causes and patients with this condition present with headache and visual obscurations along with other signs of increased intracranial pressure. It usually occurs in young, obese women; the CT or MRI reveals small ventricles and on examination the patient may have decreased vision.

Sinusitis-associated Headache
Sinusitis is wrongly thought of as a common cause for headaches. In actual practice, very few headaches are due to sinusitis. Acute sinusitis can produce a severe painful head pain in various parts of the head depending on the sinus which is involved. Sphenoid or ethmoid sinusitis usually presents with bilateral headache, can be difficult to diagnose and can be confirmed only by a special CT scan.

Medication Overuse Headache
Medication overuse headache has been variously referred to as analgesic rebound headache, ergotamine rebound headache or drug rebound headache. Simple analgesics particularly those combined with an opiate (codeine) and/or a barbiturate, and frequent doses of acetaminophen or aspirin with caffeine may also cause rebound headaches. The most significant feature is that the headache typically persists throughout the whole day, is present on waking and is described as a dull, diffuse headache. Complete withdrawal of the analgesic is the only effective treatment.[9]

EMERGENCY TREATMENT

Patients may need emergency treatment when the headache is incapacitating. The majority of patients who need emergency treatment have either an acute exacerbation of an underlying primary headache disorder, or an acute febrile disorder or some more sinister underlying neurological cause. Treatment is dictated by the specific diagnosis in patients with secondary causes of headache.

HEADACHE CLINIC

This is a new concept in the management of chronic headaches. Over the past few years, there has been a growing interest in the problem of headache.

Headache clinics differ from pain clinics in a striking way in their pharmacologic approach, as opposed to a more extensive physical and behavioral approach in pain clinics.

There are many advantages of treating patients through a headache clinic. With the help of a questionnaire and a headache diary, one can detect mixed patterns of headache. By taking a detailed history of systemic problems, prophylactic drugs can be selected suitably, side effects are detected early and drug dosages can be titrated accordingly. Drug rebound headaches are diagnosed early. Chronic headaches can at times be so debilitating and incapacitating those patients may benefit only if they are managed by a specialist experienced in headache management. The physician must, therefore, know when to refer the patient to the specialist. Continuity of care and a close patient-physician rapport are some important factors for effective treatment of headaches.[10]

CONCLUSION

The author has attempted to give you an overview of some of the more common causes of headache. There are some causes for headache in the eyes, ears, nose, and teeth that should not be overlooked. There are also treatment modalities that are non-pharmacological. Alternative therapies and traditional treatments also work well. So headache management sometimes needs a holistic approach. Given the right amount of time, interest and inclination physicians should not find headaches to be baffling or frustrating to deal with. It is "all about the art of conveying the science".

REFERENCES

1. Headache Classification Committee of the International Headache Society (IHS). The International Classification of Headache Disorders, 3rd edition (beta version). Cephalalgia. 2013;33:629-808.
2. Silberstein SD, Lipton RB, Dalessio DJ. Overview, diagnosis and classification of headache. In: Silberstein SD, Lipton RB, Dalessio DJ (Eds): Wolff's Headache and Other Facial Pain. New York: Oxford; 2001. pp. 6-26.
3. Lance JW. Mechanism and Management of Headache, 7th ed. Boston: Butterworth-Heinemann; 2005.
4. Panda S, Tripathi M. Clinical profile of migraineurs in a referral centre in India. J Assoc Physicians India. 2005; 53:111-5.
5. Diener HC, Limmroth V. Advances in pharmacological treatment of migraine. Expert Opin Investig Drugs. 2001; 10:1831-45.
6. Bigal ME, Lipton RB, Tepper SJ, Rapoport AM, Sheftell FD. Primary chronic daily headache and its subtypes in adolescents and adults. Neurology. 2004;63:843-47.
7. Chakravarty A, Mukherjee A, Roy D. Trigeminal autonomic cephalgias and variants: Clinical profile in Indian patients. Cephalalgia. 2004;24(10):859-66.
8. Dodick DW, Rozen TD, Goadsby PJ, Silberstein SD. Cluster headache. Cephalalgia. 2000;20:787-803.
9. Ravishankar K. Medication overuse headache in India. Cephalalgia. 2008;28(11):1223-6.
10. Ravishankar K. Barriers to headache care in India and efforts to improve the situation. Lancet Neurol. 2004; 3(9):564-7.

CHAPTER 14

Trigeminal Neuralgia: Causes and Treatment

Manohar L Sharma

INTRODUCTION

In the middle of 18th century, an English baroness went to stay in her palatial resort at Au Riviera, France. She started feeling excruciating pains in her right side of face. The pains were like electric shock, intermittent and were initiated by speaking, eating, drinking and even by light touch of a breeze of air or a splash of water on the face. The whole day she lay on the bed, keeping her face pressed with the palm of her hand. She was rushed to a nearby consultant physician. He introduced himself as Sir John Fothergill. As a remedy, he prescribed for her, castor oil 2 teaspoons to be taken four hourly.

The days were rainy, and the baroness had to pay frequent visits to the toilet outside, within the compound holding an umbrella in one hand. At the end of the day, she lay down exhausted in the bed. Next day when Sir Fothergill paid his morning visit and inquired how she was, she said, "I am so much exhausted I cannot appreciate any pain anymore." This account outlines the initial description of trigeminal neuralgia (TGN) though there are some other descriptions before this in literature.

Julius Andre, a French physician and a contemporary of Dr Fothergill, independently described the characteristics of this illness and named it "Tic dolorous", i.e. painful spasms of the face. Two hundred years later, i.e. in the middle of 20th century, Ciba in the name of Tegrital established the first definitive medical treatment for this illness.

Epidemiological studies show that approximately 4 to 28.9/100,000 persons worldwide experience TGN. The management for TGN can be either pharmacological or surgical treatment.[1-3] Of the surgical treatment options, microvascular decompression (MVD) is preferred option as it is almost curative and at 10 year follow-up the incidence of complete pain relief is 70–75%. It is not a neuroablative procedure (Hence no problems related to deafferentation, i.e. unpleasant dysesthesia or anesthesia dolorosa).[4] If there is no vascular compression or conflict at the trigeminal root entry zone on imaging, then, the neuroablative procedures should be considered in intractable form of the condition. Pharmacological treatment of TGN is mainly based on the antiepileptic drug carbamazepine, which will suppress the ectopic activity and is very effective, but patients may have many side effects in short and long term.[1] For this reason in Liverpool, UK, it is common practice in author's unit to offer micro vascular decompression if MR scan

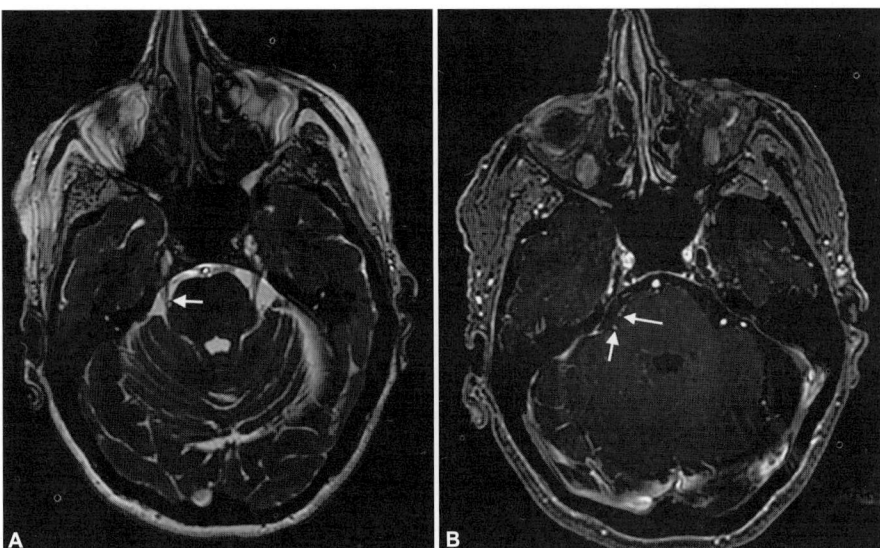

FIGS 1A and B: Neurovascular compression right side (arrows pointing to blood vessel)

demonstrates vascular compression (Fig. 1A and B) at the trigeminal nerve root entry zone.[1] However, 30% people do not get adequate pain relief after the surgical treatment (microvascular decompression) and pharmacological treatment with carbamazepine only helps about 50-60% in long term. There is large evidence base from multiple large studies to demonstrate a very good long-term outcome from these interventions.[4] Peripheral nerve blocks are not preferred as often the pain recurs soon and there is higher risk of neuritis related neuropathic pain.

CLASSIFICATION OF TRIGEMINAL NEURALGIA

Trigeminal neuralgia is a typical and classical condition of neuropathic facial pain. However, formally classifying TGN as neuropathic pain based on the grading system of the International Association for the Study of Pain is complicated by the requirement of objective signs confirming an underlying lesion or disease of the somatosensory system. Other version of the International Classification of Headache Disorders created difficulties by abandoning the term symptomatic TGN for manifestations caused by major neurologic disease, such as tumors or multiple sclerosis. These diagnostic challenges hinder the triage of TGN patients for treatment and clinical trials. In view of these issues, a new classification of TGN has been proposed.[5] It proposes three diagnostic categories. Classical TGN requires demonstration of morphologic changes in the trigeminal nerve root from vascular compression (Figs 1A and B). Secondary TGN is due to an identifiable underlying neurologic disease e.g. multiple sclerosis (Figs 2A and B). TGN of unknown etiology is labeled idiopathic. Diagnostic certainty is graded possible when pain paroxysms occur in the distribution of the trigeminal nerve branches. Triggered paroxysms permit the designation of clinically established TGN and probable neuropathic pain. Imaging and neurophysiologic tests that establish the etiology of classical or secondary TGN determine definite neuropathic pain.

DIAGNOSIS

History taking is the key to diagnosis, as this condition is not diagnosed by investigations.

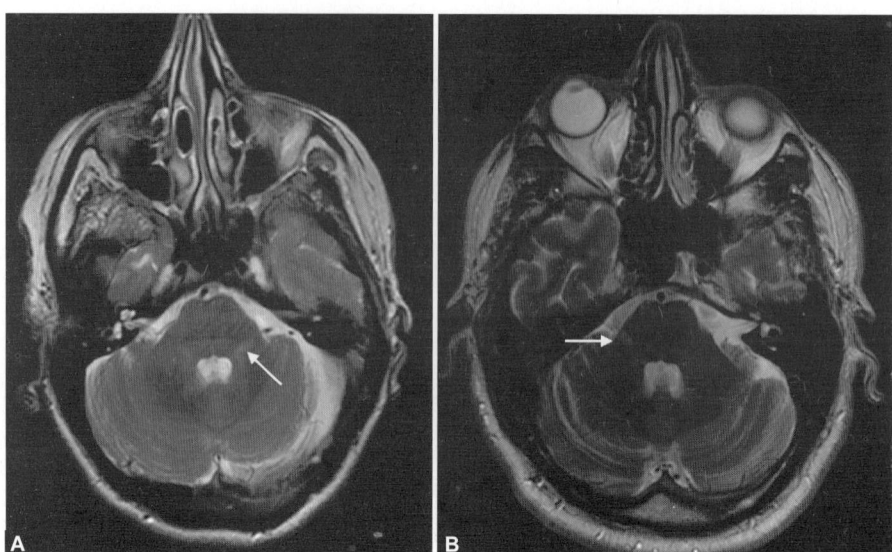

FIGS 2A and B: Multiple sclerosis-related demyelination (arrows pointing to plaque)

Investigations however help with planning medical management options.[1] Trigeminal neuralgia is the occurrence of neuralgic pains, usually described as attacks of pain over the distribution of one or more divisions of the trigeminal nerve. The pain is paroxysmal or episodic; each episode consists of a cluster of lancinating or 'electric shock' like pains, severe to excruciating in intensity lasting from a few seconds to a few minutes and keeps recurring, at a variable frequency, leaving a pain free interval ('refractory period') between the episodes.

The pains occur more frequently in the middle or later age groups, more in females than in males, more on the right than on the left side and affect the mandibular division (V3) slightly more than the maxillary (V3), with the least involvement of the ophthalmic division (V1).

The pain is usually precipitated by a sensory stimulus or a 'trigger' like a light touch, a breeze of wind or a splash of water on the face, by acts of chewing food, brushing teeth or speech. Some patients describe the pain like an attack of pain. The pains can be so severe as to induce a patient to commit suicide. Between pain free period patient and family are very anxious as to when the next attack of pain will appear. If the history is not clear or classical then patient should be reassessed another time as this may provide clearer description of pain to help diagnosis.

As current definition of neuropathic pain demands presence of a lesion or disease affecting somatosensory system, investigations are required to confirm the etiology. Although many individuals without TN will have neurovascular contact at trigeminal root entry zone, it is common to have anatomical and morphological changes in trigeminal nerve visible to imaging studies (atrophy, displacement, demyelination, etc.). Demonstration of a tumor, AV malformation or plaques related to multiple sclerosis further lends support to etiology of TGN.

ANATOMICAL PERSPECTIVE

Trigeminal nerve is a mixed nerve that consists primarily of sensory neurons. It exits the brain on the lateral surface of the pons, entering the trigeminal ganglion within a few millimeters. The trigeminal ganglion corresponds to the dorsal root ganglion of a spinal nerve. Three major branches emerge from the trigeminal ganglion. Each branch innervates a different dermatome. Each branch exits the cranium through a different foramen. The first division (V1; ophthalmic nerve) exits the cranium through the superior orbital fissure, entering the orbit to innervate the globe and skin in the area above the eye and forehead. The second division, V2, maxillary nerve, exits through the foramen rotundum, into a space posterior to the orbit, the pterygopalatine fossa. It supplies middle third of face. The third division, V3, mandibular nerve, exits the cranium through an oval hole, the foramen ovale. It supplies lower third of face. If the proposed needle trajectory is too posterior, it may enter foramen lacerum through which carotid artery passes. If the needle trajectory is too anterior, needle may enter orbital cavity leading on to retrobulbar hemorrhage. If the needle to too medial and deep, injury to cavernous sinus and cranial nerve supply to eyeball may be encountered. To minimize the risk of complications related to suboptimal needle trajectory it is preferred to undertake this procedure either in radiology suite with excellent imaging facilities (Fig. 3) or the operator should have excellent understanding of radiological anatomy of structures around foramen ovale and understanding structures which may be along the path of needle trajectory to foramen ovale.

MANAGEMENT OPTIONS

Natural History

There is large variation in natural history of TGN. Patients can have this condition on intermittent intervals for many years but usually the frequency of episodes increases with time and condition become more intractable and difficult to treat only with medications. It is still often the case that general practitioners may not be aware of this condition and of available treatment options apart from pharmacological options.

Pharmacological Management

It is fortunate that 70-80% of patients initially respond well to medical therapy and are either free from pain or relieved to a degree.[2] Carbamazepine is the drug of choice. When it fails to act, has side effects or toxicity, other drugs like oxcarbazepine, phenytoin, gabapentin, pregabalin, lamotrigine, baclofen, tricyclic antidepressants and strong opioids may be tried, but the effect is only modest and is accompanied by side effects. In acute presentation, there is role of intravenous infusion of phenytoin and lignocaine. It is very effective and buys the time to plan for definitive intervention, which may be optimization of oral intake of combination of analgesics or MVD or percutaneous intervention or stereotactic radiosurgery. The emphasis of this chapter is more on interventional techniques for TGN especially when there is poor response to pharmacological treatments or there are side effects. In later stages 25-50% of cases became refractory to the drug therapy. These medications also affect central nervous system with side effects in a substantial proportion of patients.

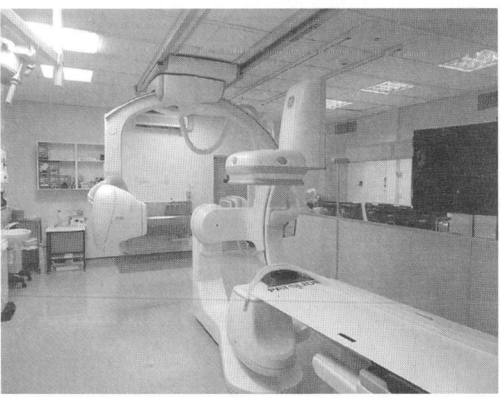

FIG. 3: Radiology biplane room as preferred by author for trigeminal interventions

The recent evidence suggests that botulinum toxin type A (BTX-A) has a clinically significant benefit in treatment of trigeminal neuralgia when compared to placebo in terms of proportion of responders, the mean paroxysms frequency per day, and the VAS score at the end of follow up. These overall outcomes consistently favor BTX-A compared with placebo across studies. The duration of effect for BTX-A seems to be at least 3 months.[6]

Neurosurgical Management Option

Microvascular decompression (MVD) remains gold standard treatment[1,4] in author's unit but this is not the case across the world because of limited access to this treatment or affordability. It essentially involves insertion of a small piece of Teflon sponge between the blood vessel and the affected nerve. Main advantage is that this does not cause any residual numbness or motor weakness or dysesthesia in face, which is otherwise seen after any neuroablative technique. Results of this surgery are better in patients who have typical history of TGN as compared to those with atypical features. Results are also better if the compression is caused by artery instead of a vein as well as if there is obvious change in the physical appearance of nerve i.e. atrophy, displacement, etc. There is very small risk of death and stroke from brain hemorrhage following this surgery (<1%). In the past sensory rhizotomy has been offered to patients with intractable form of TGN who did not have any obvious compression noted at the trigeminal root entry zone at the time of exploratory surgery. There is high cure rate and drug free rate following on from MVD. About 70–75% patients can expect to be pain free and with out need for antiepileptic as reported in many longitudinal studies over a 10-year follow-up period.

PERCUTANEOUS INTERVENTIONS

Indications for Radiofrequency/Balloon Microcompression/Glycerol Injection for Trigeminal Neuralgia

These interventions are indicated for medically refractory trigeminal neuralgia and MRI scan not showing neurovascular compression.[7-10] It may be offered to patients with positive MRI scan, if, the patient is not keen or fit to have surgery (microvascular decompression). It is very useful and effective for patients with multiple sclerosis suffering from trigeminal neuralgia, as these patients do not respond as well to microvascular decompression. Some patients may decide not to have microvascular decompression for fear of brain surgery and they usually have very good outcomes with foramen ovale based neuroablative techniques. Most patients who are offered these techniques are able to come of the medications (usually carbamezapine or other antiepileptic and strong pain killers including opioids) and this result in significant improvement in quality of life and also helps with severe anxiety for fear of neuralgia returning. There is not much difference in outcomes (pain relief and duration of effect) following various foramen ovale based techniques, though some operators and patients will have a preference of one technique over other. There are some major differences as below which may decide as which option is preferred.

SALIENT FEATURES RELATED TO EACH INTERVENTION AS RELEVANT IN PRACTICE

Radiofrequency Thermocoagulation of the Gasserian Ganglion

- In 1974, Sweet presented his method, which, by and large, is used today.[10]
- This needs patient's cooperation with sensory stimulation and retesting after the radiofrequency lesion. It means that

patient is awake and this can be very painful to patient and distressing for the theatre team, though this can be well managed by experienced anesthetist and theater team helping the operator.
- It is not preferred for first division trigeminal (ophthalmic) neuralgia for fear of causing irreversible deafferentation and consequences related to loss of corneal reflex and corneal damage.
- This technique is more likely to cause unpleasant dysesthesia including anesthesia dolorosa in comparison to other neuroablative techniques described in this chapter.
- Main advantage of this technique over other two techniques is the ability to control the degree of numbness and target the lesion based on sensory stimulation. However, there is a lot of debate on this area and some authors have published good results with this technique carried out under general anesthesia without the need of patient's cooperation. This is outside the scope of this chapter.

Balloon Microcompression of the Gasserian Ganglion

- Preferred for first division trigeminal (ophthalmic) neuralgia in comparison with radiofrequency technique.
- Patient (operator) preference to have the whole procedure under general anesthesia.
- Patients usually prefer this to radiofrequency in author's experience and the whole procedure is quicker and there is no difference in resource requirement in terms of anesthesia or theater team.
- Custom made 14g cannula and 4FG Fogarty embolectomy catheter may be used to minimize the cost of the procedure. Author has access to Mullan percutaneous trigeminal balloon microcompression set available from Cook Medical (Fig. 4). This set is more expensive but has many advantages which are outside scope of this chapter.

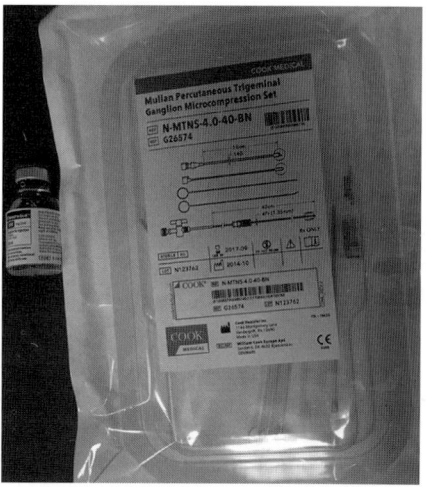

FIG. 4: Mullan percutaneous trigeminal microcompression set and water soluble contrast (omnipaque 300)

- Cannula used for balloon compression is 14G and radiological anatomy should be clearly displayed or there may be significant morbidity if the needle is introduced in the wrong foramen.

Trigeminal Glycerol Injection

- Håkansson introduced the method after a fortuitous discovery, during the development of a stereotactic technique for gamma radiation, that glycerol mixed with tantalum powder not only visualized the trigeminal cistern but also abolished pain in patients with trigeminal neuralgia. Technique and outcomes from over 2500 patients has been described in a book chapter.[11]
- This procedure may be carried out either under local anesthesia and sedation or under general anesthesia.
- Author has experience of carrying this for facial pain related to cancer in the distribution of trigeminal nerve.
- In experienced hands the results of this technique are comparable to RF

or Balloon compression. Most of the technical considerations are as for RF and Balloon compression.
- It is relatively inexpensive in comparison to above techniques as glycerol is not very expensive.

Contraindications to Rodiofrequency or Balloon Microcompression or Glycerol Injection

- Local or systemic infection
- Bleeding diathesis or anticoagulation
- Numbness in painful area (trigeminal neuropathy)
- Lack of informed consent or patient not accepting of numbness in face
- Atypical trigeminal neuralgia as results not good
- Neuropathic pain in the distribution of trigeminal nerve but features not consistent with trigeminal neuralgia.

Radiofrequency Thermocoagulation of Gasserian Ganglion

Preparation

- Consent includes discussion of likely success rate and potential complications. This is potentially neuroablative and irreversible technique and side effects may last long term and hence it is critical to have in depth discussion of pros and cons of this procedure and need for patient to co-operate at certain stages of the procedure.
- All patients must be warned about the risks of numbness, treatment failure and potential jaw weakness.
- All patients should have brain MRI to rule out neurovascular compression at the trigeminal root entry zone, tumor, multiple sclerosis or any other central causes.
- Prepare the patient as for general anesthesia and as per the local hospital policy and protocols.
- If taking aspirin then this should be stopped for seven days before the proposed date of the procedure.

- Position the patient supine on a radiolucent table with a thin pillow under the head. Thick pillow causes difficulties with visualization of foramen ovale by exaggerating neck flexion. Clear X-ray images are needed, as identification of foramen ovale is essential before inserting the needle.
- Equipment needed: radiofrequency lesion generator, 22G 100 mm, radiofrequency needle with 5 mm active tip, thermocouple probe for sensory/motor stimulation and radiofrequency lesioning, local anesthetic and simple equipment for sensory examination after the heat lesion or lesion titration.
- Strict asepsis is essential. It is usual to administer one dose of prophylactic antibiotic according to the local guidance.
- An anesthetist must be present to monitor the patient and administer general anesthesia as needed.

Technique

- The C-arm should be positioned with around a 45° caudal tilt and a 15–30° ipsilateral oblique tilt to identify the foramen ovale (Fig. 5). Minor adjustments may be needed to clearly define its margins. Usually you need to increase caudal tilt to improve visualization of foramen ovale.

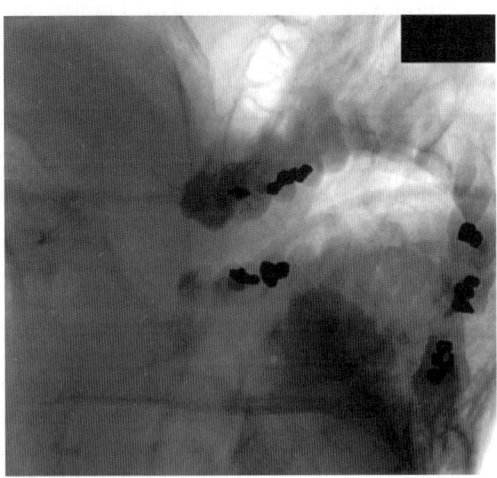

FIG. 5: Good view of foramen ovale with 38 degree caudal tilt and 24 degree oblique tilt

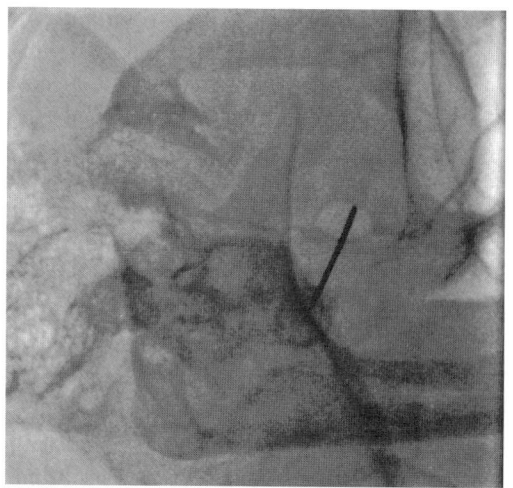

FIG. 6: RF cannula through foramen ovale

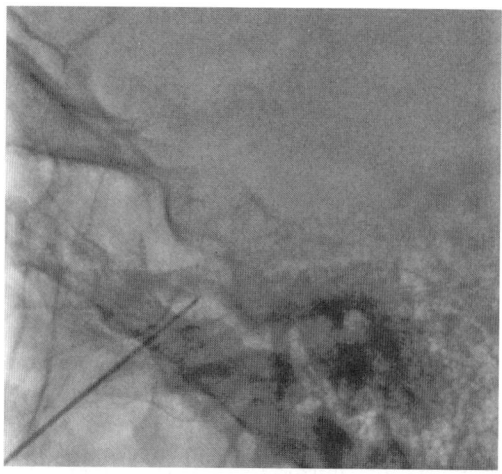

FIG. 7: Adequate insertion depth of RF cannula through foramen ovale ready for initial sensory stimulation and cannula can be inserted further by few mms if needed

- Usually the foramen ovale is visualized just medial to condyle of mandible (Fig. 6). For beginners, it may be beneficial to have experienced colleagues in theater or an experienced radiologist/radiographer.
- The needle entry point is just lateral to the angle of mouth (2–3 cm). The skin and subcutaneous tissues over this point are infiltrated with local anesthetic.
- A radiofrequency needle is advanced carefully towards foramen ovale (Fig. 6). If targeting the 2nd or 3rd division then enter at about 2 cm away from angle of the mouth aiming for the middle third of foramen ovale. If aiming for the 1st division, start about 3 cm away from angle of the mouth aiming to medial 3rd of foramen ovale. Usually it is possible to have tactile sensation while passing through foramen ovale. This can be very painful and general anesthesia or deep sedation may be needed at this stage.
- Perform motor stimulation at 2 Hz. If there are masseter movements at low sensory thresholds (<0.5 V), then advance the needle by couple of mm and retest, until these movements disappear (Fig. 7). While sensory stimulation at the times of masseter movements seen with motor stimulation will produce paresthesia in the V3 distribution, but the trigeminal ganglion will be spared of any heating effect of the procedure meaning shorter duration of pain relief. Check the needle position with a lateral X-ray view as well and the needle should not go deeper than an imaginary clival line. Stop anesthetic now, wake the patient and perform sensory stimulation at 50 Hz. Try to produce paresthesia in the affected division of the trigeminal nerve at low thresholds (0.05–0.2V). CSF may drip through the needle; this is entirely acceptable. It is usual to check for impedance at this point and essentially if it is low then it may mean the needle tip is not in the ganglion and this may mean the trigeminal ganglion may be spared of full heating effect of RF.
- If paresthesia occurs in the correct division of the trigeminal nerve, then create an RF lesion at 60° C for 90 seconds. The patient will need to be anesthetized for this lesion, as it is very painful. After the lesion, check sensory testing in the affected area of face to see whether the patient has developed

partial numbness. If not, the RF lesion will need to be repeated at 65° C and even up to 70° C, until there is objective evidence of partial numbness or hypoalgesia. Many patients find this process of repeat testing and RF inconvenient and painful, but, may not remember because of deep sedation or General anesthesia. There is variation in practice, as some practitioners prefer lesion at higher temperature. However, an author prefers lesioning at lower temperature to avoid any unpleasant dysestheisa and accepting a slightly higher risk of recurrence.
- Recently a successful technique of radiofrequency thermocoagulation of gasserian ganglion has been described under GA without the need for awakening patients for testing objective evidence of sensory loss. This may be an option in cases that otherwise may find this very painful.
- Some clinicians will use a very small dose of local anesthetic (0.2 mL of 1% lidocaine) to minimize the discomfort associated with heat lesion. Author does not use this technique but this may help reduce discomfort with out compromising ability to objectively test for sensory changes post RF lesioning.

Important Technical Considerations

- After the RF needle has been inserted through the foramen ovale, check the depth of needle insertion with a lateral view. The needle should not be inserted beyond the imaginary clival line, as this can be very dangerous and fatal.
- Try to avoid inserting the RF needle through the buccal mucosa, as it can introduce infection. Prevent this by inserting one finger into the mouth when initially inserting the RF needle.
- It may be preferable to do this procedure in radiology suite with biplane imaging facilities to help with visualization of the needle trajectory in two planes as approaching the foramen ovale.
- One needs very cooperative patient and experienced theatre team and anesthetist for this procedure.
- This procedure needs close cooperation between the operator and anesthetist, as the patient may need multiple sleep-awake cycles to produce numbness in the affected division of trigeminal nerve.

Balloon Microcompression of the Gasserian Ganglion

- This may be preferable in patients who cannot tolerate radiofrequency lesioning of the Gasserian ganglion as well as for the first division related neuralgia.
- Consent, preparation, position and image guidance to visualize the foramen ovale is as for the RF technique.
- *Equipment*: 14G cannula, 4FG Fogarty embolectomy catheter and Omnipaque 300 contrast or Mullan percutaneous trigeminal balloon micro compression set available from Cook medical as available from Cook medical. This kit has sharp and blunt trocars, which is helpful to minimise complications (Fig. 8).

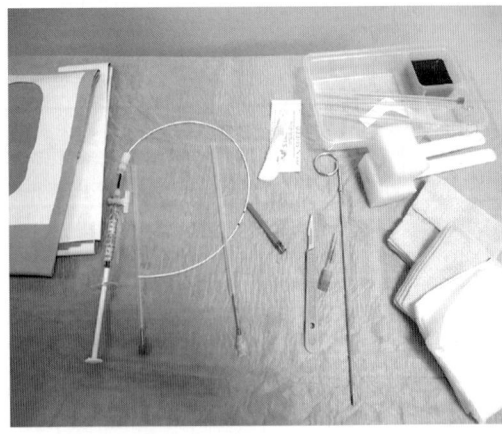

FIG. 8: Equipment set up for balloon microcompression (note a guard on the catheter) *(For color version, see Plate 9)*

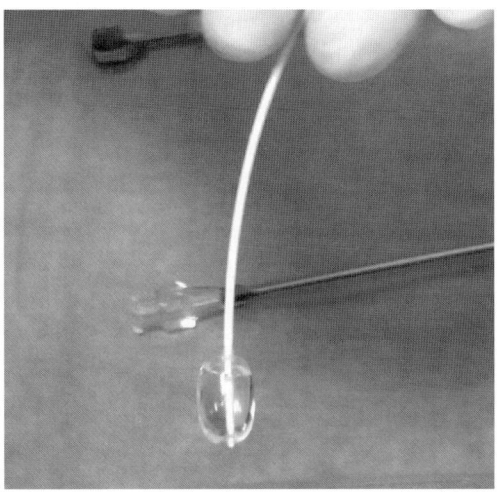

FIG. 9: Balloon being de-aired as it has air at the moment and if inflated with air the compression on ganglion is ineffective *(For color version, see Plate 9)*

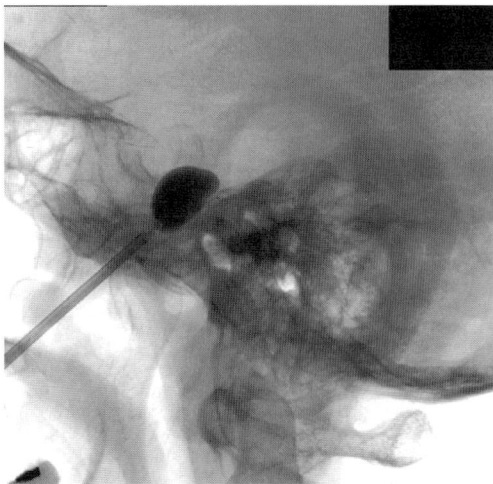

FIG. 10: Lateral view showing good pear shape of the inflated balloon-compressing ganglion against petrous part of temporal bone

- The balloon should be de-aired to facilitate effective compression of the trigeminal ganglion. This means injecting radio opaque dye into the catheter while holding the catheter vertical and aspirating back as the air in balloon shifts above the dye (Fig. 9).
- The procedure is carried out under general anaesthesia, as the patient's cooperation is not needed.
- A 14G needle is passed under X-ray guidance up to the level of foramen ovale. The needle does not go as deep as in the RF technique as the balloon reaches the point of actual compression of the trigeminal ganglion (Fig. 10). Author uses sharp trocar until reaching the base of skull at the entrance of foramen ovale. He then replaces this with blunt trocar as available in Cook Medical Kit for balloon compression to avoid any injury to structure deeper in the foramen ovale from sharper trocar.
- A 4FG Fogarty embolectomy catheter or the one in the balloon compression kit is introduced through the 14G needle. The balloon is inflated (Figs 10 to 12) with

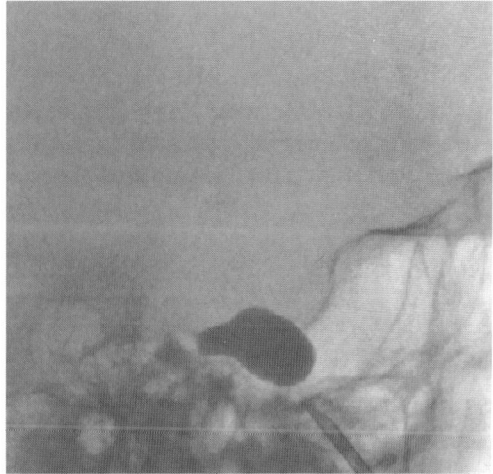

FIG. 11: Lateral view showing good pear shape of the inflated balloon-compressing but slightly excessive inflation

0.6–0.8 mL of Omnipaque 300 or equivalent water-soluble contrast for 1 minute, and then deflated for 1 minute; two more cycles of inflation/deflation are repeated. There is no proven or recommended protocol for compression

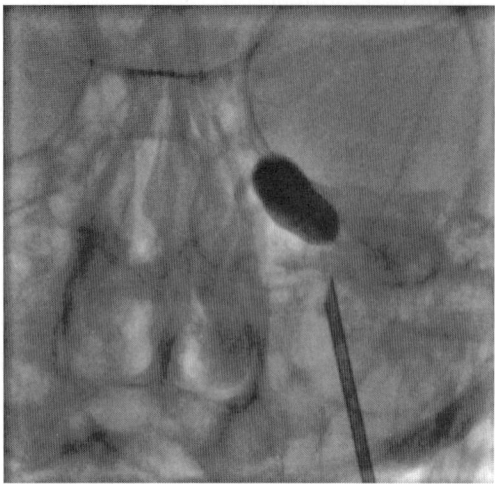

FIG. 12: Confirming good medial projection of inflated balloon in AP view

numbers and duration but this is what author has practiced as well as by his neurosurgical colleagues. On balance, it is preferred to be cautious rather than aggressive in duration of balloon compression as this may cause excessive deafferentation and associated risks. On the other hand if there is limited response or pain recurs quickly it is easier to repeat this procedure.

- A pear shape of inflated balloon reflects effective compression of gasserian ganglion (Fig. 9). It is reassuring to see medial projection of the inflated balloon on an AP view (Figs 10 and 11).
- At the end of procedure, the needle and the catheter with balloon are withdrawn together. Trying to remove the balloon catheter through the needle may result in shearing of bits of balloon and these may be left behind.

Important Technical Considerations

- The 14G needle should be introduced only up to the level of the foramen ovale and no further. However, needle may be introduced for about 5-8 mm using blunt trocar and then move back up to the entrance of foramen ovale. Doing this helps insertion of catheter, as at times otherwise insertion of catheter may be difficult.
- It is important to either mark the catheter length in advance so as not to insert too deep through the cannula or the balloon may be inflated too deep with in the brain. If the length introduced is not enough then the balloon will not inflate as part of it may still be in the cannula. Cook Medical's Mullan balloon microcompression set has a mark on the catheter informing clinician of the length to be inserted and there is a guard, which can be tightened around the catheter to prevent over insertion of catheter.
- Transient bradycardia or even asystole may be observed with balloon inflation or inserting the needle through the foramen ovale. Occasionally author will request anesthetist to administer prophylactic glycopyrrolate to counter this.
- Author prefers to check the final shape and trajectory of the inflated balloon in both the planes, i.e. anterior-posterior and lateral to ensure optimal positioning within the Meckel's cave.

Trigeminal Glycerol Injection

- Consent, preparation, position and image guidance to visualize the foramen ovale is as for the RF or balloon compression technique.
- *Equipment*: 20G needle, glycerol, luer lock syringe as otherwise it may be difficult to inject viscous glycerol through narrower gauge needle (Fig. 13).
- There is variation in anesthetic technique used for this procedure ranging from awake, sedation and under general anesthesia.
- It is usual to have head up tilt at the point of injection of glycerol to avoid spillage on to other parts of brain to avoid neurological complications. However, some operators believe that this is not essential.

Chapter 14: Trigeminal Neuralgia: Causes and Treatment

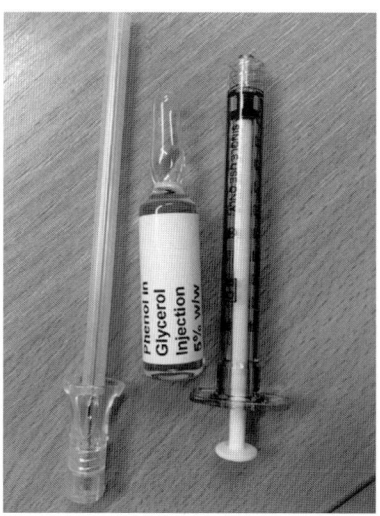

FIG. 13: Equipment needed for trigeminal glycerol injection

Technique

- Most of the technical aspects for visualization of foramen ovale and needle insertion are similar to as above for RF or balloon microcompression. Once inside the foramen ovale, it is helpful to have free flow of CSF and this may mean inserting the needle a bit further but not beyond the imaginary clival line.
- Once the 20G needle is in the correct place by observing free flow of CSF and needle not beyond the imaginary clival line, patient is asked to sit upright and patient needs to be supported by theater assistants. CSF is aspirated and 0.2–0.6 cc of glycerol is injected slowly and patient is kept in upright position for about 45 minutes to allow glycerol to be taken up by neural tissue.
- Amount of glycerol injected depends on how many divisions of trigeminal nerve need to be covered by this technique.

Important Technical Considerations

- Ensure that you have the correct preparation to inject otherwise the aqueous phenol or alcohol may have excessive spread and outcome may be adversely affected including serious catastrophe.
- It is accepted to sit up the patient at the time of injection of glycerol but there are some studies claiming this not to be absolutely essential and claiming safety.

Postprocedure Care Following Radiofrequency/Balloon/Glycerol Injection

- The patient needs the usual postoperative care and can usually be discharged the next day. With careful planning, it can be performed as day case as well. They may need simple analgesics for postoperative pain.
- It is good practice to do a neurological examination the day after and document any numbness, jaw weakness and the presence or absence of a corneal reflex. It is useful to have documentation of these finding before the procedure as well.
- It is good practice to collect outcome data in relation to pain scores, medications used for pain and any complications related to procedure and also have these documented at follow up to reflect any changes regarding efficacy and safety of the technique. In UK, it is becoming mandatory to have this data available to secure continued commissioning of services.

Side Effects and Complications of Radiofrequency/Balloon Compression/Glycerol Injection

- Temporary jaw weakness (more common with balloon microcompression) and usually resolves in 1–3 months.
- Cheek hematoma related to needle injury (settles quickly).
- Headache for few days afterwards, settles very quickly over a week or less.
- Unpleasant dysesthesia (25% with RF and 8% require medical treatment) and this may take longer to settle and often may not settle and some patients find

it unpleasant and may need treatment as for pharmacological management of neuropathic pain.
- Anesthesia dolorosa (1–4%, more common and long lasting with RF compared with balloon compression).
- Cranial nerves palsy, e.g. diplopia[12] more likely related to too medial projection of balloon or excessive spread of glycerol or RF lesioning. Author has encountered couple of cases of diplopia post balloon microcompression and these settled within three months and similar cases and recovery period is reported in literature.
- *Very rare complications*
  o Corneal ulceration
  o Retrobulbar hemorrhage and loss of vision
  o Carotid artery puncture and carotico-cavernous fistula
  o Intracranial hemorrhage
  o Meningitis
  o Facial nerve palsy (settles quickly)
  o Herpes simplex type 1 perioralis (settles quickly). There is some suggestion from literature regarding association between trigeminal neuralgia and type 1 herpes virus being latent in gasserian ganglion, though it is not widely accepted.
  o Death very rarely reported.

PATIENT REPORTED OUTCOMES FROM AN AUDIT FROM AUTHOR'S UNIT

Author performed audit of trigeminal balloon compression in his unit. A total of 43 patients were identified from review of theater records. These patients were treated with balloon microcompression performed between June 2006 and June 2008. They were followed up telephonically till August 2009, allowing a follow up of up to 38 months.

Out of total of 43 patients receiving this procedure over the 2-year-period, 95% had immediate complete pain relief (also off medications used to treat TGN) with pain relieving effect lasting in 60% patients (drug free) with mean follow up of 26 months. Allowing for repeat treatment and intake of medications, 41/43 patient's TGN related pain was very well controlled.

In this audit, there were 13/43 patients with multiple sclerosis (MS) related trigeminal neuralgia (30%). Immediate complete pain relief was seen in all the patients with MS and all were pain free in August 2009. However five of these patients, relapsed but, now all were responsive to medication (they were unresponsive to these medications before offering balloon microcompression).

Author has observed large effect size on pain relief of this treatment and it is life changing because of excellent pain relief and the ability of reduce or come off medications used otherwise to control TGN.

In conclusion, this audit shows 43 patients underwent 63 balloon microcompressions over two-year-period. 41/43 patients were pain free. 27/43 patients were off medication, which they were using before the balloon microcompression to control pain. Side effects minimal and patient were very satisfied.

There are limitations from retrospective audit and now author has set up a prospective audit to review outcomes related to trigeminal interventions and will be able to report these in due course.

BILATERAL TRIGEMINAL NEURALGIA

It is extremely rare to have bilateral trigeminal neuralgia and it is often seen in patients with multiple sclerosis related TGN. It is unusual to have TGN related pain on both side of the faces at the same time. If this is suspected then the diagnosis should be reviewed. Author has experience of offering balloon microcompression on both sides of the face but this is extremely rare and consequence of offering a neuroablative procedure on the both sides of the face should not be taken lightly and should be discussed in depth with the patient. In particular patients may find very hard to chew if they develop bilateral jaw weakness.

ALTERNATIVE NEUROABLATIVE OPTIONS

In patients who are not suitable for interventional techniques for variety of reason or technical reasons, they may be considered for gamma knife or steriotactic radio surgery to achieve similar effect as above techniques. It is noninvasive and hence avoids procedure related complications, but, the onset of effect is delayed by few weeks and there is limit on amount of radiation dose which can be used. This cannot be offered more than twice for fear of causing radiation related complications in the trigeminal root entry zone region. Author's unit is now routinely offering this to those who otherwise are high risk for interventional techniques or unsuitable for MVD or have recurrent and intractable form of TN which is otherwise poorly controlled with other treatments with good outcomes.

CONCLUSION

The TGN is usually is easy to diagnose. Close working relation in neurosurgical unit between pain services can be helpful to agree management pathway to offer a range of treatment options depending on clinical scenario and patient choice. In authors experience above mentioned percutaneous techniques are very effective to control intractable TGN which otherwise is very distressing neuropathic pain condition. Good history taking is essential to diagnosed TGN and if in doubt assess patient on another time to reassess and take history again. This usually clarifies the diagnosis. Good understanding of local anatomy and imaging facilities and theater set up and theater team are essential for a good outcome. It is helpful to collect outcomes related to these interventions on a longer-term basis to justify on going service, as there is increasing emphasis on commissioning services, which are able to demonstrate this in UK. Author find this part of his practice very rewarding, though it can be challenging in a small number of cases which may turn out to be refractory to these interventions and hence better to have access to a team with multidisciplinary approach including a neurologist, neurosurgeon, maxillofacial surgeon and a psychologist with interest in complex facial pain.

REFERENCES

1. Nurmikko TJ, Eldridge PR. Trigeminal neuralgia: pathophysiology, diagnosis and current treatment. Br J Anaesth. 2001;87:117-32.
2. Devor M, Amir R, Rappaport ZH. Pathophysiology of Trigeminal Neuralgia: The Ignition Hypothesis. The Clinical Journal of Pain. 2002;18:4-13.
3. Campbell FG, Graham JG, Zilkha KJ. Clinical trial of carbamazepine (tegretol) in trigeminal neuralgia. J Neurol Neurosurg Psychiatry. 1966;29:265-7.
4. Tatli M, Satici O, Kanpolat Y, Sindou M. Various surgical modalities for trigeminal neuralgia: literature study of respective long-term outcomes. Acta Neurochirurgica. 2008;150(3):243-55.
5. Cruccu G, Finnerup NB, Jensen TS, Scholz J, Sindou M, Svensson P, Treede RD, Zakrzewska JM, Nurmikko T. Trigeminal neuralgia: New classification and diagnostic grading for practice and research. Neurology. 2016 Jul 12; 87 (2):220-8. doi: 10.1212/WNL.0000000000002840. Epub 2016 Jun 15.
6. Morra ME, Elgebaly A, Elmaraezy A et al. Therapeutic efficacy and safety of Botulinum Toxin A Therapy in Trigeminal Neuralgia: a systematic review and meta-analysis of randomized controlled trials. J Headache Pain. 2016;17(1):63. doi: 10.1186/s10194-016-0651-8. Epub 2016 Jul 5.
7. Mullan S, Lichtor T. Percutaneous microcompression of the trigeminal ganglion for trigeminal neuralgia. J Neurosurg. 1983;59:1007–12.
8. Lichtor T, Mullan JF. A 10-year follow-up review of percutaneous microcompression of the trigeminal ganglion. J Neurosurg. 1990;72:49-54.
9. Skirving DJ, Dan NG. A 20-year review of percutaneous balloon compression of the trigeminal ganglion. J Neurosurg. 2001;94:913-7.
10. Sweet WH, Wepsic JG. Controlled thermocoagulation of trigeminal ganglion and rootlets for differential destruction of pain fibres. Part 1: trigeminal neuralgia. J Neurosurg. 1974;39:143–56.
11. Zakrewska JM. Trigeminal Neuralgia. London: WB Saunders, 1995.
12. Bergenheim AT, Linderoth B. Diplopia after balloon compression of retrogasserian ganglion rootlets for trigeminal neuralgia: Technical case report. Neurosurgery. 2008;62(2):E532-3.

CHAPTER 15

Cervical Radiculopathy Pain and Its Management

Ganesan Baranidharan

INTRODUCTION

Neurological condition characterized by dysfunction of a cervical spinal nerve, the root of the nerve or both is termed as cervical radiculopathy. It usually presents with pain in the neck and one arm with associated changes in the sensory, motor and deep tendon reflexes.[1] The most commonly affected nerves are C7 and C6.[2]

CAUSES

The cause for the nerve root irritation varies with age. In younger population, it is commonly secondary to disk herniations, whereas in the older age group, it is more degenerative changes.[3] In 70–75% of cases, it is secondary to narrowing of the foramen from adjoining structures, including decreased disk height and degenerative changes of the vertebral joints anteriorly and zygapophyseal joints posteriorly.

Herniated disk only accounts to 20–23% at the neck level (Fig. 1).

Factors that Contribute to Cervical Radiculo Pathy

- Heavy manual duties involving heavy weight
- Smoking
- Driving
- Operating vibration equipment
- Awkward neck postures at work.

Other causes include spinal tumors, expanding synovial cyst, hypertrophy to facet joints and spinal infections.

The pathophysiology is poorly understood. It could be secondary to nerve root irritation leading to an inflammatory process. Inflam-

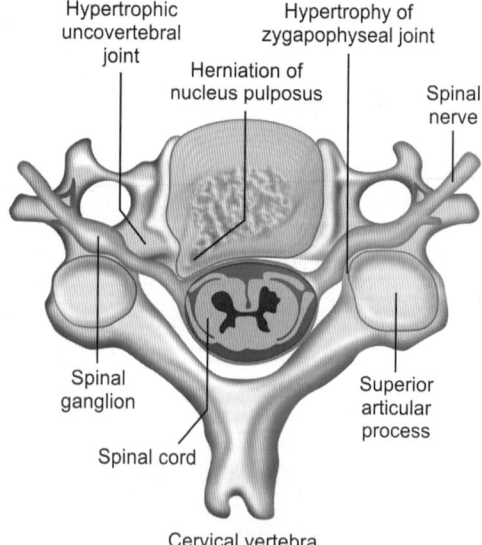

FIG. 1: Structures that can cause cervical radiculopathy (permission taken from NEJM)

matory mediators, such as nitric oxide, prostaglandin E2, interleukin-6, and matrix metalloproteinases, are released by herniated disks. Hypoxia of the nerve root and ganglion can also play a part in the symptomatology.

SYMPTOMS AND SIGNS

Patients can complain of neck and arm pain or just the arm pain. The onset can be gradual or sudden. It is typically a pins and needle, burning, shooting lancinating pain in a dermatomal pattern. Mostly its one limb affected, and can occasionally have bilateral symptoms. There will be associated history, such as injury to neck with extension and lateral rotation or slow degenerative pain as in older age patients. There can be history of weakness in some patients with loss of grip. If C1-3 is involved, can produce retro-orbital and temporal pain mimicking temporal arteritis. Holding the hand up to head on the affected side or looking down and away from the affected side can relieve the pain and rotation and bending towards the affected side can reproduce the symptoms. 'Red flag' symptoms, such as fever, unexplained weight loss, previous history of cancer, immunosuppression or intravenous drug use should warn the clinician to look for tumor or infection. Also look for symptoms of cervical myelopathy, which are diffuse hand weakness and clumsiness, difficulty with balance, urinary disturbance in the form of urgency and frequency.

CLINICAL EXAMINATION

Inspection

There will be postural asymmetry with head tilted to opposite side to expand the foramen available. Long-standing problem can lead to muscle wasting. Lateral rotation and extension will be restricted by reproduction of symptoms on the ipsilateral side. If the radiculopathy is secondary to disk prolapse, occasionally symptoms can be worsened on to the contralateral side due to exacerbation of the prolapse.

Palpation

Tenderness on the side along the paraspinal muscles and some muscle tenderness may be present as triggers in trapezius and rhomboids. Examination should involve testing sensory, motor and deep tendon reflexes. Table 1 helps us in identifying the level of the problem. Sensory testing is very subjective and can depend on individual patient.

Other tests that can be useful are:

Foraminal Compression Test (Spurling Test)

With extension and head rotated, pressure is applied on the head. If this reproduces nerve root pain, is considered positive. This is 93% specific, but not sensitive (30%).[5] It is not recommended for screening, but can help in confirming the diagnosis of cervical radiculopathy.

TABLE 1: Examination findings on different nerve root involvement[4]

Nerve root	Muscle weakness	Reflex changes	Sensory
C5	Shoulder abduction and flexion, elbow flexion	Biceps	Lateral arm
C6	Elbow flexion wrist extension	Biceps Supinator	Lateral forearm thumb, index finger
C7	Elbow extension, wrist flexion, finger extension	Triceps	Middle finger
C8	Finger flexion	None	Medial side lower forearm ring and little
T1	Finger abduction and adduction	None	Medial side upper forearm lower arm

Shoulder Abduction Test

Relief of pain on placing the symptomatic arm on the head.

Neck Distraction Test

In a supine position, application of gentle traction by placing the hands on the chin and the occiput relieves the symptom. Patients with cervical myelopathy will have hyperreflexia and hypertonia. Knee, ankle and wrist clonus can be present. Babinski, Hoffman signs (flexion and adduction of thumb on flexion of the terminal long phalanx).

DIAGNOSTIC CRITERIA

Investigations Suggested

Blood Tests

Blood tests are of limited value. CRP, ESR and white cell count can be elevated if there is an underlying infection. Plain cervical radiograph is not recommended as due to low sensitivity in detecting tumors, infection or disk herniations.[6]

Magnetic Resonance Imaging

MRI is the investigation of choice in patients with cervical radiculopathy. There are no strict guidelines on when to order these. Consider an MRI, if the symptoms are not settled in 4 to 6 weeks or if there are any red flag. There is a high incidence of radiological changes in symptomatic patients. The findings should correlate to the patient's signs, symptoms and the clinical findings (Fig. 2).

Computerized Tomography

CT is rarely indicated in cervical radiculopathy. If bony structures causing foraminal narrowing is the cause, this might show the extent. Combining this with a CT myelogram might be better than an MRI scan, but the risk and invasiveness of the procedure outweighs the benefit.

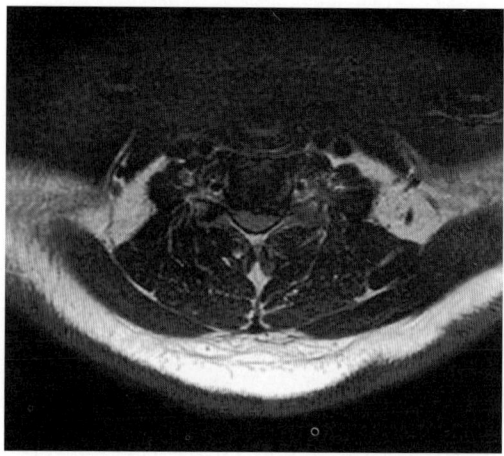

FIG. 2: MRI showing complete effacement of CSF and irritation on the left C6 nerve root

Bone scans can be used in cancer suspicion, but does not help in patients with cervical myelopathy to look at the other structures.

Electromyography

Electromyography (EMG) is a diagnostic tool; useful when clinical information and MRI are inconclusive or if there is a suspicion of peripheral entrapment. This has two-fold test, nerve conduction study and needle electrode examination. A normal study, does not exclude cervical neuropathy, if there are signs and symptoms present. The nerve conduction studies are performed by placing surface electrodes on a muscle belly and then stimulate the nerve. Both sensory and motor information can be gathered. The measured amplitude, distal latency and conduction velocity helps in finding out the demyelination. The needle EMG portion of the test involves fine needle insertion into a muscle and the electrical, voluntary contraction, spontaneous muscle unit firings are observed using an oscilloscope. This helps in finding a denervated muscle. It is useful only between 18 and 21 days after injury to the nerve.

Selective Nerve Root Block

If a particular nerve root is responsible for the patient's radiculopathy, anesthetizing this should produce resolution of the symptoms.[7] A complete resolution of the radiculopathy might be diagnostic. The down sides to these are the volume of injectate and the spread. Even small volumes have shown to spread more than one level making these investigations specificity in question.[8]

Differential Diagnosis

- Peripheral entrapment syndromes, such as carpal tunnel syndrome
  - Hypoesthesia and weakness in the nerve distribution. Tinel's sign positive in carpal tunnel syndrome.
- *Herpes zoster*: Neuropathic pain in a nerve root distribution following the typical vesicular rash.
- *Thoracic outlet syndrome*: Pain in shoulder and arm, often aggravated by the use of arm. The paresthesia is commonly seen in the C8T1 region with symptom reproduction on provocation test. The nerve conduction studies are usually normal with occasional reduction in pulse on the side of the problem.
- *Brachial plexus neuralgia*: Starts with severe pain in the neck, shoulder and arm followed by neurological weakness after few days. Both neurology and pain occurs simultaneously in cervical radiculopathy.
- *Disorders of the rotator cuff and the shoulders*: Pain in shoulder aggravated by active and passive shoulder movements.
- *Pancoast tumor*: Brachial plexus signs along with ptosis and anhydrosis (Horner's syndrome).
- *Sympathetic pain*: Diffuse pain in arm and hand associated with sympathetic changes, such as sweating, swelling, etc. No neurology.
- *Referred pain from the neck*: Could be a referred pain from cervical facet or disk, where the pain rarely goes beyond the elbows.

Treatment

The main objectives for the treatment are to relive pain, improve neurological function and to prevent further recurrences. Little is known about the natural progression of cervical radiculopathy. Some have advocated the short-term immobilization (max 2 weeks) to help pain control and also cervical pillow at night to maintain cervical spine neutrality.[9] However, there is not enough data to support these.

Medication

Most of the drugs used to control the initial pain are NSAID (2 weeks course). Occasionally opioids have been used to control the pain with not much evidence. The use of opioids should be reserved due to the complications and possible addictive and long-term effects. Short course of prednisone starting at 70 mg and tapered over few weeks have been advocated with anecdotal evidence.

Physical Therapy

The aim of physiotherapy is to restore full range of movements and flexibility of neck and shoulder movements. After a warm up, stretching and cervical muscle strengthening can be used. The scapular stabilizing muscles such as trapezius, rhomboids, serratus anterior and latissimus dorsi should also be strengthened. It is also important to maintain cardiovascular fitness by doing aerobic activity on a regular basis. Emphasis should be made on carrying this out indefinitely to avoid further recurrences.

Exercise therapy includes active range of motion exercises and aerobic conditioning followed by isometric and progressive resistive exercises after the initial pain has been controlled.

Cervical Epidural Steroid Injection

Cervical epidural steroid injection (CESI) has been used in patients who have not responded to medications, traction and well-designed physical therapy program. When properly performed by a trained person under fluoroscopy, a significant number of patients with cervical radiculopathy improve. There is a debate on the interlaminar to transforaminal approach. Due to the increased complications via a transforaminal epidural steroid injection (TFESI)[10] interlaminar approach might be preferred.

Nucleoplasty

Nucleoplasty is a percutaneous disk decompression using coblation technology. This involves passing a wand to the cervical disk, which evaporates the nucleus pulposus without producing much heat damage to the surrounding tissues. On healing, the disk shrinks and takes the pressure away from the nerve root. This is ideal for small disk bulge with corresponding nerve root symptom not responding to all conservative treatments (Figs 3A and B). There are a few case reports[11] and retrospective case series. Good RCTs are needed to support their use more widely.

Cervical Traction

Cervical traction uses a distracting force to the neck to separate the cervical segments and to relieve compression of nerve roots secondary to disks. A systematic review found that they could not get a conclusion on the efficacy due to poor methodological quality of the available data.

Surgery

In appropriate selected patient's surgery may relieve the radiculopathy. The procedures, such as diskectomy, laminectomy, and fusion, including disk replacements have been advocated in managing cervical radiculopathy.

FOLLOW-UP ADVICE

It is very important to keep up with regular physical aerobic activities and cervical muscle strengthening to prevent further recurrences.

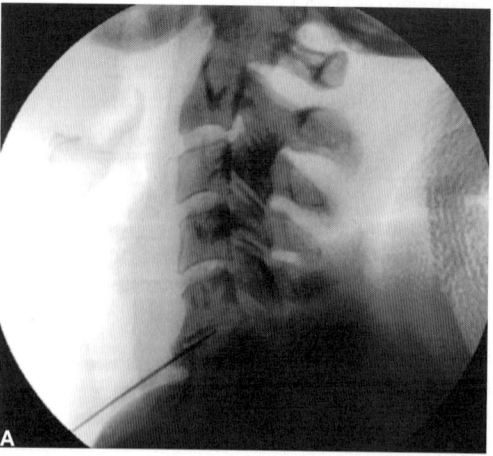 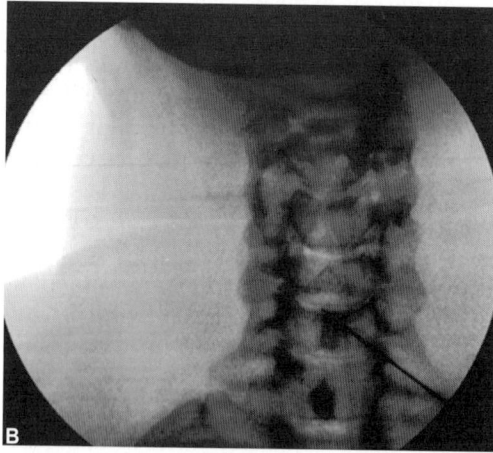

FIGS 3 A and B: Cervical nucleoplasty wand in C5, 6 disks: (A) Lateral view; (B) AP view

CONCLUSION

The multimodal approach is the key, to the management of pain due to cervical radiculopathy. It needed to be combined with physiotherapy and rehabilitation. It is preferred to use tailored approach in each patient.

REFERENCES

1. Bogduk N. The anatomy and pathophysiology of neck pain. Phys Med Rehabil Clin N Am. 2003;14(3):455-72.
2. Ellenberg MR, JC Honet, WJ Treanor. Cervical radiculopathy. Arch Phys Med Rehabil. 1994;75(3):342-52.
3. Murphey F, Simmons JC, Brunson B. Chapter 2. Ruptured cervical discs, 1939 to 1972. Clin Neurosurg. 1973; 20:9-17.
4. Barry M, Jenner JR. ABC of rheumatology. Pain in neck, shoulder, and arm. BMJ. 1995;310(6973):183-6.
5. Tong HC, Haig AJ, Yamakawa K. The Spurling test and cervical radiculopathy. Spine (Phila Pa 1976). 2002; 27(2):156-9.
6. Mink JH, Gordon RE, Deutch AL. The cervical spine: radiologist's perspective. Phys Med Rehabil Clin N Am. 2003;14:493-548.
7. Bogduk N. Lumbar spinal nerve blocks. Practice guidelines for spinal diagnostic and treatment guidelines-ISIS; 2004. pp. 3-19.
8. Datta S, et al. An updated systematic review of the diagnostic utility of selective nerve root blocks. Pain Physician 2007;10(1):113-28.
9. Carette S, Fehlings MG. Clinical practice: cervical radiculopathy. N Engl J Med. 2005;353(4):392-9.
10. Scanlon GC, et al. Cervical transforaminal epidural steroid injections: more dangerous than we think? Spine (Phila Pa 1976). 2007;32(11):1249-56.
11. Li J, Yan DL, Zhang ZH. Percutaneous cervical nucleoplasty in the treatment of cervical disc herniation. Eur Spine J. 2008;17(12):1664-9.

CHAPTER 16

Cervical Facet Joint Pain and Its Management

Sherdil Nath

INTRODUCTION

Percutaneous radiofrequency neurotomy is a technique that thermo-coagulates the nerves that supply the cervical facet joints i.e., the medial branches of the dorsal rami, by means of heat ablation.

CAUSES

Chronic neck pain with radiation to the shoulders and arms as well as to the head was shown to arise from the cervical zygapophysial (facet) joints.[1] The incidence was shown to be up to 65% in patients following car accidents causing whiplash type trauma.[2]

Other forms of trauma, strain and degenerative changes have also been considered to be responsible.[3]

SYMPTOMS AND SIGNS

The main symptom is chronic pain that may radiate to the head or down to the trapezius, shoulder, arms.[4] and sometimes even to the fingers, frequently accompanied by some subjective numbness. The pains are usually reported to be unilateral but sometimes are bilateral and are accentuated by movement especially neck extension and rotation to the painful side.

CLINICAL EXAMINATION

Inspection will often show some asymmetry as well as prominent tense muscles especially the trapezius. Movements are usually restricted and painful. Paravertebral tenderness is considered to be a reliable sign of pain arising from these joints.

DIAGNOSTIC CRITERIA

High precision local anesthetic blocks of the nerves that supply these joints are the only validated diagnostic test to confirm the diagnosis. This is the medial branch block.[5] Single blocks may result in a false-positive response, which is why it is recommended that the blocks are repeated on at least two separate occasions before the diagnosis is considered to be confirmed.[6]

INVESTIGATIONS

Although it has long been recognized that X-rays do not correlate with pain,[7] it is still customary to have X-ray studies done, often including CT and MRI. It needs to be remembered that damaged joints and discs can be asymptomatic and structures that look completely normal on X-ray may be a cause of pain. It is unfortunate that older patients with degenerative changes invariably have their pains blamed on these changes. Conversely, younger patients with no pathology on X-ray are often told that there can be nothing wrong with them. It is therefore recommended that the X-rays be interpreted with a great deal of caution. If there is paravertebral tenderness then the patient should be given the benefit of a medial branch block even if there is some other pathology on X-ray as that may well be without significance.

DIFFERENTIAL DIAGNOSIS

Neck and low-back pain are common and costly problems. In order to treat these conditions effectively, it is imperative to establish a correct diagnosis at the initial presentation. This initial diagnosis can pose some important challenges, because the clinician cannot distinguish with infallible accuracy between those patients with benign conditions and those with radicular pain or serious spinal pathology.

In the initial stage, the primary function of the history and examination is to distinguish those patients with pain of musculoskeletal origin from those with non-spinal or serious spinal pathology. Once this is accomplished, the next priority is to rule out those patients with nerve-root (radicular) pain. The patient's pain and pattern of distribution will most probably suggest whether the pain is likely to be radicular. All other cases should be classified as 'nonspecific' where radiation is most likely to be a referred pain. Although this seems quite fundamental, this diagnostic triage serves another function. By conducting a thorough history and physical examination, it is possible to evaluate the degree of pain and the functional disability of the patient. This serves to guide the clinician in a management strategy.[8]

PROBLEM DEFINITION

A simple and practical classification system for neck and low-back pain is to divide it into three categories: 1. Specific spinal pathology. 2. Nerve-root pain/radicular pain and 3. Nonspecific neck or low-back pain. The first level of diagnostic triage during the history taking is to identify 'red flags' and assess potential 'yellow flags'.[8] Red flags are signs or symptoms that should raise the suspicion of serious spinal pathology, whereas yellow flags are factors that increase the risk of developing or perpetuating chronic pain and long-term disability.[9] Clinical suspicion can be confirmed later by further investigation; however, at this point the primary goal is screening. The subsequent step is to identify those subjects with nerve-root pain. The patient's pain distribution and pattern should raise clinical suspicion, which when confirmed by the clinical examination should be a reason to refer for further evaluation. Individual red flags do not necessarily mean the presence of serious pathology; however, the presence of multiple red flags should raise clinical suspicion and indicates the need for further investigation. The incidence of spinal tumors is very low. It should be stressed that radiographs do not and should not compensate for an inadequate assessment as a result of, for example, time constraints.[8]

Medications and Interventions

Standard analgesics, such as paracetamol with or without centrally acting analgesics and physiotherapy are the first line treatment for neck pain.

By the time the patient comes to the pain therapist, these have usually been tried and the pain has not subsided, which is why diagnostic interventions are indicated.

If the clinical picture has pointed at a possible facet joint related problem then a clinical examination would have further identified the possible levels that need to be tested.

Interventional Treatment Procedures

The only reliable and validated procedure that is diagnostic for facet joint pain is the *medial branch block*, which was described in detail in 1993.[5] It is recommended that these be performed on at least two separate occasions in an effort to eliminate false-positive responders. This is primarily a diagnostic block but can also be therapeutic. Some patients do get long-term relief from repeated blocks with local anaesthetic alone but many of these will need a more definitive solution of their problem at some time, as the pain relief from facet blocks is seldom permanent. It has been shown repeatedly that there is no additional benefit of adding corticosteroids to the injections.[10-14] It is, therefore, unnecessary to add steroids to the local anesthetic injection. If the neck pain returns after a period of improvement then a radiofrequency neurotomy or denervation (Figs 1 to 3) of the facet joint will have to be performed. This is a technique for achieving neural ablation of the nerves that supply the facet joints. It requires a considerable amount of effort and dedication to learn and is not to be taken lightly. When correctly performed in the right patients the results are excellent.[15-17] When performed badly, at best it will not work and at worst the consequences can be disastrous.

The technique is described in detail.[18,19]

Follow up After Interventional Pain Treatment

After medial branch blocks it is common for the patient to experience some increased pain for a day or two after the local anesthetic wears off. This response is identical regardless of whether steroids are mixed with the local anesthetic or not (see above). This may be followed by return of pain to the usual level

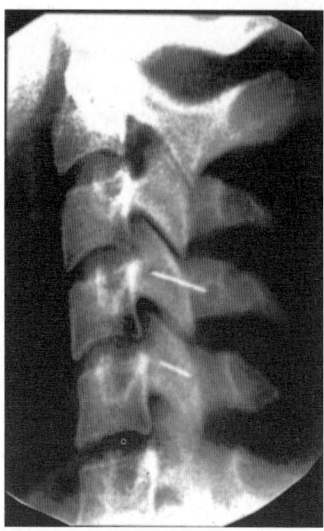

FIG. 2: Medial branch block: Needle points at centroid of the articular column

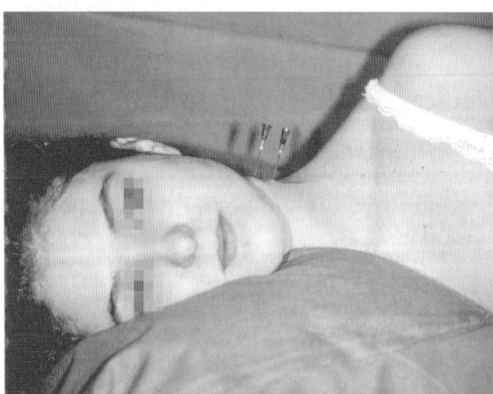

FIG. 1: Medial branch block: Patient lying on side resting on large pillow that keeps the lower shoulder pushed down to enable visualization of the lower neck

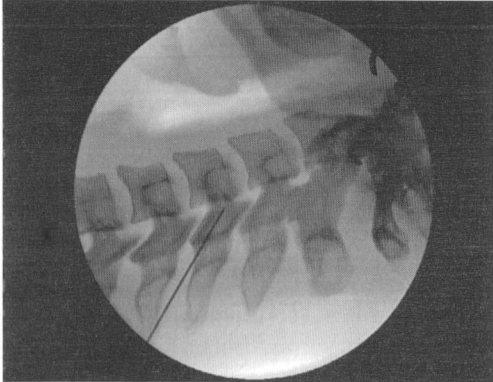

FIG. 3A: Radiofrequency denervation: Lateral view of the neck showing tip of RF cannula placed alongside the bone on the articular column. It is essential that the needle is placed parallel to the joint margins

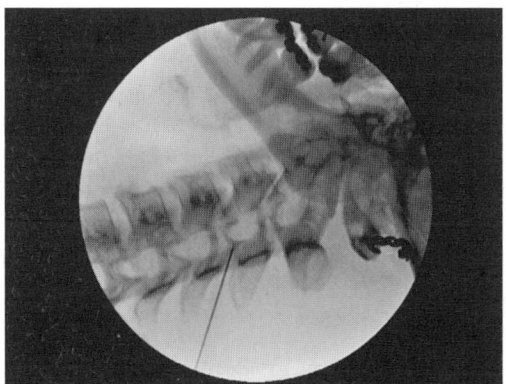

FIG. 3B: Radiofrequency denervation: Inferior oblique view showing point of cannula approaching but stopping short of the posterior border of the root foramen. The inferior oblique view is deemed perfect when the opposite pedicle is seen as a round `ball´ in the center of the vertebral body

or there may be long lasting improvement. However the pains do tend to recur after some weeks and then it is necessary to discuss the option of a radiofrequency denervation with the patient.

The other short lived problem is dizziness when the upper levels (C2- are anesthetized. The patient should be kept lying down for half to one hour and advised to not be alone. They may be so unsteady that they may fall and should definitely avoid steps except when accompanied and should avoid driving for some hours.

Following radiofrequency facet denervation, there is usually a period of increased pain that can be severe and may last a few days to a few weeks and may require strong analgesics, including opioids. It is important that the patient is aware of this. They also need to be aware that there will be some sensory loss in the skin from the neck down towards the trapezius, which usually lasts for three to six months. Normal sensations are almost always restored with time. It is not a problem that the patients find distressing, especially, if their pain has abated or disappeared.

CONCLUSION

By now it should be clear to the reader that this is not a procedure to be taken on lightly. It requires considerable skill in selecting the right patients and performing the procedure meticulously. However, when correctly performed, the results are most gratifying. Chronic neck pain with or without headache is a common affliction where the cause is often found to be from the facet joints. Successful treatment can be life changing for the patient. It is a skill well worth acquiring.

REFERENCES

1. Bogduk N, Marsland A. The cervical zygapophysial joints as a source of neck pain. Spine 1988;13:610-7.
2. Barnsley L, Lord SM, Wallis BJ, et al. The prevalence of chronic cervical zygapophyseal joint pain after whiplash. Spine 1995;20:20-6.
3. Barnsley L, Lord SM, Wall i s BJ, et al. Lack of effect of intra-articular corticosteroids for chronic pain in the cervical zygapophyseal joints. N Engl J Med 1994;330:1047-50.
4. Aprill C, Dwyer A, Bogduk N. The prevalence of cervical zygapophyseal joint pain patterns II: a clinical evaluation. Spine 1990;15:458-61.
5. Barnsley L, Bogduk N. Medial branch blocks are specific for the diagnosis of cervical zygapophysial joint pain. Reg Anesth 1993;18:343-50.
6. Barnsley L, Lord S, Bogduk N. Comparative local anesthetic blocks in the diagnosis of cervical zygapophysial joints pain. Pain 1993;55:99-106.
7. Degenerative changes seen on x-ray do not correlate with the occurrence of pain Friedenberg and Miller: J Bone Joint Surg. 1963; Gore et al: Spine, 1986.
8. Rubinstein SM, van Tulder M. A best-evidence review of diagnostic procedures for neck and low-back pain. Best Pract Res Clin Rheumatol 2008;22(3):471-82.
9. Kendall NAS, Linton SJ, Main CJ. Guide to assessing psychosocial yellow flags in acute low back pain: risk factors for long-term disability and work loss. Wellington, New Zealand: Accident Rehabilitation and Compensation Insurance Corporation of New Zealand and the National Health Committee, 1997.
10. Manchikanti L, Pampati V, Fellows B, Bakhit C. The diagnostic validity and therapeutic value of medial branch blocks with or without adjuvants. Curr Rev Pain 2000;4:337-44.

11. Bogduk N. A narrative review of intraarticular corticosteroid injections for low back pain. Pain Med 2005;6:287-96.
12. Carette S, Marcoux S, Truchon R, Grondin C, Gagnon J, Allard Y, et al. A controlled trial of corticosteroid injections into facet joints for chronic low back pain. N Engl J Med 1991;325:1002-7.
13. Barnsley L, Lord SM, Wallis BJ, Bogduk N. Lack of effect of intra articular corticosteroids for chronic pain in the cervical zygapophyseal joints. N Engl J Med 1994;330:1047-50.
14. Manchikanti L, Manchikanti Kn, Damron KS, Pampati V. Effectiveness of cervical medial branch blocks in chronic neck pain: a prospective outcome study. Pain Physician 2004;7:195-201.
15. Barnsley L. Percutaneous radiofrequency neurotomy for chronic neck pain: outcomes in a series of consecutive patients. Pain Med 2005;6:282-6.
16. Lord SM, Barnsley L, Wallis BJ, McDonald GJ, Bogduk N. Percutaneous radiofrequency neurotomy for chronic cervical zygapophyseal joint pain. N Eng J Med 1996;335:1721-6.
17. McDonald GJ, Lord SM, Bogduk N. Long-term follow-up of patients treated with cervical radiofrequency neurotomy for chronic neck pain. Neurosurgery 1999;45:61-8.
18. Bogduk N. Percutaneous radiofrequency cervical medial branch neurotomy. In: Practice Guidelines for Spinal Diagnostic and Treatment Procedures, 1st edition. International Spine Intervention Society 2004;249-84.
19. Nath S. Cervical percutaneous radiofrequency facet denervation. In: Handbook of Interventional Pain Medicine. Oxford University Press (In Print).

Cervical Diskogenic Pain and Its Management

Anil K Sharma

INTRODUCTION

There are various identifiable sources of chronic neck pain, such as cervical intervertebral disk, cervical facet joints, atlantoaxial and atlanto-occipital joints, ligaments, fascia, muscles, and nerve root. All of these structures have been shown to be capable of transmitting pain from the cervical spine resulting in symptoms of neck pain, upper extremity pain, and headaches. Yin and Bogduk[1] have demonstrated the prevalence of diskogenic neck pain to be 16%, facet joint 55%, atlantoaxial joint 9% in 143 the patients with chronic neck pain in a private practice clinic in North America. While other studies using controlled diagnostic blocks, Falco[2] have shown prevalence of facet joint pain to be ranging from 36–67% with an average of 49%. In a systematic review of cervical diskography as a diagnostic test for chronic neck pain[3], the prevalence of cervical diskogenic pain utilizing. International Association for the Study of Pain Criteria, the incidence of cervical diskogenic pain ranges from 16–20% based on three studies.[1,3,4]

CAUSES

Cervical diskogenic pain is chronic neck pain originating from cervical intervertebral disks. Intervertebral disk innervations in the cervical spine is analogous to that in the lumbar spine and can be a source of pain, with cervical disks receiving innervations posteriorly from the sinuvertebral nerves, laterally from the vertebral nerve, and anteriorly from the sympathetic trunks.[5-7]

SIGNS AND SYMPTOMS

Patients usually present as focal axial neck pain with frequent occipital headaches, also it is common to get referred pain into shoulders and between the scapular blades. Each disk has a pattern of referred pain. Patients often complain of significant tightness and muscle spasms in the neck with limitation of range of movement.

CLINICAL EXAMINATION

There is no specific clinical examination, which predicts pain from cervical diskogenic etiology. Other findings noted during clinical examination could be loss of cervical lordosis secondary to muscle spasms, trigger point in paracervical muscles, range of motion is decreased with flexion, extension and rotation. Palpation might reveal tenderness along suboccipital areas and tenderness along cervical facet joints bilaterally. These are general findings; none of them are specific for diagnosis of cervical diskogenic pain.

DIAGNOSTIC CRITERIA

MRI of the cervical spine, which might shows loss of signal in disks, degenerative changes, bulging, protrusions, and sometimes annual tears. These findings on the MRI do not necessarily means that pain is coming from disks. The only test currently available to diagnose and confirm that cervical pain is originating from abnormal looking disks on MRI is diagnostic provocative cervical diskography.

INVESTIGATIONS

Plain X-ray of cervical spine, which might show evidence of degenerative disks along with osteophytes, loss of disk height as well as loss of cervical lordosis. MRI of cervical spine, which might reveal loss of signal on disks, disk herniations, annular tear as well as evidence of degenerative changes along uncovertebral joints.

DIFFERENTIAL DIAGNOSIS

Multiple other structures can give neck pain similar to diskogenic pain. The other painful structures could be:
1. Cervical facet joints.
2. Ligaments, fascia, muscles as well as atlantoaxial and atlanto-occipital joints.

DIAGNOSIS AND TREATMENT ALGORITHM

The algorithm of investigation of chronic neck pain without a disk herniation or radicular symptoms start with clinical question, physical examination, and imaging. Various structures can give the neck pain such as cervical facet joints, atlantoaxial, atlanto-occipital joints, ligaments, fascia, muscles, etc. (Flowchart 1). After initial trial of conservative treatment which would include physical therapy, nonsteroidal anti-inflammatory medications, and muscle relaxant.

If the pain persists, attention should be focused to the next cause. If myofascial pain is being seriously considered then a trial of trigger point injections can be performed. For patients who have not responded to the

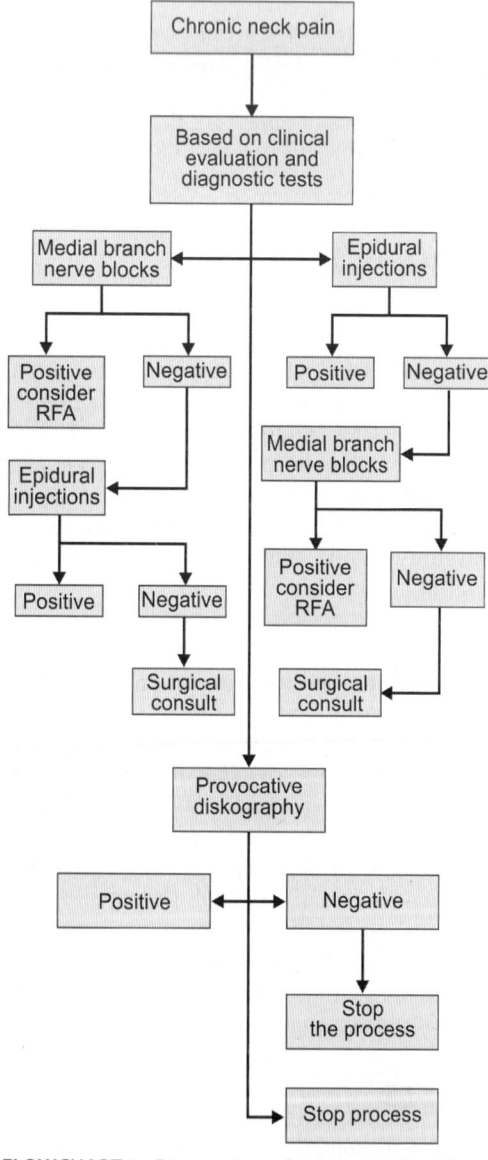

FLOWCHART 1: Diagnostic and treatment algorithm

treatment above, the next step in algorithm for chronic neck pain would be facet joint etiology. Diagnosis of facet joint pain is done by performing two diagnostic blocks of medial branches using two separate local anesthetics, each with different duration of action, which is called as controlled comparative local anesthetic block. Each block should relieve the pain by 80% and the duration of relief should coincide with the duration of anesthetic. Therapeutic facet nerve blocks can also been done in which along with the local anesthetic a steroid medication is also injected to provide with more long-term therapeutic benefit.

If the pain does not get better with diagnostic medial branch blocks, then diskogenic pain is a possible cause.

At this point, two fluoroscopy-guided cervical interlaminar epidural steroid injections should also be considered prior to proceeding with diskography. [8-10]

After carefully reviewing the MRI again, and also considering the severity of neck pain along with disability associated with pain in terms of lifestyle and ability to work. Consideration is given for cervical diskography. The patient should be willing to proceed with surgical treatment prior to considering cervical diskography.

CERVICAL DISKOGRAPHY

Multiple questions have been raised regarding the utility of cervical diskography including reported high false-positive rates in certain subpopulation; there is lack of standardization, which includes definition of concordant pain and pain intensity threshold to determine positive level. These issues have been more controversial in cervical diskography as opposed to lumbar diskography, which has been refined substantially with using volume and pressure monitoring (Figs 1A to C). However, cervical provocative diskography continues to be the only diagnostic tool capable of establishing where a particular disk is painful or not irrespective of the presence or absence of degenerative/abnormal pathology noted on the MRI. Cervical diskography carries certain risks as diskitis and infection. The incidence is low 0.2%[11,12], which is higher than lumbar diskography most likely as double needle techniques cannot be used in cervical disks. Studies have demonstrated that infection rate can be reduced significantly with use of aseptic precaution, careful needle technique and increased operative experience.[13,14] Time the needle remaining in disk during diskography, IV antibiotic

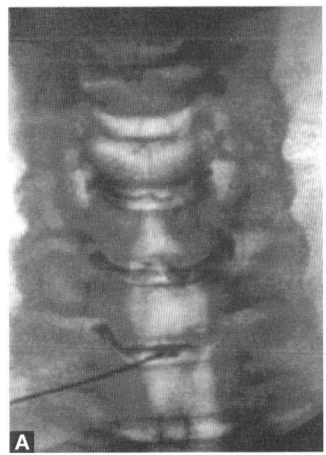
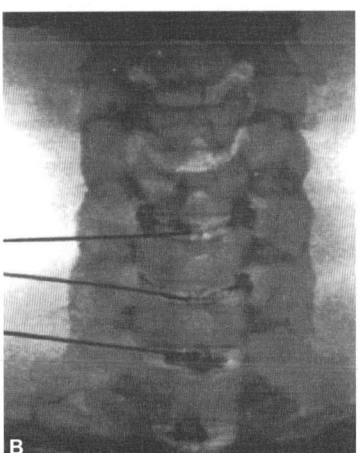
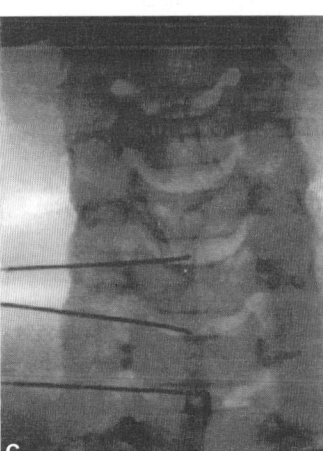

FIGS 1A to C: Cervical diskography

(the dose and timing of antibiotic can affect the incidence). It is recommended that the antibiotic be given within 60 minutes of the start of procedure and that 2 g of cefazolin be administered for adult patients.[11,15]

Also studies have shown that chlorhexidine skin preparation result in fewer bacterial colonization than povidone-iodine preparation.[13-14] Cervical diskography also carries risks of hematoma secondary to injury to major blood vessels as they are close to the trajectory of needle insertion. Recently, there have been articles suggesting acceleration of disk degeneration from needle puncture.[16]

TREATMENT

Treatment of cervical diskogenic pain is usually surgical, which can be anterior cervical diskectomy and fusion (ACDF) or artificial disk replacement. Percutaneous procedures have also been done using cobalt ion and decompression with poor results. Cervical interlaminar epidurals are not indicated for diskogenic cervical pain. Future treatment will be more biological with gene therapy so that disk can be regenerated.

CONCLUSION

Cervical diskography is a safe procedure with potential complications. Risks versus benefits should be weighed in carefully before utilizing this test to diagnose cervical diskogenic pain. Cervical diskography should also be followed by CT scan of the cervical spine within six hours.

REFERENCES

1. Yin W, Bogduk N. The nature of neck pain in a private pain clinic in the United States. Pain Med. 2008;9:196-203.
2. Falco FJE, Erhart S, Wargo BW, Bryce DA, Atluri S, Datta S, Hayek SM. Systematic review of diagnostic utility and therapeutic effectiveness of cervical facet joint interventions. Pain Physician. 2009;12:323-44.
3. Manchikanti L, Dunbar EE, Wargo BW, Shah RV, Debry R, Cohen SP. Systematic review of cervical discography as a diagnostic test for chronic spinal pain. Pain Physician. 2009:12:305-21.
4. Palit M, Schofferman J, Goldthwaite N, Reynolds J, Kerner M, Keaney D, Lawrence-Miyasaki L. Anterior disectomy and fusion for the management of neck pain. Spine 1999; 24:2224-8.
5. Bogduk N, April C. On the nature of neck pain, discography and cervical zygapophysial joint blocks. Pain 1993; 54:213-7.
6. Bogduk N, Windsor M, Inglis A. The innervation of the cervical intervertebral discs. Spine. 1989;13:2-8.
7. Grogen GJ, Baljet B, Drukker J. Nerves and nerve plexuses of the human vertebral column. Am J Anat. 1990;188:282-96.
8. Parfenchuck TA, Janssen ME. A correlation of cervical magnetic resonance imaging and discography/computed tomographic discograms. Spine. 1994;19:2819-25.
9. Deyo RA, Nachemson A, Mirza SK. Spinal-fusion surgery– The case for restraint. N Engl J Med. 2004;350:722-6.
10. Colhoun E, McCall IW, Williams L, Cassar Pullicino VN. Provocation discography as a guide to planning operations on the spine. J Bone Joint Surg Br. 1988; 70:267-71.
11. Sharma SK, Jones JO, Zeballos PP, et al. The prevention of discitis during discography. Spine J. 2009;9:936-43.
12. Simmons EH, Bhalla SK. Anterior cervical discectomy and fusion; clinical and biomechanical study with eight-year follow up. J Bone Joint Surg Br. 1969;51:225-37.
13. Sato S, Sakuragi T, Dan K. Human skin flora as a potential source of epidural abscess. Anesthesiology. 1996; 85:1276-82.
14. Yentur EA, Luleci N, Topeu I, et al. Is skin disinfection with 10% povidone-iodine sufficient to prevent epidural needle and catheter contamination? Reg Anesth Pain Med. 2003; 28:389-93.
15. Barie PS, Eachempati SR. Surgical site infections. Surg Clin North Am. 2005; 85:1115-35. viii-ix.
16. Bratzler DW, Houck PM. Antimicrobial prophylaxis for surgery: an advisory statement from the National Surgical Infection Prevention Project. Am J Surg. 2005;189:395-404

SECTION 5

Low Back Pain

CHAPTER 18

Focal Back Pain and Its Management

Sanjeeva Gupta, Shamim Haider, John A Titterington

INTRODUCTION

Focal low back pain (LBP) is a condition and not a diagnosis. Better understanding of the neuroanatomy of the spine now enables us to perform precision diagnostic techniques to diagnose specific causes of low back pain and target our treatments to treat those specific causes. Most patients with back pain can be managed conservatively and will recover with time. If back pain becomes persistent then it is important to identify the source of the back pain by clinical examination, investigations and if appropriate precision diagnostic techniques to guide further management.

CAUSES

Mechanical focal low back pain generally arises from degeneration of the various structures of the spine, most commonly the facet joints, intervertebral disks, sacroiliac joints but also the ligaments, muscles, dura mater, vertebral bodies etc. Back pain can also be a symptom of a non-mechanical pathology. These pathologies often originate from the spine but may also originate from structures around the spine, pathology distant from the spine or metabolic conditions. This chapter will discuss these pathologies in more detail predominantly under the heading "Non Mechanical Causes of Focal LBP."

MECHANICAL CAUSES OF FOCAL LOW BACK PAIN

Symptoms, Signs and Clinical Examination

The three most common causes of focal low back pain (LBP) are pain originating from the facet joints, intervertebral disks and sacroiliac joints (Fig. 1 and Box 1). Patients with focal LBP can complain of aching and/or stabbing low back pain with or without referred pain to the groin, thighs and/or sometimes into the calf muscle area. The referred pain can be unilateral or bilateral. The referred pain pattern may sometimes be difficult to differentiate from radicular pain. Patients who have had spinal surgery in the past may have burning pain in the lower back which could be neuropathic. Pain originating from facet joints is more common in older patients, increases on extension of the lumbar spine and is more prominent in the paraspinal areas at the level of the facet joints involved. Diskogenic pain is more common in patients less than 50 years of age, increases on forward flexion of the lumbar spine, increases on straining or

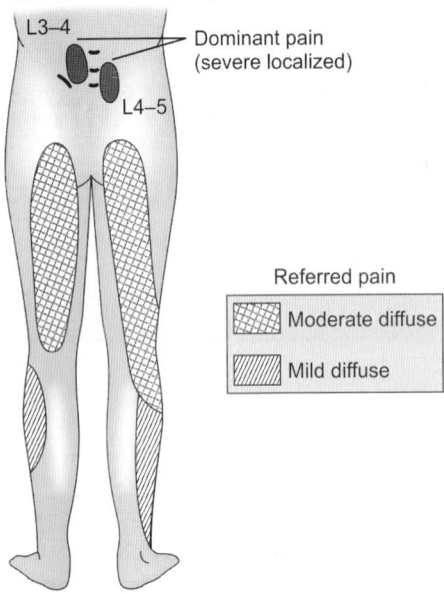

FIG. 1: Referral pattern of facet joint pain. Whilst diskogenic and SIJ pain may be referred to the groin it can mimic the above pattern for the facet joints. Hence the need for precision diagnostic techniques in carefully selected cases of persistent focal low back pain

Box 1: Some common clinical features of low back pain

Facet joint pain
- More common in patients more than 50 years of age
- Pain increases of extension of the lumbar spine
- Pain in the paraspinal areas over the facet joints causing the pain

Discogenic pain
- More common in patients less than 50 years
- Pain increases on bending forwards
- Pain increases on straining, coughing or any other activities, which increase the pressure in the disc

Sacroiliac joint pain
- More common in multiparous women
- May be unilateral or bilateral
- Maximum pain below L5 level
- Pain on pressure over the SIJ

Pain due to vertebral fracture
- History of trauma and/or osteoporosis and/or infection (Tuberculosis) and/or metastatic disease
- Focal pain at the level of the fracture

Metastatic deposits
- History of primary (Commonly prostate, breast, lungs)
- Focal pain at the vertebral levels involve
- Other signs and symptoms of primary cancer

Multiple myeloma
- Serum protein electrophoresis characteristically shows spike in the gamma globulin region. Bence-Jones proteinuria is demonstrated in 50% of subjects

coughing. Pain is more intense in the morning when the patient wakes up due to hydration of the disk, which increases the pressure in the disk and is generally most intense in the center of the spine. Sacroiliac joint (SIJ) pain can be unilateral or bilateral, more common in multiparous women, pain is predominantly below the L5 level and pressure on the SIJ will invariably reproduce concordant pain.

The referral pattern of the pain originating from any structure of the back can mimic each other. The only way of diagnosing conclusively the structure responsible for the patient's pain is by precision diagnostic techniques.

Diagnostic Criteria

As indicated above some of the signs, symptoms and the findings of the clinical examination can give us information regarding the possible sources of focal LBP but these can overlap significantly. A thorough understanding of the neuroanatomy of the spine and appropriate precision diagnostic techniques is the gold standard to diagnose the common sources of focal LBP. These techniques act as a diagnostic intervention in the immediate post procedure period due to the actions of the local anesthetic but with the addition of steroid can also provide good pain relief for several weeks in some patients. However, one of the author (SG) informs his patients that the primary aim of these procedures is diagnostic.

Facet joint pain: Median branch blocks (MBB) resulting in around 70% pain relief when performing activities of daily living for the duration of action of the local anaesthetic on at least one occasion but preferably on two separate occasions. Sometimes it is difficult for patients to quantify pain relief and in such situations one of the author (SG) finds out from the patient if the pain relief after the procedure was significant compared to the pain before the procedure before confirming the diagnosis.

Sacroiliac joint pain: Injection of local anaesthetic and steroid into the SIJ results in around 70% pain relief when performing activities of daily living for at least the duration of action of the local anaesthetic on two separate occasions.

SIJ injection may be technically challenging. The needle is placed in the lower 2 cm of the SIJ and radiocontrast dye is injected to confirm that the needle is in the SIJ before injecting local anesthetic with steroid into the SIJ. The patient should get around 70% pain relief on activities of daily living for at least the duration of action of the local anaesthetic used. In one of the authors (SG) clinical practice he injects 40 mg of triamcinalone with 2 mL of 0.25% bupivacaine. SG has described a two needle technique which in his opinion increases the chances of successful SIJ block.

Diskogenic pain: Three level lumbar provocation diskography can help diagnose the pathological disk.

Vertebral body fracture: History of trauma and/or metabolic conditions and focal tenderness.

Investigations

Full blood count, ESR, CRP, and other blood tests as appropriate.

Plain X-ray of lumbar spine: Generally not very useful. Refer to Chapter 8: Interpretation of X-ray Spine.

CT scan: Very good to identify bony pathology such as spondylolysthesis, spinal canal stenosis, fracture, etc.

Isotope bone scan: It can assist in targeting the pathological structure for further investigations

MRI scan: Good to identify soft tissue pathology with no radiation exposure. Investigation of choice for patients with focal low back pain. Useful in excluding red flags.

The findings of the radiological investigations should be compared with the clinical findings to make sense and help facilitate diagnosis. However, the gold standard investigation to diagnose persistent mechanical focal LBP is precision diagnostic techniques which can guide further management.

Differential Diagnosis

As discussed above the pain originating primarily from the spine can be diagnosed using information from the history, clinical examination, investigations and precision diagnostic techniques.

Nonmechanical causes of focal LBP are discussed further.

Treatment

Conservative Management and Pharmacotherapy

Paracetamol with or without codeine can be helpful. NSAIDs can be added if they are not contraindicated. Tricyclic antidepressants can be helpful, if the side effects are tolerated. The main aim is to provide balanced analgesia by using analgesics acting with different mechanisms of action and at different levels of the pain pathway. The aim of pain relief should be to promote physiotherapy and to return to normal activities. Other conservative measures include the use of heat/cold and transcutaneous electrical nerve stimulation. However, by the time the patient comes to the pain specialist many of these have usually been tried and the pain has not subsided therefore diagnostic interventions and treatment may be indicated.

If the clinical history has pointed to a possible source of focal LBP then the clinical examination would have further identified the possible structures, levels, and side/sides to be tested with interventions.

Interventions: It is important to identify the source of maximum pain. The patient may say that the pain is bilateral however on further questioning it often becomes apparent that the pain is more intense on one side. It is often the case that the pain starts on one side and when it becomes severe it spreads cephalad, caudal and to the contralateral side from the initial starting area of the pain. In one of the authors (SG) clinical practice before embarking on any diagnostic interventions he takes time to accurately identify the true source and side of patient's maximum pain and understand how the pain spreads as this helps him to minimize the number of structures (e.g. number of facet joints) that needs testing and reduce risk to the patient.

Facet joint pain: Some patients may gain long lasting pain relief with median branch blocks with local anaesthetic and steroid. In some cases these may be continued on a therapeutic basis. However many patients will only get temporary relief and therefore radiofrequency ablation of the relevant median branches/dorsal rami is indicated. This treatment has good evidence and is successful in greater than half of patients.

Sacroiliac joint pain: Diagnostic SIJ block with local anaesthetic and steroid. This can be repeated as therapy if the effect lasts for several weeks or months. SIJ denervation by the radiofrequency ablation of the L5 dorsal rami and lateral branches of the sacral nerves S1-3 may result in longer lasting analgesia. These nerves do not adhere to the bone as the median branches do which may explain the slightly lower success rate.

Diskogenic pain: Invasive options include: Intradiscal Electrothermal Therapy (IDET) which involves the application of heat directly to the annulus of the affected disc hoping to achieve thermal modification of collagen fibers and ablation of nociceptors; nucleoplasty; epidural steroids and spinal fusion. These interventions are considered as a last option. In the authors opinion conservative measures such as physiotherapy, regular exercise, cessation of smoking, good posture and appropriate lifting and handling techniques may be more appropriate and can make a significant difference in the management of difficult diskogenic pain.

Vertebral body fracture: Local application of lignocaine 5% plaster as described by the manufacturer may help some patients. Vertebroplasty can be helpful. However two recent publications have challenged this.

NONMECHANICAL CAUSES OF FOCAL LOW BACK PAIN

Focal low back pain can also occur due the systemic diseases, metabolic/endocrine pathologies affecting the spine, secondary tumor deposits, trauma, and diseases of the structures closely related to the spine. If these conditions are suspected patients should be referred to an appropriate specialist for further assessment and management.

There are a varied of causes of focal back pain that do not originate locally. Box 2 lists some of the important non-mechanical causes. However, the list is not exhaustive.

DESCRIPTION OF SOME COMMON CAUSES OF NONMECHANICAL FOCAL LOW BACK PAIN ENCOUNTERED IN THE PAIN CLINIC

Osteoporosis and Focal Back Pain

Osteoporosis is the most common metabolic bone disease, which occurs as a result of the rate of resorption of bone exceeding the rate of formation. Osteoporosis affects an estimated 75 million people in Europe,

> **Box 2: Nonmechanical causes of low back pain. If this condition is suspected then patient should be referred to appropriate specialist for further assessment and management**
>
> - Endocrine/metabolic
>   - Osteoporosis
>   - Osteomalacia
>   - Hyperparathyroidism
>   - Paget's disease
>   - Fluorosis
> - Bone disease
>   - Primary bone tumors, e.g. multiple myeloma, chordoma, osteoma, osteoblastoma, hemangioma
>   - Metastatic bone tumors
>   - Lymphoma
>   - Vascular malformations
> - Infectious
>   - Vertebral osteomyelitis
>   - Pyogenic
>   - Granulamatous (Tuberculous)
>   - Fungal
> - Diskitis
> - Epidural abscess
> - Sacroilitis
> - Traumatic
>   - Fracture
>   - Soft tissue injury
> - Rheumatologic
>   - Ankylosing spondylitis
>   - Psoriatic arthritis
>   - Enteropathic arthritis
>   - Reactive arthritis
>   - Rheumatoid arthritis
> - Intra-abdominal/pelvic disease (Referred pain)
>   - Abdominal aortic aneurysm
>   - Renal disease, e.g. infection, stones
>   - Pelvic tumors
>   - Fibroid of the uterus
>   - Pelvic inflammatory disease
>   - Pancreatitis
>   - Gallbladder disease
>   - Abdominal tumors
> - Others
>   - Sickle cell disease
>   - Vasculitis

USA and Japan. In 2009 the International Osteoporosis Foundation estimated the number of osteoporosis patients in India to be approximately 26 million (2003). Now the number of osteoporosis patients in India has been estimated to be 50 million (2013). It is a hugely prevalent and as the population ages it becomes an increasing problem.

Osteoporosis may be primary or secondary. Primary osteoporosis is classified as postmenopausal, senile, and idiopathic. Its incidence is higher in middle aged women; however, the male:female ratio is much more even in elderly population.

Secondary osteoporosis can be caused by wide range of conditions, including poor nutrition, endocrine abnormalities (hyperthyroidism, hyperparathyroidism, hyperadrenocorticism, hypogonadism, acromegaly), cancer related (multiple myeloma, metastatic) and drug induced (heparin, steroids, anticonvulsants).

Vertebral osteoporosis could present as constant, dull, nagging back pain, which is postulated to be due to venous stasis in vertebral bodies. Osteoporotic vertebral compression fracture is also a significant cause of back pain. It is usually first noted in thoracic spine, which may occur without a significant initial discomfort due to the support offered by the rib cage. These patients present to pain clinic with grumbling debilitating chronic back pain, punctuated with episodes of severe incapacitating pain initiated by minor mechanical events, such as lifting. Examination may additionally reveal muscle spasm in the back and thoracic kyphosis with compensatory lumbar lordosis.

Plain radiograph shows a general loss of bone density. There may be ballooning of disk into the vertebrae. Vertebral fractures and collapse may also be seen. Dual energy X-ray absorptiometry (DEXA) scan is a widely used assessment method to diagnose and assess the risk of osteoporosis. Here, bone marrow density (BMD) can be quickly assessed with minimal radiation exposure. World Health Organization's criteria for diagnosis of osteoporosis is, BMD more than 2 standard deviations below that of a young healthy adult.

Prevention is the best way to manage osteoporosis. Preventive measures include hormonal substitution when osteoporosis risk is high (especially in menopausal women), adequate calcium intake and regular exercise.

Associated back pain is treated by correcting any underlying cause, and use of non-opioid and opioid analgesics as appropriate. In patients with vertebral body collapse and significant pain not relieved by simple measures, vertebroplasty is an option.

Malignancy and Focal Back Pain

Bone pain could result from both primary and metastatic tumors. Primary neoplasms of vertebral column are rare, secondary deposits are much more common. Multiple myeloma is the most common primary malignant cancer of the spine. Metastatic vertebral pain most commonly results from cancers of the breast, prostate, and lung. Other malignancies causing vertebral lesions are renal cell carcinoma, thyroid cancer and lymphoma.

Most patients with cancerous lesions in the vertebrae experience back pain. This pain could be either nociceptive or neuropathic or mixed in nature. Mechanisms causing the back pain range from stretching of the periostium, inflammation, stimulation and injury to sensory nerves of periostium, pathological fracture of vertebrae, and spinal cord or nerve root compression.

Along with pain, presentation can include features of the primary cancer, hypercalcemia and symptoms secondary to vertebral fracture.

Diagnostic evaluation of these patients involves plain radiography to identify site of lesion and associated fractures. Computed tomography (CT) offers better resolution for evaluation of bone destruction. Magnetic resonance imaging (MRI) is especially useful in defining the soft tissue and marrow infiltration and any associated spinal cord or nerve root compression. A bone scan is used where multi-focal lesions are suspected. In patients with multiple myeloma, serum protein electrophoresis characteristically shows spike in the gammaglobulin region. Bence-Jones proteinuria is demonstrated in 50% of subjects. In patients with metastatic deposits, various tumor markers are measured serially for prognostic purposes and evaluation of progress of primary cancer (Table 1).

The focus of treatment should be directed at tumor regression, relief of cancer-related symptoms, especially pain, and preservation of functional capacity. This requires a constant and effective communication between pain, oncology, neurosurgical and orthopedic teams, as dictated by local arrangements.

Based on the nature and stage of cancer, treatment may be aimed at a cure or limiting progression of tumor or palliation. This dictates the choice of modalities for pain management. Amongst other treatments radiotherapy can be an effective treatment of spinal metastases.

Analgesics are used as per WHO pain ladder. However, conventional opioids or non-steroidal anti-inflammatory drugs (NSAIDs) may not produce adequate analgesia because of the incidental/ intermittent nature of pain and dose-limiting side effects. Therefore other more targeted pharmacotherapeutic and interventional approaches are often used. These may be used alone or in combination with traditional analgesics. They include corticosteroids, bisphosphonates, calcitonin, radionucleotides and hormonal therapy. Percutaneous vertebroplasty is a useful option for back pain related to pathological fracture of vertebrae. Minimally invasive neurodestructive techniques involving radiofrequency lesioning, cryotherapy and chemical neurolysis are also effective in well selected cases.

TABLE 1: Tumor markers for various malignancies

Cancer	Tumor marker
Colorectal	CEA (Carcinoembryonic antigen)
Breast	CA 153
Ovary	CA 125
Pancreas	CA 199
Prostate	PSA (Prostate specific antigen)
Bone	Alkaline phosphatase

Infection of Spine and Focal Back Pain

Infection in spine is an uncommon cause of back pain. It usually takes form of osteomyelitis or diskitis. The infection can be pyogenic, granulomatous or fungal.

Pyogenic osteomyelitis usually results by hematogenous spread from a distant site of infection. Common sources of infection are pelvic inflammatory disease and urinary tract infection. *Staphylococcus* is the most common infecting organism and *E. coli*, *Streptococcus* and *Pseudomonas* are implicated in minority of cases. The vertebral body of the lumbar spine is the most commonly affected site due to its rich vascularity. Often the onset is insidious with a chronic course, but occasionally the onset could be acute. Patients on immunosuppressants, diabetics and those with history of alcohol abuse are most at risk.

Tuberculous osteomyelitis is usually secondary to infection in lungs or urinary tract. The vertebral body of lower thoracic and upper lumbar spine is most commonly affected. Intervertebral disks are relatively resistant to this infection unlike pyogenic osteomyelitis. The disease has an insidious onset and chronic course. The incidence of neurological involvement is much higher in tuberculous osteomyelitis in comparison with pyogenic.

Unless there is a high index of suspicion chronic osteomyelitis with an indolent course is often difficult to diagnose. Misdiagnosis and delayed diagnosis often occur.

Spinal osteomyelitis typically causes pain that is worsened with weight-bearing and activity and is relieved only when lying down. Chronic infection is usually associated with weight loss, fatigue, fevers, and night sweats. The most common sign is localized back pain exacerbated by palpation or percussion. Patients may additionally present with radicular signs or signs of spinal cord compression. Back pain in pyogenic osteomyelitis can occasionally be severe; in tuberculosis it is rarely severe.

Intervertebral diskitis commonly occurs following idiopathic disk puncture for chemonucleolysis, diskography or percutaneous diskectomy. The clinical picture is usually that of initial pain relief from sciatica following the procedure. It is followed by severe back pain and leg cramps in the ensuing one to eight weeks. There are very few constitutional symptoms, except for a minority who run a febrile course.

Epidural abscess is a very rare infection causing back pain, most often occurring following spinal surgery. *Staphylococcus* is the most common causative organism. Typically the patient initially has localized non-mechanical pain in the night-time, followed by radicular symptoms and late features of spinal cord compression. The course is very variable.

The erythrocyte sedimentation rate is the most sensitive test for active infection. C-reactive protein level is also usually elevated. Those with signs of sepsis should have blood cultures sent to the laboratory. Needle aspiration biopsy is essential for a bacteriological diagnosis.

MRI is the most useful imaging modality for all infections of the spine. In osteomyelitis, it shows signs of disk destruction, disk space narrowing, loss of definition of the endplates and destruction of cortical margins of vertebral bodies. Additionally, MRI can differentiate between pyogenic and tuberculous infections. In diskitis, narrowing of the disk space is revealed. On the other hand, CT may be better for showing the extent of bone involvement.

An optimal outcome of vertebral osteomyelitis requires heightened awareness, early diagnosis, prompt identification of pathogens, reversal of complications, and prolonged antimicrobial therapy. It is very important to liaise closely with the spinal and/or neurosurgical teams. Urgent surgical decompression is warranted for neurological deficit.

Ankylosing Spondylitis and Focal Back Pain

Ankylosing spondylitis (AS) is the most common rheumatological condition associated with back pain. Other less common conditions with similar presentation are enteropathic arthritis (associated with inflammatory bowel disease), psoriatic arthritis and reactive arthritis. These are grouped as seronegative arthritis, as there is no association with rheumatoid factor or antinuclear antibodies.

AS causes chronic synovitis of the joints, followed by cartilage destruction, erosion, sclerosis of underlying bone and finally fibrosis/ankylosis of the joint.

AS is typically a disease of young men with women having a much lower incidence and a milder course. It usually presents as an insidious onset of a grumbling low back pain in patients below 40 years of age. Characteristically, there are remissions and exacerbations over months. Morning and post-immobility stiffness, relieved by activity or hot shower, are prominent features. Patients often experience marked night pain, initially in the low back and eventually in the entire spine. Examination reveals a limitation of lumbar motion in all planes, unlike diskogenic or facet joint pain, where limitation is marked in one plain compared to others. In the late stages of disease, when ankylosis of joints has already occurred, severe flexion deformities may occur. Extra-articular manifestations associated with AS include uveitis (common), mucosal ulcers, myocarditis, aortitis and pulmonary apical fibrosis.

Presence of HLA-B27 supports the clinical diagnosis of AS. However, its absence does not rule it out. Plain radiography in early stages demonstrates squaring of anterior vertebral body, followed by ossification of annulus fibrosis leading to bridging of disk space (syndesmophytes). In late stages, ossification of all ligaments and complete fusion of the vertebral column is seen. This pattern is referred to as 'bamboo spine.'

The principles of management are symptomatic treatment with anti-inflammatory medications, patient education and exercise programs to maintain good posture, mobility and strength of the spinal muscles. Patient should be referred to a rheumatologist for further management.

CONCLUSION

Focal low back pain (LBP) is a condition and not a diagnosis. We have discussed how a structured approach of obtaining a proper targeted history, clinical examination and investigations can guide us to the source of LBP. As discussed, precision diagnostic techniques can pin point the exact source of pain and assist in formulating an effective management plan.

Non Mechanical causes of LBP such as due to systemic diseases, metabolic/endocrine pathologies affecting the spine, secondary tumor deposits, trauma and diseases of the structures closely related to the spine should also be considered. If these conditions are suspected patients should be referred to an appropriate specialist for further assessment and management.

BIBLIOGRAPHY

1. Alan D. Kaye, S Gupta, et al. Efficacy of Epidural Injections in Managing Chronic Spinal Pain: A Best Evidence Synthesis. Pain Physician 2015; 18:E939-E1004.
2. Baheti D, Bakshi S, Gupta S, Gehdoo RP. Interventional Pain Management-A Practical Approach. New Delhi:Jaypee Medical Publishers 2008.
3. Bogduk N, Dreyfuss P, Govind J. A narrative review of lumbar median branch neurotomy for the treatment of back pain. Pain Medicine 2009;10(6):1035-45.
4. Bogduk N. A narrative review of intraarticular corticosteroid injections for low back pain. Pain Med 2005;6: 287-96.
5. Bogduk N: The innervation of the lumbar spine. Spine 1983;8:286-93.
6. Boswell MV, S Gupta, et al. A Best-Evidence systematic appraisal of the diagnostic accuracy and utility of

facet joint nerve injections in chronic spinal pain. Pain Physician 2015; 18: E497-E533.
7. Buchbinder R, Osborne RH, Ebeling PR, et al. A Randomized trial of vertebroplasty for painful osteoporotic vertebral fractures. N Eng J Med 2009;361:557-68.
8. EFFO and NOF. Who are candidates for prevention and treatment for osteoporosis? Osteoporos Int 1997;7:1.
9. Groen G, Baljet B, Drukker J. Nerves and nerve plexuses of the human vertebral colums. Am J Anat 1990;188:282-96.
10. Gupta S. Double Needle Technique for Sacroiliac Joint Injection. Submitted for Publication.
11. S Gupta, M Gupta, S Nath, Michael Hess. Survey of European pain medicine practice. Pain Physician 2012; 15: E983-E994 (Impact Factor – 4.766).
12. Lallmes DF, Comstock BA, Heagerty PJ, et al. A Randomized trial of vertebroplasty for osteoporoic spinal fractures. N Eng J Med 2009;361(6):569-79.
13. J Lee, S Gupta, C Price, AP Baranowski. Low back and radicular pain: a pathway for care developed by the British Pain Society. British Journal of Anaesthesia 2013; 111 (1): 112-120 (Impact Factor – 4.354).
14. Manchikanti L, Boswall MV, Datta S, et al. Comprehensive review of therapeutic interventions in managing chronic spinal pain. Pain Physician 2009;12:E123– E198.
15. Manchikanti L, Boswall MV, Singh V, et al. Comprehensive review of neurophysiologic basis and diagnostic interventions in managing chronic spinal pain. Pain Physician 2009;12:E71–E121.
16. Manchikanti L, Datta S, Derby R, et al. A critical review of the American Pain Society clinical practice guidelines for interventional techniques: Part 1. Diagnostic Interventions. Pain Physician 2010;13:E141-E174.
17. Manchikanti L, Datta S, Gupta S, et al. A critical review of the American Pain Society clinical practice guidelines for interventional techniques: Part 2. Therapeutic Interventions. Pain Physician 2010;13:E215-E264.
18. Manchikanti L, Pampati V, Fellows B, Bakhit C. The diagnostic validity and therapeutic value of medial branch blocks with or without adjuvants. Curr Rev Pain 2000;4:337-44.
19. Manchikanti L, S Gupta, et al. A systematic review of efficacy and best evidence synthesis of therapeutic facet joint interventions in managing chronic spinal pain. Pain Physician 2015; 18: E535-E582.
20. McGuirk BE, Bogduk N. Chronic low back pain. In: Ballantyne JC, Fishman SM, Rathmell JP (ed). Bonica's Management of Pain (4th edition). Lippincott Williams and Wilkins 2009; pp1130-41.
21. Mithal A, Bensal B, Kyer CS et al. The Asia-Pacific Regional Audit-Epidemiology, Costs, and Burden of Osteoporosis in India 2013: A report of International Osteoporosis Foundation. Indian J Endocinol Metab 2014:18(4);449-454.
22. Osteoporosis Society of India. Action Plan Osteoporosis: Consensus statement of an expert group. New Delhi 2003.
23. Patel VB, Wasserman R, Imani F. Interventional Therapies for Chronic Low Back Pain: A Focused Review (efficacy and outcomes). Anaesth Pain Med 2015;5(4):e29716.
24. R Laclaire, et al. Letter to Editor. Pain Practice 2010;10(3):261-63.
25. Ridley MG, Coppin J. Back pain: medical approach. In: Dolin SJ, Padfield NL. Pain Medicine Manual (2nd edition). Butterworth-Heinmann; 2004;pp167-76.
26. S Nath. Critiquing the critiques. Pain Physician 2011 (In Press).
27. Siemionow K, et. al. Identifying serious causes of back pain: Cancer, infection, fracture. Cleveland Clin J of Med 2008;75(8):557-66.
28. Simopoulos TT, Manchikanti L, Singh V, et al. A systemic evaluation of prevalence and diagnostic accuracy of sacroiliac joint interventions. Pain Physician 2012;15:E305-E344.
29. Stone JH. A clinicians pearls and myths in rheumatology. Springer 2009;58-59.
30. Wong DA, Transfeldt E (ed). Macnab's Backache 4th edition. Lippincott Williams and Wilkins; 2007; pp 26-59.
31. Wong DA, Transfeldt E (ed). Macnab's Backache 4th edition. Lippincott Williams and Wilkins; 2007; pp 122-32.

CHAPTER 19

Lumbar Facet Joint Pain Syndrome

Sanjay Bakshi, Gerard Grahemsen

INTRODUCTION

The lumbar facet joints are a common cause of back pain. Lumbar facet pain can be unilateral or bilateral with or without radiation to the buttocks, hips, or legs but will not typically follow a dermatomal distribution. The origin of this pain can be the result of structural damage to the joint, i.e. trauma, age related, as seen with arthritis, or inflammatory. Pain from the facet joints is often the result of damage to the joints seen with repetitive use such as frequent extension, lateral bending, or twisting of the spine. It can also result from the sudden sheering forces to the joints sustained during motor vehicle accidents, work related injuries, sports injuries, etc. In 1911, Goldthwaite recognized these joints as being a potential cause of pain.[1] Ghormley later coined the term facet syndrome in 1933, defining it as lumbosacral pain with or without sciatic pain.[2,3] In 1941, Badgley also investigated the facet joints as a cause of lower back pain, based on pathomorpologic studies of the joint.[4] Hirsch et al. in 1963 determined that injection of the zygapophysial joints reproduced a patient's back pain.[5] Rees in 1972 and later Shealy in 1974 explored and developed techniques of facet rhizolysis and radiofrequency facet denervation to treat facet mediated pain.[6–8]

Despite being a well known cause of lower back pain, lumbar facet syndrome often goes under diagnosed due to clinicians failing to recognize the clinical presentation, initiating proper workup, and instituting an appropriate treatment plan.

This chapter will focus on understanding lumbar facet syndrome and aiding clinicians to come to a timely diagnosis and treat this painful cause of lower back pain in a timely fashion to improve a patient's quality of life.

PREVALENCE AND EPIDEMIOLOGY

Chronic low back pain is common condition affecting most adults in their lifetime. However, many conditions can be the underlying cause of this complaint including disk disease, stenosis, facet mediated pain, sacroiliac joint dysfunction, etc. Manchukonda et al.[9] performed a retrospective review of 438 patients to look at the prevalence and false-positive rate of diagnostic blocks. They concluded that the prevalence of facet joint pain in the lumbar spine to be 27% and the false-positive rate with a single block to be 45% in the lumbar region. Osteoarthritis and degenerative changes of the facet joints are a common cause of back and neck pain. Therefore, the prevalence of facet mediated back pain is higher in the older population.[10] In 2008, Manchikanti et al., investigated the rate of facet related chronic low back pain in 424 patients in 6 age groups and determined the prevalence ranged from 18% in individuals aged 31-40 to 44% in persons aged 51-60 years.[11] Schwarzer and colleagues reported a higher positive rate to diagnostic injections in older adults and noted the average age of patients was 59 years.[12]

ANATOMY

The facet joints, also known as zygapophysial joints, are a pair of joints located on the posterior aspect of the spine. The facet joint is comprised of the superior articular process and inferior articular process of adjacent vertebrae and is lined with cartilage, allowing the joint to move or glide smoothly. A sac like capsule filled with synovial fluid surrounds the joint. Therefore, the facet joints are synovial joints. This capsule is innervated by the nervous system and supports the idea of the facet joint as a pain generator. Accessory ligaments unite the laminae, transverse process, and spinal processes and help stabilize the joint. The facet joints provide stability and allow the spine to flex, extend, and rotate.[13]

The facet joints are innervated by the articular branches of the medial branches. At each level, the dorsal ramus provides a medial branch that exits the intertransverse space crossing over the top of the transverse process in a groove at the point where the transverse process joins the vertebrae. The nerve then travels inferiorly and medially across the posterior surface of the ventral laminae where it gives off branches to innervate the facet joint. Each facet joint receives its innervation from a medial branch nerve of two posterior primary rami.[14] One branch arises from the nerve at the same level as the joint, and the other from the segmental level above.[15] For example, L2 and L3 medial branches innervate the L3-4 facet joint. Also keep in mind that the numbering of the medial branches differs from their location. Thus the L4 medial branch courses over the L5 transverse process and the L3 medial branch courses over the L4 transverse process.[16] This explains the lack of specific clinical symptoms related to facet mediated pain and explains the rationale of why the dorsal nerve from the vertebral level above the symptomatic level must also be blocked or denervated to provide pain relief.

CAUSES

Facet mediated pain is typically seen in the elderly, in persons with occupations requiring repetitive hyperflexion, hyperextension, twisting, or bending of the spine, or following an accident. The typical causes of facet mediated lumbar pain are osteoarthritis, rheumatoid arthritis, ankylosing spondylitis, bony overgrowth of the facets, erosions of the adjacent bone margins, degenerative conditions resulting in reduction or loss of the facet cartilage, disk degeneration, or acute causes such as instability of the joint itself after trauma such as a motor vehicle accident. These conditions can cause high stress and strain leading to tissue damage and the release of chemicals resulting in irritation or inflammation of the nerves innervating the facet joint leading to back pain. In some cases infection can also lead to facet mediated pain, however for the purposes of this chapter we will focus on noninfectious etiologies.

Since the facet joint is a synovial joint, there are cases where chronic inflammation can lead to the synovial joints filling with fluid and distend. This will lead to a synovial cyst that can cause compression of a nerve root in the neural foramen. If this occurs a patient may experience facet mediated back pain with a radicular component.

SIGNS AND SYMPTOMS

When evaluating a patient with back pain it is imperative to take an extremely detailed history and thorough physical examination. This is crucial in assessing a patient with suspected facet mediated pain because radiological imaging studies may be within normal limits. The history should begin with details of pain including; location, quality, radiation, severity, duration, an accurate depiction of any traumatic event, and a detailed social history including occupation and activities. The detailed history will guide you in composing a differential diagnosis of the many causes of back pain.

Patients presenting with facet mediated lumbar pain will typically present complaining of focal back pain that may be unilateral or bilateral. The pain is often poorly localized and in some cases may radiate to the hip, buttock, or posterior thigh. The patient may have history of an accident resulting in hyperextension of the spine, such as with a motor vehicle accident or fall. If there is no history of trauma they may have an occupation that requires repetitive movements of the spine seen with construction or sports. In some cases just age alone may lead to the cause of the facet problem. In 2002, to help aid in the diagnosis of facet mediated pain, Windsor et al.,[17] used electrical stimulation of the right L1 through L4 medial branch of the posterior primary ramus and the right L5 dorsal ramus to induce medial branch referral patterns. They mapped the subject's referral sites, creating a well defined composite drawing.

The patient may describe stiffness in the back frequently in the morning. The pain will often be reproduced or increase in intensity with extension of the spine, seen with arising from a seated position, lateral bending or twisting. The patient's pain may be chronic due to the slow onset of most of the age related causes of facet pain.

If the previously mentioned signs and symptoms are present a clinician may suspect facet mediated pain. However, a differential diagnosis must be established to include other causes of back pain that may overlap or mimic facet mediated pain. Lumbar conditions that should be part of the differential diagnosis include; lumbar disk herniation, diskogenic pain, sacroiliac joint syndrome, spinal stenosis, spondylosis, spondylolisthesis, vertebral compression fracture, and ankylosing spondylitis. The clinician should also inquire about recent weight loss, fatigue, and fever to rule out more serious cause of focal back pain that include malignancy, osteomyelitis, epidural abscess, and diskitis.

CLINICAL EXAMINATION

The physical examination should be focused on neurological, musculoskeletal, and vascular findings. The examination should begin with vital signs to rule out any fever. Palpation of the pulses in the lower extremities should be preformed to rule out vascular insufficiency that may cause claudicative symptoms. Next, neurological examination of the lower extremities should be done to determine if there are any changes in sensation in the back or extremities along a dermatome or changes in reflexes. The musculoskeletal exam will give you the most information to establish the diagnosis of facet syndrome. The clinician should assess the patients strength in all muscle groups of the lower extremities, perform straight leg testing, assess gait, including toe and heel walking, assess range of motion in the lumbar spine including, flexion, extension, right and left rotation, and lateral bending, and thoroughly palpate all components of the posterior lumbar spine, including the spinal process (midline), facet joints (lateral to midline), sacroiliac joints, and hips.

The clinical examination of a patient with suspected lumbar facet mediated pain will demonstrate reproduction or increased pain with extension and lateral bending to the affected side. Upon palpation tenderness will often be described over the affected joints. There typically will be no changes in gait, motor function, reflexes, or sensation. In rare cases, if facet overgrowth or a synovial cyst is compromising the neural foramen, there may be possible changes in the above examination.

DIAGNOSTIC CRITERIA

Once the diagnosis of lumbar facet mediated pain is suspected by history and physical examination, one must decide what imaging studies should be preformed to aid in the diagnosis. Imaging studies may be helpful but are often an unreliable indicator of facet pain.[18] Lumbar plain radiographs are typically not useful in diagnosing facet mediated pain because they will often show facet joint arthritis at the same rate in asymptomatic and symptomatic individuals. Computed tomography and magnetic resonance imaging are helpful in ruling out other causes of lumbar pain that may mimic facet pain or may show bony overgrowth, erosion of the joint, or a synovial cyst but may fail to diagnose a facet problem. SPECT/CT (single photon emission computed tomography) imaging of the lumbar spine may also play a role in the diagnosis of lumbar facet mediated pain. SPECT/CT is a nuclear medicine test in which the images of a SPECT scan and a traditional CT scan are combined to more precisely evaluate the affected body part.

SPECT is commonly used to assess mechanical back pain using an injection of a radiopharmaceutical for bone scans. These whole body scans are very sensitive but are poorly specific to study bone disorders. SPECT combined with CT scanning is thought to allow for a more precise localization and improved diagnosis of low back pain improving its specificity by creating a three dimensional reconstruction. This can be used to allow for more accurate localization of metabolically affected facet joints to aide in the selection of specific facet joints to treat or proceed with diagnostic injection. Matar H Navalkissoor S, et al., studied SPECT/CT imaging as an adjunct in the management of suspected facet joint arthropathy.[19] They performed a retrospective consecutive study looking at 72 patients with chronic neck or back pain from outpatient spinal clinics with clinical features suggestive of facetogenic pain. They concluded hybrid SPECT/CT imaging identified potential pain generators in 92% of cervical spine scans and 86% of lumbar spine scans. The scans precisely localized SPECT positive facet joints targets in 65% of the referral population and a clinical decision to inject was made in 60% of those cases. Although, SPECT/CT scan is currently not routinely used to diagnosis facet mediated pain we do feel this should be investigated further and additional clinical studies are necessary to determine the reliable of this testing to accurately help guide therapy and improve treatment outcomes.

Multiple studies have shown a lack of correlation between the results of conventional clinical examination and the response to controlled blocks.[20-22] Therefore the most accurate way to confirm the diagnosis of lumbar facet mediated pain is by anesthetizing the nerves that innervate the facet joint.[23] (Fig. 1). This procedure is called a diagnostic lumbar medial branch block and is typically performed under fluoroscopic or ultrasound guidance. A response of 80% reduction of the patient's preprocedure pain is considered a positive response. Placebo response to

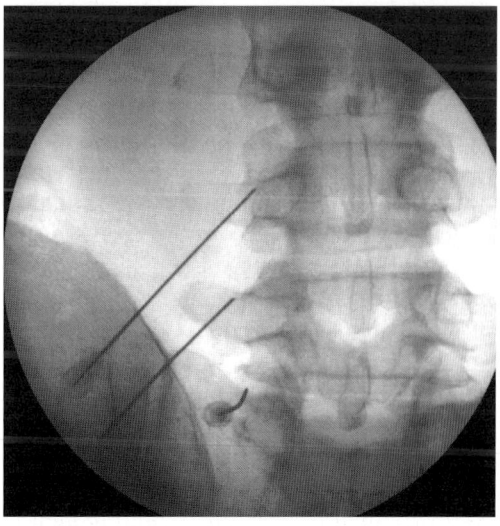

FIG. 1: Needle position lumbar medial branch L 3, 4, 5 AP view

the injections should always be considered and a repeat test should be performed using a different local anesthetic paying careful attention to the duration of desired effect to rule out a false positive response. Pampati et al.,[24] published an observational report of outcomes assessment to determine the accuracy of controlled diagnostic blocks in managing lumbar facet pain at the end of 2 years. The authors concluded that controlled diagnostic lumbar facet joint nerve blocks are valid utilizing the criteria of 80% pain relief and the ability to perform previously painful movements, with a sustained diagnosis of lumbar facet joint pain in at least 89.5% of the patients at the end of a 2-year follow-up period. Another accepted method to confirm the diagnosis is stimulation of the lumbar facet joints with injections of hypertonic saline or contrast medium. This will in turn produce back pain and somatic referred pain identical to that seen in patients.[25]

Indications to proceed with a diagnostic interventional procedure, such as a medial branch block, to confirm facet mediated pain include: Low back pain present for greater than 3 months, pain score greater than 5, failure to respond to more conservative therapies, and other causes of lumbar pain have been ruled out such as lumbar disk herniation, etc. The patient should also be aware that the procedure is being done purely for diagnostic purposes to determine if the facet joints are the origin of their back pain. The patient should be educated on how to record the results of the procedure on a pain diary and the importance of a follow up appointment to discuss the results should be stressed.

The American Society of Interventional Pain Physicians (ASIPP) published revised Guidelines for Interventional Techniques in April 2013 including the workup and management of lumbar facet joint pain. The guidelines discussed and reviewed literature on the various ways to confirm the diagnosis of lumbar facet mediated pain, including diagnostic lumbar facet joint blocks, therapeutic facet joint nerve blocks, and intra-articular injections.

Controlled diagnostic blocks of the lumbar facet or zygapophysial joint can be performed by anesthetizing the joint via injection of local anesthetics intra-articularly or in close proximity to the medial branches of the dorsal rami that innervate the target joint. ASIPP's analysis of the evidence of controlled diagnostic blocks of the lumbar facet joint revealed good evidence for diagnostic facet joint nerve blocks with 75–100% pain relief as the criterion standard with dual blocks based on 13 controlled diagnostic block studies with fair evidence with 50–74% relief based on 5 studies with limited evidence for 75–100% pain relief as the criterion standard with a single block based on 4 studies and poor based on a single study with 50–74% pain relief as the criterion standard with a single block.[26]

Lumbar facet joint nerve blocks are often utilized to diagnosis facet mediated pain. These blocks are often done in pairs and the patient is given a pain diary to record the results to confirm the accuracy of the blocks. The injections are done prior to initiate treatment with radiofrequency ablation to these nerves. ASIPP's analysis of the evidence of lumbar facet joint nerve blocks determined that based on 2 high quality studies and one moderate quality study, the evidence for the lumbar facet nerve blocks using local anesthetics with or without steroid for managing chronic low back pain of facet origin is fair to good for short- and long-term improvement.[26]

Intra-articular facet injection of steroids with or without local anesthetic is thought to be beneficial to reduce facet mediated pain due to inflammation of the joint. ASIPP's analysis of the evidence of intra-articular facet injections based on the one moderate quality study with weakly positive or undetermined results and 5 observational studies,[26] the evidence for intra-articular injections is limited.

TREATMENT

Initial treatment of lumbar mediated facet pain should be conservative. Often, physical therapy in conjunction with oral medications is very effective in alleviating a patient's symptoms. Nonsteroidal anti-inflammatory drugs are effective in most cases in reducing the inflammation in the joint; however, in some cases the patient may require muscle relaxers or opioid pain medication if the pain is severe.

If conservative measures fail to adequately alleviate a patient's pain, intra-articular facet joint injections may be considered (Figs 2 and 3). In this case, the clinician will place a needle into the facet joint itself and inject it with a corticosteroid, such as triamcinolone, to reduce the irritation and inflammation of the nerve roots. This procedure may be repeated in some cases, depending on the duration of effect. If intra-articular facet joint injections fail to produce long term benefit and the diagnosis of facet mediated pain has been establish with diagnostic medial branch blocks, radiofrequency denervation (rhizotomy) can be considered for long term benefit. The patient

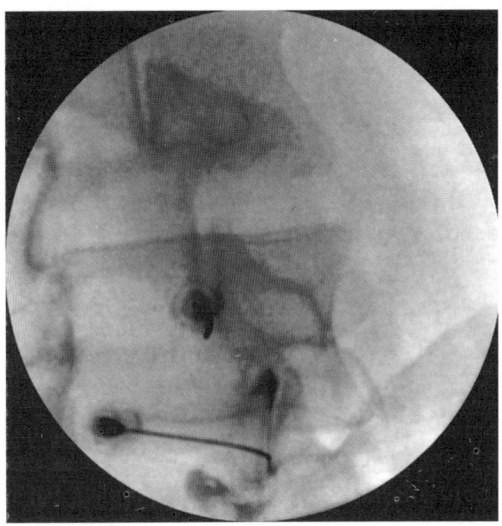

FIG. 3: Needle position lumbar facet joint L 3, 4, 5 – lateral view

should be educated that the radiofrequency denervation may take several weeks before the benefit of the procedure is seen.

Radiofrequency ablation of the lumbar facet nerves (medial branches) can be performed either by a heat (thermal) lesion or pulsed mode radiofrequency. Radiofrequency acts by denaturing the nerves and the pain may return when the axons regenerate requiring repeating the radiofrequency. Thermal radiofrequency lesioning is performed at 80–85°C, allowing for a larger lesion to be made. Pulsed mode radiofrequency is performed by administering a strong electric field to the tissue that surrounds the electrode and the temperature of the tissue surrounding the tip of the electrode does not exceed 42°C and heat is dissipated during the silent period.

ASIPP's analysis of the evidence of radiofrequency ablation of the lumbar facet nerves based on 6 positive randomized trials and 10 positive observation studies, the evidence for conventional radiofrequency neurotomy in managing chronic low back pain of facet joint origin in the lumbar spine is good for short and long term pain relief. Based on

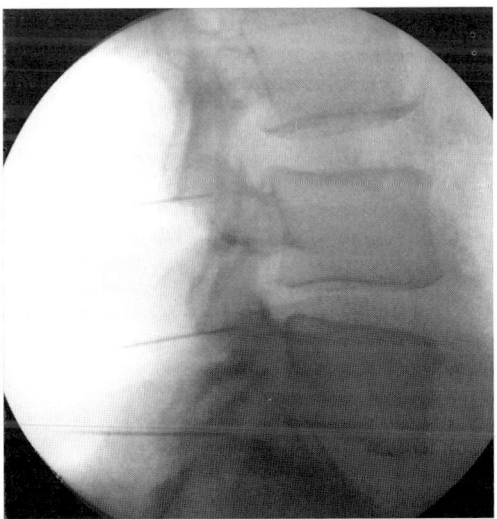

FIG. 2: Needle position lumbar facet joint L 3, 4, 5 – AP view

one randomized trial and one observational study meeting inclusion criteria, the evidence is limited for pulsed radiofrequency neurotomy for managing chronic low back pain of facet joint origin.[26]

Techniques and details of these procedures can be found in: (1) Interventional Pain Management: A Practical Approach, 2nd Edition Jaypee 2016; (2) Interventional Techniques in Chronic Spinal Pain, ASIPP, 2007: (3) Interventional Pain Management, 2nd Edition; W Saunders, 2000.

If conservative treatment and interventional pain management procedures fail to control a patient's pain, surgery may be indicated. Typically, a lumbar fusion will be performed to immobilize the facet joint to alleviate any pain that may occur with motion at the affected level. However, the surgeon will determine the appropriate surgery and a referral should be made.

CONCLUSION

Navigating the complexities of chronic low back pain is often a challenging and frustrating task of a clinician. Being well versed in spinal anatomy, taking an accurate history, performing a thorough neuromuscular physical examination, utilizing proper imaging and performing diagnostic procedures will aid in this challenge. Establishing the diagnosis of facet mediated chronic low back pain will require the clinician to utilize all these tools and this chapter can be used a guide to establish this diagnosis.

REFERENCES

1. Goldthwaite JE. The lumbosacral articulation: an explanation of many causes of lumbago, sciatica, and paraplegia. Boston Med Surg J. 1911;164:365-72.
2. Manchikanti L, Singh V, et al. Interventional techniques in chronic spinal pain: lumbar facet interventions. ASIPP. 2007;18:253-76.
3. Ghormley RK. Low back pain. With special reference to the articular facets, with presentation of an operative procedure. JAMA. 1933;101:1773-77.
4. Badgley CE. The articular facet in relation to low back pain and sciatic radiation. J Bone Joint Surg. 1941; 23:481.
5. Hirsch C, Ingelmark BE, Miller M: The anatomical basis for low back pain: Studies on the presence of sensory nerve endings in ligamentous, capsular and intervertebral disc structures in the human lumbar spine. Acta Orthop Scand. 1963;33:1-17.
6. Rees WE: Multiple bilateral subcutaneous rhizolysis of segmental nerves in the treatment of the intervertebral disc syndrome. Ann Gen Pract. 1971;26:126-7.
7. Shealy CN: Percutaneous radiofrequency denervation of the spinal facets: Treatment for chronic back pain and sciatica. J Neurosurg. 1975;43:448-51.
8. Shealy CN: Facet denervation in the management of back and sciatic pain. Clin Orthop. 1976;115:157-64.
9. Manchukonda R, Kavita KN, Cash KA. Facet joint pain in chronic spinal pain: an evaluation of prevalence and false- positive rate of diagnostic blocks. J Spinal Disord Tech. 2007;20(7):539-45.
10. Gelhorn AC, Katz JN. Osteoarthritis of the spine: the facet joints. Nat Rev Rheumatol. 2013;9(4):216-24.
11. Manchikanti L, Manchikanti KN, Cash KA, et al. Age-related prevalence of facet-joint involvement in chronic neck and low back pain. Pain Physician. 2008;1:67-75.
12. Schwarzer AC, Wang SC, Bogduk N, et al. Prevalence and clinical features of lumbar zygapophyseal joint pain: a study in an Australian population with chronic low back pain. Ann Rheu Dis. 1995;54(2):100-6.
13. Moore KL, Dalley AF, et al. Clinically Oriented Anatomy, 4th edition. Lippencott Williams and Wilkens, 1999.
14. Waldman S. Interventional Pain Management, 2nd edition. W Saunders; 2001.pp.454.
15. Mooney V. Facet syndrome: Clinical entities. Weinstein JN, Weisel SW. The Lumbar Spine. (The International Society for the Study of the Lumbar Spine) Philadelphia. W Saunders; 1990.pp.422-41.
16. Bakshi S, Abrahamsen A. Lumbar Facet and Medial Branch Block. Interventional Pain Management: A Practical Approach. Jaypee; 2009.pp.190-7.
17. Windsor RE, King FJ, et al. Electrical stimulation induced lumbar medial branch referral patterns. Pain Physician. 2002;5:347-53.
18. Schwarzer AC, Wang SC, O'Driscoll D, et al. The ability of computed tomography to identify a painful zygapophysial joint in patients with chronic low back pain. Spine. 1995;20:907-12.
19. Matar H, Navalkissoor S, Berovic, Shetty R, Garlick N, Casey A, Quigley A. Is hybrid imaging (SPECT/CT) a useful adjunct in the management of suspected facet joints arthropathy. 2013;37:865-0.

20. Schwarzer AC, Wang S, Bogduk N, McNaught PJ, Laurent R. Prevalence and clinical features of lumbar zygapophysial joint pain: A study in an Australian population with chronic low back pain. Ann Rheum Dis. 1995; 54:100-6.
21. Schwarzer AC, Derby R, Aprill CN, Fortin J, Kine G, Bogduk N. Pain from the lumbar zygapophysial: A test of two models. J Spinal Disord. 1994;7:331-6.
22. Revel M, Poiraudeau S, Auleley GR, Payan C, Denke A, Nguyen M, Chevrot A, Fermanian J. Capacity of the clinical picture to characterize low back pain relieved by facet joint anesthesia. Proposed criteria to identify patients with painful facet joints. Spine. 1998;23:1972-77.
23. Mooney V, Robertson J. The facet syndrome. Clinical orthopedics. 1976;115:149-56.
24. Pampati S, Cash KA, Manchikanti L. Accuracy of diagnostic lumbar facet joint nerve blocks: a 2-year follow up of 152 patients diagnosed with controlled diagnostic blocks. Pain Physician. 2009;12:855-66.
25. Manchikanti L, Singh V, et al. Interventional techniques in chronic spinal pain: lumbar facet interventions. ASIPP. 2007;18:253-76.
26. Manchikanti L, et al. An update of comprehensive evidence-based guidelines for interventional techniques in chronic spinal pain. Part II: Guidance and recommendations. Pain Physician. 2013;16:S115-S132.

CHAPTER 20

Lumbar Spinal Stenosis

Steve M Aydin, Thomas P Lione

INTRODUCTION

Lumbar spinal stenosis (LSS) is a common cause of pain and disability due to narrowing of the spinal canal and/or neuroforamen, especially in older adults. The prevalence and overall burden of LSS continues to grow due to an increase in the aging population.[1,2] It is considered a chronic disease caused primarily by age related degenerative narrowing of the spinal canal leading to compression and ischemia of the spinal nerves. LSS typically manifests as unilateral or bilateral buttock, lower extremity pain, heaviness, numbness, tingling or weakness, often exacerbated by walking and standing, but relieved by sitting and forward flexion.[1] LSS can be the result of a primary or secondary cause. Primary causes typically result from congenital anatomical variants and development, whereas secondary causes are more commonly related to acquired anatomy and other etiologies that may result in spinal canal or neuroforaminal narrowing.[2-4]

CAUSES

Lumbar spinal stenosis can be classified according to anatomical etiology and can be characterized as: central, lateral, and/or foraminal stenosis.[2-4]

Central canal stenosis may result from a decrease in the anteroposterior or transverse space, or a combination due to disk height loss. This can occur with or without herniation of the intervertebral disk and hypertrophy of the facet joints and the ligamentum flavum.[5] Typically, it is fibrosis that causes ligamentum flavum hypertrophy secondary to mechanical stress. A similar process of decreased disk height, facet joint hypertrophy and/or vertebral endplate osteophytosis can also result in lateral recess stenosis.[5] The foraminal stenosis can be either anteroposterior or vertical and typically results from a combination of disk space narrowing and overgrowth anterior to the facet joint capsule, and/or from posterolateral osteophytes from vertebral endplates protruding into the foramen or a herniated disk compressing a nerve root.[5]

Primary LSS is the result of idiopathic, congenital, or achondroplastic causes. Secondary stenosis occurs as a result of degenerative processes such as spondylosis, spondylolisthesis, and/or scoliosis. Hypertrophy or ossification of ligaments can also cause LSS. Other causes of secondary LSS may include infections, neoplasms, rheumatologic conditions, traumas, endocrine, or iatrogenic causes.[6-8]

LSS can affect one or multiple levels of the lumbar spine and its development is usually multifactorial. Research has shown that higher levels of circulating inflammatory factors also contribute to LSS. Specifically, high levels of interleukin-1β have been found in inflamed and arthritic lumbar facet joints, which is postulated to diffuse into the spinal canal and to the stabilizing surrounding lumbar ligaments.[9-11]

The majority of patients presenting with symptoms of lumbar spinal stenosis will be older than 50 years of age and most commonly have symptoms related to secondary causes of LSS.[12] As the spinal canal and neuroforaminal space diminishes, the pressure on the spinal cord and other nervous system structures becomes more compromised. The available space may fluctuate depending on patient positioning.[13] It has been demonstrated that epidural pressure increases in extension of the lumbar spine and static standing. Contrastingly, flexion and sitting unloads the epidural space allowing for the spinal canal to widen. This is in contrast to the load and pressure felt by the lumbar disks.[14-17]

This notion of increased pressure on the spinal cord and nervous system structures in LSS further contributes to the understanding of neurogenic claudication, also known as pseudoclaudication.[1] This term refers to pain from lumbar spinal stenosis referring down from the lumbar area into the extremities while ambulating or during functional tasks. Clinical presentation will include pain, cramping, and burning worsened by ambulation or extension positions. These symptoms will often resolve after a few minutes (usually >5 minutes) of rest.[2,15-18]

The narrowing or increased pressure on the nervous structures in the canal and neuroforamen are also thought to cause a reduction in arterial blood flow resulting in transient ischemia. Venous congestion can also develop. The symptoms of pain are also believed to be the result of an autonomic deregulation of the vascular system for the lower extremity, as a result of more proximal insult at the spinal level.[2,10-11]

SIGNS AND SYMPTOMS

Although LSS is a clinical diagnosis that relies on anatomic description, the assessment of the severity of LSS depends on the patient's description of symptoms and on physical examination.

Lumbar spinal stenosis can present with a myriad of symptoms. It is most often seen in the aging population greater than 50 years of age. It can present slowly and progressively, worsening over time. Typically, it will initially present with lower back pain that will get worse with ambulation or certain positioning.[19]

Symptoms can be coupled with paresthesias into the lower lumbar region, the buttocks, and eventually down the legs. The distribution of pain in the lower extremities is dependent on the location of stenosis. Occasionally a cramping like sensation will be described as well.[2,20]

Symptoms may be unilateral or bilateral, and do not have to be present in a symmetrical pattern. Neurogenic claudication (also known as pseudoclaudication) will be described as pain in the leg with cramping, which worsens with ambulation. Patients will often complain of pain in the lower extremities that worsens with prolonged ambulation. They will also provide a history of pain that inhibits them from walking as far as they used to. Upon sitting, resting, or leaning forward the pain will improve and dissipate over minutes.[2,19]

Patients may complain of a heavy feeling in the legs, weakness in the extremities, as well as, in severe cases, bowel or bladder dysfunction. They will often have precipitous decline in daily functioning, activities of daily living, and/or ambulation. Severe cases may also present with balance and proprioceptive impairment.[2,16-19]

CLINICAL EXAMINATION AND FINDINGS

As with all patient encounters, the history and physical is a critical part of the diagnosis of any medical problem. In the cases of lumbar spinal stenosis specific questions regarding the history should be asked and focused on.

History should focus on questions regarding duration, onset, quality, location, intensity, improvement/worsening actions, function, and prior treatments. Questions regarding patient's ambulation history, with specific distances that can be walked should be asked. Inquire about whether or not pain improves with the use of a rolling walker or shopping cart. History regarding bowel and bladder incontinence or retention should also be obtained.

For the physical exam, observation of the patient ambulating and sitting should be done at the start of the encounter. Palpation of the spine and extremities should also be done. Inspection of the skin as well as the posture of the lumbar region should be checked. The range of motion, of the lumbar spine and lower extremities is followed by sensation and reflexes. Strength testing of the bilateral lower extremities should also be checked. Examination of the lower back may reveal reduced mobility with extension being more limited than flexion.[5] Hamstring tightness may also be described.

Inspection of the spine should also assess lordosis. With loss of lumbar lordosis, the spinal canal may widen, and the neuroforamen are more open. When the patient is sitting, and has a forward posture or leaning forward onto their knees supported by their arms, the patient is unloading the spine and maintaining a flexed position to open the spinal canal and neuroforamin.

Reflexes may be normal or depressed. However, in certain cases of lumbar spinal stenosis, hyperreflexia with clonus and/or spasticity may be noted, as this may be a sign of myelopathy. Sensation may be normal, or have some areas of decreased sensation, as well as loss of proprioception. A uniform pattern is not necessarily seen in all cases.

Strength testing should be done in all the key muscle groups of the bilateral lower extremities; hip flexors, knee extensors, ankle dorsiflexors, ankle plantar flexors, and great toe extensors. Muscle strength may be normal or weakened. Many patients may have normal strength at time of examination; however, with ambulation they may develop weakness with symptoms of neurogenic claudication.[4,19]

Observation of the patient's gait, balance, and endurance is important as well. Gait will often be coupled with a broad based gait, with slightly flexed knees and hips, allowing for the patient to flatten the lumbar lordosis, opening the spinal canal and neuroforamen. In many cases, the patient will adapt to using a shopping cart or functional rolling walker to allow for prolonged ambulation and support. When inspecting range of motion of the lower extremities, the pelvis will be anteriorly rotated, while the hamstring will be tight and popliteal angles will be increased. A Romberg's maneuver will often be done to appreciate the patient's proprioceptive function. The Romberg's test can sometime be positive, if the dorsal columns of the spinal cord become compromised by the stenosis in the central canal.[2,4]

The combination of a good history and physical exam will facilitate an appropriate, accurate diagnosis and work-up for the patient. Special attention should be given to ambulation, function, as well as overall patient safety.

DIAGNOSTIC CRITERIA AND IMAGING

Lumbar spinal stenosis does not have a specific classification system to diagnosis severity of disease. Symptoms can be categorized into anatomic or primary versus secondary causes. History and physical exam is the most important diagnostic tool in most cases. Imaging and electrodiagnostic testing (EMG) may aid in confirming the diagnosis.

Imaging may include X-ray, CT scan, MRI, and myelogram. Electrodiagnostic and nerve conduction studies (NCS) may also be obtained to help assist in making the diagnosis. The primary purpose of imaging is to assess the diameter of the spinal canal. Absolute stenosis is noted when the diameter is less than 10 mm, while relative spinal stenosis is noted to be between 10 mm and 12 mm.

Central canal and neuroforaminal stenosis can best be assessed with MRI (Figs 1 and 2) and CT scan (Figs 3A to C). This will provide both an axial and sagittal view of the spine.

CT myelogram may be employed to illustrate bony details as well as the nerve root anatomy, but this is a more invasive type of procedure (Figs 4A and B).

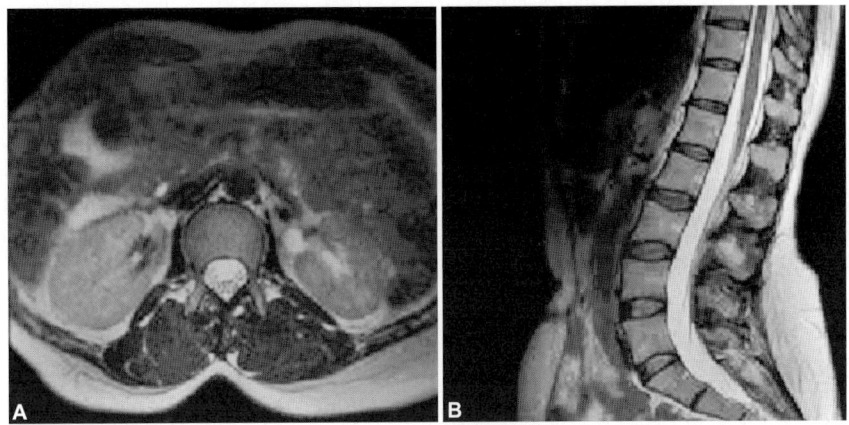

FIGS 1 A and B: MRI of lumbar spine T2 sagittal axial view-A nonstenotic tumor spine, showing good amount of space for spinal cord and nerve roots

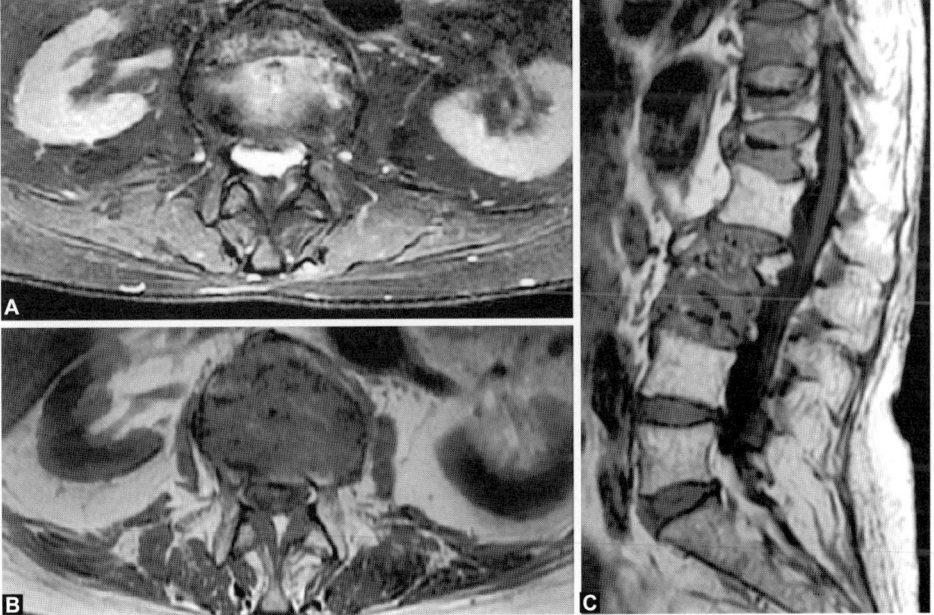

FIGS 2A to C: MRI of lumbar spine and axial views-note narrowing at multiple levels on the sagittal T1 view. The axial view of T1, 2 and shows narrowing of spinal canal relative to the figures in 1A and B

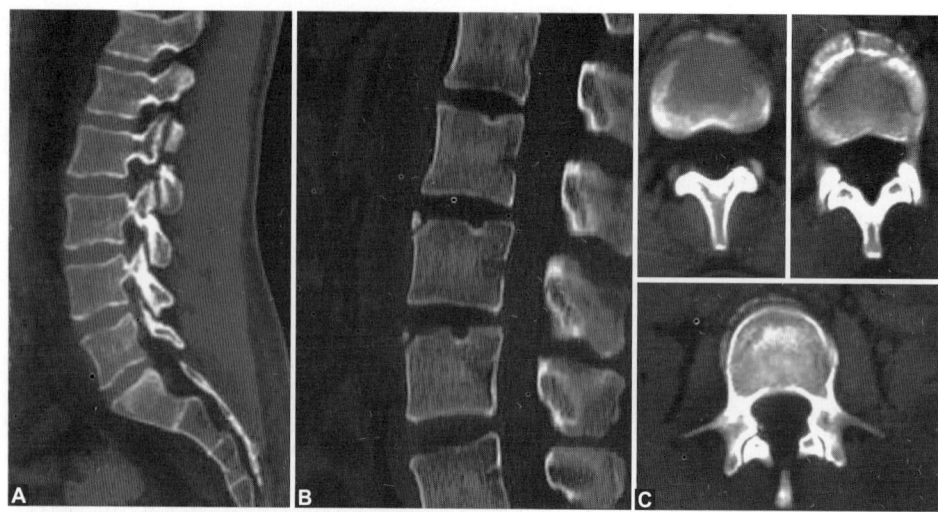

FIGS 3A to C CT scan of lumbar spine axial and sagittal views. This represents nonstenotic spinal view

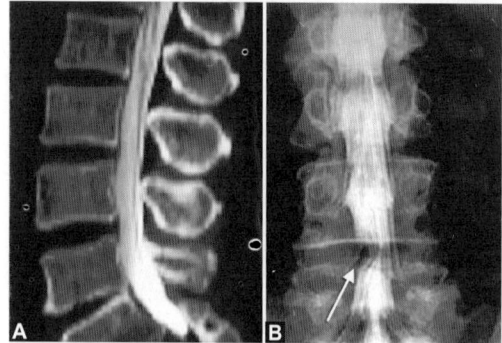

FIGS 4A and B: CT myelogram showing an abnormal flow-where the arrow is, indicating spinal canal stenosis at that level

EMG/NCS is often used to help determine if a coexisting peripheral neuropathy may be present in addition to symptoms of spinal stenosis.

TREATMENT OPTIONS

For pain resulting from lumbar spinal stenosis, conservative treatments should be attempted initially. Physical therapy, range of motion exercises, and home exercise regimens should be employed to improve and optimize strength and flexibility. Focus on improving endurance to slow the sequelae of deconditioning should also be emphasized.[5]

In the case of LSS, the most common complaint from patients is a decline in ambulation distance and radiating pain into the lower extremities.

First-line conservative treatments for LSS pain include analgesics, NSAIDs, opioids, and muscle relaxants. Typically, a pain reducer such as acetaminophen is tried initially. Caution should be exercised to ensure doses do not exceed 2–3 g daily. If pain continues, nonsteroidal anti-inflammatory drugs (NSAIDs) may also be employed. NSAIDs should also be used with caution due to gastrointestinal, cardiovascular, and renal side effects. Opioid medication and muscle relaxants may also be considered in some cases, but should be reserved for more refractory cases when pain is severe.[2,4,19]

Neuropathic membrane stabilizing medicines such as gabapentin and pregabalin may also be utilized. Additionally, tricyclic antidepressants have also been shown to be helpful; however, caution must be used due to their anticholinergic side effects, especially in the elderly.

Interventional procedures have been used with success to treat symptoms and alleviate pain. Commonly, epidural steroid injections are done via different approaches such as interlaminar, transforaminal, or caudal to reduce inflammation.[20-22] Typically, local anesthetic is also used in combination with steroid, and aids in symptomatic relief beyond the time of the half-life of the local anesthetic. This is postulated to be related to the sympathetic blockade that occurs.

Minimally invasive procedures have also been used by some interventional pain physicians. For lumbar central canal stenosis, a procedure known as minimally invasive lumbar decompression (MILD) exists and may be appropriate in certain cases. This procedure involves a percutaneous laminectomy and thinning of the ligamentum flavum resulting in an increased canal diameter, therefore decreasing the severity of stenosis on the neural structures.[23]

Alternative treatment options such as manipulation, acupuncture, and alternative medicines can also be helpful for some patients.

In cases refractory to more conservative treatments such as medications, therapy, and interventions, surgical evaluation may be appropriate. The risks and benefits for every patient should be considered, as well as other premorbid medical issues. Surgery may be an option to relieve pressure on the neural structures and help relieve symptoms in severe cases with increasing pain, decreasing function, and/or neurologic compromise.

CONCLUSION

Lumbar spinal stenosis is a condition that can profoundly limit both function and mobility. Patients with LSS will often present with a decline in ambulation and pain radiating into the legs, which typically improves with rest. A detailed history and physical are essential for diagnosis, along with appropriate imaging. Many patients will respond to conservative treatment, however, interventional options may be employed to improve function and quality of life.

REFERENCES

1. Ammendolia C. Degenerative lumbar spinal stenosis and its imposters: three case studies. J Can Chiropr Assoc. 2014;58(3).
2. Katz MD, et al. lumbar spinal stenosis. N Eng J Med. 2008;358:818-25.
3. Katz JN, et al. Degenerative Lumbar spinal stenosis: Diagnostic value of history and physical examination. Arthritis Rheum. 1995;38:1236-41.
4. Siebert E, et al. Lumbar spinal stenosis: Syndrome, diagnostic and treatment. Nat Rev Neurol. 2009;5:392-403.
5. Genevay S, et al. Lumbar spinal stenosis. Best Practice & Research Clinical Rheumatology. 2010;24:253-65.
6. Fogel GR, et al. Spinal epidural lipomatosis: case reports, literature review and meta-analysis. Spine J. 2005;5: 202-11.
7. Atlas SJ & Delitto A. Spinal stenosis: surgical versus nonsurgical treatment. Clin Orthop Relat Res. 2006;443: 198-207.
8. Kobayashi S, et al. Blood Circulation of cauda equina and nerve root [Japanese]. Clin Calcium. 2005;15:63-72.
9. Porter RW. Spinal stenosis and neurogenic claudication. Spine. 1996;21:2046-52.
10. Igarashi A, Kikuchi S, Konno S. Correlation between inflammatory cytokines released from the land symptoms in degenerative lumbar spinal disorders. J Orthop Sci. 2007;12(2):154-60.
11. Chosa E, Sekimoto T, Kubo S, Tajima N. Evaluation of circulatory compromise in the leg in lumbar spinal canal stenosis. Clin Orthop Relat Res. 2005;431:129-33.
12. Danielson B, Willén J. Axially loaded magnetic resonance, image of the lumbar spine in asymptomatic individuals. Spine. 2001;26:2601-6.
13. Adamova B, Vohanka, S. Dusek L. Dynamic electrophysiological examination in patients with lumbar spinal stenosis: is it useful in clinical practice? Eur Spine J. 2005;14:269-76.
14. Weinstein JN, et al. Surgical versus nonsurgical therapy for lumbar spinal stenosis. N Engl J Med. 2008;358: 794-810.
15. Ciricillo SF, Weintein PR. Lumbar spinal stenosis. West J Med. 1993;158:11-7.
16. Schonstrom N, Lindahl S, Willen J, et al. Dynamic changes in the dimensions of the lumbar spinal canal: an experimental study in vitro. J Orthop Res. 1989; 7(1):115-21.

17. Bridwell KH. Lumbar spinal stenosis. Diagnosis, management, and treatment. Clin Geriatr Med. 1994; 10(4):677-701.
18. Mazanec DJ, et al. Lumbar canal stenosis: Start with nonsurgical therapy. Cleveland Clinic of Journal of Medicine. 2002;69:909-17.
19. Seung—Yeop L, et al. Lumbar stenosis: A recent update by review of literature. Asian Spine Journal. 9.5;2015.pp.818-28.
20. Friedly J, Chan L, Deyo R. Increases in lumbosacral injections in the medicare population: 1994 to 2001. Spine. 2007;32(16):1754-60.
21. Ng LC, Sell P. Outcomes of a prospective cohort study on periradicular infiltration for radicular pain in patients with lumbar disc herniation and spinal stenosis. Eur Spine J. 2004;13(4):325-9.
22. Gibson JN, Waddell G. Surgery for degenerative lumbar spondylosis. Cochrane Database Syst Rev. 2005;4: CD001352.
23. Deer TR, Karural L. New image-guided ultra minimally invasive lumbar decompression method: The mild procedure. Pain Physician. 2010;13:35-41.

Lumbar Diskogenic Back Pain

Selaiman Noori, Sudhir Diwan, Neel Mehta

INTRODUCTION

Low back pain is a major cause of pain and disability in the industrialized nations, and therefore, a significant economic and public health burden. It is the leading cause of work absenteeism and lost productivity, far exceeding any other medical condition. In 2012, low back symptoms accounted for 1.4 percent of principal reasons for office visits in the United States.[1] It has been estimated to result in 175.8 million days of restricted activity annually in the United States, and at any given time, 2.4 million Americans are disabled from low back pain (LBP).[2] In most industrialized nations, the lifetime prevalence of LBP is estimated to be as high as 84 percent,[3] with up to 12% of the population being disabled by it.[4] Although most cases of LBP are self-limited, approximately 20% recur within six months and a subset of patients will develop chronic pain.[5] In approximately 40% of LBP complaints in adults, the etiology of pain can be attributed to a diskogenic origin.[6,7] In a 2006 review by Katz, the total costs of spinal disorders in the United States were estimated to be in excess of $100 billion per year. Two-thirds of these costs were attributable to lost wages and productivity.[8] Therefore, LBP is not only a major healthcare problem; it is a socioeconomic challenge, as well.

CAUSES

Lumbar disk pain is a very complicated, multifactorial process in which a detailed characterization remains elusive. However, biological, mechanical, and environmental factors are widely considered as key contributors to the degenerative process.[9] Although there are differences that can be seen between normal and degenerative lumbar disks, disk degeneration is part of the normal aging process and the vast majority of degenerative disks are asymptomatic.

Causes of internal disk derangement, also referred to as degenerative disk disease (DDD), usually involve an accumulation of traumatic events ranging in severity and ultimately causing degeneration of the annulus fibrosus. During the process of degradation, there is development of annular fissures, allowing for migration of nucleus pulposus content. The inner nucleus pulposus has no nerve supply, however, the outer third of the surrounding annulus is innervated. Leaked nuclear proteins incite an autoimmune reaction involving upregulation of several proinflammatory cytokines, including interleukin-1 beta and tumor necrosis factor alpha, which can lead to sensitization of annular sensory nerves.[10] Furthermore, tiny blood vessels in the disk

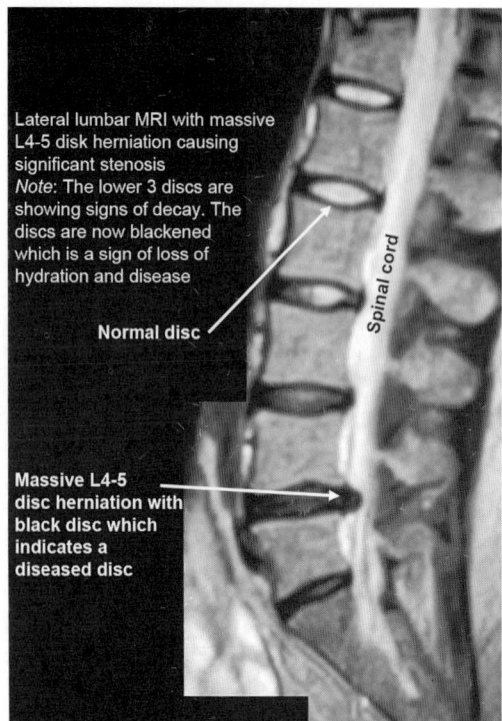

FIG. 1: Comparison of normal disk vs. disk herniation

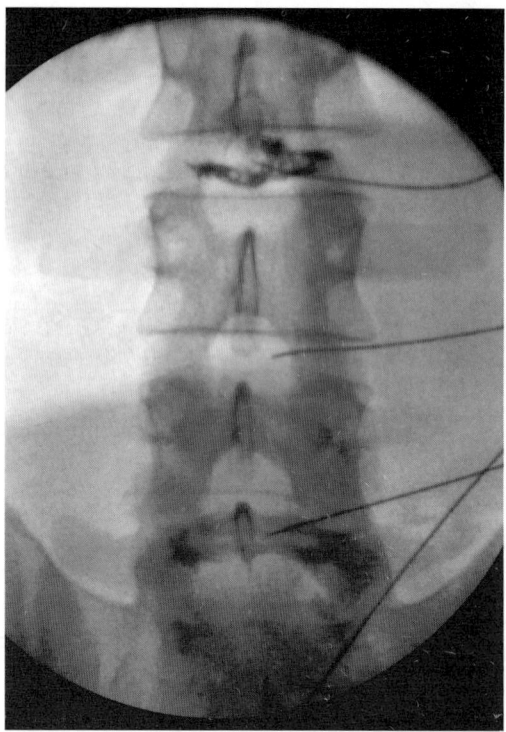

FIG. 2: 3 Level diskogram showing healthy L3/4 and L4/5 disk, but leak at L2/3 disk

become obliterated over time, leaving the intervertebral disk an avascular structure supported only through extracellular fluid osmosis. With the aging process, there is net loss of proteoglycans and water content from the gelatinous nucleus, leading to impairment of nutrition and healing ability, and a reduction in hydrostatic pressure and intervertebral disk height. Secondary to the combination of these events, any mechanical turbulence, such as that caused by twisting or weight-bearing, provokes pain and leads to chronic symptoms.[11]

The deterioration process also leads to a stiffening of the intervertebral disk, which alters the axial load distribution and in turn overloads the surrounding annulus.[12] Axial rotation of the spine or rotation of a flexed spine may isolate some of the annular fibers and cause further annular tears. These annular injuries may or may not be symptomatic, but over time, they can coalesce to weaken the annulus fibrosus. The increased stress on the annulus can lead to structural failures, such as disk bulging, disk space narrowing, or even frank herniation. In addition, the loss of disk space height may lead to segmental instability and increased forces on zygapophyseal joints, resulting in sclerosis and hypertrophy. Ultimately, this degenerative cascade can lead to a narrowing of the spinal canal and intervertebral foramen, producing an acquired spinal stenosis.

SIGNS AND SYMPTOMS

Herniated disks occur primarily in the second through fifth decades of life and have a slight male preponderance. The L4-5 disk has been shown to be the most commonly herniated disk (closely followed by the L5-S1 disk), resulting in an L5 radiculopathy.[13] Over 85% of patients who present to primary care, however, have nonspecific LBP—that is, LBP in which a specific disorder or anatomical abnormality cannot reliably be identified.[14] There are no specific characteristics in the patient history that confirm or disprove the diagnosis of diskogenic LBP. Diskogenic pain is typically aggravated by upright sitting, lumbar flexion, coughing, sneezing, or activities that increase intradiskal pressure.[15] Pain eventually may radiate into the leg, characterized as achy, burning, or electrical shock and is often described as a shooting or stabbing pain. Common features of radiculopathy are leg pain in a dermatomal distribution, exacerbation of pain with a sitting position, and amelioration of pain during standing or ambulation. Higher herniations (third or fourth lumbar levels) can radiate into the groin or anterior thigh. Lower radiculopathies (first sacral level) cause pain in the calf and bottom of the foot. Fifth lumbar radiculopathy, which occurs most commonly, causes lateral and anterior thigh and leg pain. Often, accompanying numbness or tingling occurs with a distribution similar to the pain. Associated muscle weakness may be unrecognized if the pain is incapacitating. Lying supine with legs slightly elevated usually alleviates pain. Short walks can bring relief, however, long walks often aggravate the pain.

CLINICAL EXAMINATION

Despite the enormous resources devoted to it, diskogenic pain lacks clear diagnostic criteria as there are no disease defining characteristics in the history or physical examination. Patients may be neurologically normal, may have a profound radiculopathy, or may even demonstrate a cauda equina syndrome. A positive straight leg raising sign is almost always present, however, a crossed straight leg raising sign may be even more predictive of a lumbar disk herniation. The back may appear scoliotic, gait is often abnormal, and muscle weakness may be present when testing heel and toe walking. Pain as a result of pressure on the spinous process is considered characteristic of diskogenic LBP. Together, these symptoms often correlate to axial back pain or lumbar sprain/strain. Examination findings may aid in treatment planning or monitoring patient progress, but for the majority of patients, exam features will not provide a diagnosis.[16]

DIAGNOSTIC CRITERIA

The use of diagnostic imaging is prevalent in the workup of suspected diskogenic pain. Imaging techniques used include computed tomography (CT), magnetic resonance imaging (MRI), plain radiographs (X-rays), myelography, and CT-myelography. A 2013 review by Malik et al. found that MRI was the most frequently used imaging modality, followed by X-rays and CT.[17] MRI is helpful in visualizing disk pathologies, such as degeneration, desiccation, and loss of height, however, radiographic findings commonly correlate poorly with clinical presentation. It is well known that asymptomatic disks may appear abnormal on MRI, while normal appearing disks have been shown to be abnormal on provocation.[18] The inconsistency between radiographic findings and clinical presentation leaves open the critical question of causality. In many cases, provocative diskography may provide the link in diagnosing suspected diskogenic origins of back pain. It is the only imaging technique that directly relates the morphologic abnormalities seen on MRI with clinically observed pain.[19]

INVESTIGATIONS SUGGESTED

Plain radiographs can detect underlying structurally pathologic conditions. However, these studies generally are not recommended during the first month of symptoms unless there are correlating worrisome symptoms or suspicion for fracture. X-rays allow visualization of facet joints, neuroforamen, and the pars interarticularis, helping to detect degenerative changes of the spine. In some cases, there can be evidence of certain features that are pertinent to localizing the site of pain.

CT of the lumbar spine provides superior anatomical imaging of the osseous structures of the spine, as well as good resolution for detecting disk herniation. As with MRI, the frequency of false-positive findings in asymptomatic patients is high. Therefore, CT is best used when a fracture is suspected, although it can be used in the detection of disk injury in patients who cannot undergo MRI. In addition, CT is recommended when more detailed imaging of the bony architecture is important.

A myelogram involves penetration of the subarachnoid space and is often performed in conjunction with a CT scan. Myelography is generally reserved as a preoperative test to assist in surgical planning. It provides a detailed anatomic picture, particularly of spinal osseous elements, which allows correlation with examination findings. Myelography is rarely used in the nonoperative evaluation of patients with acute LBP, except in cases in which the clinical picture supports a progressive neurologic deficit and MRI and electromyogram have been nondiagnostic.

MRI provides high-resolution imaging that allows accurate description of intervertebral disk pathology. In T2-weighted MRI sequences, compartments with high water content appear bright, correlating positively with signal intensity. Therefore, T2 MRI is sensitive to disk degeneration where there is reduction in signal intensity of the nucleus pulposus secondary to altered hydration status.[20] Sagittal sections reveal the vertebral column, intervertebral disks, spinal canal, and spinal cord. Axial views show disks, vertebral bodies, the spinal cord, and spinal roots. Neural element encroachment seen on the sagittal view can be confirmed on axial view. MRI is also useful for assessment of canal encroachment and spinal stenosis. As with CT, MRI can increase the identification of clinically irrelevant abnormalities that may cause harm if a cascade of unnecessary tests and/or treatments is triggered.[21] Therefore, each study must be correlated to the patient's history, physical examination, and other diagnostic tests.

Areas known as high-intensity zones (HIZs) are bright white signals present in the posterior annulus fibrosus of lumbar disks on T2-weighted MRI. The HIZ is clearly demarcated from the nucleus pulposus in that it is surrounded on all sides by the low-intensity (black) signal of the annulus fibrosus and is appreciably brighter than the signal of the nucleus. Histologic examination of the HIZ revealed it to be a site of highly vascularized granulation tissue in annular tears of painful disks.[22] It is suggested that the inflammatory process leading to HIZ formation causes irritation of pain fibers.[23] HIZs are not a sign of back pain because they occur in asymptomatic individuals, as well. However, studies have shown that HIZs have high specificity, occurring in about 30% of patients with chronic LBP. Therefore, if a suspected disk has an HIZ present, it is very likely to be the source of pain.[24]

Electrodiagnostic studies, including nerve conduction studies, needle electromyography, and somatosensory evoked potentials, are helpful when the diagnosis remains unclear in patients with limb pain. They also aid in excluding other causes of sensory and motor disturbances, such as peripheral neuropathy and motor neuron disease. Additionally, electrodiagnostics can provide useful prognostic information by quantifying the extent and acuity of axonal involvement in radiculopathies. Electrodiagnostic studies performed less than 3 weeks after the onset of symptoms may result in a false-negative study since evidence of denervation does not appear until 2 to 3 weeks postinjury. When imaging studies reveal multiple abnormalities, which are common in older individuals with degenerative changes, electrodiagnosis can assist in localizing the etiology of the patient's symptoms.

Lumbar diskography is the second most frequently used test to diagnose diskogenic pain and can be helpful in patients who have not responded to a well-coordinated rehabilitation program or have normal or equivocal MRI findings. In such cases, provocative diskography may have some benefit in localizing a symptomatic disk as the etiology of nonradicular back pain. A positive diskogram must include reproduction of symptoms upon injection of a symptomatic disk, a nonpainful response upon injection of control disks, and observed annular pathology on postdiskography CT scan. Diskography offers a more precise technique for delineating diskovertebral pathology, with sensitivities similar to or better than MRI and CT with or without myelography.[25] However, provocative diskography has been associated with controversy due to unproven validity and multiple studies of small sample sizes demonstrating low specificity and a high rate of patient-specific false-positive responses.[26,27] Certain groups of patients also tend to over report pain during diskographic injection, and practitioners should have a screening tool seeking out those with financial gain, malingering, and somatization. A 2008 systematic review of all studies on disk stimulation, however, increased the sample size of study subjects and found the false-positive rate to be less than 10%.[28]

Still, diskography is an invasive procedure and long-term follow-up of diskography patients has demonstrated acceleration of disk degeneration.[29] Although it has yet to be demonstrated that any targeted intervention can reliably treat disks identified as the anatomic source of pain by provocative diskography, some authors argue there is diagnostic utility in disk stimulation.[30,31] Namely, it gives the patient a source for their pain, protects them from inappropriate testing and treatment, and allows delivery of more appropriate therapy.

DIFFERENTIAL DIAGNOSIS

The differential diagnosis is first and foremost directed at ruling out red flags, such as trauma and fractures, infection, tumors, and neurological complications. Thereafter, one strives to rule out visceral pain. Before making a decision about the interventional treatment plan, it is important to demonstrate that the diskus intervertebralis is the cause of the (pseudo-) radicular pain. Common associated diagnoses included lumbosacral facet syndrome, radiculopathy, pars interarticularis injury, sacroiliac joint injury, lumbosacral spine acute bony injuries, spine strain/strain injuries, and spondylolysis. Furthermore, practitioners must be careful to investigate spinal stenosis, piriformis syndrome, peripheral vascular disease, cauda equina syndrome, abdominal aortic aneurysm, renal calculi, pelvic inflammatory disease, infective processes (e.g., epidural abscess, osteomyelitis), rheumatoid arthritis, and ankylosing spondylitis.

TREATMENT PROTOCOL

Although it is considered a "degenerative" or aging process, patients with diskogenic back pain often improve over time. During the acute phase of a rehabilitation program, treatment focuses on reducing pain symptoms. Instruction in posture and body mechanics in activities of daily living is aimed at protecting injured structures, reducing symptoms, and preventing further injury. Patients should be instructed to avoid positions that increase intradiskal pressure, such as sitting, bending, and lifting. A short course of bed rest (1–2 days) may provide some beneficial effects via pain modulation and reduction of intradiskal pressure, but longer courses of bed rest yield detrimental effects on bone, connective tissue, muscle, and cardiovascular fitness. There is no evidence for the combination of treatments such as traction, manipulation, hot packs, or corsets.[32] Modalities, such as electrical stimulation, should be limited to the initial stages of treatment so that patients can quickly progress to more active treatment that includes restoration of motion and strengthening.

Immediate surgical consultation is warranted in the setting of acute diskogenic back or leg pain associated with progressive neurologic loss. Urgent surgical decompression is necessary in patients presenting with cauda equina syndrome, characterized by saddle anesthesia (i.e., perineal numbness) and bowel or bladder dysfunction. Other indications for surgical intervention are less well defined, and there is inconclusive data showing that operative intervention restores neurologic function more rapidly than nonoperative treatment. Patients who recover without surgery usually demonstrate signs of improvement within the first 3-6 weeks from the time of onset. Many authors suggest that it is reasonable to operate on patients with significant neurologic loss (e.g., a foot drop) that has not improved by 6 weeks post-injury.

Various medications have been used in the treatment of LBP from DDD, including acetaminophen, nonsteroidal anti-inflammatory drugs (NSAIDs), muscle relaxants, opioid analgesics, oral corticosteroids, and antidepressants. Before prescribing these medications, the physician should be aware of the contraindications, common adverse effects, and mode of action of each agent. There are no known studies that have demonstrated that long-term antinociceptive medication has any significant positive effect in patients with diskogenic low back pain. Generally, medication such as NSAIDs and weak opioids are recommended for a limited duration of use (maximum of three months). [33]

Nonopioid analgesics, such as NSAIDs and acetaminophen, are widely regarded as first-line agents. NSAIDs offer additional anti-inflammatory effects compared with acetaminophen and have been shown by several studies to be slightly better for chronic pain relief.[34,35] Risks are associated with NSAIDs, especially in the elderly population and in those with a history of peptic ulcer disease, hypertension, or renal insufficiency. Cyclooxygenase (COX)-2 selective inhibitors are newer generation NSAIDs that have lower risk of gastrointestinal side effects, however, their long-term use is precluded by an increased risk of myocardial infarction. Adult doses include ibuprofen 400-600 mg four times daily with food or celecoxib, a COX-2 inhibitor, 200 mg daily, or alternatively, 100 mg twice daily.

Although there is a scarcity of high-quality or long-term trials studying the efficacy of opioid use specifically for chronic back pain, the use of short-term opioids may be appropriate for LBP that is unresponsive to alternative medication.[36,37] On the other hand, opioids should be used with caution for long-term treatment.[38] Opioids can be prescribed for acute disk herniation or severe acute exacerbations of LBP to facilitate participation in an active rehabilitation program. They should be used on a defined dosing schedule and not on an as-needed basis. In addition, adequate baseline levels should be established to achieve analgesia. If opiate medication is deemed necessary, a trial of oxycodone 5-10 mg every 4-6 hours can be used. The use of non-opioid analgesics, such as tramadol (Ultram), is also an option. Tramadol inhibits the reuptake of synaptic serotonin and norepinephrine, causing inhibition of ascending pain pathways, which ultimately alters the perception of and response to pain. Adult doses are 50-100 mg every 4-6 hours, not to exceed 400 mg per day.

Tricyclic antidepressants (TCAs) are useful analgesics in patients with pain of neurogenic origin. If taken at bedtime, the sedating effects of TCAs can also be beneficial in chronic LBP patients who suffer from sleep disturbances. Furthermore, TCAs may concomitantly treat depression, which is common in patients with chronic LBP. Initial doses should be low and subsequent doses slowly increased to minimize adverse effects. One example, Amitriptyline (Elavil) works by inhibiting reuptake of serotonin and/or norepinephrine in the presynaptic neuronal membrane, which may increase the synaptic concentration of serotonin in the CNS. Amitriptyline is dosed 30-100 mg at bedtime.

Skeletal muscle relaxants may be helpful adjunctive therapy to analgesics in some patients with LBP. They can be used as short-term adjunctive medications, but are generally not recommended for long term use.[39] A sample medication, such as Cyclobenzaprine (Flexeril), acts centrally and reduces motor activity of tonic somatic origins influencing both alpha and gamma motor neurons. It is structurally related to tricyclic antidepressants and thus carries some of the same liabilities. A trial of 10 mg three times a day initially, not to exceed 60 mg per day, can be used.

Oral steroids are potent anti-inflammatory medications that, in theory, represent useful agents in the treatment of patients with radiculopathy due to local inflammation resulting from disk injury or herniation. No standard doses have been established for oral prednisone in the treatment of lumbar radicular pain. An example is prednisone (Deltasone, Sterapred, Orasone), which decreases inflammation by suppressing migration of polymorphonuclear leukocytes and reversing increased capillary permeability. Dose at 60-80 mg per day in 1-2 divided doses initially, followed by tapering off the medication over 8 to 10 days.

Lumbar epidural injection, with or without steroids, is a simple and common procedure that is frequently used to treat a variety of low back conditions. Controlled studies have evaluated their effectiveness in the treatment of lumbar conditions, with some authors reporting success in certain subgroups of patients with diskogenic back pain. Nonradicular pain has been shown to be predictive of poor treatment response rates to epidural injection. On the other hand, patients presenting with radicular features tend to respond better, which, in turn, allows further benefit from participation in a comprehensive rehabilitation program. Importantly, most studies indicate that epidural injection is most likely to be successful in patients who have had symptoms for less than 6 months.[40] In older populations, however, radiculopathy is more likely to result from spinal stenosis (spinal canal or foramina), and in such settings, epidural injection has not been found to be nearly as effective. When compared with surgical interventions, there is a paucity of data and no randomized controlled trials, however, a systematic review of comparative analysis with lumbar fusion showed epidural injections to have superior long-term efficacy in managing chronic lumbar diskogenic pain.[41]

Surgical intervention commonly involves different methods of fusing the lumbar spine and intervertebral disk replacement. Few studies have found surgical intervention to be beneficial in the treatment of LBP and there remains a general lack of consensus regarding the indications in patients with DDD.[16] A significant morbidity associated with lumbar fusions involves painful juxtafusional joint pains, which may require reoperation within approximately 10 years of a successful fusion surgery. Destruction of healthy tissue and increased stress on contiguous vertebra can hasten degeneration of spinal functional units adjacent to the fused vertebrae. Furthermore, fusion may cause limited range of motion as a consequence.[42]

Total lumbar disk replacement surgery, also known as disk arthroplasty, may be useful to treat low back pain while avoiding the limitations of surgical fusion, including limitations in range of motion, segmental instability, and degeneration of adjacent spinal segments. Candidates for disk arthroplasty are limited to patients without significant facet joint dysfunction, which has been associated with poor outcomes.[43]

Nucleus pulposus replacement increases disk space height in the degenerating disk, decreasing the transmission of forces onto the annulus, facet joints, and other stabilizing structures. Compared with total disk replacement, this surgical option involves less surgical exposure, potentially provides spine biomechanics similar to native disks, and offers the advantage of allowing for revision with fusion should nucleus pulposus replacement fail. Nevertheless, there remains a lack of evidence showing a long-term clinically significant improvement in pain and function after disk replacement.[44,45] Disk prostheses currently under investigation are primarily composed of water absorbing hydrogels that release water when loaded. Limitations in implant materials include toxicity of the materials and the danger of their extrusion from the disk space.[46]

Intradiskal electrothermal therapy (IDET) is directed at annular tear pathology and attempts to alter tears and associated neural components. It involves the insertion of an electrothermal catheter into a painful intervertebral disk under fluoroscopic guidance. Thermal energy delivered by the catheter results in breakdown and restructuring of collagen fibers in the posterior annulus. Indication for IDET includes positive diskography study, radial fissure detected in post-diskography CT, and sufficient intervertebral disk height to allow introduction of an electrode. Thermocoagulation by IDET seals annular tears, stiffens the intervertebral disk, and ablates nerve endings in the annulus. Trials for IDET have been small and few have rendered applicability and firm conclusions.[47] Furthermore, a high failure rate limits the utility of IDET, but those patients who respond positively to treatment report significant improvement in pain.[48]

Intradiskal biacuplasty (IDB) is a thermal annular procedure that was developed to improve upon the deficiencies of IDET. IDB utilizes two thin radiofrequency electrodes to deliver thermal energy within a painful disk. Internal cooling of the bipolar probes allows a larger volume of annular tissue to be heated while simultaneously avoiding excessive disk charring and injury to adjacent vertebral nerves.[49] In a prospective, randomized, crossover trial, IDB was shown to have a greater proportion of treatment responders when compared with conventional medical management (CMM).[50] IDB has a greater performance consistency and lower complication rate than previous minimally invasive thermal procedures, and may offer a promising alternative to open surgical intervention.

Currently, the goal of most treatments available for diskogenic pain is symptom reduction, but none actually aims to restore and maintain the structure of degenerated disks. Attempts are being made toward this end with investigations into regenerative therapies such as stem cells and specific growth factor injections. One such biological approach is cell therapy, a minimally invasive technique aimed at regenerating the intervertebral disk through the intradiskal injection of exogenous disk cells, nondisk chondrocytes, or undifferentiated stem cells. Cell therapy has shown a lot of promise in preclinical research and multiple *in vivo* studies have demonstrated proliferation and long-term survival of transplanted mesenchymal stem cells in disk degeneration models.[51] However, few clinical trials have investigated the regenerative potential of cell therapy. In the Eurodisc study, postdiskectomy patients were treated with culture-expanded autologous disk chondrocytes, and at two-year follow up, reported greater pain reduction than non-treatment group.[52] Another investigational drug is NuQu, which consists of culture-expanded, allogeneic, juvenile chondrocytes delivered percutaneously. Currently in an on-going phase II clinical trial, NuQu demonstrated significant clinical and radiographic improvement at the 12-month report from a phase I study in fifteen patients with single level DDD.[53] Ideally, cell therapy should be instituted in the early stages of disk degeneration, before structural changes have occurred, to optimize the synthesis of new extracellular matrix by injected cells.

Platelet-rich plasma (PRP) injection is another biologic therapy aimed at regenerating the intervertebral disk. This approach consists of the intradiskal injection of PRP, an autologous injectate concentrated with platelets from the patient's own whole blood. PRP contains high levels of growth factors and cytokines, such as platelet-derived growth factor (PDGF), epithelial growth factor (EGF), and insulin-like growth factor (IGF-1). These factors promote healing by stimulating tissue repair, collagen synthesis, and angiogenesis.[54] In vitro and animal studies have shown promising results[55] and a recent prospective, double-blind, RCT reported clinically significant improvement sustained at two years.[56] The preliminary results of another recent prospective trial demonstrated a 47% categorical success rate at 6 months in 22 patients with diskogenic lumbar back pain.[54] Although more clinical studies are needed, regenerative therapies, such as PRP and cell therapy, may have a future role in augmenting surgical interventions or even preventing surgery in many patients.

CONCLUSION

Lumbar diskogenic back pain is among the most common causes of LBP and there are a number of diagnostic and treatment modalities available. Therefore, treating physicians should take steps to thoroughly assess a patient before deciding on an interventional pain procedure.

REFERENCES

1. Centers for Disease Control and Prevention. National Ambulatory Medical Care Survey: 2012 Summary Tables. [Online]. [cited 2016 August 27. Available from: http://www.cdc.gov/nchs/data/ahcd/namcs_summary/2012_namcs_web_tables.pdf.
2. Hicks G, Morone N, Weiner D. Degenerative lumbar disc and facet disease in older adults: prevalence and clinical correlates. Spine (Phila Pa 1976). 2009;34(12):1301-16.
3. Cassidy J, Carroll L, Cote P. The Saskatchewan health and back pain survey. The prevalence of low back pain and related disability in Saskatchewan adults. Spine (Phila Pa 1976).1998;23(17):1860-6.
4. Balague F, Mannion A, Pellise F, Cedraschi C. Non-specific low back pain. Lancet. 2012;379(9814):482-91.
5. Schwazer A, Aprill C, Bogduk N. The prevalence and clinical features of internal disc disruption in patients with chronic low back pain. Spine. 1995;20(17):1878-183.
6. Schwarzer A, Aprill C, Derby R, Fortin J, Kine G, Bogduk N. The relative contributions of the disc and zygapophyseal joint in chronic low back pain. Spine (Phila Pa 1976). 1994;19(7):801-6.
7. DePalma M, Ketchum J, Saullo T. What is the source of chronic low back pain and does age play a role? Pain Med. 2011;12(2):224-33.
8. Katz J. Lumbar disc disorders and low-back pain: socioeconomic factors and consequences. J Bone Joint Surg Am. 2006;88(Suppl 2):21-4.
9. Peng B. Pathophysiology, diagnosis, and treatment of discogenic low back pain. World J Orthop. 2013;4(2): 42-52.
10. Hoyland J, Le Maitre C, Freemont A. Investigation of the role of IL-1 and TNF in matrix degradation in the intervertebral disc. Rheumatology. 2008; 47(6): 809-14.
11. Coppes M, Marani E, Thomeer R, Groen G. Innervation of "painful" lumbar discs. Spine (Phila Pa 1976).1997;22(20):2342-29.
12. Adams M, Roughley P. What is intervertebral disc degeneration, and what causes it? Spine (Phila Pa 1976). 2006;31(18):2151-61.
13. DeCandido P, Reinig J, Dwyer A, Thompson K, Ducker T. Magnetic resonance assessment of the distribution of lumbar spine disc degenerative changes. J Spinal Disord. 1998;1(1):9-15.
14. van Tulder M, Assendelft W, Koes B, Bouter L. Spinal radiographic findings and nonspecific low back pain. Spine (Phila Pa 1976).1997;22(4):427-34.
15. Navar D, Zhou B, Lu Y, Solomonow M. High-repetition cyclic loading is a risk factor for a lumbar disorder. Muscle Nerve. 2006;34(5):614-22.
16. Fishman S, Ballantyne J, Rathmell J. Bonica's management of pain. 4th ed. Philadelphia: Lippincott Williams & Wilkins; 2009.
17. Malik K, Cohen S, Walega D, Benzon H. Diagnostic criteria and treatment of discogenic pain: a systematic review of recent clinical literature. Spine J. 2013;13(11):1675-189.
18. Linson M, Crowe C. Comparison of magnetic resonance imaging and lumbar discography in the diagnosis of disc degeneration. Clin Orthop Relat Res. 1990;250: 160-3.

19. Zhou Y, Abdi S. Diagnosis and minimally invasive treatment of lumbar discogenic pain: a review of the literature. Clin J Pain. 2006;22(5):468-81.
20. Samartzis D, Borthakur A, Belfer I, Bow C, Lotz J, Wang H, et al. Novel diagnostic and prognostic methods for disc degeneration and low back pain. Spine J. 2015;15(9):1919-132.
21. Deyo R. Cascade effects of medical technology. Annu Rev Public Health. 2002;23:23-44.
22. Peng B, Hou S, Wu W, Zhang C, Yang Y. The pathogenesis and clinical significance of a high-intensity zone (HIZ) of lumbar intervertebral disc on MR imaging in the patient with discogenic low back pain. Eur Spine J. 2006;15(5):583-7.
23. Aprill C, Bogduk N. High-intensity zone: a diagnostic sign of painful lumbar disc on magnetic resonance imaging. Br J Radiol. 1992;65(773):361-39.
24. Carragee E, Paragoudakis S, Khurana S. 2000 Volvo Award winner in clinical studies: Lumbar high-intensity zone and discography in subjects without low back problems. Spine (Phila Pa 1976). 2000;25(23):2987-292.
25. Ito M, Incorvaia K, Yu S, Fredrickson B. Predictive signs of discogenic lumbar pain on magnetic resonance imaging with discography correlation. Spine (Phila Pa 1976). 1998;23(11):1252-8.
26. Carragee E, Tanner C, Khurana S, Hayward C, Welsh J, Date E, et al. Rates of false-positive lumbar discography in select patients without low back symptoms. Spine (Phila Pa 1976). 2000;25(11):1373-81.
27. Carragee E, Alamin T, Carragee J. Low-pressure positive discography in subjects asymptomatic of significant low back pain illness. Spine (Phila Pa 1976). 2006;31(5):505-9.
28. Wolfer L, Derby R, Lee J, Lee S. Systematic review of lumbar provocation discography in asymptomatic subjects with a meta-analysis of false positive rates. Pain Physician. 2008;11(4):513-38.
29. Carragee E, Don A, Hurwitz E, Cuellar J, Carrino J, Herzog R. 2009 ISSLS Prize Winner: Does discography cause accelerated progression of degeneration changes in the lumbar disc: a ten-year matched cohort study. Spine (Phila Pa 1976). 2009;34(21):2338-45.
30. Cohen S, Larkin T, Barna S, Palmer W, Hecht A, Stojanovic M. Lumbar discography: a comprehensive review of outcome studies, diagnostic accuracy, and principles. Reg Anesth Pain med. 2005;30(2):163-83.
31. Bogduk N, Aprill C, Derby R. Lumbar discogenic pain: state-of-the-art review. Pain Medicine. 2014;14(6):813-36.
32. Luijsterburg P, Verhagen A, Ostelo R, van den Hoogen H, Peul W, Avezaat C, et al. Physical therapy plus general practitioners' care versus general practitioners' care alone for sciatica: a randomised clincal trial with a 12-month follow-up. Eur Spine J. 2008;17(4):509-17.
33. Koes B, van Tulder M, Peul W. Diagnosis and treatment of sciatica. BMJ. 2007;334(7607):1313-7.
34. Wegman A, van der Windt D, van Tulder M, Stalman W, de Vries T. Nonsteroidal antiinflammatory drugs or acetaminophen for osteoarthritis of the hip or knee? A systematic review of evidence and guidelines. J Rheumatol. 2004;31(2):344-54.
35. Hickey R. Chronic low back pain: a comparison of diflunisal with paracetamol. NZ Med J. 1982;95(707):312-4.
36. Chaparro L, Furlan A, Deshpande A, Mailis-Gagnon A, Atlas S, Turk D. Opioids compared to placebo or other treatments for chronic low-back pain. Cochrane Database Syst Rev. 2013;8:CD004595.
37. Abdel Shaheed C, Maher C, Williams K, Day R, McLachlan A. Efficacy, tolerability, and dose-dependent effects of opioid analgesics for low back pain: a systematic review and meta-analysis. JAMA Intern Med. 2016;176(7):958-68.
38. Deyo R, Von Korff M, Duhrkoop D. Opioids for low back pain. BMJ. 2015;350:g6380.
39. van Tulder M, Touray T, Furlan A, Solway S, Bouter L. Muscle relaxants for nonspecific low back pain: a systematic review within the framework of the cochrane collaboration. Spine (Phila Pa 1976). 2003;28(17):1978-92.
40. Phillips F, Lauryssen T. The lumbar intervertebral disc, 1st ed. New York: Thieme Medical Publishers; 2009.
41. Manchikanti L, Staats P, Nampiaparampil D, Hirsch J. What is the role of epidural injections in the treatment of lumbar discogenic pain: a systematic review of comparative analysis with fusion. Korean J Pain. 2015;28(2):75-87.
42. Barrick W, Schofferman J, Reynolds J. Surgery anterior lumbar fusion improves discogenic pain at levels of prior posterolateral fusion. Spine (Phila Pa 1976). 2000;25(7):853-7.
43. David T. Clinical case series long-term results of one-level lumbar arthroplasty: minimum 10-year follow-up of the CHARITE artifical disc in106 patients. Spine (Phila Pa 1976). 2005;32(6):661-6.
44. Jacobs W, van der Gaag N, Kruyt M, Tuschel A, de Kleuver M, Peul W, et al. Spina (Phila Pa 1976). 2013;38(1):24-36.
45. Hellum C, Johnsen L, Storheim K, Nygaard O, Brox J, Rossvoll I, et al. Surgery with disc prothesis versus rehabilitation in patients with low back pain and degenerative disc: two year follow-up of randomised study. BMJ. 2011;342:d2786.
46. Sasso R, Foulk D. Radomized trial prospective, randomized trial of metal-on-metal artifical lumbar disc replacement: initial results for treatment of discogenic pain. Spine (Phila Pa 1976). 2006;33(1):123-31.

47. Assietti R, Morosi M, Block J. Intradiscal electrothermal therapy for symptomatic internal disc disruption: 24-month results and predictors of clinical success. J Neurosurg Spine. 2010;12(3):320-36.
48. Pauza K, Howell S, Dreyfuss P, Peloza J, Dawson K, Bogduk N. A randomized, placebo-controlled trial of intradiscal electrothermal therapy for the treatment of discogenic low back pain. Spine J. 2004;4(1):27-35.
49. Kapural L, Mekhail N, Hicks D, Kapural M, Sloan S, Moghal N, et al. Histological changes and temperature distribution studies of a novel bipolar radiofrequency heating system in degenerated and nondegenerated human cadaver lumbar discs. Pain Medicine. 2009;9(1):68-75.
50. Desai M, Kapural L, Petersohn J, Vallejo R, Menzies R, Creamer M, et al. A prospective, randomized, multicenter, open-label clinical trial comparing intradiscal biacuplasty to conventional medical management for discogenic lumbar back pain. Spine (Phila Pa 1976). 2016;41(13):1065-74.
51. Benneker L, Andersson G, Iatridis J, Sakai D, Hartl R, Ito K, et al. Cell therapy for intervertebral disc repair: advancing cell therapy from bench to clinics. Eur Cell Mater. 2014;27:5-11.
52. Meisel H, Sioldla V, Ganey T, Minkus Y, Hutton W, Alasevic O. Clinical experience in cell-based therapeutics: disc chondrocyte transplantation a treatment for degenerated or damaged intervertebral disc. Biomol Eng. 2007;24(1):5-21.
53. Coric D, Pettine K, Sumich A, Boltes M. Prospective study of disc repair with allogeneic chondrocytes presented at the 2012 Joint Spine Section Meeting. J Neurosurg Spine. 2013;18(1):85-95.
54. Levi D, Horn S, Tyszko S, Levin J, Hecht-Leavitt C, Walko E. Intradiscal platelet-rich plasma injection for chronic discogenic low back pain: preliminary results from a prospective trial. Pain Med. 2016;17(6):1010-22.
55. Monfett M, Harrison J, Boachie-Adjei K, Lutz G. Intradiscal platelet-rich plasma (PRP) injections for discogenic low back pain: an update. Int Orthop. 2016;40(6):1321-28.
56. Tuakli-Wosornu Y, Terry A, Boachie-Adjei K, Harrison J, Gribbin C, LaSalle E, et al. Lumbar intradiscal platelet rich plasma (PRP) injections: a prospective, double-blind, randomized controlled study. PM R. 2015;8(1):doi: 10.1016/j.pmrj.2015.08.010.

CHAPTER 22

Sacroiliac Joint Pain Syndrome and Its Management

Andrew R Cooper

INTRODUCTION

The sacroiliac joint (SIJ) is an important cause of low back pain, being the largest weight-bearing joint in the body, with a prevalence of between 15% and 40%.[1,2] The paired SIJs distribute body weight across the pelvis and lower limbs following the curvature of the pelvis in a double shape.

They are classified as complex diarthrodial joints (Fig. 1). The upper and anterior part is a true synovial joint between sacrum and ileum. While the lower and posterior part is a fibro-cartilaginous connection between sacrum and ileum with only a small synovial part to it. It is only the posterior part of the SIJ, which is accessible to injection because of the close connection with the hip joint, gluteal and piriformis muscles.

The clinical picture as to the exact pain generator is often unclear from the history and examination. The SIJ has an extensive and variable sensory innervations pattern arising from the lumbar plexus anteriorly and sacral

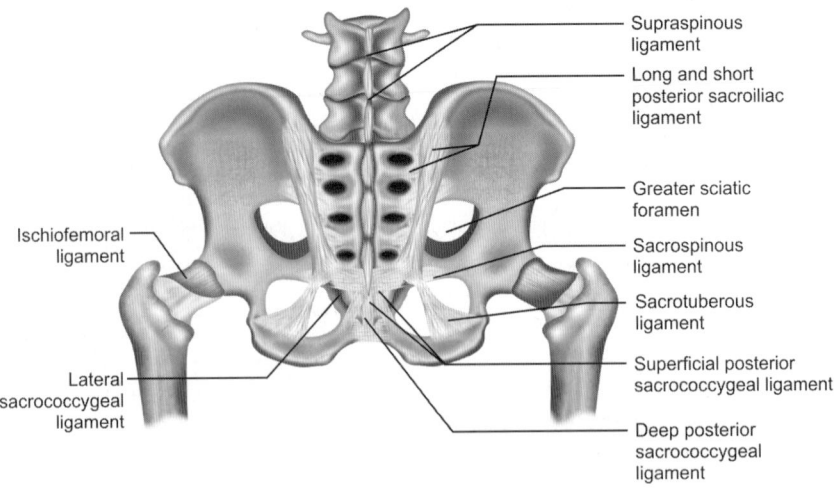

FIG. 1: Anatomy of sacroiliac joint

plexus posteriorly with contributions from S1 to S4 posterior primary rami predominating.

The function of the SIJ is to prevent rotation of the spine at the pelvis while transmitting axial loads and to facilitate parturition.

CAUSES OF SACROILIAC JOINT PAIN SYNDROME

Several causes of SIJ pain syndrome include:
- *Intra-articular*: Arthritis, infection, metabolic diseases spondyloarthropathies, idiopathic.
- Reiter's syndrome, inflammatory bowel diseases, and ankylosing spondylitis are strongly associated with SIJ pain.
- *Extra-articular*: Fractures, myofascial pain, ligament injury, attachment injury, etc.
- *Shear forces*: Postlumbar fusion surgery, pelvic fractures, abnormal gait associated with leg shortening, etc. In late pregnancy, the lax ligaments in the pelvis and weight gain put extra strain on the spine, and may lead to mechanical changes, this can result in SIJ pain.

SIGNS AND SYMPTOMS

Typically pain from the sacroiliac joint is experienced in the gluteal area over the SIJ and into the buttock with referral patterns to the high, and occasionally below the knee, although it can occur anywhere along the leg below L5. It is reproduced by stressing the joint and relieved by blocking the joint with local anesthetic.
- It is usually unilateral being described as a dull aching pain, which can radiate into the hip or groin, or anywhere down the leg and can mimic sciatica. Straight leg raising tests can help differentiate being unaffected in SIJ pain.
- Pain is often exacerbated by turning over in bed, putting on shoes and socks and leg lifting to get into or out of a car or out of bed in the morning.
- Prolonged sitting or standing can exacerbate the pain and stiffness, which is not helped by walking, unlike Z-joint pain, which can be eased, by walking.

CLINICAL EXAMINATION

It is often unreliable due to the immobility and location of the joint. Around 50 various tests for SIJ pain have been described, suggesting that there is not good reliability or specificity for so many tests.

They can be grouped into:
- Positional palpation tests
- Motion palpation tests
- Adaptive shortening tests
- Pain provocation tests—SIJ-PPTs.

Generally the pain provocation tests are most often employed in clinical practice, and range from applying gentle palpation over the joint looking for localized tenderness in the upright position, to more forceful "thrusts" with the patient prone. The Fortin "Finger test" described the localized tenderness from light finger pressure over the upper part of the joint at the posterior superior iliac[3] crest. Unreliable findings can occur by stressing other adjacent structures either instead, or in addition to the SIJ and findings of clinical examination should be interpreted cautiously.

Other useful tests include Patrick's or Faber's test (Fig. 2). Gaenslen's test (Fig. 3),

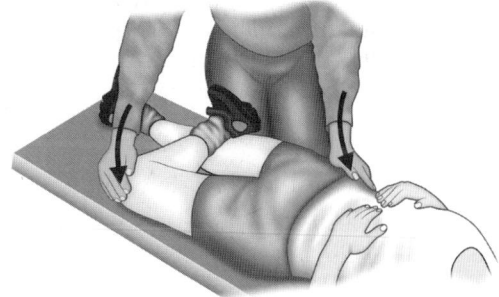

FIG. 2: Patrick's or Faber's test (Flexion, abduction, external rotation at the hip)

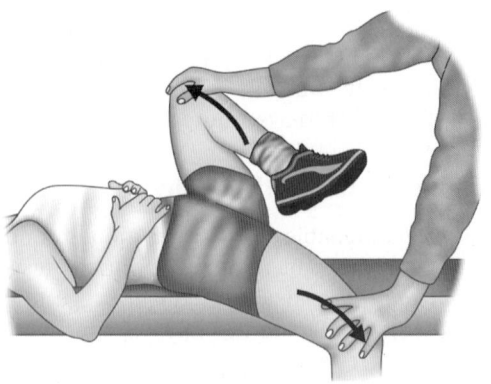

FIG. 3: Gaenslen's test. Stresses both SIJs simultaneously. Patient is supine with the sore side one edge of table. The unaffected side is flexed at both knee and hip joints bringing the unaffected leg towards the abdomen while the sore side is gently extended

shear test, and forced hip abduction tests are felt to be more useful.[1,4,5] The individual clinical examination tests have low predictive value but this is improved when more than one different test is positive.[2]

DIAGNOSTIC CRITERIA

It is very important in chronic pain that there is cognizance regarding the role of psychological factors and secondary gain issues that may exist, particularly, if interventional procedures of an invasive nature are being considered. While physical examination alone cannot diagnose SIJ pain, being affected by examiner technique and individual patient variability, the sensitivity and reliability is improved when more than one test is positive approaching 94% and 78%, respectively when three or more tests are positive.[5,7]

When none of the provocation tests fail to reproduce the patient's pain then SIJ pain is very unlikely. In multiparous women, maximum pain below L5 vertebral body level along with tenderness on examination over the SIJ and/or posterior superior iliac spine is highly suggestive of SIJ pain.

INVESTIGATIONS

In making, the diagnosis it is important to exclude other causes of low back pain and in particular traumatic, infective or neoplastic etiologies. Onset of SIJ pain is often insidious over several years and can present very similar to hip joint pain, when both conditions can sometimes coexist. Z-Joint pain and diskogenic pain should also be excluded, if necessary by performing specific diagnostic blocks.

Laboratory Tests

Which may be helpful when inflammatory, metabolic, or neoplastic diseases are suspected include:
- Full blood picture (FBP)
- Erythrocyte sedimentation rate (ESR)
- C-reactive protein (CRP)
- Antinuclear antibody (ANA) profile
- Human leukocyte antigen (HLA)-B27-status
- Rheumatoid factor (RF)
- Prostate specific antigen (PSA)
- Plasma protein electrophoresis (PPE) and other tests for malignancy.

Imaging Studies

Owing to the wide variability in joint anatomy of patients, imaging studies is not helpful in examining the SIJ. They are more useful when investigating for other causes of pain such as neoplastic, metabolic or infective ("red flags"). The anterior posterior (AP) pelvis and lumbar spine plain X-rays while they may demonstrate sclerosis or gross degenerative changes cannot determine if the joint is the pain generator for that particular patient. CT, MRI or bone scanning have similar limitations in practice but are helpful in identifying disk pathology presenting with similar symptoms.

Diagnostic Blocks

Injection of local anesthetic into the SIJ is the most useful diagnostic investigation and is usually performed using fluoroscopy

Chapter 22: Sacroiliac Joint Pain Syndrome and Its Management

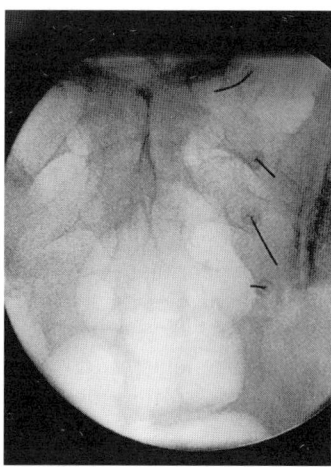

FIG. 4A: Contrast has been injected into the right SIJ—sacral foramen have been marked

(Figs 4A and B). CT is not required unless difficulty is found in viewing SIJ with fluoroscopy. There may be a future role for ultrasound-guided blocks to reduce X-ray exposure. Both false-positive and negative results can occur with blocks and good attention to detail is required to reduce these errors. There is an associated placebo effect with single injections and repeated blocks are usually needed. Repeating these blocks with long-and-short acting LA can enhance their value. Reference should be made to the literature for detailed descriptions of individual techniques.[7-9]

An alternative approach is to perform lateral branch nerve blocks whereby the nerves are blocked on route from the sacral foramina to the SIJ. However, while useful in practice for therapeutic purposes, they are likely to have more false-positives in comparison to intra-articular blocks, which are considered the gold standard for diagnosis. This is because larger volumes of local anesthetic are used compared to the intra-articular block (5–10 mL versus 0.51.5 mL), with more likelihood for spread beyond the targeted area.

Schwarzer reported in a study looking at pain provocation, analgesia and image pattern from intra-articular injection that groin pain was the only pain referral pattern found to be associated with response to sacroiliac joint block.[1]

DIFFERENTIAL DIAGNOSIS

- Osteoarthritis (OA) hip joint pain
- Diskogenic pain
- Z-joint pain
- Myofascial pain syndrome
- Piriformis pain syndrome

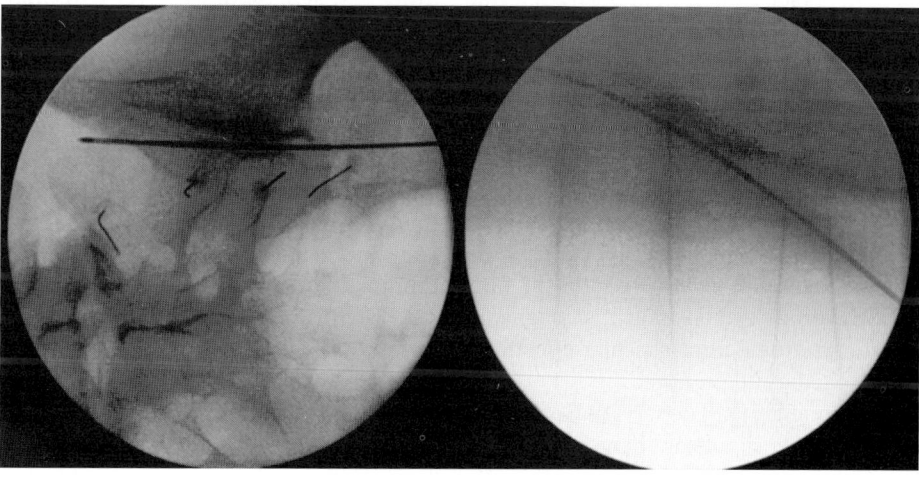

FIG. 4B: Electrode position for performing a radiofrequency thermocoagulation procedure in AP and lateral views which must be clearly identified before starting the procedure

- Ankylosing spondylitis
- Reiter's syndrome
- Psoriatic arthritis
- Inflammatory arthritis.

TREATMENT PROTOCOL

It commences with the least invasive therapies, before moving onto, the more invasive interventional and potentially more harmful techniques. If there is a specific entity, such as inflammatory arthropathies, rheumatoid disease, inflammatory bowel diseases, ankylosing spondylitis, Reiter's syndrome, etc. primary therapy for the condition is employed, which may help to settle the symptoms of SIJ pain with beneficial effects for many patients.

The rest, avoiding activities, which aggravate the pain, physiotherapy, heat and manipulative therapy may be useful and will benefit many. The massage, stretching exercises, hydrotherapy can be helpful in some cases a multidisciplinary approach may be useful when the condition becomes chronic. The analgesic drugs, cognitive behavior therapy, physiotherapy and rehabilitation may be useful for many patients.

There are many alternative therapies, which patients have often tried before referral to the specialist pain clinic, which is usually only when chronicity has been established.

Interventional therapy includes SIJ injections with local anesthetic and steroids. In practice often there is no difference between results after intra-articular or periarticular injections. The significant pain reductions can be expected for repeated injections with benefit lasting from several months to one year. However, in establishing the diagnosis of SIJ pain syndrome intra-articular injections are more specific and preferred.

Radiofrequency (RF) denervation of the SIJ is performed after significant benefit has been demonstrated after repeated SIJ blocks with the aim of producing effective long-term pain reduction and depending on the technique used variable results can be expected.

Ferrante reported a study on 30 patients who underwent 50 RF lesions in the postero-inferior aspect of joint using, "leap frogging, technique at <1 cm intervals.[10] He found 36% obtained better than 50% pain reduction for at least 6 months (mean duration of pain relief 12+/-1.2 months). Yin obtained over 50% reduction in pain in 64% of[14] patients and complete relief in 36% following deep interosseous ligamentous RF lesions.[11] This suggested that most of the sensory innervations was from S1 to S4.

Based on these and other studies the technique of cooled radiofrequency (CRF) was developed in order to address the large variability in the sensory nerve supply, which can travel up to 10 mm above the sacrum on route from the sacral foramen to the SIJ capsule. This technique by cooling the active RF electrode permits a much larger circumferential lesion than can be obtained by standard RF and should ensure a larger thermal neurolytic zone around the electrode. Cohen reported a study using combined traditional RF and CRF in 28 patients, with significant improvement over placebo (more than 50% reduction in pain) from 79% at 1 month to 57% at 6 months.[12] Cheng compared outcomes after either traditional RF ablation or cooled RF ablation of the lateral branches in a comparative retrospective observational study and did not observe a difference in pain reduction at 6 months following treatment between the groups, with > 50% pain reduction being achieved in both groups at 6[13] months. Bellini reported good results in pain reduction of >50% with improved disability scores up to 6 months after using a single strip lesion multi electrode device (Simplicity 3 probe) for SIJ denervation.[14] Investigations a recurrently under way comparing the Single multi channel electrode device (Simplicity 3 electrode) to the CRF technique.

FOLLOW-UP ADVICE

It is important to review the patients, after interventional procedures to establish, that, they do obtain the benefit beyond possible placebo response and also to ensure that any possible complications are recorded. The potential complications of injection and RF procedures include:[15]

- Flare-up of pain is often experienced following RF procedures and this usually settles within 7–10 days. Additional strong analgesics, such as codeine, tramadol, oxycontin or nonsteroidal analgesics may be needed for nociceptive pain flare-up. Neuropathic pain and dysthesia, if present are disturbing can be helped with use of regular anticonvulsants, such as gabapentin, pregablin or carbamazepine, may be prescribed for a few months. The tricyclic agents, such as amitriptyline or duloxetine may also be required for burning type pain.
- Infection is rarely seen.
- Motor weakness should also be rare.
- Bleeding is unlikely as there are no major blood vessels in the area for treatment.
- Occasionally, bladder disturbance has been reported for a few hours in the immediate post-RF period.
- Topical ice packs or anti-inflammatory agents may be useful.
- Bathing or swimming should be avoided for a few days to reduce the risk of infection for needle tracks.
- Corticosteroid associated effects of facial flushing; fluid retention mastalgia, leg edema; menstrual upsets; hyperglycemia and polyuria or transient hypertension are often found but usually only require explanation and reassurance in most patients. The diabetics may need to read just their insulin for a few days.

CONCLUSION

Sacroiliac joint pain is one of important cause of low back pain referred to buttock area. The use of multimodal approach is the key to the success of maximum pain relief.

REFERENCES

1. Schwarzer AC, April CN, Bogduk N. The sacro iliac joint in chronic low back pain. Spine. 1995;20(1):31-7.
2. Maigne JY, Aivaliklis A, Pferer F. Results of sacroiliac joint double block and value of sacroiliac pain provocation tests in 54 patients with low back pain. Spine. 1996;21: 1889-92.
3. Fortin JD, Falco FJ. The Fortin finger test: an indicator of sacroiliac joint pain. Am J Orthop (Belle Mead NJ). 1997; 26(7):477-80.
4. Slipman CW, Sterenfield EB, Chou LH, et al.The predictive value of provocative. Sacro iliac joint stress man oeuvres in the diagnosis of sacro iliac joint syndrome. Arch Phy Med Rehabil. 1998;79:288-92.
5. Laslett M, Williams M. The reliability of selected pain provocation tests for sacro iliac joint pathology. Spine. 1994;19:1243-9.
6. Dreyfuss MD. Practice guidelines and protocols for sacro iliac joint blocks. In: International Spine Intervention Society. ISIS 9th Annual Scientific Meeting. San Francisco, CA: ISIS; 2001.pp.35-49.
7. Van der Wurff P, Buijs E, Grohen G. A multi-test regimen of pain provocation tests as an aid to reduce unnecessary minimally invasive saceoiliac joint procedures. Arch Phys Med Rehabil. 2006;87:10-4.
8. Manckikanti L, et al. Evaluation of the relative contributions of various structures in chronic low back pain. Pain Physician. 2001;4:308-16.
9. Rosenberg JM, Quint TJ, De Rosayro AM. Computerized tomographic localization of clinically guided sacroiliac joint injections. Clin J Pain. 2000;16:18-21.
10. Ferrante FM, King LF, Roche EA, et al. Radio frequency sacroiliac joint denervation for sacroiliac syndrome. Reg Anesth Pain Med. 2001;26:137-42.
11. Yin W, Willard F, Carreiro J, Dreyfuss P. Sensory stimulation guided sacroiliac joint radiofrequency neurotomy: technique based on neuroanatomy of the dorsal sacralplexus. Spine. 2003;28:2419-25.
12. Cohen SP, Hurley RW, Buckenmaier CC 3rd, et al. Randomized placebo controlled study evaluating lateral branch denervation lateral branch radiofrequency denervation for sacroiliac joint pain. Anesthesiology. 2008;109:279-88.
13. Cheng J, Pope J, et al. Comparative outcomes of cooled versus traditional radiofrequency ablation of the lateral branches for sacroiliac joint pain. Clinical Journal of Pain. 2013;29(2)132-7.
14. Bellini M, Barbeiri M. Single strip lesions radiofrequency denervation for treatment of sacroiliac joint pain: two years' results. Anaesthesiology Intensive Therapy. 2016; 48(1):19-22.
15. Rathmell JP. Sacroiliac joint injection. Atlas of Image-guided Intervention in Regional Anesthesia and Pain Medicine. Lippincott Williams and Wilkins; 2006.pp.93-100.

Coccygodynia and Its Pain Management

Yashwant L Nankar

INTRODUCTION

Coccyx is the term derived from the Greek word "Cuckoo" due to its resemblance to the beak of this bird. Coccygodynia, is pain in the region of the coccyx, typically is triggered by or occurs while sitting. It is five times more prevalent in women than men and the average age is 40 years.[1]

It occurs after direct trauma to the coccyx from a kick or a fall directly on coccyx and can also occur after difficult vaginal delivery. In most cases, abnormal mobility is seen on dynamic standing and seated radiographs.

It is a readily treatable condition and a multidisciplinary approach employing physical therapy and nonsteroidal anti-inflammatory drugs is useful in most of the patients. The fluoroscopy-guided injections and surgery for selected patients lead to the greatest chance of improvement and satisfaction in such patients.[2]

This chapter provides an overview of the pathoanatomy, etiology, clinical features, and treatment of coccydynia.

CLINICAL ANATOMY

The coccyx is a triangular bone that comprises the most distal aspect of the vertebral column. It consists of three to five fused rudimentary vertebral units. The ventral surface of the coccyx is slightly concave with transverse grooves that demarcate the regions where the vestigial coccygeal units had previously fused. The dorsal aspect is slightly convex and displays similar transverse markings as well as multiple paired tubercles known as the coccygeal articular processes, the most superior of which are referred to as the coccygeal cornu. These structures articulate with the sacral cornu either as a symphysis or as a true synovial joint.

The sacrococcygeal joint has a limited amount of movement in flexion and extension, ranging from approximately 5° to 15° in either direction.[3] The flexion occurs when moving from a standing to a sitting position, which is thought to enable optimal force absorption in the seated position and reverse occurs when moving from a seated to a standing position. In addition the movements occur during defecation, where flexion controls descent of feces and extension allows release. The coccyx also provides positional support to the anus.

ETIOLOGY

The exact cause is unknown in over 70% of cases. The most common cause of coccydynia is single direct axial trauma such as a fall directly onto the coccyx or, during parturition. The cumulative trauma that occurs due to sitting awkwardly, prolonged bicycle riding, use of "keep-fit" rowing machine, obesity, prolonged sitting and during defecation.

The other causes include myofascial trigger points in pelvic muscles, hypermobile coccyx, scoliotic deformity, coccygeal disc degeneration, lumbar disc pathology, tumor, infection, bursitis of the coccygeal adventitia and prolonged surgical operation in lithotomy position.

SIGNS AND SYMPTOMS

These patients complains of pain in and around the coccyx: The onset of pain may be insidious resulting in a possibly long delay from onset to diagnosis, and the pain is associated with sitting and is exacerbated when rising from a seated position.

The severity of the pain is dependent on various predisposing factors, such as the duration of time spent sitting. Patients may report relief of their pain when they sit on their legs or on one buttock or some patients have frequent need to defecate or pain with defecation. The women report an exponential increase in pain during the premenstrual period or sexual intercourse. The history of constipation and blood in the stool is suggestive of the tumor or metastasis.

PHYSICAL EXAMINATION

Inspection of the sacrococcygeal region may show pilonidal cysts.

Palpation often reveals localized tenderness and may be greatest at the sacrococcygeal joint rather than at the coccygeal tip with associated swelling.[2]

In addition, a mass such as representing a bone spicule or causative tumor may occasionally be palpated. The rectal examination or manipulation of the coccygeal segments or sacrococcygeal joint will elicit pain.

DIAGNOSTIC AND IMAGING WORK-UP

Laboratory investigations is to check the inflammatory conditions. The occult blood in stool is to confirm the gastrointestinal (GI) pathology.

Imaging

X-ray: Anteroposterior and lateral radiographs of the sacrococcygeal region to find out curvature of coccyx and rule out fracture if any.

Dynamic radiographs obtained in both the sitting and standing positions. A comparison of sitting and standing films will yield radiographic abnormalities in up to 70% of symptomatic coccydynia cases.[1] Anterior hypermobility, subluxation or posterior displacement of the mobile segment of the coccyx is seen when the patient is seated (Fig. 1). A spicule of the distal tip is seen most commonly with an immobile coccyx.[2]

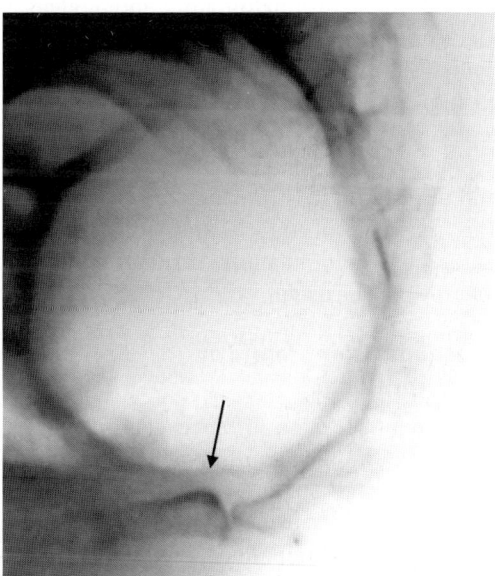

FIG. 1: Lateral radiographic seated view of a 45-year-old woman with increased flexion coccygodynia (arrow)

The magnetic resonance imaging (MRI) and technetium Tc-99m bone scans may demonstrate inflammation of the sacrococcygeal area indicative of coccygeal hypermobility.[1] Dynamic MRI by assessing the difference between coccyx position at maximum contraction and during straining or evacuation. These tests can also be used to exclude certain forms of underlying pathology such as chordoma.

Provocative discography has been found to be a more promising investigation in the assessment of coccydynia.[4]

Diagnostic block: Injection of local anesthetic under fluoroscopic guidance may also be useful in diagnosis.[5]

TREATMENT STRATEGY

Nonsurgical Management

Nonsurgical strategies remain the gold standard treatment for coccydynia. They consist of use of medications such as laxatives, nonsteroidal anti-inflammatory and analgesic medications, opioids, topical creams, rest, hot baths (Sitz bath), reduced sitting and use of cushion to protect the coccygeal region from repetitive trauma.

Physical therapy consisting of diathermy and ultrasound may provide temporary relief. The massage of the levator muscles and intrarectal manipulation through physical therapy may be useful.

Injections Using Steroid or Local Anesthetic[6]

The patient selection for coccygeal injections is crucial. The rectal and or pelvic pathology should be ruled out and patients should have intact skin with no evidence of pilonidal cyst.

Wray[7] recommended administering a mixture of steroid (40 mg methylprednisolone) and long-acting anesthetic (10 mL 0.25% bupivacaine) which may be repeated if necessary.

Coccygeal Nerve Block

This block may be used for therapeutic and diagnostic purposes to confirm the presence of coccygodynia.

It is done where a needle is inserted alongside of the coccyx under the fluoroscopy. This procedure is site specific and selectively blocks perineal pain. The technique is simple, there is no danger of infection in the intrathecal or extradural space, there is no need to keep the patient immobilized for a long time after the procedure and can be repeated, if required.[8]

Ganglion Impar Block

It has been shown to benefit patients with coccygodynia.[9] It is done with local anesthetic and has pain reduction ranging from 75 to 100%, with efficacy lasting for more than 1 year. Radiofrequency ablation is recommended in selected patients.[10] It can be used for the treatment of severe pain due to carcinoma.

Pulsed Radiofrequency

Caudal epidural pulsed radiofrequency (PRF) may be an alternative to surgery for coccygodynia patients.[11]

Dextrose Prolotherapy

Dextrose prolotherapy is an effective treatment option in patients with chronic, recalcitrant coccygodynia and should be used before undergoing coccygectomy.[12]

Spinal Cord Stimulation

Data on the use of spinal cord stimulation are limited, but a case report of success with this modality was presented.[13]

Coccygeoplasty

Injection of polymethyl methacrylate cement in a patient with a coccygeal fracture.[14]

Surgical Management

Patients who fail to respond to conservative therapies, advanced degeneration such as coccygeal instability (e.g. subluxation or hypermobility) or spicule formation, may be considered for surgical intervention.

The surgical management generally involves either excision of the mobile segment or a total coccygectomy. The most frequent complication of coccygectomy is wound infection; rectal injury, anal sphincter injury and incontinence have been rarely reported.[15]

CONCLUSION

Coccygodynia condition should be taken seriously and treated sympathetically. It is a readily treatable condition and deserves better attention.

A multidisciplinary approach employing physical therapy and nonsteroidal anti-inflammatory drugs should be employed first; fluoroscopic-guided injection and surgery lead to the greatest chance of improvement and satisfaction in chronic coccygodynia patients.

REFERENCES

1. Fogel G, Cunningham P, Esses S. Coccygodynia: evaluation and management. J Am Acad Orthop Surg. 2004;12:49-54.
2. Maigne JY, Doursounian L, Chatellier G. Causes and mechanisms of common coccydynia: Role of body mass index and coccygeal trauma. Spine. 2000;25:3072-9.
3. Woon JT, Stringer MD. Clinical anatomy of the coccyx: a systematic review. Clin Anat. 2012;25:158-67.
4. Maigne JY, Guedj S, Straus C. Idiopathic coccygodynia: lateral roentgenograms in the sitting position and coccygeal discography. Spine. 1994;19:930-4.
5. Galhom A, Mohammad al-Shatouri, El-Fadl SA. Evaluation and management of chronic coccygodynia: Fluoroscopic guided injection, local injection, conservative therapy and surgery in non-oncological pain. Egyptian J Radiol Nucl Med. 2015;46:1049-55.
6. Mitra R, Cheung L, Perry P. Efficacy of fluoroscopically guided steroid injections in the management of coccydynia. Pain Physician. 2007;10:775-8.
7. Wray C, Easom S, Hoskinson J. Coccydynia: aetiology and treatment. J Bone Joint Surg. 1991;73:335-8.
8. Foye PM, Patel SI. Paracoccygeal corkscrew approach to ganglion impar injections for tailbone pain. Pain Pract. 2009;9:317-21.
9. Buttaci C, Foye PM, Stitik TP. Coccygodynia successfully treated with ganglion impar blocks: a case series. Am J Phys Med Rehabil. 2005;85(9):783-4.
10. Demircay E, Kabatas S, Cansever T, Yilmaz C, Tuncay C, Altinors N. Radiofrequency thermocoagulation of ganglion impar in the management of coccydynia: preliminary result. Turk Neurosurg. 2010;20(3):28-33.
11. Atim A, Ergin A, Bilgic S, Deniz S, Kurt–E. Pulsed radiofrequency in the treatment of coccygodynia. Agri. 2011;23(1):1-6.
12. Khan SA, Kumar A, Varshney MK, Trikha V, Yadav CS. Dextrose prolotherapy for recalcitrant coccygodynia. J Orthop Surg (Hong Kong). 2008;16(1):27-9.
13. Haider N. Coccydynia treated with spinal cord stimulation: A case report. Amer Acad Pain Med. 24th Annual Meeting. 2008. Poster 144.
14. Dean LM, Syed MI, Jan SA, Patel NA, Shaikh A, Morar K, et al. Coccygeoplasty: treatment for fractures of the coccyx. J Vasc Interv Radiol. 2006;17:909-12.
15. Trollegaard AM, Aarby NS, Hellberg S. Coccygectomy: an effective treatment option for chronic coccydynia: retrospective results in 41 consecutive patients. J Bone Joint Surg Br. 2010;92:242-5.

CHAPTER 24

Piriformis and Iliopsoas Pain Syndromes and Its Pain Management

Dwarkadas K Baheti

PIRIFORMIS SYNDROME

Introduction

Piriformis (PF) syndrome has been described by Yeoman W[1] in 1928 and since then it has a controversial diagnosis. The piriformis is a deep-seated muscle and irritate or compress the proximal sciatic nerve due to spasm or contracture. The piriformis muscle runs from the sacrum to the greater trochanter, which is the outer part of upper femur (thigh). The sciatic nerve runs either through or under the piriformis muscle as it leaves the spine.

Pain may be felt in the affected buttock, thigh and leg because the pain travels within the distribution of the sciatic nerve. The piriformis syndrome/deep glutei syndrome is a neuromuscular disorder[2] that occurs when the sciatic nerve is compressed or otherwise irritated by the piriformis muscle causing pain, tingling and numbness in the buttocks and along the path of the sciatic nerve descending down the lower thigh and into the leg.

Piriformis syndrome is also referred to as pseudo-sciatica, wallet sciatica, and hip socket neuropathy. The condition which can mimic diskogenic sciatica usually is caused by neuritis of the proximal sciatic nerve. PF affects many different people, such as athletes, patients who have undergone surgery in or near the area of the piriformis muscle.

Anatomy

The piriformis muscle is flat, pyramid-shaped, and oblique. This muscle originates to the anterior of the S2-S4 vertebrae, the sacrotuberous ligament, and the upper margin of the greater sciatic foramen. Passing through the greater sciatic notch, the muscle inserts on the superior surface of the greater trochanter of the femur. With the hip extended, the piriformis muscle is the primary external rotator; however, with the hip flexed, the muscle becomes a hip abductor. The piriformis muscle is innervated by branches from L5, S1, and S2.

Etiology

Piriformis can be due to various etiology such as hyperlordosis, muscle anomalies with hypertrophy; fibrosis (due to trauma), partial or total nerve anatomical abnormalities; pseudoaneurysms of the inferior gluteal artery adjacent to the piriformis syndrome; bilateral piriformis syndrome due to prolonged sitting during an extended neurosurgical procedure; cerebral palsy; total hip arthroplasty; fibrodysplasia ossificans progressiva (myositis ossificans); vigorous physical activity and leg length discrepancy.[3]

Etiopathology

The muscle trauma or over use leads to shortening or spasm of piriformis muscle. This may compress or strangle the sciatic nerve beneath the muscle. This is commonly known as nerve entrapment or as entrapment neuropathies. In 17% of an assumed normal population the sciatic nerve passes through the piriformis muscle, rather than underneath it and in 16.2% of patients undergoing surgery for a suspected piriformis syndrome such an anomaly was found leading to doubt about the importance of the anomaly as a factor in piriformis syndrome.[4] At times inactive glutei muscles ex-bedridden patient can develop the piriformis syndrome.

Differential Diagnosis

Differential diagnosis can be, herniated disk, hip arthritis, stress fracture, snapping hip syndrome, diskogenic origin, facet joint syndrome, spinal canal stenosis, sacroiliac dysfunction, and sacroiliac (SI) syndrome. The computed tomography (CT) may show asymmetrical enlargement of the piriformis muscle.

Diagnostic Criteria

The diagnosis is largely clinical and is one of exclusion mentioned above in differential diagnosis. In physical examination, attempts are made to stretch the irritated piriformis and provoke sciatic nerve compression, such as the Freiberg, the Pace, and the FAIR (flexion, adduction, and internal rotation) maneuvers (Fig. 1).

The tenderness is in the area of the sciatic notch. The pain is exacerbated with activity, prolonged sitting, or walking.

The diagnostic modalities, such as CT, magnetic resonance imaging (MRI), ultrasound, electromyography (EMG) are useful. The magnetic resonance neurography[5] can show the presence of irritation of the sciatic nerve at the level of the sciatic notch where the nerve passes under the piriformis muscle. The neurography can determine whether or not a patient has a split sciatic nerve or a split piriformis muscle this may be important in getting a good result from injections or surgery.

Image-guided injections carried out in an open MRI scanner, or other 3D image guidance can accurately relax the piriformis muscle to test the diagnosis.

Treatment Plan

The multimodal approach, such as medications, interventional treatment procedure and rehabilitation are best one. The medications include either singly or in combination of nonsteroidal anti-inflammatory drugs (NSAIDs), analgesics, muscle relaxants, antidepressants and neuropathic medications are necessary. The piriformis injection is

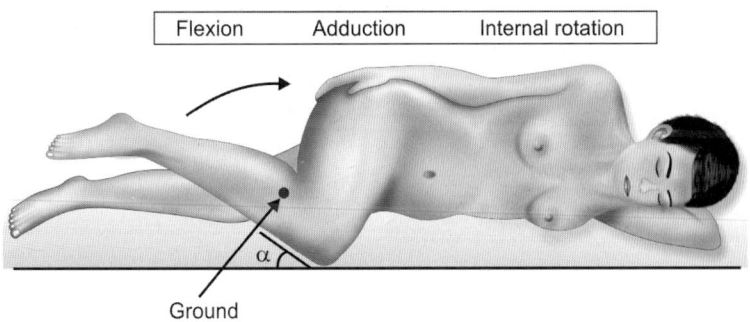

FIG. 1: FAIR test—flexion, adduction, and internal rotation

performed under guidance of fluoroscopy, CT, or MRI. The use of fluoroscopy or high frequency ultrasound or EMG guidance is useful.

Fluoroscopy-guided Piriformis Injection Technique

Step 1: The patient in prone position under fluoroscopy, anteroposterior view, of affected side. The sacrum and greater trochanter are used as medial and lateral bony landmarks. The greater trochanter and lateral border of sacrum are identified. A line may be drawn from the posterior inferior iliac spine to the greater trochanter. The skin entry site is at the midpoint of this line.

Under local anesthesia, a 3½ inch 23 gauge spinal needle is directed to bony endpoint, and then withdraws. In most of the cases paresthesia is felt.

Step 2: After negative aspiration; inject inj. omnipaque 3 cc to 5 cc to confirm the needle placement. It should delineate the contour of the piriformis muscle (Fig. 2).

Step 3: Now inject inj. aurocort (preservative free triamcinolone acetate) 40 mg with inj. bupivacaine 0.25% 5 cc or inj. ropivacaine 0.5% 3 cc into the muscle. For long-term pain relief then paralyzing agent inj. botulinum type A5 100 units injected.

The rehabilitation program includes physical therapy such as teaching of stretching techniques, massage, and strengthening of the core muscles (abs, back, etc.) to reduce strain on the piriformis and increase range of motion. The use of ice and/or heat can be helpful when the pain starts, or immediately after an activity that causes pain.

In selected cases, custom foot orthotics also help with both treatment and prevention. The gait correction will allow the muscle to relax and heal itself. The ultrasound provides deeper heat than heat packs alone. The surgery by sectioning piriformis at its origin, release of any fibrous bands and external sciatic neurolysis.[6]

Piriformis syndrome complications:[7]
- Sciatic nerve palsy
- Vascular injury
- Infection
- Hematoma.

Ultrasound Guidance for Piriformis Block (Fig. 3)

Ultrasound-guided procedures has advantage over the fluoroscopy. In comparison to fluoroscopy it improves the visualization of tissues and in addition avoids exposure to radiation. It also improves correct needle placement.

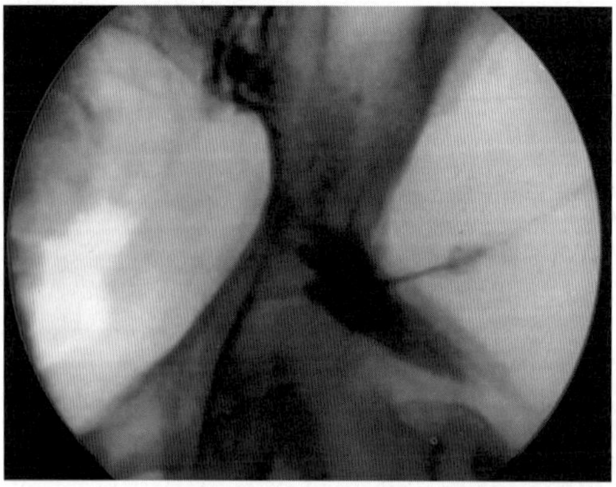

FIG. 2: Needle in piriformis muscle with spread of dye
Courtesy: Dr YL Nankar

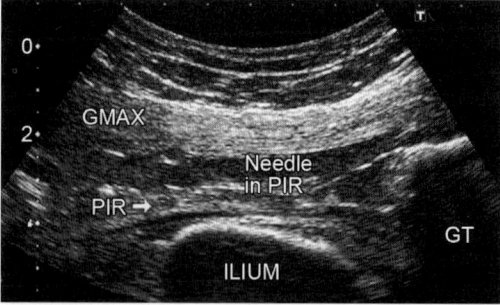

GMAX, Glueteus Maximus; PIR, piriformis; GT, greater trochanter.

FIG. 3: Ultrasound-guided landmarks

PSOAS OR ILIOPSOAS SYNDROME

Introduction

Iliopsoas (IP) syndrome is one of several conditions that affect the hip joint. The iliopsoas muscles include the psoas major, psoas minor, and the iliacus and lie in front of the hip joint. Its main movement is flexion of the hip. The iliopsoas tendon attaches to the thigh bone to the muscle and iliopsoas bursa is the largest bursa in the body.

The chronic lower back pain involving the hips, legs, or thoracic regions can often be traced to an iliopsoas muscle spasm. The groin pain can present a difficult therapeutic and diagnostic dilemma. The source of pain in this region can be from abdominal wall hernias to muscle abnormalities; primary hip disorders (i.e. osteoarthritis); tight iliopsoas; iliopsoas bursitis or tendinitis; ilioposoas tendinitis often seen in rheumatoid arthritis; and secondary mechanical wear or impingement from indwelling orthopedic hardware (i.e. total hip replacements).

The iliopsoas bursitis/tendonitis is caused by overuse and friction as the tendon rides over the iliopectineal eminence of the pubis. This condition is associated with lifting, unloading trucks, and participating in sports requiring extensive use of the hip flexors (e.g. soccer, ballet, uphill running, hurdling, jumping).

Symptoms

The pain in the hip and thigh region, hip stiffness and a clicking or snapping feeling in the hip are signs of iliopsoas injuries. The snapping hip syndrome may be caused by the iliopsoas tendon catching on the pelvis when the hip is flexed. This may cause, a 'snap' and that may or may not cause pain. There is the achy lower back for a few days. Then, the pain seems to spread to the rest of the low back, lower thoracic and even the buttocks (glutei muscles) and hip. The initial pain happens when rising from a seated position even standing, walking or lying down is not comfortable and extending the leg while driving can cause pain too. The patient is unable to stand straight due to uni or bilateral psoas spasm.

Diagnosis

It is best done with a clinical "hands-on" examination will give much needed information and helps in treatment. The X-rays are always negative for findings of IP syndrome. The sonograms may assist with diagnosis. The MRI is most helpful of any imaging tests.

Treatment

The multimodal therapy includes use of NSAIDs, analgesic and injection into iliopsoas. The site of injection depends upon the clinical symptoms, physical examination and MRI.

Iliopsoas Injection Technique

Step 1: The patient in prone position under local anesthesia and C-arm confirm an anteroposterior (AP) view. A 23-gauge, 3.5-inch spinal needle was directed to the affected side and advanced on the left in the inferior portion of the transverse process of the lumbar spines of L2, L3 and L4. Then confirm in the lateral view and advance the needle in the mid-point of the vertebral body.

Step 2: The needles position are confirmed in AP view the tips should be at the level of the transverse process of L2, L3, and L4, then an injection with 2 mL of inj. omnipaque will outlines the iliopsoas muscle (Fig. 4).

Step 3: After negative aspiration inject, the mixture of inj. bupivacaine 0.25% or inj. ropivacaine 0.2% 10–15 cc and inj. triamcinolone 80 mg (Aurocort-preservative free triamcinolone) at all three levels in divided dosage. For long-term pain relief, 100 units of inj. botulinum toxin type A is injected in the divided dosage at three sites.

Iliopsoas Bursa Injection Procedure

Step 1: The patient is in supine position after preparing of the area; feel the pulsation of the femoral artery at the midpoint of the

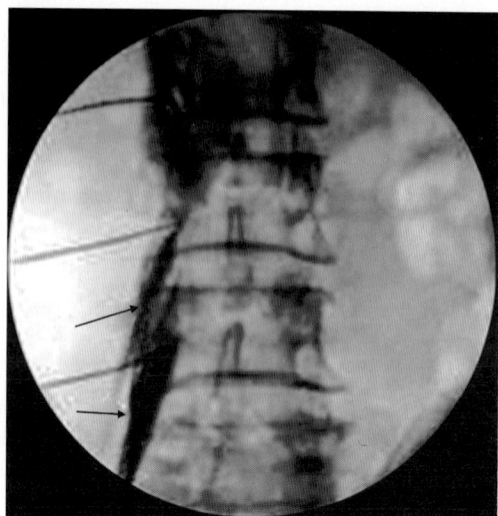

FIG. 4: Outline of iliopsoas muscle—anteroposterior view

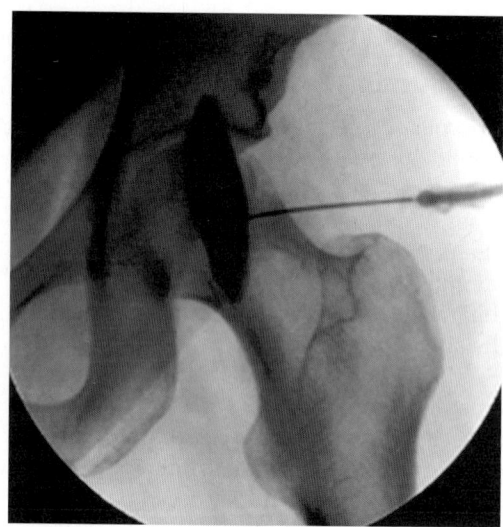

FIG. 6: Spread of contrast into the iliopsoas bursa—AP view

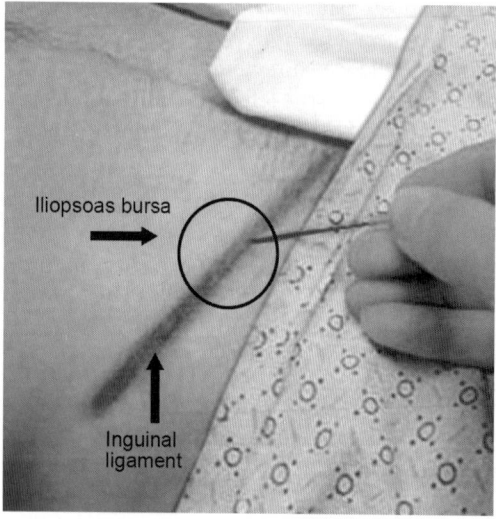

FIG. 5: Needle entry point below inguinal ligament for iliopsoas bursa injection

inguinal ligament is identified. The entry point of needle at a point 2½ inches down and 2½ inches lateral to these femoral arterial pulsations (Fig. 5). In anteroposterior (AP) view of the hip and aim for the superomedial aspect of the femoral head (11 o'clock on the left and 1 o'clock on the right), touch the overlying acetabulum, and pull back.

Step 2: After negative aspiration inject 2 cc of inj. omnipaque, a contrast and confirm the spread of dye (Fig. 6).

Step 3: Again after negative aspiration the mixture of inj. bupivacaine 0.25% or inj. ropivacaine 0.2% plus preservative free inj. triamcinolone acetate 40 mg (Aurocort) injected in to the bursa. For long-term pain relief 100 units of inj. botulinum toxin type A, can be injected.

Iliopsoas Tendon Injection Procedure

Step 1: The entry point of the needle is same as for iliopsoas bursa injection. The patient is supine position and under fluoroscopy visualizes the lesser trochanter and directs the needle on the lesser trochanter.

Step 2: Now confirm the tip of the needle on lesser trochanter, after negative aspiration Inj. Omnipaque 3 cc and visualize the spread of the dye.

Step 3: Again after negative aspiration the mixture of inj. bupivacaine 0.25% or inj. ropivacaine 0.2% plus preservative free inj. triamcinolone acetate 40 mg (Aurocort) injected in to the bursa. For long-term pain relief 100 units of inj. botulinum toxin type A, can be injected. It should be followed with rehabilitation of the deficient muscle functions. If the muscle is weak, strengthen it and a type of crunch is a good tool. There are variations that can customize these exercises for distance runners and individual needs. If the muscle is tight, stretching is paramount.

CONCLUSION

Piriformis and iliopsoas syndromes are different clinical entity in diagnosis of low back pain. A proper history and clinical examination along with investigations, such as MRI, neurography, EMG and nerve conduction studies to rule out these two conditions are of prime importance. This will provide excellent pain relief in many chronic low back pain patients and will avoid unnecessary interventional spine pain procedures and cost effective too.

The back pain sufferers know all too well the agony of simple movement. For many, spinal adjustments, massage or the more drastic measure—back surgery—are ineffective because the real issue could be iliopsoas syndrome.

REFERENCES

1. Yeoman W. The relation of arthritis of the sacroiliac joint to sciatica. Lancet. 1928;2: 1119-22.
2. Wyant GM. Chronic pain syndromes and their treatment. III. The piriformis syndrome. Can Anaesth Soc J. 1979;4: 305-8.
3. Kirschner JS, Foye PM, Cole JL. Piriformis syndrome, diagnosis and treatment. Muscle Nerve. 2009;40(1):10-8.
4. Popovac H, Bojanic I, Smoljanovic T. Leg length discrepancy as a rare cause of a piriformis syndrome. J Back Musculoskelet Rehabil. 2012;25(4):299-300.
5. AG, Haynes J, and Jordan SE, et al. Sciatica of nondisk origin and piriformis syndrome: diagnosis by magnetic resonance neurography and interventional magnetic resonance imaging with outcome study of resulting treatment. J Neurosurg Spine. 2005;2(2):99-115.
6. Smoll NR. Variations of the piriformis and sciatic nerve with clinical consequence: review. Clin Anat. 2010;23(1):8-17.
7. Benzon HT, Katz JA, Benzon HA, Iqbal MS. Piriformis syndrome: anatomic considerations, a new injection technique, and a review of the literature. Anesthesiology. 2003;98(6):1442-8.

SECTION 6

Urogenital and Pelvic Pain

CHAPTER 25

Nonmalignant Urogenital Pain Management

Ashish Gulve, John Hughes

INTRODUCTION

Chronic urogenital pain is a complex, perplexing problem involving a significant number of patients and invariably needing multidisciplinary management. The patients frequently come with poorly defined symptoms and significant psychosocial changes. Patients affected with urogenital pain pay huge personal costs in terms of years of suffering, disability, sexual dysfunction, marital discord and loss of employment. In women approximately 10% of referrals to gynecologists and 44% of laparoscopies are performed to evaluate chronic pelvic pain.[1,2] The pelvic and perineal area has a complex neurophysiology. There are contributions from somatic, visceral, sympathetic and parasympathetic nerves. The pain could therefore be nociceptive, visceral, and neuropathic or mixed in nature.

A comprehensive, multidisciplinary approach involving gynecologist, urologist, obstetrician, gastroenterologists, general surgeons, psychologists, physiotherapist and pain physicians are essential.

Patients presenting with urogenital pain (Box 1) can be divided into two broad groups:
1. Those with well-defined conditions that have a clear treatment pathway (e.g., urinary tract infection, renal stones).
2. Those with poorly defined conditions for which there is no clearly defined diagnosis or curative treatment. These are often best described as chronic pelvic pain syndromes (Table 1).[3] No proven infection or other obvious pathology. It also includes conditions described as **'Chronic Pelvic Pain Syndrome' (Fig. 1)**.

These syndromes are associated with changes in the central nervous system that may allow for the persistent perception of pain in the absence of ongoing acute changes. There may also be central sensitization, which amplifies the perception of a stimulus such that nonpainful stimuli become perceived as painful.[4] These changes occur throughout the nervous system and may influence the psychological changes seen in these patients.

NEUROANATOMY OF PELVIS AND PERINEUM

The pelvic structures receive thoracolumbar sympathetic (T12-L1) and visceral innervations via the superior hypogastric plexus. The parasympathetic and further visceral innervations via the pelvic splanchnic nerves and somatic innervations from the pudendal nerve (S2-4), obturator nerve (L2-4) and coccygeal plexus (S4-5).

Box 1: Diseases that may cause or contribute to urogenital pain

Female genitilia
- Vulvodynia
- Vulvar Vestibulitis Syndrome
- Clitorial Pain

Male genitilia
- Prostatitis
- Prostadynia
- Orchialgia
- Epididymitis
- Balanitis
- Congenital seminal vesicle obstruction

Gynecologic-extrauterine
- Adhesions
- Adnexal cysts
- Chronic ectopic pregnancy
- Chlamydial endometritis or salpingitis
- Endometriosis
- Endosalpingiosis
- Ovarian retention syndrome
- Ovarian remnant syndrome
- Ovarian dystrophy or ovulatory pain
- Pelvic congestion syndrome
- Postoperative peritoneal cysts
- Residual accessory ovary
- Subacute salpingo-oophoritis
- Tuberculous salpingitis

Gynecologic-uterine
- Adenomyosis
- Atypical dysmenorrhea or ovulatory pain
- Cervical stenosis
- Chronic endometritis
- Endometrial or cervical polyps
- Intrauterine contraceptive device
- Leiomyomata
- Genital prolapse

Urologic
- Bladder neoplasm
- Chronic urinary tract infection
- Interstitial cystitis
- Radiation cystitis
- Recurrent, acute cystitis
- Recurrent, acute urethritis
- Stone/urolithiasis
- Uninhibited bladder contractions
- Detrusor-sphincter dyssynergia
- Urethral diverticulum
- Urethral caruncle
- Urethral Syndrome

Continued

Continued

Anorectal pain
- Levator Ani Syndrome
- Proctalgia Fugax
- Anal Fissures
- Thrombosed Hemorrhoids
- Rectal Prolapse

Gastrointestinal
- Carcinoma of the colon
- Chronic intermittent bowel obstruction
- Colitis
- Constipation
- Diverticular disease
- Inflammatory bowel disease
- Irritable bowel syndrome

Musculoskeletal
- Abdominal wall myofacial pain
- Coccygodynia
- Compression of lumbar vertebrae
- Degenerative joint disease
- Disk
- Faulty or poor posture
- Fibromyositis
- Hernias: ventral, inguinal, femoral, Spigelian
- Ischial Spine and Pudendal Nerve Entrapment
- Low back pain
- Muscular strains and sprains
- Neoplasia of spinal cord or sacral nerve
- Neuralgia of iliohypogastric ilioinguinal, and/or genitofemoral nerves
- Piriformis syndrome
- Rectus tendon strain
- Spondylosis
- Symphysis Pubis Dysfunction
- Sacroiliac Joint Pain

Other
- Abdominal cutaneous nerve entrapment in surgical scar
- Abdominal epilepsy
- Abdominal migraine
- Bipolar personality disorder
- Depression
- Familial Mediterranean fever
- Neurologic dysfunction
- Porphyria
- Post-surgical Neuromas
- Shingles
- Sleep disturbances
- Somatic referral

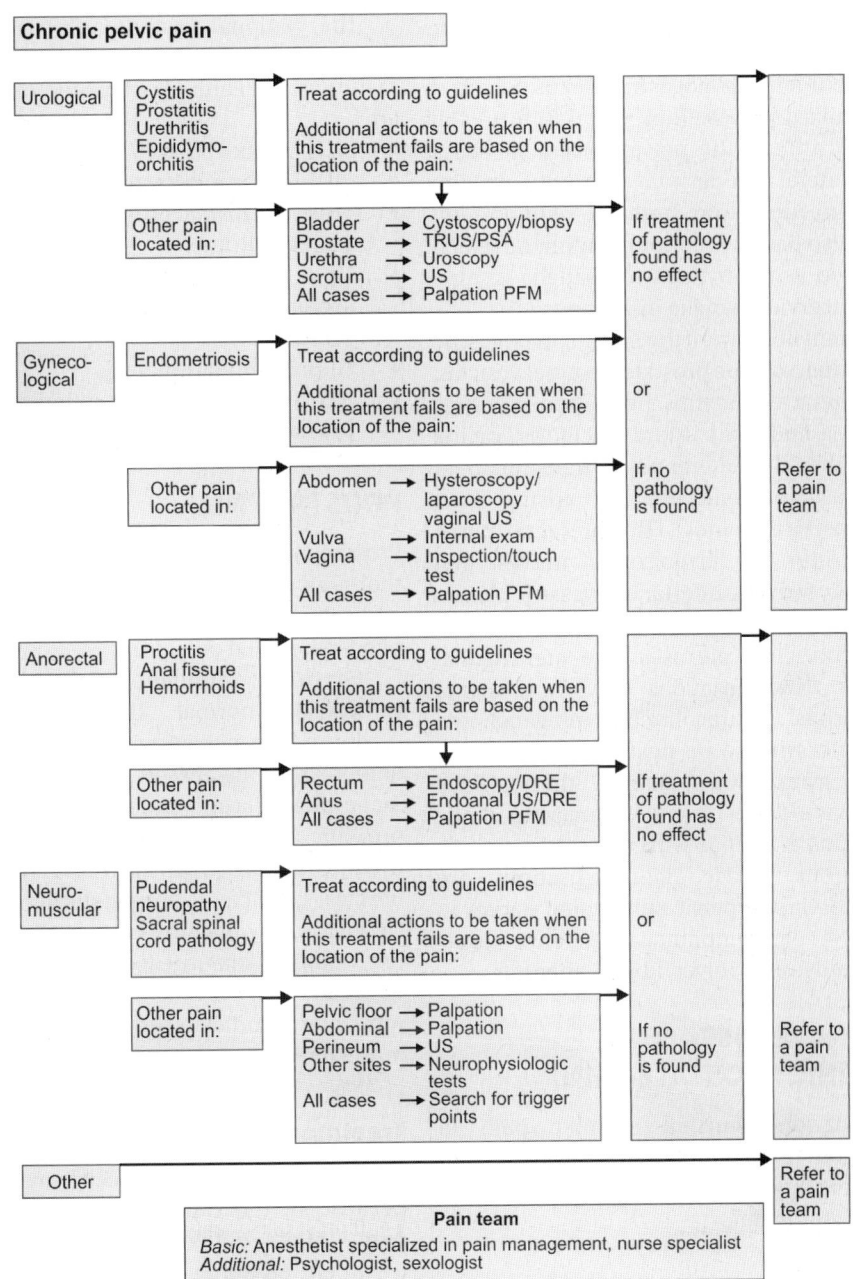

FIG. 1: An algorithm for diagnosing and managing chronic pelvic pain (CPP)

Source: From Fall M, et al. EAU guidelines on chronic pelvic pain. Eur Urol. 2010, with permission.

The pelvic splanchnic nerves and associated visceral nerves join the sympathetics to form the inferior hypogastric plexus, which is thus a mixed plexus. They go on to form sub plexuses around the pelvic viscera. It has a posterolateral retroperitoneal component with interconnections from both the right and left side. It also has an anterior component, which is referred as the hypogastric ganglia in men and paracervical ganglia in women.

Efferent fibers from the inferior hypogastric plexus innervate the prostate, seminal vesicles, vas deferens, epididymis, penis, penile corpus cavernosa and the corpora of clitoris, vagina and urethra. The lateral pelvis transmits pain via parasympathetic neurons arising from S2-S4 (nervi erigentes). The presacral nerve divides into the hypogastric nerves that eventually form the inferior hypogastric plexus. This plexus divides into vesicle, middle rectal and uterovaginal plexuses. The uterovaginal plexus carries sensations only from vagina and corpus. Thoracolumbar preganglionic fibers also synapse on postganglionic nerves in the sympathetic ganglia that mingle with autonomic sacral parasympathetic projections as well as with the pelvic somatic innervations. Pelvic floor sensations are mediated via the pelvic splanchnic nerves to the S2-S4 parasympathetic afferents. Testis and epididymis involves T10-L1 afferents.

CHRONIC PROSTATITIS (CHRONIC PROSTATE PAIN)

Persistent or recurrent episodic pain in the region of the prostate, associated with symptoms suggestive of urinary tract and/or sexual dysfunction.

Symptoms

Symptoms may include persistent urinary urgency, dysuria, poor urinary flow, perineal discomfort and pain. Pain can radiate to the lower back, suprapubic area and groin. Patient may also complain of pain with ejaculation.

The National Institute of Diabetes and Digestive and Kidney Diseases of the National Institutes of Health classification of prostatitis are:

- NIH I: Acute bacterial prostatitis.
- NIH II: Chronic bacterial prostatitis.
- NIH III: Chronic prostatitis/chronic pelvic pain syndrome.
- III A: Inflammatory (expressed prostatic secretion, urine after prostatic massage, semen);
- III B: Noninflammatory.
- NIH IV: Asymptomatic inflammatory, e.g. prostatitis confirmed by histology.

PROSTADYNIA

Prostadynia is a diagnosis of exclusion. A thorough urological examination is essential, and referred pain from, colorectal structures need to be ruled out.

Physical examination of the prostate is typically normal. There would be no tenderness on palpation. Urodynamic studies demonstrate decreased urinary flow rates, incomplete relaxation of the bladder neck and prostatic urethra, as well as abnormally high urethral closure pressure at rest. The external urethral sphincter is normal during urination.

Laboratory diagnosis by a two-glass test or pre- and post-massage test (PPMT).[5]

In an extensive analysis of both tests, PPMT was able to indicate the correct diagnosis in more than 96% of patients.[6]

Treatment

Many therapies are based on anecdote because of the unknown cause of prostate pain. Most patients require multimodal treatment aimed at the main symptoms and taking comorbidities into account (Fig. 2).

Alpha-blockers such as terazosin, alfuzosin, doxazosin, tamsulosin, reduce urinary symptoms and pain. An alpha-blocker should be given for at least 3–6 months before assessing treatment. Empirical antibiotic therapy

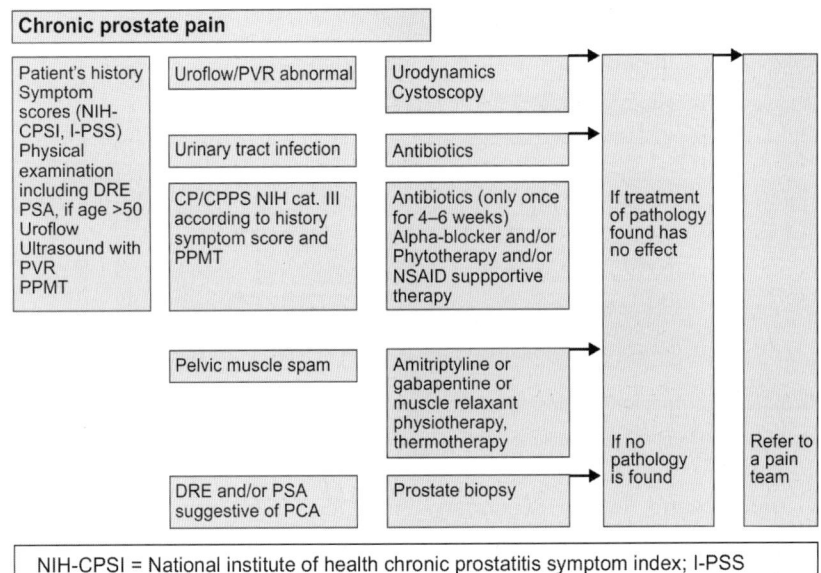

FIG. 2: General diagnostic and treatment algorithm for chronic prostate pain

Source: From Fall M, et al. EAU guidelines on chronic pelvic pain. Eur Urol. 2010, with permission.

is widely used because some patients have improved with antimicrobial therapy. Patients responding to antibiotics should be maintained on medication for 4–6 weeks or even longer. Nonsteroidal anti-inflammatory drugs may be of benefit in some patients. Immunomodulation using cytokine inhibitors or other approaches may be helpful. Corticosteroids are generally not effective.

Opioids produce modest pain relief in some patients with refractory prostate pain syndrome and should be used in collaboration with pain clinics and other treatments. 5-α-reductase inhibitors such as finasteride may improve voiding and pain. The alternate therapies such as biofeedback, relaxation therapy, has improved lifestyle and may improve symptoms. The transrectal and transurethral heat therapy is helpful.

Surgery

Surgery processes such as transurethral incision of the bladder neck,[7] radical transurethral resection of the prostate[8,9] or in particular radical prostatectomy, has a very limited role with specific indication.[10] The transurethral needle ablation of the prostate (TUNA) was only comparable to sham treatment.[11]

ORCHIALGIA/TESTICULAR PAIN

Repeated episode of testicular pain could be due to urinary tract or sexual dysfunction without any epididymo-orchitis or other obvious pathology.

Like many urogenital pains, it has a wide differential diagnosis. Many patients cannot

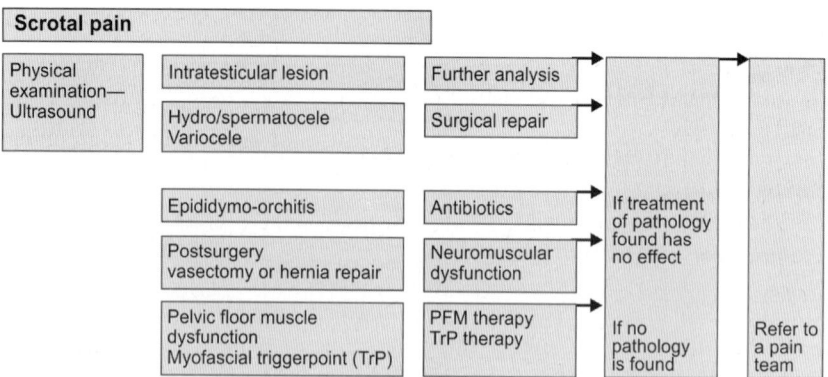

FIG. 3: An algorithm for diagnosing and managing scrotal pain
Source: From Fall M, et al. EAU guidelines on chronic pelvic pain. Eur Urol. 2010, with permission.

recall any precipitating event. Secondary causes include infection, tumor, testicular torsion, varicocele, hydrocele, spermatocele, trauma, including repetitive microtrauma. Previous surgeries, such as vasectomy, inguinal hernia repair or testicular surgery can lead to altered sensation and neuropathic pain or a chronic inflammatory process. Referred pain from ureters, hip, lumbar facet joints or disks should be ruled out in addition to entrapment neuropathies of ilioinguinal or genitofemoral nerves (Fig. 3).

Treatment is based on generalized management of urogenital pain.

BLADDER PAIN SYNDROME (INTERSTITIAL CYSTITIS)

The European Society for the Study of bladder pain syndrome/Interstitial cystitis calls the disease bladder pain syndrome (BPS), including a history of more than 6 months of pelvic pain, pressure, or discomfort perceived to be related to the urinary bladder, accompanied by at least one other urinary symptom, such as persistent urge to void or urinary frequency.

Bladder pain syndrome (BPS) is a symptom complex affecting urinary bladder and is characterized by pelvic pain, urinary urgency, frequency and nocturia. It is a severely debilitating syndrome with poorly understood etiology. It is more common among Caucasians and there is a female predominance of about 10:1. Associations between BPS and inflammatory bowel disease, systemic lupus erythematosus, irritable bowel syndrome, fibromyalgia and panic disorders have been reported.[12-15]

Bladder pain syndrome may result from complex interactions between nervous, immune and endocrine systems. Factors contributing to its pathogenesis include infections, inflammation, mast cell activation, urothelial dysfunction, autoimmune mechanisms, nitric oxide synthetase-dependent nitric oxide production, increased sympathetic outflow, toxic constituents in urine and decreased bladder perfusion leading to cellular hypoxia.

The diagnosis is made using symptoms, examination, urine analysis, cystoscopy with hydrodistension and biopsy. Cystoscopy can reveal destructive inflammation (ulcerations) with some patients eventually developing a small-capacity fibrotic bladder or upper urinary tract outflow obstruction. Reddened mucosal areas often associated with small vessels and a characteristic waterfall-type of bleeding will be present in classic interstitial cystitis.

Treatment

It is empiric with simple analgesics, weak or strong opioids. Corticosteroids can be useful in patients with ulcerative interstitial cystitis. Antihistaminics (H1 and H2 blockers), tricyclic antidepressants, pentosanpolysulfate sodium, long-term antibiotics, immunosuppressant's, such as azathioprine, anticonvulsants (pregabalin and gabapentin), immunoregulators (sulplatast tosilate), bioflavonoids (quercetin) and recombinant human nerve growth factor.

Intravesical treatment with local anesthetics, pentosanpolysulfate sodium, heparin, hyaluronic acid, chondroitin sulfate, dimethyl sulfoxide, BCG, and vanilloids has been used (Fig. 4).

The transurethral resection, coagulation and Laser aims to remove urothelial lesions. Intravescial botulinum toxin injection may have antinociceptive effects. TENS, physical therapy and sacral neuromodulation in intractable patients have also been recommended.

Surgical Treatment

Surgical treatment in the form of supratrigonal cystectomy, subtriagonal cystectomy or radical cystectomy including resection of urethra has been suggested but multidisciplinary involvement with a pain management unit is strongly recommended.

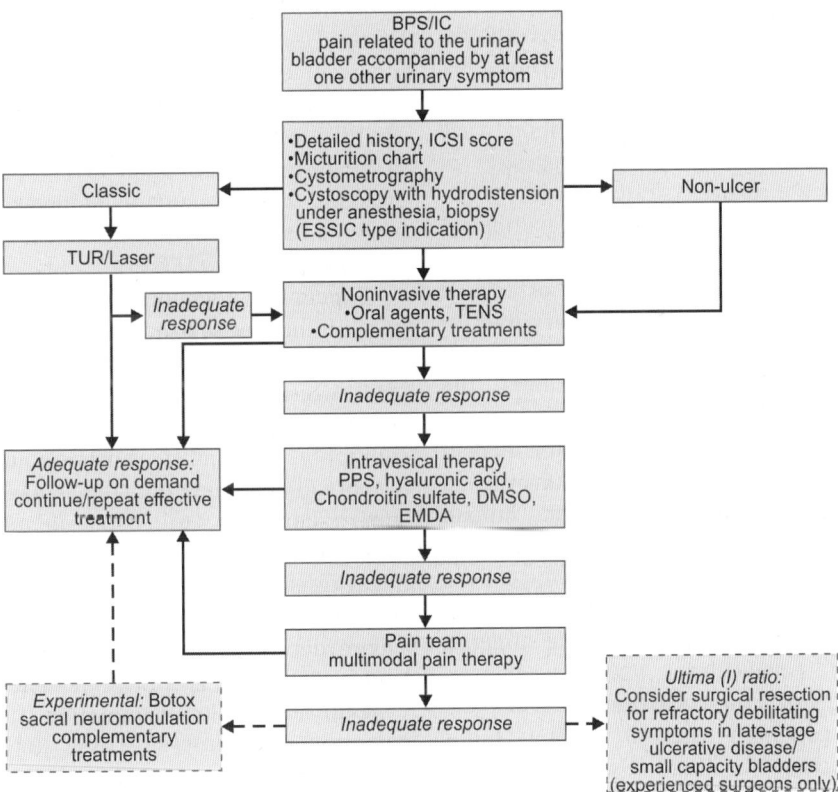

FIG. 4: Flowchart for the diagnosis and therapy of bladder pain syndrome/interstitial cystitis
Source: From Fall M, et al. EAU guidelines on chronic pelvic pain. Eur Urol. 2010, with permission.

VULVAR PAIN SYNDROME (VULVODYNIA)

Within this syndrome, several clinical entities are described. Vulvodynia is defined as vulval burning or pain that cannot be consistently and tightly localized by point pressure 'mapping' by probing with a cotton-tipped applicator or similar instrument. The vulvar vestibule may be involved but the discomfort is not limited to the vestibule.

Clinically, the pain may occur with or without provocation (touch, pressure or friction). In localized vulvar pain syndrome, pain is consistently and tightly localized by point-pressure mapping to one or more portions of the vulva while in vulvar vestibulitis pain is localized by point-pressure mapping to one or more portions of the vulvar vestibule. Other entities include vulvar pain syndromes. (Persistent or recurrent episodic vulvar pain either related to the micturition cycle or associated with symptoms suggestive of urinary tract or sexual dysfunction without any proven infection or other obvious pathology) and vaginal pain syndrome (Persistent or recurrent episodic vaginal pain associated with symptoms suggestive of urinary tract or sexual dysfunction without any proven vaginal infection or other obvious pathology). The incidence is as high as 5%.[16] The women are typically Caucasian, nulliparous with median age of 32 years. Bartholin's abscess, vulvovaginal candidiasis, herpes, herpes-zoster, human papilloma virus, *Trichomonas* and molluscum contagiosum infections are some of the causes. Trauma due to sexual assault, vaginal deliveries, episiotomy, hymenectomy or vaginal surgeries can result in vulvodynia. Vulvar dermatoses are a frequent cause of chronic vulvar pain. Systemic conditions such as systemic lupus erythematosus, Crohn's disease, Behçet's disease, Sjögren's syndrome, allergic dermatitis, urethral syndrome and interstitial cystitis, local neoplasms can cause vulvodynia.

Medical management often required a multimodal approach and includes supportive measures such as proper vulvar hygiene, sitz bath, topical local anesthetics, antivirals, antifungals, antihistaminics, topical estrogen, steroids and anti-inflammatory. Hormone replacement therapy, tricyclic antidepressants, anticonvulsants, capsaicin are useful in some patients. Biofeedback, psychological and behavioral pain management should be considered. Surgical intervention, such as perineoplasty, vestibuloplasty, partial or total vestibulectomy with vaginal advancement should only be considered as part of a multidisciplinary approach.

URETHRAL PAIN SYNDROME

Urethral pain syndrome is characterized by recurrent episodic urethral pain, usually on voiding, with daytime frequency and nocturia. The diagnosis is one of exclusion upon absence of proven infection or other obvious pathology. Systemic diseases, such as diabetes mellitus, multiple sclerosis and collagen diseases should be ruled out (Fig. 5).

Subclinical infections, chronic inflammation of the periurethral glands or urethral spasticity with periurethral muscle fatigue has been suggested as possible etiologies.

Patients would present with dysuria, suprapubic discomfort, urinary frequency and dyspareunia. Voiding difficulties may occur in some patients.

A careful examination to rule out anatomical causes for pain should be performed. Urethral infections, such as syphilis, gonorrhea, Chlamydia or Mycoplasma stones, tumors, cysts or diverticuli should be excluded.

Pain and tenderness may be present on palpation. Urethrocystoscopy may reveal slightly inflamed mucosa. Treatment includes empirical antibiotic therapy followed by low dose long-term antibiotic therapy. Anti-inflammatories, muscle relaxants and

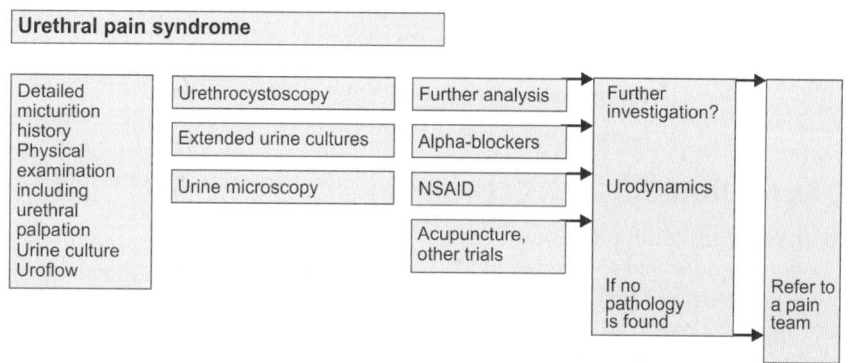

FIG. 5: An algorithm for diagnosing and managing urethral pain syndrome
Source: From Fall M, et al. EAU guidelines on chronic pelvic pain. Eur Urol. 2010, with permission.

α-antagonists are useful in some patients. Vaginal estrogen for peri- and postmenopausal women are recommended.

ANORECTAL PAIN SYNDROMES

Anorectal pain syndromes involve persistent or recurrent, episodic rectal pain with associated rectal trigger points/tenderness related to symptoms of bowel dysfunction in the absence of proven infection or other obvious pathology. Levator ani syndrome and proctalgia fugax are the two most common functional disorders. When the pain is continuous it is called as proctodynia while a paroxysmal pain would be proctalgia fugax.

Levator Ani Syndrome

Levator ani syndrome is also known as puborectalis syndrome, chronic proctalgia or pelvic tension myalgia. The symptoms are typically dull, aching or pressure like discomfort in the rectum that lasts several hours. Prolonged sitting and defecation precipitate the pain. There may be a sensation of incomplete defecation in some patients. The pain episodes are chronic and recurrent lasting for 20 minutes or longer.

On rectal examination, there may be tenderness on palpation due to levator ani muscle spasm. The muscle is palpated by moving the examining finger from the coccyx posteriorly to the pubic symphysis on either side. The tenderness is usually asymmetric.

Other organic conditions, such as inflammatory bowel disease, cryptitis, anal fissures, hemorrhoids, coccygodynia, ischemia and intersphincteric abscess should be ruled out.

Treatment is symptomatic and involves digital massage to the levator ani muscle three to four times per week. The duration of massage depends on individual patient's tolerance. Muscle relaxants, such as benzodiazepines, methocarbamol can be useful. Sitz bath can help some patients.

Proctalgia Fugax

Proctalgia fugax is characterized by sudden, severe, aching, cramping, gnawing or stabbing rectal pain lasting seconds to minutes that seems to arise in the rectum. It is intermittent pain occurring at irregular intervals and patients are completely asymptomatic until the next episode. The frequency of these episodes varies. The duration is generally less than 5 minutes but occasionally can last up to 30 minutes. There may be associated anal sphincter spasm or contractions of the puborectalis and external anal sphincter. It is more common in females. Treatment involves clonidine, salbutamol or nitrates inhalation, diltiazem and caudal epidural injection of local anesthetic and steroids.

PUDENDAL NEURALGIA

In some patients with pudendal neuralgia, there may be pudendal nerve entrapment. Pudendal nerve entrapment (PNE) may causes neuropathic pain in the region supplied by the pudendal nerve. The pudendal nerve being chronically compressed in the ischiorectal fossa. In men with pudendal nerve entrapment, aberrant development and subsequent malpositioning of the ischial spine appear to be associated with athletic activities during their youth.[17] The changes occur during the period of development and ossification of the spinous process of the ischium. Pudendal nerve is entrapped between the sacrotuberous and sacrospinous ligaments and may engage the falciform process of the sacrotuberous ligament. The stretching of the pudendal nerve from chronic constipation causes neuropathy.[18] The normal vaginal delivery causes measurable neuropathy lasts approximately three months.[19] Patients with PNE typically present with pain in the penis, scrotum, labia, vagina, perineum, or anorectal region. The pain may be in the form of numbness or burning, sharp shooting kind of pain that is aggravated by sitting, relieved by standing, and absent when recumbent or when sitting on a toilet seat. The pain is usually unilateral.

Pudendal nerve entrapment is a clinical diagnosis of conditions in patients with the typical history. Neurological examination of the perineum is invariably normal.

Prostatitis like urogenital pain and voiding and sexual dysfunction are commonly seen in patients with pudendal neuropathy. Men with urogenital pain or rectal pain or both, with or without voiding symptoms and with or without ejaculatory pain, may have chronic pelvic pain syndrome. Prostatitis (reproductive tract infection) is ruled out by the absence of infection or inflammatory cells in the prostatic secretions. These patients have National Institutes of Health (NIH) category IIIB chronic prostatitis and chronic pelvic pain syndrome.[20]

The patients can be divided into 5-symptom groups: [21]

1. Short-term pain preceded, by voiding complaints; usual onset is after 2–5 months of identifiable trauma.
2. Insidious, long-standing symptoms with many past consultations and treatments or surgical procedures.
3. Sudden onset of pain while squatting and lifting. Often this pain precipitates a visit to an emergency department, but no pathologic features are identified. This pain is often wrongly treated as epididymitis or testicular torsion.
4. Pain after pelvic radiation therapy, typically for carcinoma of the prostate.
5. Pain from inflammatory processes after perineal surgery or drainage of phlegmon.

The MRI is not adequate for diagnosis of PNE. Specialized neurophysiological testing may reveal sacral reflex latency and the pudendal nerve distal motor latency. The value of the clinical neurophysiological investigations is debatable. Imaging techniques that permit 3-dimensional reconstruction of the pelvis have been used to evaluate pudenda artery abnormalities[22] with 3-dimensional reconstruction one may be able to measure the positional variation of the Ischial spine over the ischial tuberosity and the distance between the ischial spine and the sacrococcygeal notch.

The diagnostic and therapeutic pudendal nerve block can be useful.

Surgical decompression of the pudendal nerve in the Alcock's canal will result in pain relief in patients who had short-term relief with diagnostic block.

Pulsed radiofrequency of the pudendal nerve has also been useful in some patients.[23]

Nonsurgical management should be in the form of specific physiotherapy targeted towards pelvic floor muscles, simple analgesics, weak and strong opioids. Anticonvulsants and antidepressants are useful in patients with neuropathic symptoms.

COCCYGODYNIA

Pain localized to the coccyx is a common cause of perineal pain. It is more common in women and elderly debilitated patients. Coccygodynia is characterized by pain and tenderness in the area of coccyx, typically worse with sitting for prolonged time. A transient exacerbation of the pain when standing up from sitting can occur in patients with posterior subluxation of coccyx.

A history of an acute event (e.g. trauma or childbirth) may be present in some while in others a history of repetitive microtrauma may be present. There may be no identifiable cause. Only injuries sustained within the month before the onset of coccygodynia will significantly increase the risk of instability (especially of posterior luxation), and that only this recent trauma has an established effect in terms of precipitating coccygodynia. The same time limit applies to childbirth.[24] If more than a month has elapsed since the traumatic event, the percentage of patients with instability will not differ significantly from that in patients without a history of trauma.

On examination, there may be pain at the coccyx or sacrococcygeal junction. Before making a diagnosis of coccygodynia, a thorough history, examination and investigations to rule out other pathologies causing referred pain is important. Pain from lumbo-sacral spine, sacrum, anus, rectum, pelvis and genitourinary tract can be referred to the coccyx. Inflammatory arthritic conditions should be ruled out.

Investigations with lateral dynamic radiographs of the sacrum and pelvis may reveal pathologies, such as posterior or anterior subluxation, hypermobility of coccyx and bony spicules. The comparison of standing versus sitting radiographs allows the measurement of sagittal rotation of the pelvis (pelvic tilt) and of the coccygeal angle of incidence, which are characteristic features of the subject's way of sitting down. These angles are related to the subject's BMI and determine the type of coccygeal lesion.

Coccygodynia from anterior luxation or from spicules was seen to occur in leaner and slightly younger patients while posterior subluxation is common in obese patients and post-traumatic coccygodynia.

Treatment

Initial conservative treatment of coccygodynia should include modified sitting position to avoid further irritation of coccyx due to pressure. A donut-shaped pillow will help take pressure off the coccyx when sitting. The manipulations under anesthesia, stretching the ligaments attached to the coccyx can be helpful.

Nonsteroidal aniti-inflammatory drugs NSAIDs (such as diclofenac, ibuprofen, naproxen and COX-2 inhibitors) may help to reduce inflammation and pain. It often takes many weeks, or even months, for the pain to subside. If the pain is persistent or severe, additional treatments may include local anesthetic and steroid injection at the sacro-coccygeal junction or Ganglion Impar block.

Patients getting short-term pain relief with Ganglion Impar block may get longer relief with pulsed or thermal radiofrequency of ganglion impar or chemical neurolysis. Physical therapy with ultrasound can also be helpful.

For people who have persistent pain that is not alleviated or well-controlled with conservative treatment, surgical removal of the coccyx (coccygectomy) is an option. The results of coccygectomy are extremely variable and there are significant risks and complications.

GENERALIZED TREATMENT OF UROGENITAL PAIN

There is very little specific evidence for the role of analgesic and coanalgesic drugs in CPP, with one systematic review in women suggesting that further research is required.[25]

Medications

Paracetamol

It should be considered on its own. It has analgesic and antipyretic activity and is used in acute and chronic painful conditions.[26]

There is evidence for its use in somatic pain and arthritic pain in particular,[27,28] but the benefits are limited. There is little evidence about its role in urogenital pain.

NSAIDs

For practical purposes, the NSAIDs may be divided into:
- Nonselective, low potency (e.g. salicylic acid, ibuprofen, mefenamic acid)
- Nonselective, high potency (e.g. ketoprofen, diclofenac, ketorolac)
- COX2 selective drugs (e.g. celecoxib, etoricoxib).

There is very little evidence for NSAIDs to be used in the management of CPP and even less evidence for COX2 selective drugs. Most analgesic studies have investigated dysmenorrhea, in which NSAIDs were found to be superior to placebo and possibly paracetamol.[29]

Tricyclic Antidepressants TCAs

There is very little evidence in CPP for TCAs in humans.

Saarto and Wiffen[30] concluded that TCAs are effective for neuropathic pain suggested dose of amitriptyline and nortriptyline was 150 mg once daily.

Anticonvulsants

Gabapentin and pregabalin have been used for pain management and produce a more natural sleep state at night than antidepressants. Pregabalin has been studies in large, long duration studies, and in four neuropathic pain conditions, including fibromyalgia.

It has useful levels of efficacy in all the conditions, with NNTs of 3 to 5 in neuropathic pain, and around 9 in fibromyalgia.[34] Pregabalin has NNH of 6 to 8.[31]

N-methyl-D-aspartate (NMDA) Antagonists

The NMDA receptor channel complex is known to be an important channel for the development and maintenance of chronic pain. It is felt to be particularly important when there is evidence of central sensitization and opioid tolerance.[32-36]

Ketamine

It is useful chronic pain states such as peripheral neuropathies with allodynia, stump and phantom pain, central pain, and cancer-related pain, with and without a neurological component but its long-term role remains unclear.[37] Ketamine is primarily at the NMDA receptor, is used for nerve injury or central sensitization.

Sodium Channel Blockade

It is useful for patients with urogenital pain, nerve injury and neuropathic change. The sodium channels underlie the mechanisms of mechano-, thermo-, and chemosensitivity.[38] It is demonstrated that intravenous lidocaine reduces neuropathic pain and allodynia. The positive response to intravenous lignocaine does not indicate that mexiletine will work.[39]

Opioids

There is now a general acceptance that opioids have a role in the management of chronic nonmalignant pain.[40] The use of opioids in urogenital pain is poorly defined. Their use in neuropathic pain remains equivocal but a meta-analysis suggests clinically important benefits.[41] Generally, slow-release preparations are preferred for chronic pain. The titrating of the dose should be closely monitored to assess both benefit and side effects. Rotating from one opioid to another also requires close monitoring as there are no exact dose equivalents. Assessing benefit from opioids should include objective improvements in function.

Morphine, oxycodone, transdermal fentanyl and methadone can be used. Methadone is a strong analgesic with a long track record of use. It has opioid and NMDA-antagonistic activity.[42] The Canadian Pain Society[41] supports its use as a fourth-line agent in treating neuropathic pain in a consensus document. Rotating from other opioids to methadone is not an exact science because dosing ratios are not clearly understood.[43]

Metabolite accumulation and cardiac side effects can be a problem.

Buprenorphine and pentazocine both have agonist and antagonist properties and can induce withdrawal symptoms in patients used to opioids. Buprenorphine topical patches may offer a similar advantage to topical fentanyl. Codeine and dihydrocodeine are effective for the relief of mild-to-moderate pain. They are limited by side effects (notably constipation) and genetic variance of metabolism that affects analgesic efficacy. Tramadol produces analgesia by two mechanisms, an opioid effect and an enhancement of serotoninergic and adrenergic pathways.[44,45] A Cochrane review suggests that there is a role for tramadol in neuropathic pain management.[46]

The decision to start long-term opioid therapy should be made by an appropriately trained specialist in consultation with another physician only after all other reasonable treatments have been tried and failed.

General guidelines for the use of opioids in chronic pain should be followed.[47,48]

Interventional Procedures

These blocks are initially done diagnostic with local anesthetic block followed by neurolytic

Table 1: Interventional treatments for urogenital pain

Intervention	Indications	Comments
Bilateral lumbar sympathetic block	Orchialgia, testicular/scrotal pain syndromes, post-hernia repair pain and renal pain.	No controlled studies
Neurolytic blocks should be avoided in nonmalignant pain.		
Superior hypogastric plexus block	Orchialgia, prostadynia, penile/clitorial pain, interstitial cystitis, vulvodynia and renal pain	
	Diagnostic and prognostic tool before presacral neurectomy, to rule out referred low back pain from abdominal/pelvic pain. Neurolytic blocks should be avoided in nonmalignant pain.	
Ganglion impar block	Coccygodynia, intractable neoplastic perineal pain	
Pudendal nerve block	Penile, clitorial, vulvar and perineal pain syndromes possibly pelvic floor muscle spasm and pudendal nerve injury related pain.	
Coccygeal, ileoinguinal and genitofemoral nerve blocks	Scrotal/testicular pain syndromes, neuropathic pain associated with nerve damage, such as following hernia repairs	
Sacral neuromodulation	Refractory urinary voiding disorders, interstitial cystitis	

are preferred. The variety of interventional procedure includes bilateral lumbar plexus block, hypogastric, lumbar sympathetic blocks pudandal nerve block, ganglion of impar block, coccygeal, genitofemoral, ileoinguinal, sacral neuromodulation (Table 1).

Other interventional procedures include repeated bladder over distension, electromotive drug administration are useful in some patients.

CONCLUSION

Nonmalignant urongenigtal pain is an entity with many syndromes. Pain in this entity has many facets such urological, gynecological, vulvar, prostatic factors.

The multimodal pain relief in association of tackling of psychological issues will help in maximum pain relief.

REFERENCES

1. Howard FM. The role of laparoscopy in chronic pelvic pain: Promise and pitfalls. Obstet Gynecol Surv .1993;48: 357-87.
2. Reiter RC. A profile of women with chronic pelvic pain. Clin Obstet Gynecol. 1990;33:130-6.
3. Fall M, et al. EAU guidelines on chronic pelvic pain. Eur Urol. 2010;57(1):35-48.
4. Maria Adele G, et al. Viscero-visceral hyperalgesia: Characterization in different clinical models. Pain 2010;151(2):307-22.
5. Nickel JC. The Pre- and post- massage test (PPMT): A simple screen for prostatitis. Tech Urol. 1997;3(1): 38-43.
6. Nickel JC, Shoskes D, Wang Y, Alexander RB, Fowler JE Jr, Zeitlin S, O'Leary MP, Pontari MA, Schaeffer AJ, Landis JR, Nyberg L, Kusek JW, Propert KJ. How does the pre-massage and post-massage 2-glass test compare to the Meares-Stamey 4-glass test in men with chronic prostatitis/chronic pelvic pain syndrome? J Urol. 2006;176(1):119-24.
7. Kaplan SA, Te AE, Jacobs BZ. Urodynamic evidence of vesical neck obstruction in men with misdiagnosed chronic nonbacterial prostatitis and the therapeutic role of endoscopic incision of the bladder neck. J Urol. 1994;152(6 Pt 1):2063-5.
8. Barnes RW, Hadley HL, O'Donoghue EP. Transurethral resection of the prostate for chronic bacterial prostatitis. Prostate. 1982;3(3):215-9.
9. Sant GR, Heaney JA, Meares EM. Radical transurethral prostatic resection in the management of chronic bacterial prostatitis. J Urol. 1984;131:184A.
10. Nickel JC. Prostatitis: Evolving management strategies. Urol Clin North Am. 1999;26(4):737-51.
11. Leskinen MJ, Kilponen A, Lukkarinen O, Tammela TL. Transurethral needle ablation for the treatment of chronic pelvic pain syndrome (category III prostatitis): A randomized, sham-controlled study. Urology. 2002;60(2):300-4.
12. Alagiri M, Chottiner S, Ratner V, Slade D, Hanno PM. Interstitial cystitis: unexplained associations with other chronic disease and pain syndromes. Urology. 1997;49(5A suppl):52-7.
13. Clauw DJ, Schmidt M, Radulovic D, Singer A, Katz P, Bresette J. The relationship between fibromyalgia and interstitial cystitis. J Psychiatr Res. 1997;31(1):125-31.
14. Erickson DR, Morgan KC, Ordille S, Keay SK, Xie SX. Nonbladder related symptoms in patients with interstitial cystitis. J Urol. 2001;166(2):557-61; discussion 561-2.
15. Myrna M. Weissman, Raz Gross, Abby Fyer, Gary A. Heiman, Marc J Gameroff, Susan E. Hodge, David Kaufman, Steven A. Kaplan, Priya J Wickramaratne. Interstitial Cystitis and Panic Disorder—A Potential Genetic Syndrome. Arch Gen Psych. 2004;61:273-9.
16. Goetsch MF. Vulvar vestibulitis: Prevalence and historic features in a general gynecologic practice population. Am J Obstet Gynecol. 1991;164:1609-16.
17. Antolak SJJ, Hough DM, Pawlina W, Spinner RJ. Anatomical basis of chronic pelvic pain syndrome: the ischial spine and pudendal nerve entrapment. Med Hypotheses. 2002;59(3):349-53.
18. Amarenco G, Lanoe Y, Perrigot M, Goudal H. A new canal syndrome: compression of the pudendal nerve in Alcock's canal or perineal paralysis of cyclists (French). Presse Med. 1987;16:399.
19. Tetzschner T, Sorensen M, Lose G, Christiansen J. Pudendal nerve function during pregnancy and after delivery. Int Urogynecol J Pelvic Floor Dysfunct. 1997;8:66-8.
20. Krieger JN, Nyberg L Jr, Nickel JC. NIH consensus definition and classification of prostatitis. JAMA. 1999; 282:236-7.
21. Antolak SJ Jr, Hough DM, Pawlina W, Spinner RJ. Anatomical basis of chronic pelvic pain syndrome: The ischial spine and pudendal nerve entrapment. Med Hypotheses. 2002;59(3):349-53.

22. Kawanishi Y, Lee KS, Kimura K, Kojima K, Yamamoto A, Numata A. Feasibility of multi-slice computed tomography in the diagnosis of arteriogenic erectile dysfunction. BJU International. 2001;88:390-5.
23. Rhame EE, Levey KA, Gharibo CG. Successful treatment of refractory pudendal neuralgia with pulsed radiofrequency. Pain Physician. 2009;12(3):633-8.
24. Maigne J, Doursounian L, Chatellier L. Causes and mechanisms of common coccydynia. Role of body mass index and coccygeal trauma. Spine. 2000;25:3072-9.
25. Stones W, Cheong YC, Howard FM. Interventions for treating chronic pelvic pain in women. Cochrane Database System Rev. 2005;(2):CD000387.
26. Bannwarth B, Pehourcq F. Pharmacologic basis for using paracetamol: Pharmacokinetic and pharmacodynamic issues. Drugs. 2003;63 Spec No 2:5-13 (French)
27. Bradley JD, Brandt KD, Katz BP, Kalasinski LA, Ryan SI. Treatment of knee osteoarthritis: Relationship of clinical features of joint inflammation to the response to a nonsteroidal anti-inflammatory drug or pure analgesic. J Rheumatol. 1992;19(12):1950-4.
28. Williams HJ, Ward JR, Egger MJ, Neuner R, Brooks RH, Clegg DO, Field EH, Skosey JL, Alarcon GS, Willkens RF, et al. Comparison of naproxen and acetaminophen in a two-year study of treatment of osteoarthritis of the knee. Arthritis Rheum. 1993;36(9):1196-206.
29. Marjoribanks J, Proctor ML, Farquhar C. Nonsteroidal anti-inflammatory drugs for primary dysmenorrhoea. Cochrane Database Syst Rev. 2003;(4):CD001751.
30. Greco CD. Management of adolescent chronic pelvic pain from endometriosis: a pain center perspective. J Pediatr Adolesc Gynecol. 2003;16(3 Suppl):S17-9.
31. Moore R, Straube S, Wiffen PJ, Derry S, McQuay H. Pregabalin for acute and chronic pain in adults. Cochrane Database Syst Rev. 2009;8(3):CD007076.
32. Price DD, Mayer DJ, Mao J, Caruso FS. NMDA-receptor antagonists and opioid receptor interactions as related to analgesia and tolerance. J Pain Symptom Manage. 2000;19(1 Suppl):S7-S11.
33. Eide PK, Jørum E, Stubhaug A, Bremnes J, Breivik H. Relief of post-herpetic neuralgia with the Nmethyl-D-aspartic acid receptor antagonist ketamine: A double-blind, cross-over comparison with morphine and placebo. Pain. 1994;58(3):347-54.
34. Guirimand F, Dupont X, Brasseur L, Chauvin M, Bouhassira D. The effects of ketamine on the temporal summation (wind-up) of the R (III) nociceptive flexion reflex and pain in humans. Anaesth Analg. 2000;90(2):408-14.
35. Laurido C, Pelissier T, Pérez H, Flores F, Hernández A. Effect of ketamine on spinal cord nociceptive transmission in normal and monoarthritic rats. Neuroreport. 2001;12(8):1551-54.
36. Mikkelsen S, Ilkjaer S, Brennum J, Borgbjerg FM, Dahl JB. The effect of naloxone on ketamine induced effects on hyperalgesia and ketamine-induced side effects in humans. Anaesthesiology. 1999;90(6):1539-45.
37. Visser E, Schug SA. The role of ketamine in pain management. Biomed Pharmacother. 2006;60(7):341-8.
38. Cummins T, et al. Sodium channels as molecular targets in pain. In: Devor M, Rowbotham M, Wiesenfeld-Hallin Z (Eds): Proceedings of the 9th World Congress on Pain. Seattle: IASP; 2000.pp.77-91.
39. Baranowski AP, De Courcey J, Bonello E. A trial of intravenous lidocaine on the pain and allodynia of postherpetic neuralgia. J Pain Symptom Manage. 1999; 17(6):429-33.
40. Galer BS, Harle J, Rowbotham MC. Response to intravenous lidocaine infusion predicts subsequent response to oral mexiletine: A prospective study. J Pain Symptom Manage. 1996;12(3):161-7.
41. McQuay H. Opioids in pain management. Lancet. 1999;353(9171):2229-32.
42. Moulin DE, Clark AJ, Gilron I, Ware MA, Watson CP, Sessle BJ, Coderre T, Morley-Forster PK, Stinson J, Boulanger A, Peng P, Finley GA, Taenzer P, Squire P, Dion D, Cholkan A, Gilani A, Gordon A, Henry J, Jovey R, Lynch M, Mailis-Gagnon A, Panju A, Rollman GB, Velly A. Canadian Pain Society. Pharmacological management of chronic neuropathic pain–consensus statement and guidelines from the Canadian Pain Society. Pain Res Manag. 2007; 12(1):13-21.
43. Hewitt DJ. The use of NMDA-receptor antagonists in the treatment of chronic pain. Clin J Pain. 2000;16(2 Suppl):S73-9.
44. Fredheim OM, Borchgrevink PC, Klepstad P, Kaasa S, Dale O. Long-term methadone for chronic pain: A pilot study of pharmacokinetic aspects. Eur J Pain. 2007;11(6):599-604.
45. Sagata K, Minami K, Yanagihara N, Shiraishi M, Toyohira Y, Ueno S, Shigematsu A. Tramadol inhibits norepinephrine transporter function at desipramine-binding sites in cultured bovine adrenal medullary cells. Anaesth Analg. 2002;94(4):901-6.
46. Desmeules JA, Piguet V, Collart L, Dayer P. Contribution of monoaminergic modulation to the analgesic effect of tramadol. Br J Clin Pharmacol. 1996;41(1):7-12.
47. Hollingshead J, Du hmke RM, Cornblath DR. Tramadol for neuropathic pain. Cochrane Database Syst Rev. 2006;(3):CD003726.
48. Kalso E, Allan L, Dellemijn PL, Faura CC, Ilias WK, Jensen TS, Perrot S, Plaghki LH, Zenz M. Recommendations for using opioids in chronic non-cancer pain. Eur J Pain 2003;7(5):381-86.

49. The Pain Society, Recommendations for the appropriate use of opioids for persistent non-cancer pain. A consensus statement prepared on behalf of the Pain Society, the Royal College of Anaesthetists, the Royal College of General Practitioners and the Royal College of Psychiatrists. London: The Pain Society, 2010.
50. Goetsch MF. Vulvar vestibulitis: Prevalence and historic features in a general gynecologic practice population. Am J Obstet Gynecol 1991;164:1609-16.
51. Antolak SJJ, Hough DM, Pawlina W, Spinner RJ. Anatomical basis of chronic pelvic pain syndrome: the ischial spine and pudendal nerve entrapment. Med Hypotheses, 2002;59(3):349-53.
52. Rhame EE, Levey KA, Gharibo CG. Successful treatment of refractory pudendal neuralgia with pulsed radiofrequency. Pain Physician. 2009;12(3):633-8.

CHAPTER 26

Chronic Nonmalignant Pelvic Pain

Kyriacos Kyriakides

INTRODUCTION

Chronic pelvic pain (CPP) is a significant and perplexing problem in current medical practice. Its pathogenesis is poorly understood, often investigations reveal no obvious cause and more often than not there is little correlation between the patient's pain severity and degree of any documented tissue pathology. These patients have often consulted doctors from various specialties, had numerous investigations and quite often have undergone surgery without any benefit.

This chapter focuses mainly on nonmalignant CPP in women, and their management from the pain clinic perspective. However, one needs to be aware that there are other causes of pelvic pain, which are not gender-specific, arising from the bowel, urinary tract and the musculoskeletal system. In addition, the general principles of management of CPP, transcends gender differences.

DEFINITIONS

Two definitions must follow, which are interrelated. The first, is that of pain itself by the International Association for the study of Pain (IASP), which defines pain as "an unpleasant sensory and emotional experience due to actual or potential tissue damage, or expressed in terms of such damage".[1] The second definition is that of CPP itself, which can be defined as "noncyclical pain in the lower abdomen or pelvis of at least 6 months duration and which is severe enough to interfere with the quality of life of the woman".

What this means in practice is that CPP is a symptom, not a diagnosis. The patient's report of pain is valid even if no pathology is demonstrated, a quite common finding in patients suffering from CPP, and consideration of psychosocial factors can be as important as biomedical factors.

EPIDEMIOLOGY

Studies using various definitions estimated that the prevalence of CPP ranges from 2.1 to 24% of the female population worldwide.[2] Population surveys in the USA revealed that CPP has a prevalence of about 12%, with a lifetime incidence of 33%.[3] It accounts for 10% of gynecological consultations and up to 33% of laparoscopies,[4] while in the UK it accounts for up to 40-52% of laparoscopies.[5] It also accounts for 12-16% of hysterectomies, with questionable efficacy since it is reported that 25% of CPP referrals have had hysterectomies previously for CPP.[6]

Chronic pelvic pain is a common presentation in UK primary care, with 38/1000 women affected annually—a rate comparable to those of migraine, asthma (37/1000) and back pain (41/1000).[7]

The economic burden of CPP is difficult to establish, and no recent data is available. However, it is clear that CPP is associated with massive direct (healthcare) and indirect (work related) costs. These combined costs were estimated, in 1990 in the US, at 2 billion dollars annually.[8] In the UK, using hospital episode data, it has been estimated that the combined costs of CPP in 1992 totalled £182 million.[9] The full scale of the problem is unimaginable, when one takes into consideration the full impact to the individual in terms of pain, distress and disability as well as the impact on spouses/partners and their immediate family.

ETIOLOGY

Chronic pelvic pain has been attributed to a variety of conditions (Table 1). The following should be borne in mind when dealing with CPP:

- Often no pathological cause is found
- A pathological cause may be present but cannot be demonstrated
- Where a 'cause' is found it may be an incidental finding
- Where a 'cause' is treated there may be no improvement as the pain may be due to another as yet undiagnosed cause.

ASSESSMENT

Women with CPP want to feel they are being taken seriously, desire reassurance, and attach importance to having an explanation for their pain. Often, they already have a theory or a concern about the origin of their pain. These ideas should be discussed in the initial consultation. It has been shown that consultations that elicit the woman's own ideas will result in a better doctor-patient relationship and improved concordance with investigation and treatment.

TABLE 1: Differential diagnosis of chronic pelvic pain

Gynecological	Urological	Gastrointestinal	Musculoskeletal/ neurological	Psychological
Endometriosis	Chronic urinary tract infection	Irritable bowel	Low back pain (Referred)	Somatization
Pelvic inflammatory disease	Urethral syndrome	Inflammatory bowel disease	Myofascial pain	Depression
Adhesions	Calculi	Diverticulitis	Neuropathy/Nerve entrapment	Anxiety
Pelvic congestion	Interstitial cystitis	Malabsorption	Malignancy	Eating disorders
Retroverted/prolapsed uterus	Prostadynia	Abdominal angina		Post-traumatic
Fibroids	Testicular pain	Chronic constipation		
Intrauterine devise	Malignancy	Malignancy		
Ovarian remnant syndrome				
Broad ligament defect				
Malignancy				

History

A good history is essential and should include a chronological account of previous other specialty referrals, investigations and treatments, with outcomes thereof. Prior other specialist assessments do not exempt the pain clinician from taking a full history and examination. Where this does not occur prior to referral to the Pain Clinic, other clinicians with a 'pelvic interest', e.g. urologists and gastroenterologists, should be consulted as necessary. However, unnecessary inter-specialty referrals should be avoided at all cost as they encourage the patient to remain in a 'seek a diagnosis and get a cure' mindset.

A detailed description of the pain (site, radiation, character, severity, exacerbating and relieving factors, periodicity and associated symptoms) and its impact on the patient (sleep, mood and function) should be elicited.

Systemic review should be particularly directed to gynecological, gastroenterological, urological and musculoskeletal areas. A potential cause may thus be revealed. Multiple visceral organ involvement may be explained by the phenomenon of viscero-visceral hyperalgesia, where hypersensitivity in one pelvic viscus (e.g. uterus) may trigger hypersensitivity in another pelvic viscus (e.g. bladder) due to convergent overlapping afferent innervation at the same spinal cord level.[10] On the other hand, pelvic visceral pain can give rise to referred somatic pain in the low back/abdomen, with or without hyperalgesia through the mechanisms of convergence/facilitation (plus activation of viscero-somatic/sympathetic reflex arcs) and convergence-projection, respectively.[11] Equally skeletal structures of the spine and pelvis (e.g. facet and sacroiliac joints) can give rise to referred pain in the pelvic area, which can be perceived as pelvic visceral pain.

A number of studies on patients with CPP have demonstrated the prevalence of pathology in the psychosocial/sexual domains[12-17] and treatment strategies directed to this pathology have resulted in improved patient outcomes. Therefore, detailed psychological assessment, preferably by a trained psychologist experienced in the area of sexual function, should also be undertaken.

Examination

Many patients come to the pain clinic expecting a full examination. The examination should entail body habitus, posture and gait. Obvious signs of distress while moving or being superficially examined, such as grimacing and crying are noted, as are behavioral elements to the pain presentation.

Detailed pelvic examination, including internal examination, is clearly beyond the remit of a pain clinician's expertise. Most patients with CPP will already have had a full gynecological (urological or gastroenterological, depending on the symptoms) work-up. An internal examination by a pain clinician should only be undertaken with appropriate training in how to interpret findings and, of course, with good reason to believe that it will add to the diagnosis.

An external abdominal examination can yield useful information as well as providing reassurance to the patient. Following inspection, gentle abdominal palpation can reveal a number of sources of pain, which might not have been considered prior to referral to the pain clinic. These include:

- Pain due to the presence of a peripheral neuropathy (genitofemoral, ilioinguinal and iliohypogastric neuralgias) related to either previous surgery or idiopathic in origin
- Pain arising from the presence of a myofascial trigger point (MTP)
- Pain due to muscular dysfunction, which is referred pain generated by the viscero-somatic reflex

A rectal examination should be performed in males.

Another system that needs to be carefully examined is the musculoskeletal system. This may reveal skeletal structures of the spine or pelvis such that the facet joints and the sacroiliac joints giving rise to referred pain, which is perceived as visceral pain.

Investigations

It should have been carried out prior to pain clinic referral, include:
- Full blood count
- Erythrocyte sedimentation rate (ESR)
- C-reactive protein (CRP)
- Urea and electrolytes
- Urine for microscopy and culture
- Cervical smear for culture and cytology
- Plain abdominal film and
- Abdominal ultrasound.

Laparoscopy is regarded as the gold standard[18,19] although many target conditions cannot be diagnosed in this way. It appears that approximately two-thirds of women with CPP have laparoscopically detectable pathology and approximately one-third have a normal laparoscopy. Although its accuracy is not perfect, the use of magnetic resonance imaging (MRI) for the differential diagnosis of CPP has the potential to replace diagnostic laparoscopy in a proportion of women.[20,21]

MANAGEMENT/TREATMENT OPTIONS

There are a number of randomized controlled trials in the management of CPP in women. Unfortunately, the quality of the studies is not always the best. There is scope for much more comprehensive studies which should include measures of function as well as pain scores in accordance with IMMPACT guidelines.[22]

Recently, the British Pain Society in the UK has published a patient pathway map for the management of Chronic Pelvic Pain in both men and women.[23] This pathway has the intention of "improving and streamlining the delivery of timely, evidence-based and individualized care".

Multidisciplinary Team Approach

Chronic pelvic pain can be a diagnostic and therapeutic dilemma, and it has proved difficult to manage using an unprofessional model. A biopsychosocial model in a multidisciplinary setting should be followed from the outset. The aim should be to develop a partnership between clinician and patient to plan a management programme. The patient should be encouraged to see their role as an active participant in the road to recovery. As with most other chronic pains, the main aim of treatment is not cure but to maximize function and improve quality of life.

A meta-analysis has established the effectiveness of a multidisciplinary team approach to assessment and treatment of chronic pain.[24] More specifically, one randomized controlled trial[25] and one controlled cohort study[26] described in the literature attest to the benefit of this approach in CPP. Although the multidisciplinary approach has been strongly advocated in the management of CPP[27,28] and fits with the biopsychosocial model of pain, such clinics are few and far between, leading to lack of a holistic approach. The construction of the team will vary, but should ideally involve clinicians (gynecology and pain medicine), a psychologist, a physiotherapist and a nurse specialist with an interest and/or training in CPP. The nurse can provide an all-important general supportive role for the patient, acting as 'glue' between the other practitioners.

Specific Treatment

The evidence for other interventions in the treatment of CPP is remarkably sparse, although pharmacotherapy may follow general chronic pain management lines.

Pharmacotherapy

Analgesics are often the first line of management, and women often try to manage their pain with over the counter painkillers before consulting with their general practitioner.

Currently, there is no robust evidence for the use of any pain pharmacotherapy in the treatment of CPP. However, it is reasonable to prescribe analgesics along the World Health Organization analgesic ladder guidelines (WHO, 1990). Although this tool was primarily developed for cancer pain, its general principles can be adapted to noncancer pains. However, use of strong opioids in CPP, like any other chronic nonmalignant pain, is the subject of much current controversy, in terms of appropriateness and effectiveness, especially in the long term.

The WHO guidelines also provide for the use of adjuvants/coanalgesics (antidepressant and anticonvulsant drugs) at any point. Despite current lack of robust objective evidence that they are effective in CPP, antidepressants may be useful for their anti-neuropathic and/or sleep effects. Amitriptyline is of course the most common to be prescribed. Even a 10 mg dose can improve sleep, but for its anti-neuropathic effect, the dose should be gradually increased to a range of up to 75–100 mg nocturnally.

Studies investigating the use of co-analgesics in the treatment of CPP are gradually emerging. One small randomized controlled trial, comparing sertraline with placebo in the treatment of CPP, showed no evidence of improvement in pain scores.[29] Another randomized controlled trial of gabapentin,[30] which is frequently used for neuropathic pain, assessed this drug either alone or in combination with amitriptyline. All women who took part in the study reported improvements in pain, but gabapentin alone or with amitriptyline was superior to amitriptyline alone in the reduction of pelvic pain reported on a visual analogue scale. However, as there were design faults in the study (randomization method not stated, lack of blinding) the result should be substantiated in a larger, higher quality trial.

Stimulation/Modulation

The evidence for the use of nonpharmacological modalities (e.g. acupuncture, transcutaneous nerve stimulation) in the treatment of CPP, is not convincing. However, a trial may be appropriate in some patients, especially if given as part of a multidisciplinary clinic regime, as these therapies appear to help some chronic visceral pains.

Interventional Procedures

The principles of neural blockade have been applied to chronic pain management for many years. Such interventional procedures are now used with much less enthusiasm, as the results in chronic pain are temporary and partial at best in most cases (with the exception perhaps of targeted precise injections for the treatment of spinal pain). There are three main reasons as to why neural blockade can fail to relieve chronic pain:

1. There can be multiple pain pathways from putatively pain-generating tissues.
2. Central sensitisation changes take place (at the level of the spinal cord and brain) which occur proximal to the site of the peripheral block.
3. Presence of important psychosocial factors.

Caudal epidural injections have been used in CPP often with disappointing results, mainly for the above listed reasons. Superior hypogastric plexus block (SHPB)[31] is another interventional procedure that has been used in the management of CPP. However, there is insufficient evidence to support its use in the routine treatment of nonmalignant CPP. From the author's personal clinical experience, a trial of SHPB may be indicated in carefully selected group of patients when all other conservative therapy has failed (unpublished data). SHBP could be useful in the treatment of malignant pelvic pain, as a neurolytic procedure.

Despite all these limitations, interventional procedures may have a role to play in the treatment of MTPs, peripheral neuralgias and referred pelvic pain arising from skeletal structures such as facet and/or sacroiliac joints.

CONCLUSION

Chronic pelvic pain is common, affecting perhaps one in six of the adult female population. Much remains unclear about its etiology and pathophysiology. CPP should be seen as a symptom with a number of contributory factors rather than a diagnosis in itself. The multifactorial nature of CPP should be discussed and explored from the start. The aim should be to develop a partnership between patient and clinicians to plan a management programme. Such a program is best delivered within a multidisciplinary CPP clinic. Further research is needed to identify which are the essential components of interdisciplinary approaches in order to achieve optimum outcome for the individual patient.

REFERENCES

1. International Association for the Study of Pain. Pain terms: A current list with definitions and notes on usage: pain. Pain. 1986; Suppl 3:S217.
2. Latthe P, et al. WHO systematic review of prevalence of chronic pelvic pain: a neglected reproductive health morbidity. BMC Public Health. 2006;6:177.
3. Walker EA, et al. The prevalence of chronic pain and irritable bowel syndrome in two university clinics. J Psychosom Obstet Gynaecology. 1991; Suppl 12:65.
4. Reiter RC, et al. Demographic and historical variables in women with idiopathic chronic pelvic pain. Obstet Gynaecol. 1990;75:428.
5. Campbell F, Collett B. Chronic pelvic pain. Nr J Anaesth. 1994;73:574-8.
6. Slocumb JC. Operative management of chronic abdominal pelvic pain. Clin Obstet Gynaec. 1990;33:196.
7. Zondervan KT, et al. Prevalence and incidence of chronic pelvic pain in primary care: evidence from a national general practice database. Brit Jour Obstet & Gynaecol. 1999;106(11):1149-55.
8. Reiter RC, et al. Chronic Pelvic Pain. Clin Obstet Gynaecol. 1990;33:117-8.
9. Davies L, et al. The economic burden of intractable gynaecological pain. J Obstet Gynaecol. 1992;12(S2):54-6.
10. Giamberardino M. Urogenital pain and phenomena of viscero-visceral hyperalgesia. In: Giamberardino M (Ed.). Pain 2002–An Updated Review. Seattle: IASP Press. 2002.pp.413-22.
11. Giamberardino MA, Constantini R. Visceral pain phenomena in the clinical setting and their interpretation. Visceral Pain: clinical, pathophysiological and therapeutic aspects. Oxford University Press. 2009.pp.9-19.
12. Walker EA, et al. Relationship of chronic pelvic pain to psychiatric diagnoses and childhood sexual abuse. Am J Psychiatry. 1988;145:75-80.
13. McGowan LP, et al. Chronic pelvic pain: a meta-analytic review. Psycho Health. 1998;13:937-51.
14. Rosendanthal RH. Psychology of chronic pelvic pain. Obstet Gynaecol Clin North Am. 1993;20:627-42.
15. Reiter RC, et al. Correlation between sexual abuse and somatisation in women with somatic and non-somatic chronic pelvic pain. Am J Obstet Gynaecol. 1991;165:104-9.
16. Walker EA, ct al. Sexual victimisation and chronic pelvic abuse in women with chronic pelvic pain. Obstet Gynaecol Clin North Am. 1993;20:795-807.
17. Rapkin AJ, et al. History of physical and sexual abuse in women with chronic pelvic pain. Obstet Gynaecol. 1990;79:92-6.
18. Howard FM. The role of laparoscopy in chronic pelvic pain: promise and pitfalls. Obstet Gynaecol Surv. 1993;48:357-87.
19. Howard FM. The role of laparoscopy as a diagnostic too in chronic pelvic pain. Best Pract Res Clin Obstet Gynaecol. 2000;14:467-94.
20. Cody J, et al. Diagnostic value of radiological tests in chronic pelvic pain. Baillieres Best Pract Res Clin Obstet Gynaecol. 2000;14:433-66.
21. Bazot M, et al. Imaging of chronic pelvic pain. J Radiol 2008;89(1 Pt 2):107-14.
22. Dworkin RH, et al. Core outcome measures for chronic pain clinical trials: IMMPACT recommendations. Pain. 2005;115:9-19.
23. AP Baranowski, et al. Pelvic Pain: a pathway for care developed for both men and women by the British Pain Society. British Journal of Anaesthesia. 2014;112(3):452-9.
24. Flor H, et al. Efficacy of multidisciplinary pain treatment centres: a meta-analytic review. Pain. 1992;49:221-30.
25. Peters AA, et al. A randomised clinical trial to compare two different approaches in women with chronic pelvic pain. Obstet Gynaecol. 1991;77:740-4.
26. Kames LD, et al. Effectiveness of an interdisciplinary pain management programme for the treatment of chronic pelvic pain. Pain. 1990;41:41-6.
27. Stones RW, et al. Interventions for treating chronic pelvic pain in women (Cochrane Review). Cochrane Database Syst Rev. 2000;(4)CD000387.
28. Stones RW, et al. Health services for women with chronic pelvic pain. J R Soc Med. 2002;95:531-5.
29. Engel CC, et al. A randomised, double-blind crossover trial of setraline in women with chronic pelvic pain. J Psychosom Res. 1998;44(2):203-7.
30. Sator-Katzenschlager SM, et al. Chronic pelvic pain treated with gabapentin and amitriptyline: a randomised controlled pilot study. Wien Klin Wochenschr. 2005;117(21-22):761-8.
31. P Prithvi Raj, et al. Hypogastric plexus block and neurolysis. Radiographic Imaging for Regional Anaesthesia and Pain Management. Churchill Livingstone; 2003.pp.231-7.

SECTION 7

Cancer Pain

CHAPTER 27

Head and Neck Cancer Pain Management

Manohar L Sharma

INTRODUCTION

Cancer-related pain in the head and neck region is common and is typically associated with significant psychological and physical suffering. Apart from pain, many patients with head and neck cancer experience problems with speech, swallowing, taste, hearing, cosmetic appearance, breathing, and airway control.

Head and neck cancer usually refers to malignant tumors that arise in the mucosa of the oral cavity, pharynx, larynx, nasal cavity, and paranasal sinuses. More than 90% of the head and neck tumors are squamous cell carcinoma. Worldwide, more than 500,000 new cases of head and neck squamous cell carcinomas are projected annually. The recent cancer estimates show that each year, 0.675 million patients suffer from head and neck cancer and 60% of all head and neck cancer occur in less developed countries.[1] Many patients present in late or advanced stages. A tumor-infiltrated lymph node can act as a source for further dissemination into the surrounding lymphatic's or the blood stream, the latter resulting in distant metastases.

Usually patients with early stage disease are treated with surgery or radiotherapy and patients with advanced stage disease are treated by a combination of surgery, radiotherapy, and/or chemotherapy. In all treatment modalities, progress has been made over the last decade. Surgical techniques are still evolving, with greater focus on minimally invasive procedures to minimize postsurgical chronic pain and improved functional and cosmetic outcomes.

Most of those who have head and neck cancer have uncontrolled local disease irrespective of the presence of metastasis. Distant metastasis arises in lung, liver and bone in a small number of patients particularly, if there is involvement of multiple lymph nodes. The 5-year survival rate of multimodal chemoradiotherapy is below 20%, with a median survival of less than 12 months.[2] In the vast majority of cases, pain is directly related to the malignancy or is a consequence of curative or palliative treatment. In some cases, pain may be coincidental and unrelated to cancer. Pain is common in patients with head and neck cancer and is reported by approximately half of patients prior to cancer therapy, 81% during therapy, 70% at the end of therapy, and by 36% at 6 months after treatment. Pain is experienced beyond the 6-month period by approximately one-third of patients and is typically more severe than pretreatment cancer-induced pain.[3]

PREVALENCE OF PAIN IN HEAD AND NECK CANCER

Two recent systematic reviews of nearly 100 published studies on the prevalence of pain in cancer patients and the adequacy of analgesic treatment in such patients have indicated that cancer-related pain is still a major problem, despite recent advances in analgesic treatments. Van den Beukenvan Everdingen et al.[4] reported an overall pain prevalence of greater than 50% in patients with all cancer types; the highest cancer subtype was head and neck cancer, with pain prevalence of 70%.

Various published studies report pain prevalence in head and neck cancer between 40% and 94%, between different clinical settings (oncology clinic or palliative care), types of cancer, its treatment and including developing countries.[5] Forty to sixty two percent of patients with head and neck cancer related pain receive inadequate pain relief as shown in various studies.[6] It may be very important to define cancer-related pain risk factors to target resources to "at risk" group.

High prevalence of neuropathic (34%), breakthrough (50–60%) and pain of non-malignant origin (25%) has been found in patients with head and neck cancer. In a study by Epstein et al. 57% of patients reported continuous pain, and combined continuous and intermittent pain was reported by 79% of patients.[7] This study specifically evaluated patients' pain experience, who had head and neck cancer and were undergoing radiotherapy. This study provides evidence that those patients with head and neck cancer experience nociceptive and neuropathic pain during radiotherapy despite ongoing pain management. Twenty-nine percent of the patients were not satisfied with cancer-related pain treatment despite its ongoing management. It is important to identify different pain types as treatment for neuropathic pain may be quite different from the pain of nonmalignant origin. Severe breakthrough pain (BTP) is an indicator of poor prognosis. Inadequate management of breakthrough pain may result in poor function, depression and hospital admission. Severe uncontrolled breakthrough or incident pain may be life-threatening, if patients are treated with escalating doses of opioids, without recourse to specific treatment strategy targeted to cause of pain.

ETIOLOGY OF HEAD AND NECK CANCER-RELATED PAIN

Pain can be caused by cancer itself. It can be due to cancer invading bone, nerve, muscle, mucosal damage, and tumor pressure. It can be caused by cancer treatments, including surgery, radiotherapy, and chemotherapy. One of the common manifestations is mucositis-related pain. At times, the pain may be unrelated to cancer and may be myofacial or related to temporomandibular joint dysfunction. It is important to understand pathogenesis of cancer-related pain, so as to develop novel approaches to treat cancer-related pain and improve patient outcome.

Pain Due to Head and Neck Cancer

Tumor-related pain is often present at the time of diagnosis of head and neck cancer (85%). Intensity of pain is related to tumor stage and bone involvement. Pain usually occurs with treatment of head and neck cancer, increases in intensity during course of radiotherapy and persists after treatment. Cancer cells may invade and compress pain sensitive structures and cause inflammation. Bone pain may be caused by stretching of periosteum, compression and invasion of nerves, vascular damage, microfractures, and muscle spasm. Cytokines and other algogenic molecules cause pain in tumor environment of hypoxia and low pH. Inflammation is major cause of pain in head and neck cancer. This is initiated by reactive oxygen species and release of mediators from tumor cells, circulating leukocytes, platelets, endothelial cells, and immune cells normally present in affected tissue and nerve tissues. The low pH in solid tumors is possibly due to inflammation, tumor cell metabolism, and death of cancer cells with release of contents, which may cause pain by activation of sensory neurons through acid sensing ion channels. Cancer cells also cause activation of osteoclasts leading on to lower pH for dissolution of bone minerals. Tumor necrosis factor (TNF) is central in activation of cytokines and growth factors and plays role in inflammation, neuropathic pain and is very important in generation of mucositis-related pain. Prostaglandins are induced in peripheral tissues by inflammatory cytokines and growth factors. Increased levels are seen in head and neck cancers and in metastasis. Prostaglandins cause sensitization of C-polymodal nociceptors and A-delta mechano-nociceptors to mediate hyperalgesia.

Modulation of pain is further influenced by balance of different nerve fiber input at spinal cord level, including descending inhibition. It can be affected by learned behavior, stress, and acute pain. Perception of pain eventually can be influenced by attention, expectation, anxiety, and depression. Interaction between the sympathetic nervous system and nociceptors are thought to be important mechanism for some components of neuropathic pain.

Pain Due to Chemotherapy and Radiotherapy

A number of chemotherapy agents, including vinca alkaloids (vincristine, vinblastin) cause neurotoxicity. Cisplatin and associated compounds are linked with neuronal death leading on to loss of large myelinated nerve fibers. Other agents used in cancer treatment or supportive care (Interferon, thalidomide, amphotericin-B) can induce sensory neuropathies.

Bisphosphonates have established role in treatment of cancer involving bones. These are commonly employed in multiple myeloma, metastatic breast, prostate, lung, and colon cancer. Main benefits include prevention of bone-related events, less incidence of hypercalcemia, and less bone pain related to cancer. Bisphosphonates act by reducing osteoclast activity related to cancer. This reduces resorption of bone due to normal remodeling and malignancy. One of the problems with bisphosphonate use has been acute pain mimicking bone pain, dental pain, or jaw pain.[8] Bisphosphonates may be associated with non-healing bony lesions involving dentoalveolar bone. Patients on bisphosphonates are considered at higher risk for osteonecrosis, if they undergo dental surgery. Pain caused by osteonecrosis is usually related to secondary infection of soft tissue surrounding the areas of exposed bone. Chronic osteonecrosis can spread to involve nerve bundles (e.g. the inferior alveolar nerve) and generate numbness and pain.[9]

Radiotherapy-associated mucositis is the most feared complication in patients undergoing radiotherapy for head and neck cancer. Mucositis-related pain from radiotherapy usually settles in 1–2 months, but mucosal discomfort may last more than 12 months. Patients may be left with mucosal atrophy, temporomandibular joint disorder, and neurologic injury in the form of deafferentation, if the field of irradiation involves these structures. Studies have reported residual problems; xerostomia (57%), jaw pain involving muscles or joint (27%), and increased dental caries rate (10%).[10]

Pain Due to Surgery

Surgical treatment (removal) of cancer may be expected to relieve pain. Usually pain initially increases after surgery and then improves gradually over period of time. Neck surgery to remove cancer is usually associated with shoulder and arm pain afterwards. Cervical metastatic disease is usually treated by radical neck dissection, originally described by Crile in 1906.[11] Radical neck dissection is implicated in poorer quality of life, health status and shoulder-related disabilities.[12] More recent trend has been to be relatively conservative and this has had positive impact on quality of life and health status in patients requiring neck dissection for cancer. It is not known why patient undergoing neck dissection, suffer from postoperative neck and shoulder pain. Mechanisms could be the mechanical overload of the shoulder caused by changed scapular position and denervation of trapezius muscle leading on to reduced stabilization. Trapezius muscle may be denervated, if spinal accessory nerve is removed during neck dissection. However, even if spinal accessory nerve is preserved during surgery, patients still can have shoulder pain afterwards. There is some evidence to suggest that if cervical sensory nerve is not removed during surgery, then, there is less postoperative pain and sensory deficit. There is also evidence that removal of lymph nodes from the posterior triangle of neck is associated with neck and shoulder pain.[13]

ASSESSMENT OF HEAD AND NECK CANCER-RELATED PAIN

Effective management requires accurate diagnosis of the etiology of pain. The process would consist of an elaborate pain history, a biopsychosocial overview, history of previous treatments, examination and review of investigations including imaging. This is best done if a multidisciplinary team is involved. At our center, this is done by means of a joint clinic led by the Consultants in Palliative Medicine and Pain Medicine. These consultants have easy access to other specialist who may be involved in treating these patients (oncologist, maxillofacial surgeon or general surgeon). The patients' notes and investigations are available prior to consultation. Besides doctors, nurses, pharmacists, social care workers, psychologist, and physiotherapists, it is useful to have dental hygienists on board. This is to have someone knowledgeable in oral medicine on board.

It is vital to assess pain and its impact on daily function and quality of life. Various questionnaires exist (brief pain inventory, hospital anxiety and depression scale, EQ-5D, etc.) and can be adapted from chronic nonmalignant pain practice. Frequent reassessment is vital to judge impact of pain treatments on pain levels, side effects, function and quality of life. Sometimes, in patients with head and neck cancer, pain assessment is difficult due to tracheostomy tube placement, loss of speech function, or severe oral pain causing difficulty in communication.

MANAGEMENT OF HEAD AND NECK CANCER-RELATED PAIN

Usually treatment of cancer in the form of curative or palliative surgery, chemo- and/or radiotherapy may have useful impact on pain. However, in many cases, this may also cause the pain.

Role of Surgery

Sentinel node biopsy most commonly is the first surgical procedure. If the node is positive then invasive neck dissection is undertaken. Minimal invasive techniques like endo-nasal endoscopic, robotic surgery and image-guided surgery are used in selected patients.[14] In postoperative period, patients report highest pain scores following oral cancer surgery, followed by larynx, oropharynx and nasopharynx surgery.[15] When patients were reviewed at more than 6 months postsurgery, impairment due to moderate or severe pain was found in 34.3% of patients.[16] Pain develops following surgery due to musculoskeletal syndromes and TMJ disorders (muscle fibrosis, scar, and limited jaw opening). Resection of mandible may lead to regional hyperalgesia and allodynia.[17] At 3 years post-surgery, patients suffer more pain and disability than matched subjects.[18] There is shift towards less radical approach for neck dissection, to improve patient satisfaction and quality of life.

Chemotherapy and Radiotherapy-induced Pain

Oral Mucositis

The most common pain problem following chemotherapy and radiotherapy is due to oral mucositis (OM).[19] Oral mucositis is defined as inflammation of oral mucosa resulting from cancer therapy typically manifesting as swelling, erythema, ulceration and atrophy. The prevalence ranges from 10% to 100%. Chemotherapy-induced OM occurs within a few days where as postradiotherapy OM takes a few weeks to develop.[20] Combined chemotherapy and radiotherapy has been reported to result in increased frequency, severity and duration of mucositis. Secondary infection further aggravates the pain. From pain management perspective, it is worth keeping in mind that these patients are frequently fed by nasogastric tube and hence limitations in route and formulations of analgesic delivery.

Various management strategies include basic oral hygiene care, bland oral ringes (normal saline or bicarbonate), topical anesthetics and analgesics (lignocaine viscous solution, benzocaine, diphenhydramine, topical morphine, coating agents such as milk of magnesia, loperamide, etc.), topical antimicrobials (poor evidence), and systemic analgesics. Other therapies, which have been tried include topical ketamine and capsaicin.

Pharmacological Management of Pain in HNC

Systemic Medications

The WHO analgesic ladder has been successfully used to treat cancer related pain.[21] To maintain freedom from pain, drugs should be given "by the clock", that is every 3–6 hours, rather than "on demand." This three-step approach of administering the right drug in the right dose at the right time is inexpensive and effective in 80–90% of the patients.[22]

Opioids may be administered by mouth, rectally, transdermally, subcutaneous, intravenous, intrathecally and epidurally. The less invasive routes are preferred before escalating to parenteral therapy. To calm fears and anxiety, additional drug—adjuvants—should be used. Adjuvant drugs may not be primarily analgesic in their mechanism of action, but have analgesic effects in certain pain conditions.

Patient-controlled analgesia (PCA) has been shown to be useful for mucositis pain.[23] Transdermal fentanyl patches are widely used, if oral route is not available and cause less constipation than morphine. However, 20–30% of patients do not achieve satisfactory analgesia despite using the WHO ladder and opioid rotation.

Breakthrough Pain (BTP)

Breakthrough pain may occur in 50–95% of patients.[24] This is characterized by rapid onset of pain occurring once to four times a day lasting from seconds to hours. BTP can be incident (coughing, sneezing), end of dose or idiopathic (progressive cancer). Treatment options include titrating short-acting opioids along with increasing long-acting opioids till tolerated or switching to subcutaneous infusion, if there are concerns with bioavailability of opioids. Other approaches would include opioid rotation. Interventional pain procedures should be considered early to derive maximum benefit.

Adjuvant Analgesics

It is important to use adjuvant analgesics as part of a multimodal approach to treat pain. Amitriptyline has been found to be useful in addition to morphine in a RCT.[25] Additionally Amitriptyline improves sleep. Gabapentin, pregabalin have been approved by NICE for treatment of neuropathic pain and can be useful to treat the neuropathic components of the cancer-related pain.[26] It is important to prescribe medications for restorative sleep (anxiolytics or hypnotics) as lack of sleep intensifies pain. Other agents which are useful include steroid, cannabinoids, alpha 2 adrenergic receptor agonist, topical lidocaine and ketamine.

Interventional Pain Management

Interventional procedures can be very effective in head and neck cancer related pain for patients poorly responsive to conservative methods. Peripheral neurolytic nerve blocks using 6–10% aqueous phenol can be very effective. Various nerve blocks include but are not limited to—supraorbital, infraorbital, inframental nerve, occipital nerve, maxillary, mandibular nerve block, sphenopalatine ganglion,[27] gasserian ganglion; RF, glycerol injection or balloon compression. These are very effective in cancer-related facial pain. Other blocks may include cervical dorsal root ganglion radiofrequency, cervical epidural, stellate ganglion block for selective indications. It may be good practice to carry out diagnostic block before proceeding to definitive neurolytic block as some patients may be unhappy with numbness or dysesthetic symptoms resulting from de-afferentation. In very complex head and neck cancer related pain patients, neurosurgical help may be requested to consider intracranial sensory rhizotomy of cranial nerves, however, the results can be borderline. Intrathecal or intraventricular morphine infusion can be considered in intractable cases, if local expertize and infrastructure support exists.[28]

Cognitive and Other Pain Management Options

Pan et al.[29] in a review of 11 controlled and two noncontrolled trials reported that acupuncture, transcutaneous nerve stimulation, group therapy, self-hypnosis, relaxation, imagery, cognitive behavioral therapy and massage therapy were useful in management of pain in terminally ill patients. It is vital for these patient to have access to community-based, easily accessible service (community drug/IV team, district or McMillan nurses, general practitioner for home visit if needed, day care hospice for patient to visit/ access complementary therapies, etc.) as first point of contact, should they get in to problems with poor pain control.

Noninvasive MR-guided Neuroablative Technique

MR-guided focused ultrasound has received much attention of late and is being used with in research setting. Concept of this treatment is to create ultrasound-mediated destruction of tumor or metastasis or the neural pathway to provide pain relief. Patient is treated with in MR scanner and ultrasound beam is focused with guidance of MR scan precisely to the area in question. This leads on to rise in temperature and hence destruction of the tissue in precise location. Patients can stay awake for this procedure though it is painful and they require analgesia for the procedure. This has become popular in gynecology field to treat fibroids, in neurosurgical field to treat tremor by neuroablation of central neural pathways and in oncology to treat bony metastasis-related pain.[30,31] This is highly likely to be useful for pain related to bony metastasis linked to head and neck cancer.

CONCLUSION

Pain in head and neck cancer patients is a significant problem. A multidisciplinary assessment is advocated for evaluation of these patients. Treatment modalities like surgery, chemotherapy and radiotherapy are often helpful, but can also cause pain. Pain management includes pharmacotherapy and interventional pain management techniques. Increasingly early escalation to strong opioids and early application of interventional techniques is being advocated for symptomatic control of pain in head and neck cancer patients.

REFERENCES

1. Parkin DM, Bray F, Ferlay J, Pisani P. Estimating the world cancer burden: Globocan 2000. Int J Cancer. 2001;94(2):153-6.
2. Carvalho AL, Salvajoli JV, Kowalski LP. A comparison of radio therapy or chemotherapy with a symptomatic treatment alone in advanced head and neck carcinomas. Eur Arch Otorhinolaryngol. 2000;257:164-7.
3. Epstein JB, Hong C, Logan RM, et al. A systematic review of orofacial pain in patients receiving cancer therapy. Supportive Care Cancer. 2010;18:1023-31.
4. Van den Beuken-van Everdingen MHJ, Rijke JM de, Kessels AG, et al. Prevalence of pain in patients with cancer: a systematic review of the past 40 years. Ann Oncol. 2007;18:1437-49.
5. William JE, Yen JTC, Parker G, et al. Prevalence of pain in head and neck cancer out-patients. Jay Laryngol Otol. 2010;124:766-73.
6. Deandrea S, Montanari M, Moja L, Apolone G. Prevalence of undertreatment in cancer-related pain. A review of published literature. Ann Oncol. 2008;19:1985-91.
7. Epstein JB, Wilkie DJ, Fischer DJ, Kim YO, Villines D. Neuropathicc and nociceptive pain in head and neck cancer patients receiving radiation therapy. Head Neck. Oncol. 2009;1:26.
8. Lazarovici T. Oral bisphosphonate-related osteonecrosis of the jaw: incidence, clinical features, prevention, and treatment recommendations. Clin Rev Bone Miner Metab. 2010;8(1):27.
9. JB Epstein, et al. Pain caused by cancer of the head and neck and oral mucositis. Bonica's management of pain, 4th edition. Lippincott Williams and Wilkins; 2010.pp.618-29.
10. Cacchillo D, Barker GJ, Barker BF. Late effects of head and neck radiation therapy and patient/dentist compliance with recommended dental care. Spec Care Dent. 1993;13:159-62.
11. Crile G, III. On the technique of operations upon the head and neck. Annal Surgery. 1906;44(6):842-50.
12. Terrell J, Ronis D, Fowler K, et al. Clinical predictors of quality of life in patients with head and neck cancer. Arch Otolaryngol Head Neck Surg. 2004;130(4):401-8.
13. CM Townsend, et al. The biological basis of modern surgical practice. Sabiston Text Book of Surgery, 17th edition. Philadelphia: Saunders; 2004.vol 25:p.2388.
14. Bree RD, Leemans CR. Recent advances in surgery for head and neck cancer. Curr Opin Oncol. 2010;22:186-93.
15. Terrell JE, Nanavati K, Esclamado RM, Bradford CR, Wolf GT. Health impact of head and neck cancer. Otolaryngol Head Neck Surg. 1999;120:852-9.
16. Gellrich NC, Schimming R, Schramm A, Schmalohr D, Bremerich A, Kugler J. Pain, function, and psychologic outcome before, during, and after intraoral tumor resection. J Oral Maxillofac Surg. 2002;60(7):772-7.
17. Chow HT, Teh LY. Sensory impairment after resection of the mandible: a case report of 10 cases. J Oral Maxillofac Surg. 2000;58:629-35.
18. Hammerlid E, Taft C. Health-related quality of life in long-term head and neck cancer survivors: a comparison with general population norms. Br J Cancer. 2001;84:149-56.
19. Benoliel R, Epstein J, Eliav E, Jurevic R and Elad S. Orofacial pain in cancer: Part I– Mechanisms. J Dent Res. 2007;86:491.
20. Raber-Durlacher JE, Elad S, Barasch A. Oral mucositis. Oral Oncology. 2010;46(6):452-6.
21. Grond S, Zech D, Lynch J, Diefenbach C, Schug SA, Lehmann KA. Validation of World Health Organisation Guidelines for pain relief in head and neck cancer. A prospective study. Ann Otol Rhinol Laryngol. 1993;102:342-8.
22. Zech DF, Grond S, Lynch J, Hertel D, Lehmann KA. Validation of World Health Organisation guidelines for cancer related pain relief: a ten-year prospective study. Pain. 1995;63(1):65-76.
23. Pillitteri LC, Clark RE. Comparison of a patient-controlled analgesia system with continuous infusion for administration of diamorphine for mucositis. Bone Marrow Transplant. 1998;22:495-8.
24. Lossignol DA, Dumitrescu C. Breakthrough pain: progress in management. Current Opinion in Oncology. 2010;22(4):302-6.
25. Mercadante S, Fulfaro F, Casuccio A. A randomised controlled study on the use of anti-inflammatory drugs in patients with cancer related pain on morphine therapy: effects on dose-escalation and a pharmacoeconomic analysis. Eur J Cancer. 2002;38:1358-63.
26. Free full text access at www.nice.org.uk/guidance/CG96.
27. Varghese BT, Koshy RC. Endoscopic transnasal neurolytic sphenopalatine ganglion block for head and neck cancer related pain. J Laryngol Otol. 2001;115(5):385-87.
28. Appelgren L, Janson M, Nitescu P, Curelaru L. Continuous intracisternal and high cervical intrathecal bupivacaine analgesia in refractory head and neck pain. Anaesthesiology. 1996;84:256-72.
29. Pan CX, Morrison RS, Ness J, Fugh-Berman A, Leipzig RM. Complementary and alternative medicine in the management of pain, dyspnea, and nausea and vomiting near the end of life. A systematic review. J Pain Symptom Manage. 2000;20:374-87.
30. Rodrigues DB, Stauffer PR, Vrba D, Hurwitz MD. Focused ultrasound for treatment of bone tumors. Int J Hyperthermia. 2015;31(3):260-71.
31. Napoli A, Anzidei M, Marincola BC, Brachetti G, Noce V, Boni F, Bertaccini L, Passariello R, Catalano C. MR Imagingguided Focused Ultrasound for Treatment of Bone Metastasis. Radiographics. 2013;33:1555-68.

Breast Cancer: Pain and Its Management

PN Jain

INTRODUCTION

According to GLOBOCAN 2008 cancer fact sheet, incidence of breast cancer was approximately 1.38 million (23% of all cancers).[1,2] The developed countries have a higher incidence of breast cancers (>80 for every 100,000 persons) as compared to developing nations (<40 for every 100,000 persons. Breast cancer is one of the most prevalent types of cancer in developed world resulting in approximately 500,000 deaths worldwide annually and now becoming increasingly prevalent in developing countries also.[3] According to a WHO estimate, about 70% of new cases of breast cancer by 2020 shall be reported in developing countries.[4] Risk factors for breast cancer include longer lifespan, a high-fat diet and obesity, lack of exercise, genetics, and various reproductive changes.

According to estimate by International Association for the Study of Pain, breast cancer is on rise and ranging 40–89%. About 20–50% women has pain especially neuropathic one is a common symptom in patients following surgery even after radiotherapy and axillary node dissection.[5]

Patients can suffer significant pain during the course of breast cancer which may either be related to the disease or its treatment.

The prognosis is heavily dependent on the stage of disease at the time of presentation. If diagnosed early, by an early physical examination by a trained professional or a mammogram, then 5-year survival is 97%, but after metastases it is only approximately 25%. The treatment of breast cancer may involve surgery (including lumpectomy or mastectomy, usually with axillary node biopsy or dissection), radiotherapy (external-beam or interstitial implants), chemotherapy, or adjuvant hormonal therapy (e.g. tamoxifen or an aromatase inhibitor in hormone-dependent breast cancer), and if HER2/neu (erbB2) receptor positive, then trastuzumab therapy.[6]

SYMPTOMATOLOGY

Pain may be a late symptom in later stage, may be due to involvement of muscles, ribs. They may develop neuropathic pain following surgery, radiotherapy, plexopathy or scar pain. Brain and/or meningeal spread[7] of cancer can lead to headache or pain in the distribution of a cranial nerve which may be refractory to opioids and adjuvant drugs.

According to report 2–83% breast cancer survivors have lymph edema of chest or arm.[8]

Pain Due to Tumor

Breast cancer can cause pain at the site of the primary tumor, particularly when the tumor invades the local skin. The most common sites of metastatic spread of breast cancer are the bones, lungs, and liver. Approximately 25% of breast cancers spread to the bones first; the spine, ribs, pelvis, and long bones are most commonly affected. Patients may experience dull and constant pain at the site of metastases. The intensity may worsen during standing posture, or during activity, or on palpation of the affected area. Pathological fractures or vertebral collapse can lead to sudden onset of intense pain. Dry cough due to lung metastases may exacerbate preexisting bone pain. Liver involvement can lead to visceral pain, including right upper-quadrant abdominal pain that is frequently referred to the right shoulder.

TREATMENT-RELATED PAIN

Surgery

Biopsies or surgical procedures can produce acute pain. In a systematic review of pain after breast cancer surgery, pain in the breast or axilla ranged from 12% to 51%, with significant reduction in range of motion and in hand grip strength. About 25% of patients in these studies reported phantom sensations. In a prospective study of women undergoing breast surgery, most reported tightness in the breast and axillary incisions, along with axillary edema at 6 months which may persist. In a prospective study designed to identify risk factors predictive of the development of chronic pain after breast cancer surgery, younger age, more invasive surgery, postoperative radiation therapy, and clinically meaningful postoperative pain were found to be predictive.[8] Emotional factors may not be associated with chronic pain.[9,10]

Radiation Therapy

Radiotherapy can cause painful skin reactions during active treatment to significant moist desquamation. Long-term reactions, such as cervical or brachial plexopathies[13] due to radiotherapy have also been reported. For pain due to bone metastasis external beam radiotherapy; radioisotopes are useful. The single[8-10] Gy and fractionated (20–30 Gy in 5-10 fractions) radiotherapy provides good pain relief. The bisphosphonates give pain relief and also reduces fracture risk. External beam radiotherapy is useful.

Chemotherapy

Most commonly chemotherapeutic agents include anthracyclines (e.g. doxorubicin), alkylating agents (e.g. cyclophosphamide), and taxanes (paclitaxel, docetaxel). Anthracyclines and alkylating agents can cause mucositis or painful mouth sores. Acute paclitaxel syndrome, consisting of arthralgias and myalgias, may begin shortly after infusion and may last several days. Intensity of pain may be mild to debilitating. Painful peripheral neuropathy is a known adverse effect that can occur in up to 60% of patients receiving taxanes may resolve in most patients but some continue to have persistent pain. Tamoxifen has been known to cause bone pain and Aromatase inhibitors also lead to significant arthralgias and myalgias in some patients.

Pain Management Strategies

Assessment of pain is of paramount importance to determine the underlying etiology, which will guide the appropriate pain management. According to WHO, pharmacotherapy constitutes the main treatment for cancer pain. The analgesics are used as per five principles—'by mouth', 'by the clock', 'by the ladder', 'for the individual' and 'attention to detail'. The WHO analgesic ladder provided excellent guidelines for use of various drugs from weak to strong opioids for different types of pain.

Standard analgesic therapies, such as non-steroidal anti-inflammatory drugs, opioids, and adjuvant agents are essential. Tricyclic antidepressants[11] may be particularly useful in treating postmastectomy pain syndrome which may establish few weeks after surgery or many months later. Radiotherapy can be extremely beneficial for bone metastases from breast cancer. Radiotherapy to painful metastatic bone lesions can be given over several weeks or in a single fraction of 8 Gy. Relief may begin within days of treatment, and may take several weeks after treatment to provide maximum effect. In some cases of multifocal metastatic bone disease that have moderate to severe pain and unresponsive to analgesics, radiopharmaceuticals such as strontium-89 or samarium-153 may be used. Radionuclide therapy may especially be rewarding in patients who have good general condition with Hb >10 g% and normal platelets count. Bisphosphonates have shown benefit in relieving pain from bone metastases, as well as preventing skeletal fractures and also the nerve compression. Splinting and immobilization can be less invasive approaches, yet surgical stabilization should be considered in appropriate patients. Vertebroplasty is a good minimally invasive option used when metastasis occurs in the vertebral bodies, leading to collapse and resultant compression of nerve roots. These patients complain of movement-related gravity dependent pain and may become bedridden. Physiotherapy can be essential for maintenance of range of motion[12,13] and for prevention and treatment of lymphedema.

Interventional pain therapies, including nerve blocks, can be useful in selected individuals. Palliative care, with attention to pain and other symptoms, is appropriate from the time of diagnosis, also during the course of this disease till the end of life.

Management of Breakthrough Pain

Breakthrough pain (BTP) can be controlled by treating the underlying etiology, optimizing around the clock medications and using specific medications. In patients with well-controlled baseline pain having BTP episodes, increase in baseline opioid dose results in better pain relief. For BTP episodes, about one-sixth (17%) of the daily dose of morphine can be used. Fentanyl in various forms such as Oral Transmucosal Fentany Citrate (OFTC); fentanyl buccal tablet (FBT); Sublingual fentanyl (SLF); Fentanyl Buccal Soluble Film (FBSF) provide faster and effective analgesia and is well tolerated.

Noble Pharmacological Therapies

CB2 Agonist

Cannabinoid receptor 2 (CB2) is novel approach to manage neuropathic pain.[14] The higher doses may have side effects dizziness, blurred vision. Johnson et al.[15] reported that tetrahydrocannabinol: cannabidiol (THC: CBD) extract provides good pain relief for cancer patients refractory to opioids.

Tetrodotoxin

Upregulation of voltage-gated sodium (Na$^+$) channels has been seen in metastatic cancers including breast cancer.[16] It produces good analgesia by blocking action potential propagation or ectopic discharges.

Botulinum Toxin

Botulinum toxin has ability to suppress the release of neurotransmitters involved in transmission of pain impulses/nociception, i.e. endothelin-1, substance P, and calcitonin gene-related peptide (CGRP) and neuropeptide Y. It has been used to control postmastectomy pain and has potential to reduce cancer-induced bone pain.[17]

Caffeine

Caffeine is an antagonist of adenosine receptors-A [1], A [2A], A [2B].

It is beneficial as an adjuvant with NSAIDs and opioids. A successful clinical trials have established the efficacy of caffeine as an adjuvant to opioids for relief of postoperative pain after breast surgery.[18]

Soy Isoflavones

Shown analgesic after surgery for breast carcinoma.[19]

Key Points

- The effective treatment options have increased life expectancy in breast cancer patients.
- Chronic pain has depreciated quality of life of breast cancer survivors.
- The variety of medications and its accessibility has provide satisfactory analgesia and decreased its side effects.
- More research is needed to manage breast cancer, and maximum pain relief with minimum side effects.

CONCLUSION

Life expectancy in breast cancer patients has increased due to availability various treatment options. Most patients with pain can be successfully treated after a thorough assessment delineating the possible mechanism of inferred pain syndrome. Most common causes of pain are brachial plexopathy, bone metastasis, post-mastectomy pain syndrome, lymphedema, and in last stages brain and liver metastasis. Novel therapies need further confirmation after phase III and IV studies to further strengthen the pharmacological therapies available including NSAIDs and opioids. More research is warranted to provide the most effective pain relief with minimum side effects.

REFERENCES

1. Hortobagyi GN, de la Garza Salazar J, Pritchard K, Amadori D, Haidinger R, Hudis CA, et al. The global breast cancer burden: variations in epidemiology and survival. Clin Breast Cancer. 2005;6:391-401.
2. GLOBOCAN 2008, Cancer Fact Sheet. Breast Cancer Incidence and Mortality Worldwide in 2008. [accessed on July 20, 2011.
3. American Cancer Society. Global cancer facts and figures 2007. American Cancer Society 2007.
4. World Health Organization. Global cancer rates could increase by 50% to 15 million by 2020. Available at 3. http://www.who.int/mediacentre/news/releases/2003/pr27/en/. Accessed February 28, 2009.
5. Jung BF, Ahrendt GM, Oaklander AL, Dworkin RH. Neuropathic pain following breast cancer surgery: proposed classification and research update. Pain. 2003;104:1-13.
6. Turner NC, Jones AL. Management of breast cancer: part II. BMJ. 2008;337:540.
7. Jain PN, Kavishwar N, Jalali R. Refractory Headache in a Patient with Breast Cancer and Carcinomatous Meningitis Unresponsive to Analgesics: Case Report Journal of Pain & Palliative Care Pharmacotherapy. 2005;19(2).
8. Riesman JS, Dijkstra PU, Hoekstra HJ, Eisma WH, Szabo BG, Groothoff JW, Geertzen JH. Late morbidity after treatment of breast cancer in relation to daily activities and quality of life: A systematic review. Eur J Surg Oncol. 2003;29:229-38.
9. Poleshuck EL, Katz J, Andrus CH, Hogan LA, Jung BF, Kulick DI, Dworkin RH. Risk factors for chronic pain following breast cancer surgery: A prospective study. J Pain. 2006;7:626-34.
10. Katz J, Poleshuck EL, Andrus CH, Hogan LA, Jung BF, Kulick DI, Dworkin RH. Risk factors for acute pain and its persistence following breast cancer surgery. Pain. 2005;119:16-25.
11. Kalso E, Tasmuth T, Neuvonen PJ. Amitriptyline effectively relieves neuropathic pain following treatment of breast cancer. Pain. 1996;64:293-302.
12. Kärki A, Simonen R, Mälkiä E, Selfe J. Impairments, activity limitations and participation restrictions 6 and 12 months after breast cancer operation. J Rehabil Med. 2005;37:180-8.
13. Stubblefield MD, Custodio CM. Upper-extremity pain disorders in breast cancer. Arch Phys Med Rehabil. 2006;87(Suppl 1):S96-9.
14. Noyes R Jr, Brunk SF, Avery DA, Canter AC. The analgesic properties of delta-9-tetrahydrocannabinol and codeine. Clin Pharmacol Ther. 1975;18:84-9.
15. Johnson JR, Burnell-Nugent M, Lossignol D, GanaeMotan ED, Potts R, Fallon MT. Multicenter, double-blind, randomized, placebo-controlled, parallel-group study of the efficacy, safety, and tolerability of THC: CBD extract and THC extract in patients with intractable cancer-related pain. J Pain Symptom Manage. 2010;39:167-79.
16. Onkal R, Djamgoz MB. Molecular pharmacology of voltagegated sodium channel expression in metastatic disease: clinical potential of neonatal Nav 1.5 in breast cancer. Eur J Pharmacol. 2009;625:206-19.
17. Layeeque R, Hochberg J, Siegel E, Kunkel K, Kepple J, Henry-Tillman RS, et al. Botulinum toxin infiltration for pain control after mastectomy and expander reconstruction. Ann Surg. 2004;240:608-13.
18. Sawynok J. Methylxanthines and pain. Handb Exp Pharmacol. 2011;200:311-29.
19. Borzan J, Tall JM, Zhao C, Meyer RA, Raja SN. Effects of soy diet on inflammation-induced primary and secondary hyperalgesia in rat. Eur J Pain. 2010;14:792-8.

Carcinoma Lung: Pain and Its Management

Arun K Bhaskar

INTRODUCTION

Primary cancer of the lung is one of the most common cancers in the world; additionally, it is also a common site for metastatic disease.[1] Pain is not a common presenting symptom of lung cancer, but about a half of patients have pain whilst undergoing treatment of the disease and nearly all patients with advanced lung cancer would be requiring treatment for their pain. Lung cancers can invade local structures including chest wall, spine and the brachial plexus giving rise to severe pain.[2] Neuroendocrine tumors and pleural mesotheliomas also affect the lung and give rise to painful symptoms.[3] Additionally, the treatment of lung cancers, be it surgery, radiotherapy and chemotherapy can lead to chronic pain states that may pose a difficult problem for the pain clinician.[4] The experience of pain from other causes and preexisting chronic pain conditions can also be worsened and the psychological distress of dealing with cancer can also make the pain feel worse.[5] All in all, a multimodal, multidisciplinary approach to pain management should be adopted to provide symptomatic relief for these patients.[6]

CAUSES

Pain due to the disease itself:
- Chest wall involvement
- Pleural disease—mesotheliomas, invasion from lung parenchyma
- Metastatic disease to bone—ribs, vertebra, sternum, scapula
- Invasion of brachial plexus from Pancoast's tumor
- Pain from distance metastasis like liver
- Referred pain to the shoulder due to diaphragmatic involvement
- End of life issues complicated by cough, hemoptysis and breathlessness.[7]

Pain due to the treatment of the cancer:
- Post-thoracotomy pain[8]
- Post-irradiation pain and plexopathy[9]
- Chemotherapy-induced peripheral neuropathy.[10]

SIGNS AND SYMPTOMS

The most common symptom a patient complains of at the time of diagnosis is cough and expectorated sputum may contain blood; it may be also associated with loss of appetite, weight loss and fatigue.[11] Patients may also complain of shortness of breath and reduced exercise tolerance; this can be early in the disease if there is pleural effusion. The above symptoms can get worse as the disease progresses and are particularly distressing towards the end of life. Symptoms and signs of pain very much depends on the structures affected by the disease and it can give rise to pain of varying intensities.[12]

Involvement of the pleura, chest wall including the ribs give rise to pain that is triggered or worsened on deep inspiration, coughing, or sneezing.[2] The patient can usually identify the exact point where he or she feels the pain. Bone pain can vary anywhere from a dull ache to severe sharp pain, worse at night and also can have a sudden increase in intensity on movement.[13] Tenderness may be elicited if there are bony lesions in the sternum, ribs, or vertebra. Patients may also have a band-like pain around the chest if there is cord compression due to spinal disease and this may be associated with signs and symptoms of cord compression. The scapular and shoulder involvement causes movement at the joint restricted and could be very painful.

Pain in the shoulder could also be a sign of phrenic nerve or direct diaphragmatic involvement or due to affection of basal pleura with or without pleural effusion.[2] Early involvement of the intercostal nerves can cause specific dermatomyotomal pain that can be much localized and made worse on deep inspiration and coughing. Infiltration of the brachial plexus from Pancoast's tumors can cause severe neuropathic pain rendering the affected limb extremely painful to move; it may cause motor loss and progressive lymphedema. Stridor, difficulty in swallowing and shortness of breath can occur, if there is tumor infiltration of the vagus or recurrent laryngeal nerve. Mediastinal lymphadenopathy can also cause shortness of breath and difficulty in swallowing due to obstruction of the bronchi and esophagus.[12]

The various treatment modalities of lung cancer by itself can give rise to chronic pain conditions. The post-thoracotomy pain is a well-known painful condition and affects more than half the patients; more than 30% of the patients may have this even after five years.[14] The pain is a combination of neuropathic and myofascial pain that can be present at all times or provoked and the scar pain may be associated with allodynia and hyperpathia.[15]

External beam radiotherapy and radiosurgery with gamma knife can cause neuropathic pain associated with allodynia and hyperpathia over the skin of the affected area. Treatment of Pancoast's tumors with high dose radiotherapy can cause brachial plexopathy and associated neuropathic pain.[9]

Chemotherapy drugs used in the treatment of lung cancers like taxanes (paclitaxel, docitaxel) and platinum compounds like cisplatin are implicated in chemotherapy-induced peripheral neuropathy causing pain and numbness in the feet and hand that can get progressively worse as the treatment cycles progress.[16]

CLINICAL EXAMINATION

Assessment of pain involves the general assessment of the intensity of the pain using visual analogue scores, but clinical examination often can reveal the cause of the pain.[17] Eliciting allodynia and/or hyperpathia over the affected area could identify focal neuropathic pain on the chest wall.[15]

Exquisite tenderness may be provoked on palpation at areas where there is an underlying bony metastasis in the ribs, sternum (Fig. 1) and spine. The rib fractures may be palpated during chest wall examination. Associated symptoms like breathlessness may be caused by pleural effusion or collapse of the lung due to tumor infiltration of the bronchi-dullness on percussion, rhonchi and crackles on auscultation should raise suspicion[3] and may need confirmation with appropriate imaging techniques.

Patients would need a neurological examination to identify and also to monitor

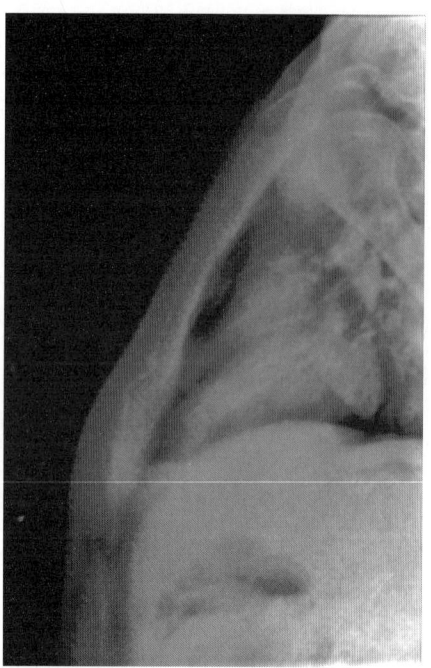

FIG. 1: Sternal metastasis from Ca lung

progression of the deficit if there is involvement of spinal or brachial plexus infiltration.[18] Signs of muscle wasting, motor weakness and Horner's syndrome on the affected side could point towards a Pancoast's tumor.

Signs of peripheral neuropathy may be elicited by sensory testing in patients with chemotherapy-induced neuropathy.[18]

DIAGNOSTIC CRITERIA

It is often important to identify the mechanism of the pain to make the appropriate management plan based on the patient's condition and available resources. A correlation of the signs and symptoms supported by the relevant investigation findings would point towards a starting point for the management of most painful conditions.[2] Additions and amendments to the initial management plan can be made based on the patient's response and disease state and the oncological management plan.

INVESTIGATIONS

A chest X-ray may show a rib fractures, pleural effusion, presence of pneumothorax or collapse of the lung; they can also show calcified pleural plaques in mesotheliomas (Fig. 2).[18] Most patients would need a CT scan or MRI scan to specifically identify the exact location of the problem so as to plan an intervention to alleviate the pain. Bone scans and positron emission tomography (PET) scans can be used for early identification of the lesions.[11]

Ultrasonogram of the liver may show liver metastasis and basal deposits involving the diaphragm. The blood tests for hormonal assays and specific markers would identify paraneoplastic syndromes and neuroendocrine tumors.[3] Routine blood tests including full blood count (FBC), urea and electrolyte (U and E) and coagulation profile would be needed before planning any interventional procedures for obvious reasons.

DIFFERENTIAL DIAGNOSIS

- Chest wall pain
  - Neuropathic
  - Post-thoracotomy pain
  - Rib fractures; rib metastasis

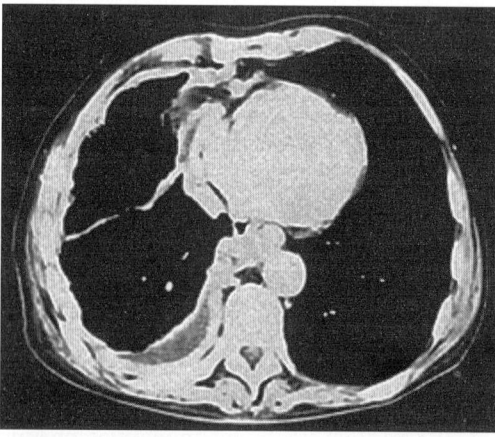

FIG. 2: Pleural mesothelioma

- o Musculoskeletal
- Pleural disease
  - o Mesotheliomas
  - o Invasion from lung parenchyma
  - o Pleural effusion
  - o Post-pleurodesis pain
- Metastatic disease to bone
  - o Ribs, vertebra, sternum, scapula
- Brachial plexopathy
  - o Pancoast's tumor, secondaries
  - o Post-irradiation
- Liver capsular pain
- Diaphragmatic pain.

TREATMENT

Treatment of lung cancer pain can be broadly divided to:
- Management of the pain symptomatically with analgesics and adjuvants,
- Specific management of the underlying cause of the pain or the mechanism of pain either by the oncological management of the tumor (Figs 3A and B), or by pain interventional procedures that block the pain pathways.

Most patients would have been started on simple analgesics like paracetamol and NSAIDs early on when the painful symptoms develop.[19]

Patients may be also on weak opioids like tramadol or codeine phosphate and the main reasons for referral are inadequate pain control or undesirable side-effects causing distress and poor compliance.[20] So also, some patients are reluctant to take strong opioids like morphine or oxycodone due to the stigma attached to them and their concerns of getting addicted to these drugs.[21] Patient education and optimizing the pain management plan would be the first step to establish the confidence of the patient and also to pave the way for further progression to stronger analgesics.[22] It is to be impressed upon the patients that regular analgesia would be more efficacious in controlling the pain rather than taking it on demand.[23]

The WHO pain ladder recommends paracetamol 1 gram four times a day with the maximum daily dose of 4 grams not to be exceeded.[24] Concomitant use of NSAIDs,[25] if not contraindicated, like ibuprofen, mefanamic acid or diclofenac would be better tolerated if taken after food and if this is to be continued for a prolonged period, an addition of a proton pump inhibitor (PPI) like omeprazole or lansoprazole may be advisable. Alternatively, patient may be commenced on a COX 2 inhibitor like celecoxib, if conventional NSAIDs are not tolerated due to its' side effects.

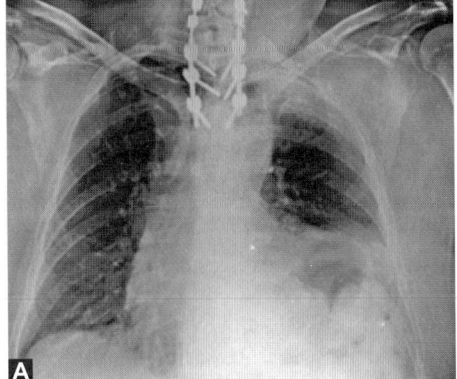 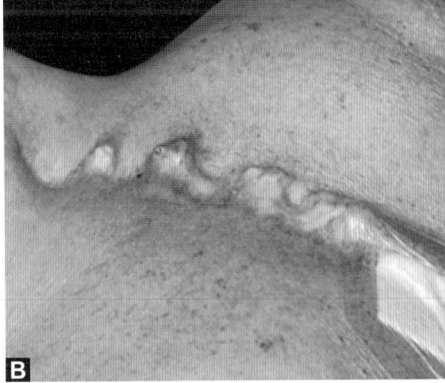

FIGS 3A and B: Patient with Ca lung with spinal metastasis requiring spinal fixators. He had undergone resection by radiosurgery using gamma knife

Weak opioids like tramadol 50 to 100 mg four times a day or codeine phosphate 30 to 60 mg four times a day could be sufficient to control pain in the early stages, but if the pain is not adequately controlled, it may be best to switch to a strong opioid like morphine or oxycodone at a smaller dose rather than increase the weak opioids at a higher dose.[26]

Compliance may be better if a laxative is added to avoid troublesome constipation, which is a common side effect that makes people avoid taking these medications.[27]

Morphine, oxycodone and hydromorphone by mouth are the commonly used strong opioids.[28] These are usually given twice a day as sustained-release or modified release preparations,[29] e.g. morphine slow release tablet (MST), oxycontin, palladone SR, etc. and the dose can be titrated up to response or until a ceiling limit is reached due to undesirable and unacceptable side effects.[30]

Traditionally, patients are also prescribed short-acting preparations (oramorph, oxynorm) at 1/6th dose of their 24 hour dose of long-acting opioids for management of breakthrough pain;[31] however, more recently these are being superseded by fentanyl preparations[32] delivered transmucosally via the buccal (Actiq, Effentora Cephalon), sublingual (abstral prostrakan) and intra-nasal routes (Instanyl Nycomed, PecFent Archimedes pharma) as it is quicker acting and is better suited to the breakthrough pain profile.[33] Transdermal fentanyl patches and subcutaneous syringe drivers of various opioids are better suited if patients cannot tolerate the oral route or the absorption from the gut is not reliable.[34]

Patients can also benefit from interpleural catheters[35] for bupivacaine infusions and also intrathecal lines[36] using morphine, clonidine and ziconotide[37] to manage pains not responding well to systemic opioid therapy.[38]

Neuropathic pain should be ideally managed with specific neuropathic pain agents along with other analgesics.[39] Gradual titration allows the patient to adapt to the drug without having troublesome side effects like sedation, drowsiness and lethargy. Anticonvulsants like gabapentin or pregabalin and antidepressants like amitriptyline, nortriptyline and duloxetine are among the commonly used systemic neuropathic pain medications. Gabapentin is commonly used at doses of 300 to 600 mg three to four times a day, but doses as high as 3600 to 4800 mg in a twenty-four hours period.[40] Pregabalin has the advantage of twice daily dosing and most patients require a dose of 75 to 300 mg twice daily for controlling the pain.[41]

Amitriptyline has more side-effects like dry mouth and sedation, hence it is best titrated up slowly in 10 to 25 mg increments as tolerated and doses higher than 75 mg are unlikely to be beneficial and are more likely to cause side-effects.[42] Duloxetine, a selective noradrenaline reuptake inhibitor, at doses of 60 mg once or twice daily can also be used for neuropathic pain.[43] Ketamine,[44,45] cannabinoids,[46] and methadone have also been used in the management of resistant pains, but should be used with caution when higher doses are considered.

Chest wall pain or thoracotomy scar pain, which is focal or localized, could be managed with local therapies that does not cause any significant side effects. 5% Lidocaine plasters applied for a period of 12 hours during a 24-hour period can provide good analgesia for the focal neuropathic pain.[47]

Capsaicin cream at strengths of 0.025–0.075% applied three to four times a day for several weeks has been shown to be beneficial, but it has poor compliance due to difficulty in repeated application several times a day for several weeks. An 8% capsaicin patch as a single application for 60 minutes after pretreatment with local anesthetic cream could give lasting pain relief for more than 3 months at a time.[48]

Post-thoracotomy scar pain and post-irradiation allodynia can be successfully managed with percutaneous electrical nerve stimulation therapy (PENS-Algotech corporation) for alleviation of the focal neuropathic pain (Figs 4 and 5)

Pain interventional procedures like intercostal blocks[49] and thoracic paravertebral blocks[50] (Fig. 6) can be used effectively in managing chest wall pain due to tumor infiltration or involvement of the ribs.

Diagnostic blocks with local anesthetic may be carried out to check the effectiveness of the block prior to using neurolytic agents like phenol or alcohol neurolysis for multiple rib metastasis from Ca lung can be also carried out selectively at the sensory roots using intrathecal absolute alcohol (Fig. 7) using the hypobaric property to float it up in the CSF.

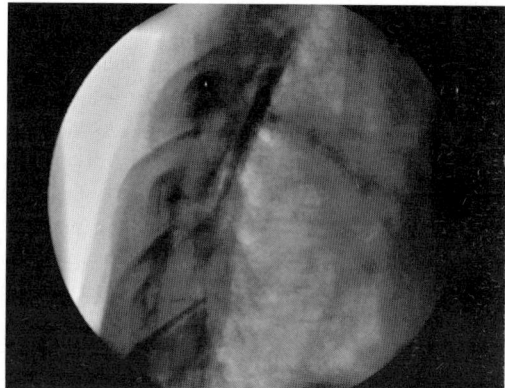

FIG. 6: Thoracic paravertebral block for multiple rib metastasis from Ca lung

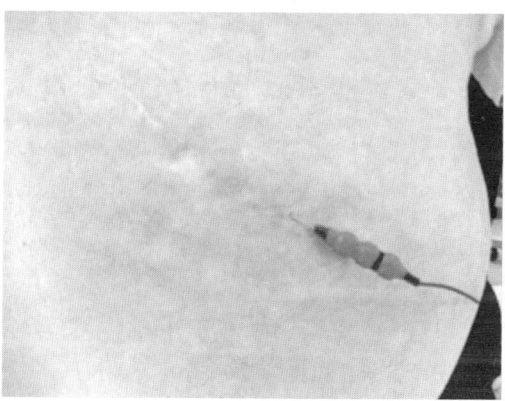

FIG. 4: PENS therapy for post-thoracotomy pain
(*Courtesy*: Algotech Ltd., United Kingdom)

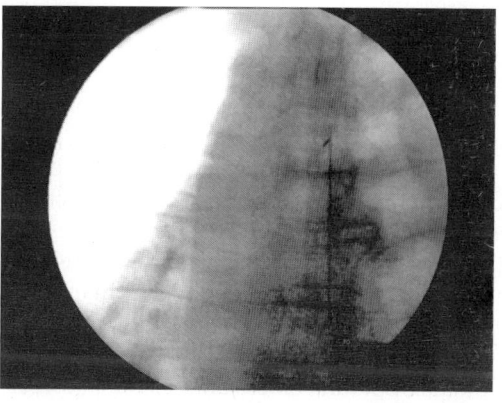

FIG. 7: Thoracic selective sensory intrathecal neurolysis for rib metastasis involving pedicle

This is particularly beneficial if the tumor infiltration is at the costovertebral junction involving the spinal roots.

Intrapleural Block (Fig. 8)

Injection of tetracycline 8–10 cc via intrapleural catheter helps in relief of pain by causing pleurodesis.[50]

Patients may develop frozen shoulder due to disease involvement or due to treatment or even due to prolonged immobility due to involvement of neighboring structures; the pain can be alleviated by a simple suprascapular nerve block[51,52] with or without trigger point injections and this would

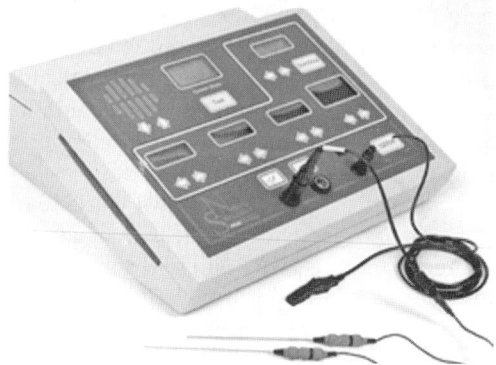

FIG. 5: PENS generator, Algotech corporation

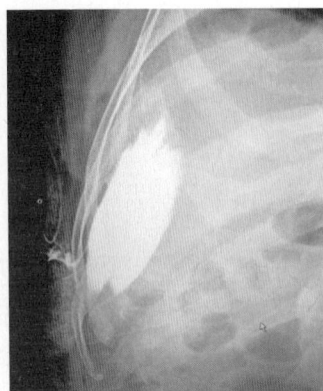

FIG. 8: Intra pleural block-dye spread
(*Courtsey:* Dr DK Baheti)

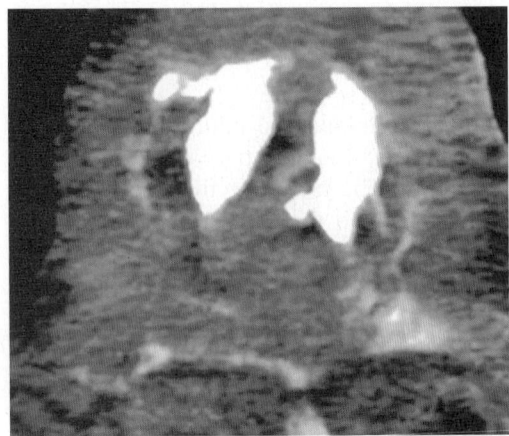

FIG 9: Coblation of vertebral body metastasis

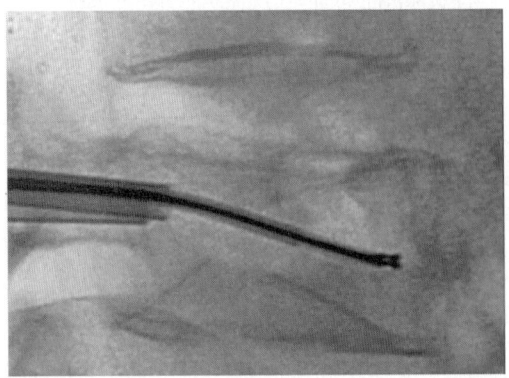

FIG 10: Injection of PMMA cement
(*Courtesy:* Arthrocare Ltd)

also enable to carry out physiotherapy and mobilization of the joint.

Spinal metastasis needs to be managed urgently not just for the pain, but also as it poses risk of spinal cord compression. External beam radiotherapy as a single or multiple fractions to the affected site also arrests the progression of the disease and provide good pain relief;[53] however, it may take a few weeks to have that effect and alternative pain relief measures may have to be put in place in the meantime. Thoracic epidural blocks and bilateral thoracic dorsal root ganglion radiofrequency ablation[54] can give adequate analgesia at the affected level. However, if the stability of the spine is in question, they may need to undergo spinal fixation or vertebroplasty[55] to provide stability and this gives good analgesia as well.

The tumor inside the vertebral body can be debulked using coblation prior (Fig. 9) to injecting bone cement (Fig. 10). If there are neurological signs and there is significant risk of cord compression, patients may need to be given high dose steroids[3] and urgent consultation by the spinal or spinal fixators (Fig. 11) to stabilize the spine following multiple metastasis neurosurgeons should be sought for spinal fixation to prevent further deterioration. The residual pain after the procedure may be managed symptomatically.

Targeted radiotherapy to bone metastasis in ribs can have dramatic reduction in bone pain.[56] Bisphosphonates[57] like zolendronic acid can cause significant reduction of the bone pain and also pain due to hypercalcemia in paraneoplastic syndromes.[58] Calcitonin has also been used successfully in alleviating bone pain.[59]

Brachial plexopathy is particularly difficult to treat with medical management alone, as there is a big difference in the pain intensity at rest and on movement. Selective sensory neurolysis of the cervicothoracic roots of the brachial plexus with intrathecal absolute alcohol (Fig. 12) can give excellent

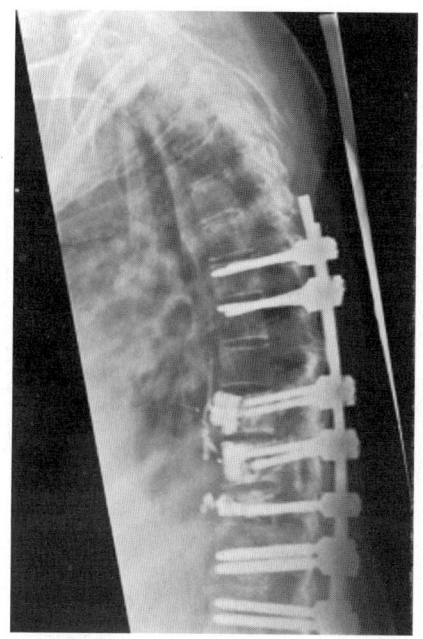

FIG 11: Spinal fixators to stabilize the spine following multiple metastasis

analgesia, but preserving whatever residual motor function in that upper limb. Stellate ganglion blocks have also been used in managing sympathetically mediated pain. The disruption of the lateral spinothalamic tract on the contralateral side by percutaneous cordotomy[60] is a well-known technique for the management of intractable unilateral chest pain particularly of pleuritic origin associated with mesotheliomas[61] (Fig. 13).

In addition to all of the above, it should be noted that treatment, be it curative or palliative, of the underlying pathology with surgery, radiotherapy or chemotherapy also helps towards alleviating the pain.[62]

However, these treatment options can also give rise to various pain states that may require the input of the pain physician. Epidural infusions and patient-controlled analgesias (PCAs) are used in the management of acute postoperative pain and chemotherapy-induced oral mucositis pain[63] could be quite challenging to manage due to the nature of the symptoms.[64]

Complementary therapies[64] like acupuncture,[65] massage and aromatherapy[66] have been shown to be of some benefit to alleviate patients' pain and other symptoms. With advancing disease, end of life care brings in additional problems like breathlessness and intractable cough, which may be managed with opioids like morphine for symptomatic relief; this may have to be delivered via a continuous infusion subcutaneously via a syringe driver as the patient may not be in a state to take oral medications.[67]

Benzodiazepines like diazepam and midazolam are also used to alleviate anxiety and also in the management of death-rattle as part of end of life care. If there is obstruction due to the tumor, insertion of stents to maintain the patency of the trachea, bronchus and esophagus can provide appropriate symptomatic relief.

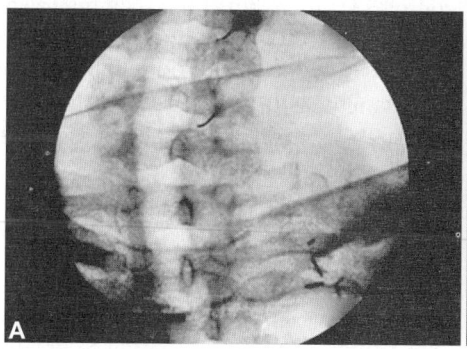 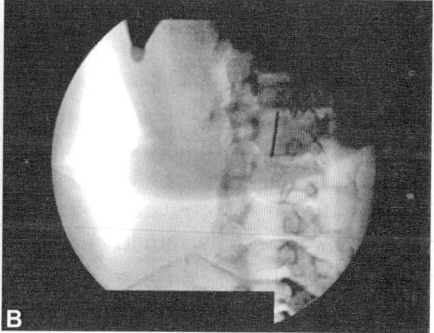

FIGS 12A and B: Cervical selective sensory neurolysis with absolute alcohol for brachial plexus infiltration and diaphragmatic

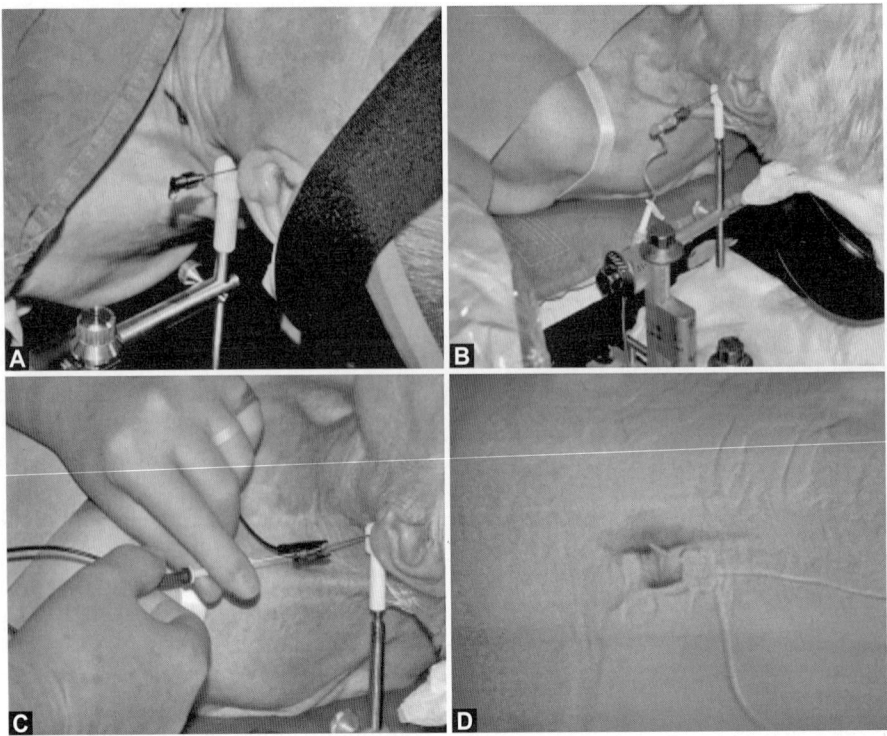

FIGS 13A to D: Percutaneous cervical cordotomy for intractable pain from pleural mesothelioma
(*Courtesy:* Dr Paul Cook, Oldham, United Kingdom)

FOLLOW-UP ADVICE

Patients are to be followed-up as required depending on the stage of the disease for ensuring that the symptoms are controlled adequately and also to monitor for potential side effects. Frequent follow-ups may be required during the dose titration phase of opioids and neuropathic pain medications to ensure compliance and also to reassure the patient, till stable doses are achieved. Once adequate pain control is achieved, follow-ups can be arranged at appropriate frequencies depending on the patients' needs and conveniences in an outpatient setting. However, patient and carers should be aware of a contact point either in person or over the telephone in case of urgency to ensure that continuity of care is maintained. Most pain interventional procedures may be carried out as a day case procedure; patients undergoing percutaneous cordotomy are best observed for at least 24 hours in the hospital prior to discharge as there is a risk of developing delayed complications like respiratory depression and neurological deficits due to cord edema. Patients who are on high dose of opioids for managing their pain may also need to be observed overnight as they can develop increased sedation and potentially respiratory depression due to the disproportionally high dose of the opioids once excellent analgesia has been achieved following the pain interventional procedure. During the end of life stage, frequent follow-ups are required to ensure that the needs of the patient and relatives are addressed promptly; the role of the palliative care teams in the hospital and in the community are invaluable to ensure that these needs are appropriately met.

CONCLUSION

The cancer pain is a multifaceted problem, which can be due to tumor or secondaries. It also has nociceptive and neuropathic components. Cancer pain is managed with multidisciplinary approach.

REFERENCES

1. GLOBOCAN 2008. Cancer incidence and mortality worldwide; IARC 2010 http://globocan.iarc.fr.
2. Pass HI. Lung Cancer: Principles and Practice, 3rd edition. Lippincott Williams and Wilkins, 2005.
3. Cassidy J, Spence RAJ, Payne M. Oxford Handbook of Oncology, 2nd edition. Oxford: Oxford University Press; 2006.
4. Portnenoy RK, Lesage P. Management of cancer pain. Lancet. 1999;353(9165):1695-700.
5. Zara C, Baine N. Cancer pain and psychosocial factors: a critical review of the literature. J Pain and Symptom Manage. 2002;24:526-42.
6. The British Pain Society: Cancer Pain Management-A perspective from the British Pain Society, supported by the Association for Palliative Medicine and the Royal College of General Practitioners; 2010.
7. Watson M, et al. Oxford Handbook of Palliative Care. Oxford University Press; 2005.
8. Maguire MF, Ravenscroft A, Beggs D, Duffy JP. A questionnaire study investigating the prevalence of the neuropathic component of chronic pain after thoracic surgery. Eur J Cardiothorac Surg. 2006;29:800-5.
9. Galecki J, Hicer-Grzenkowicz J, Grudzien-Kowalska M, Michalska T, Zalucki W. Radiation-induced brachial plexopathy and hypofractionated regimens in adjuvant irradiation of patients with breast cancer-a review. Acta Oncologica. 2006;45:280-4.
10. van den Beuken-van Everdingen MH, de Rijke JM, Kessels AG, Schouten HC, van Kleef M, Patijn J. Prevalence of pain in patients with cancer: a systematic review of the past 40 years. Ann Oncol. 2007;18(9):1437-49.
11. Kufe DW, et al. Cancer Medicine, 6th edition. BC Decker, 2003.
12. Caraceni A, Portenoy RK. An international survey of cancer pain characteristics and syndromes. Pain 1999;82(3):263-74.
13. Davies A. Cancer related breakthrough pain. Oxford Pain Library, OUP. Farquhar-Smith WP 2008. Anaesthetic/interventional techniques. In: Davis A (Ed). Cancer related Bone Pain, Oxford Pain Library, OUP.
14. Karmakar MK, Ho AM. Post-thoracotomy pain syndrome. Thoracic Surg Clin. 2004;14:345-52.
15. Woolfe CJ, Mannion RJ. Pain: Neuropathic pain: aetiology, symptoms, mechanisms and management. Lancet. 1999;353:1959-64.
16. Quastoff S, Hartrung HP. Chemotherapy induced peripheral neuropathy. J Neurol. 2002;249(1):9-17.
17. WHO (1990) Cancer pain relief and palliative care. WHO Tech Rep Ser 804.WHO, Geneva.
18. Longmore M, Wilkinson IB, Davidson EH, Foulkes A, Mafi AR. Oxford University Press, 2010.
19. Stockler M, Vardy J, Pillai A, Warr D. Acetaminophen (paracetamol) improves pain and well-being in people with advanced cancer receiving a strong opioid regimen: a randomized, double-blind, placebo controlled cross-over trial. J Clin Oncol. 2004;22(16): 3389-94.
20. Wilkie D, Keefe F. Coping strategies of patients with lung-cancer related pain. Clin J Pain. 1991;7:792-9.
21. Breivik H, Cherny N, Collett D, de Conno F, Filbet M, Foubert AJ, Cohen R, Dow L. Cancer-related pain: a pan-European survey of prevalence, treatment and patient attitudes. Ann Oncol. 2009;20(8):1420-33.
22. Allard P, Maunsell E, Labbe J, Dorval M. Educational interventions to improve cancer pain control: a systematic review. J Palliat Med. 2001;4(2):191-203.
23. Ahmedzai SH, Boland J. The total challenge of cancer pain in supportive and palliative care. Curr Opin Support Palliat Care. 2007;1:3-5.
24. Meldrum M. The ladder and the clock: cancer pain and public policy at the end of the twentieth century. J Pain Symptom Manage. 2005;29(1):41-54.
25. McNicol E, Strassels SA, Goudas L, Lau J, Carr DB. NSAIDs or paracetamol, alone or combined with opioids, for cancer pain. Cochrane Database Syst Rev. 2005; Issue 2. Art. No: CD005180. DOI: 10.1002/14651858. CD005180.
26. Ferreira SL, Kimura M, Teixeira MJ. The WHO analgesic ladder for cancer pain control, twenty years of use. How much pain relief does one get from using it? Support Care Cancer. 2006;14:1086-93.
27. Mercadante S, Arcuri E. Pharmacological management of cancer pain in the elderly. Drugs and Aging. 2007; 24(9):761-76.
28. Wiffen PJ, McQuay HJ. Oral morphine for cancer pain. Cochrane Database of Systematic Reviews. 2007; Issue 3. Art. No: CD003868.
29. Lauretti GR, Oliveira GM, Pereira NL. Comparison of sustained-release morphine with sustained-release oxycodone in advanced cancer patients. Br J Cancer. 2003;89(11):2027-30.

30. McCarberg BH. The Treatment of breakthrough pain. Pain Med. 2007;8(1):S8-S13.
31. Hanks GW, de Conno F, Cherny N, Hanna M, Kalso E, McQuay HJ, Mercadante S, Meynadier J, Poulain P, Ripamonti C, Radbruch L, Casas JR, Sawe J, Tycross RG, Ventafridda V. Morphine and alternative opioids in cancer pain: the EAPC recommendations. Expert Working Group of the Research Network of the European Association for Palliative Care. Br J Cancer. 2001;84:587-93.
32. William L, Macleod R. Management of breakthrough pain in cancer patients. Drugs. 2008;68(7):913-24.
33. Bennett DS, Burton AW, Fishman S, Fortner B, McCarberg W, Miasskkowski C, Nash DB, Pappagallo M, Payne R, Ray J, Viscussi ER, Wong W. Consensus panel recommendations for the assessment and management of breakthrough pain. Pharmacy and Therapeutics. 2005;30(5):296-301.
34. Clark AJ, Ahmedzai SH, Allan LG and Camacho F. Efficacy and safety of transdermal fentanyl and sustained-release oral morphine in patients with cancer and chronic non-cancer pain. Curr Med Res Opin. 2004;20(9):1419-28.
35. Amesbury B, O'Riordan J. The use of interpleural analgesia using bupivacaine for pain relief in advanced cancer. Palliat Med. 1999;13(2):153-8.
36. British Pain Society. Intrathecal drug delivery for the management of pain and spasticity in adults; recommendations for best clinical practice. Br Pain Soc. 2008.
37. Staats P, Yearwood T, Wallace MS, Byas-Smith M, Fisher R, Bruce DA, Mangieri EA, Luther RR, Mayo M, McGuire D, Ellis D, Charapata SG, Presley RW, Wallace MS. Intrathecal ziconotide in the treatment of refractory pain in patients with cancer or AIDS. J Am Med Assoc. 2004; 291:63-70.
38. Smith TJ, Coyne PJ, Staats PS, Deer T, Stearns LJ, Rauck RL, Booryz-Marx RL,Buchser E, Catala E, Bryce DA, Cousins M, Pool GE. An implantable drug delivery system (IDSS) for refractory cancer pain provides sustained pain control, less drug related toxicity and possibly better survival compared with comprehensive medical management (CMM). Ann of Oncol. 2005;16:825-33.
39. Dworkin RH, O'Connor AB, Backonja M, Farrar JT, Finnerup NB, Jensen TS. Pharmacological management of neuropathic pain: evidence-based recommendations. Pain. 2007;132(3):237-51.
40. Caraceni A, Zecca E, Bonezzi C, Arcurib E, Yaya Tur R, Maltoni M, Visentin M, Gorni G, Martini C, Tirelli W, Barbieri M, de Conno F. Gabapentin for neuropathic cancer pain: a randomized controlled trial from the gabapentin cancer pain study group. J Clin Oncol. 2004;14:2909-17.
41. Dickinson AH, Matthews EA, Suzuki R. Neurobiology of neuropathic pain: mode of action of anticonvulsants. Eur J Pain. 2002;6(Suppl A):51-60.
42. Sindrup SH, Otto M, Finnerup NB, Jensen TS. Antidepressants in the treatment of neuropathic pain. Basic Clin Pharmacol and Toxicol. 2005;96:399-409.
43. Finnerup NB, Otto M, McQuay HJ, Jensen TS, Sindrup SH. Algorithm for neuropathic pain treatment: an evidence based proposal. Pain. 2005;118:289-305.
44. Bell R, Eccleston C, Kalso E. Ketamine as an adjuvant to opioids for cancer pain. Cochrane Database. Syst Rev. 2003.1:CD003351.
45. Okon T. Ketamine: an introduction for the pain and palliative medicine physician. Pain Physician. 2007;10: 493-500.
46. Campbell FA, Tamer MR, Carroll D, Reynolds DJ, Moore RA, McQueen HJ. Are cannabinoids an effective and safe treatment option in the management of pain? A qualitative systematic review. Br Med J. 2001;323:13-6.
47. Davies PS, Galer S. Review of Lidocaine patch 5% studies in the treatment of post herpetic neuralgia. Drugs. 2004;64(9):937-47.
48. Davis MP. What is new in neuropathic pain? Support Care Cancer. 2007;15:353-72.
49. Wong FCS, Lee TW, Yuen KK, Lo SH, Sze WK, Tung SY. Intercostal nerve blockade for cancer pain: effectiveness and selection of patients. Hong Kong Med J. 2007;13:266-70.
50. Baheti DK. Intrapleural Block. Interventional pain management: A practical approach. In: Baheti, Bakshi, Gupta, Gehdoo (Eds). Jaypee Medical Publisher; 2010. pp.130-6.
51. Raj PP, et al. Interventional pain management: image-guided procedures. 2nd edition, Saunders/Elsevier.
52. Lipton S. Relief of pain in clinical practice. Blackwell Scientific Publications, Oxford: England. 1979.
53. Sze WM, Shelley MD, Held I, Wilt TJ, Mason MD. Palliation of metastatic bone pain: single fraction versus multifraction radiotherapy a systematic review of randomized trials. Clin Oncol. 2003;15(6):345-52.
54. Gauci CA. Manual of RF Techniques, 2nd edition. Flivopress.
55. Hentschel SJ, Burton AW, Fourney DR, Rhines LD, Mendel E. Percutaneous vertebroplasty and kyphoplasty performed at a cancer centre: refuting proposed contraindications. J Neurosurg-Spine. 2005;2(4):436-40.
56. McQueen H, Carroll D, Moore RA. Radiotherapy for painful bone metastases: a systematic review. Clin Oncol. 1997;9:150-4.
57. Ross JR, Saunders Y, Edmonds PM, Patel S, Broadley KE, Johnston SR. Systematic review of role of bisphos-

phonates on skeletal morbidity in metastatic cancer. Br Med J. 2003;327:469-72.
58. Wong RKS, Wiffen PJ. Bisphosphonates for the relief of pain secondary to bone metastases. Cochrane Database of Syst Rev. 2002; 2. Art. No.: CD002068. DOI:10.1002/14651858.CD002068.
59. Martinez-Zapata MJ, Roque M, Alonso-Coello P, Catala E. Calcitonin for metastatic bone pain. [Update of Cochrane Database Syst Rev. 003; 3:CD003223; PMID: 12917954]. [Review] [27 refs] [Journal Article. Meta-Analysis. Review] Cochrane Database Syst Revs. 3:CD003223.
60. Crul BJP, Blok LM, Van Egmond J, Van Dongen RTM. The present role of percutaneous cordotomy for the treatment of cancer pain. J Headache Pain. 2005;6(1):24-9.
61. Jackson MB, Pounder D, Price C, Mathews AW, Neville E. Percutaneous cervical cordotomy for the control of pain in patients with pleural mesothelioma. Thorax. 1999; 54:238-41.
62. Clarkson JE, Worthington HV, Eden TOB. Interventions for treating oral mucositis for patients with cancer receiving treatment. Cochrane Database of Syst Rev 2007, Issue 1. Art. No: CD001973. DOI: 10. 1002/14651858.
63. Sonis ST. The pathobiology of mucositis. Nature Rev Cancer. 2004;4(4):277-84.
64. Ernst E, Pittler MH, Wider B, Boddy K. Complementary therapies for pain management. London: Elsevier/Mosby 2007.
65. Lee H, Schmidt K, Ernst E. Acupuncture for the relief of cancer-related pain-a systematic review. Eur J Pain. 2005;9:437-41.
66. Fellowe D, Barnes K, Wilkinson S. Aromatherapy and massage for symptom relief in patients with cancer. The Cochrane Database of Syst Rev 2004; 3. Art. No: CD002287.
67. Ahmedzai SH. Window of opportunity for pain control in the terminally ill. Lancet. 2001;357(9265):1304-5.

30
CHAPTER

Upper Abdominal Malignancy: Pain and Its Management

Dwarkadas K Baheti

INTRODUCTION

The upper abdominal pain is one of the most common symptoms in contrast to other areas of the body. The abdominal organs have poorly developed sensory systems and are relatively insensitive to many stimuli compared with a more sensitive organ such as the epidermis. In addition to the relative, paucity of sensory nerve endings, as the same group of nerves may supply several viscera. There are very few well known nociceptive triggers in the abdominal cavity. The visceral pain is transmitted from nociceptors found on the walls of the abdominal viscera via sympathetic and parasympathetic pathway.

The upper abdominal visceras are innervated by celiac plexus. These include pancreas, liver, gallbladder, omentum, mesentery, and alimentary tract from stomach to the transverse portion of large colon.

The tumor can be detected on MRI of abdomen such as pancreatic tumor, duodenal mass, secondaries in liver and kidney tumor (Figs 1 to 4).

CAUSES OF CHRONIC UPPER ABDOMINAL PAIN

- Tumors arising from stomach, liver, gallbladder, kidney, spleen, pancreas, aortic lymph adenopathy, omental mass,

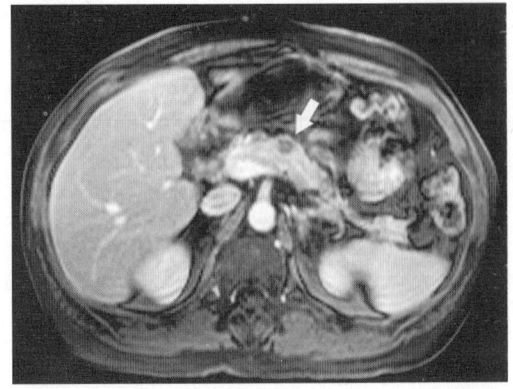

FIG. 1: Pancreatic tumor
(*Courtesy*: Dr Makarand Kulkarni)

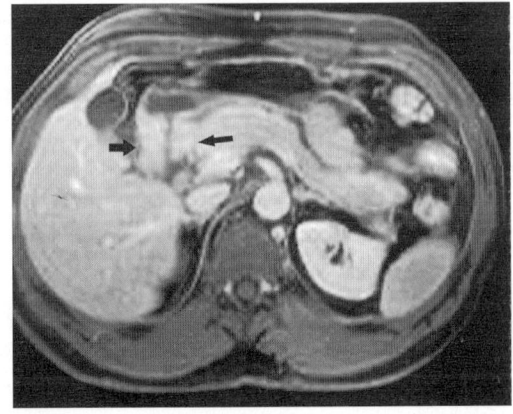

FIG. 2: Duodenal tumor
(*Courtesy*: Dr Makarand Kulkarni)

Chapter 30: Upper Abdominal Malignancy: Pain and Its Management

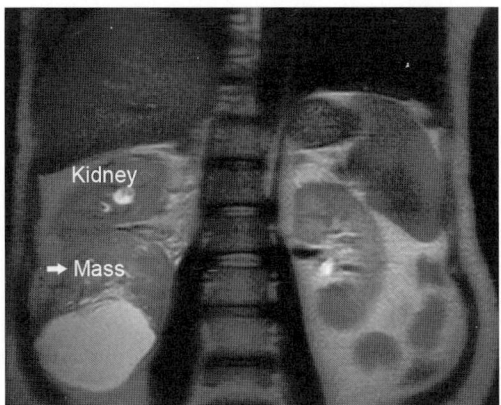

FIG. 3: Kidney tumor
(*Courtesy*: Dr Makarand Kulkarni)

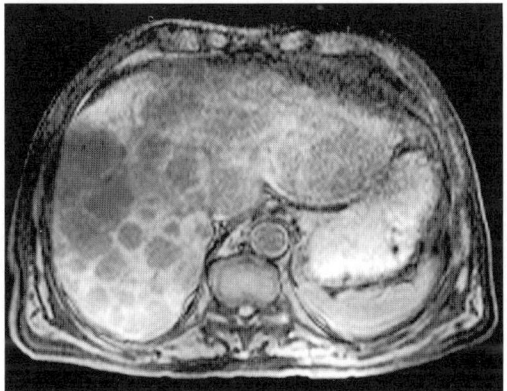

FIG. 4: Liver mass
(*Courtesy*: Dr Makarand Kulkarni)

- retroperitoneal tumors or metastatic spread.
- Chronic pancreatitis, alcoholic pancreatitis.
- GERD or chronic duodenal ulcer.[1]
- Any chronic upper abdominal pain of unknown origin.

SYMPTOMS AND SIGNS

- Pain in epigastrium, right or left hypochondrium referred to back is common symptom. Pain is usually vague, deep, squeezing, crampy, or colicky, stretching, compressing due to invading or distention of visceral structures, burning sensation or sharp stabbing
- Pain in epigastrium is referred to back or to left or right shoulder, e.g. shoulder pain that appears when the diaphragm is invaded with tumor
- Inability to lie down on the back.
- Nausea/vomiting
- Constipation
- Yellowish discoloration of skin
- Insomnia
- Irritability, depression or anxiety.

DIAGNOSTIC CRITERIA

A thorough clinical examination is necessary to evaluate the severity of pain and associated medical illness.

General Examination

The examination of cardiovascular and respiratory system is done to know the hemodynamic status and respiratory insufficiency. This will help to assess the additional risk of performing of celiac plexus or splanchnic plexus block.

Examination of Abdomen

Inspection

- Distention of epigastrium or abdomen
- There may be edema over legs
- Yellowish discoloration of skin, sclera.

Palpation

- Tumor or mass in epigastrium, right or left hypochondrium, kidney can be palpable
- There may be free fluid in abdomen due to ascites
- Abdominal wall palpation for trigger points
- Pitting edema.

Auscultation

- Auscultation of cardiac system for any associated disease and of respiratory system for bronchospasm, rales or rhonchi.

INVESTIGATIONS

- *X-ray*: Chest and abdomen to know the extent of tumors.
- *Abdominal ultrasound*: This is a non-invasive test (just like a prenatal ultrasound) that examines each specific organ in the abdomen for certain problems as well as abdominal tumors.
- *CT scan of thorax and abdomen*: This will suggest the bony spread into the ribs and vertebrae.
- *MRI thorax, dorsal, abdomen and pelvis*: This will confirm the diagnosis, extent and spread of the disease. In some cases of liver tumor or secondary's primary can be detected. The spread and extent of involvement of tumor will suggest the neuropathic component of pain.

Blood Tests

CBC: To know the Hb concentration, serum proteins. Bleeding and clotting time, HIV, HCV, HbSAg.

Other Tests

- *Kidney function test*: For serum creatinine level
- *Urine tests*: Routine urine—to know for any infection or blood in urine.

TREATMENT PROTOCOL

Aim is to provide total pain management by using multimodal therapy includes medication, interventional treatment procedure and palliative care as life expectancy is limited so precise plan of treatment will provide maximum pain relief and improve quality of life.

Pharmacological

The dosage and route of drug depend upon body weight and the clinical condition of patient.

Analgesics

Non-narcotics analgesic: Paracetamol (oral, intramuscular) 10–15 mg/kg; Inj. Tramadol hydrochloride 1–2 mg/kg; Inj. Ketamine sulfate 1–2 mg/kg.

Narcotic analgesic
- Codeine phosphate 15, 30 mg
- Morphine sulfate—oral (10, 30 mg); Inj. 15 mg/cc IM; epidural infusion 2–3 mg/day; Intrathecal testing—Inj. morphine sulfate 1–2 mg (depending upon dose of oral morphine)
- Fentanyl—Injectable, lollypop, Transdermal patch (12.5; 25, 50, 75, 100 µg)
- Inj. pethidine—1 mg/kg body wt.
- Butrum—nasal spray one puff every 12 hours
- Proxyvon—paracetamol + dextropropoxyphene
- NSAIDs—diclofenac, ketorolac.

For breakthrough pain
- Inj. Paracetamol 10–15 mg/kg over 15–20 minutes
- Inj. Tramadol hydrochloride 50 mg diluted in 10 cc normal saline IV slowly over 5–10 minutes
- Inj. Ketamine hydrochloride 0.1 mg/kg IV.

Antispasmodics

- Antimuscarinics such as dicycloverine, hyoscine, atropine, propantheline.
- Smooth muscle relaxants such as alverine, mebeverine and peppermint oil.

Laxatives

- Bulk-forming laxatives, such as wheat bran and ispaghula husk
- Osmotic laxatives, such as lactulose and macrogols

- Stimulant laxatives, such as senna and glycerol suppositories
- Enema as and when necessary.

Hyperacidity drugs (preferably given empty stomach)

- Tab. Ranitidine—150-300 mg—twice daily
- Cap. Omeprazole—20-40 mg—twice daily
- Cap. Pantoprazol—20-40 mg—twice daily
- Cap. Rabiprazol—40 mgm twice daily.

It is advisable to add Tab. Domperidone 15-30 mg along with above drugs. (*See* Recommended Ref No. 1).

Interventional Treatment Procedures

Neurolytic blocks such as splanchnic[2] or celiac plexus[3-5] are effective in controlling visceral cancer pain. These techniques have a low undesirable effects and improves gastric motility.

A detailed description of the techniques for these blocks is beyond the scope of this chapter and is available (*See* Recommended for Ref. No. 2).

Basic Procedures

- Epidural-continuous drug—Inj. morphine sulfate
- Neurolytic procedures done are either splanchnic plexus—block (Fig. 5) or celiac plexus block fluoroscopy guided (Fig. 6), CT guided (Fig. 7)
- These procedures can be done either by posterior, transdiskal, transaortic[6] or anterior approach and are done either under fluoroscopy, CT[7] or ultrasound guidance (Fig. 8)
- The neurolysis is done with 50% alcohol or by radiofrequency ablation.[8]

Advanced

Intrathecal drug delivery system—implantable pump (Fig. 9) is implanted into the abdominal wall for chronic upper abdominal pain due to pancreatic cancer.

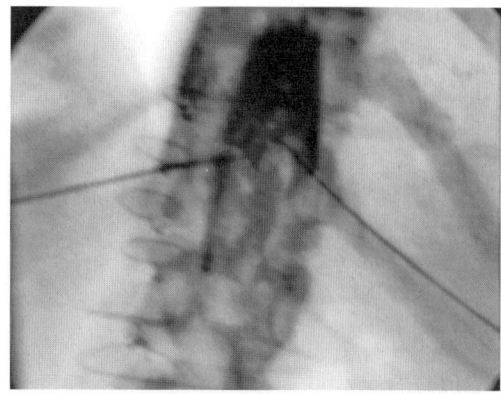

FIG. 6: Celiac plexus needle position—fluoroscopy

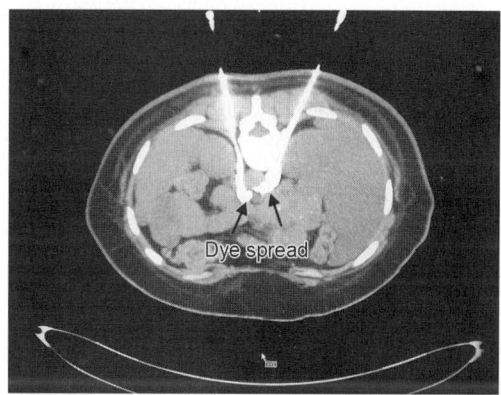

FIG. 7: Celiac plexus—CT guided dye spread

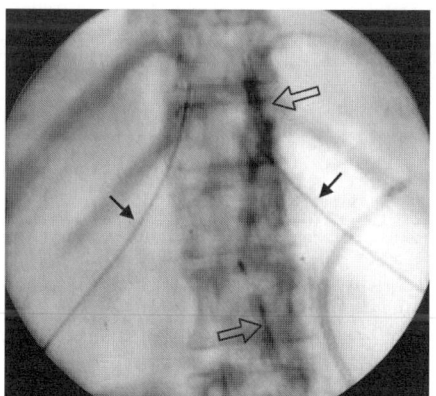

FIG. 5: Needles at splanchnic plexus—AP view

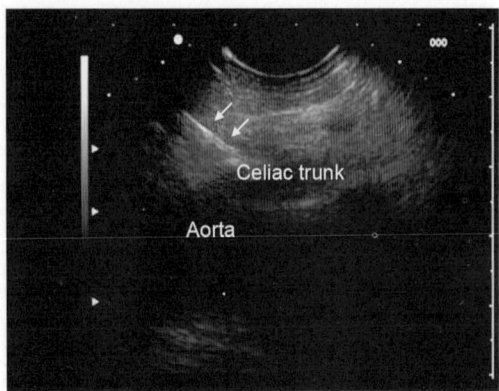

FIG. 8: US guided celiac plexus

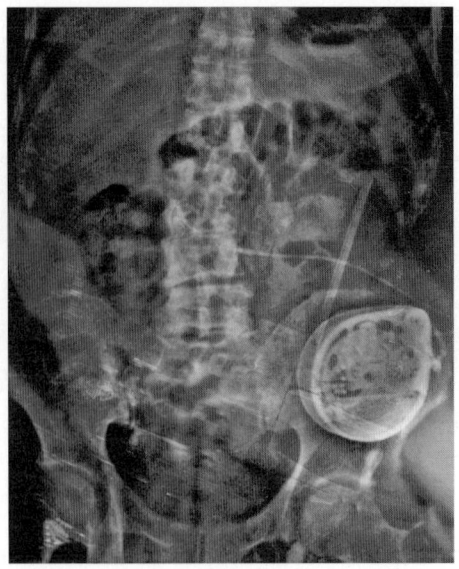

FIG. 9: Implantable pump *in situ*

Nutritional Supplements

The general condition of patient usually demands nutritional supplements and is done in consultation with primary physician and/or nutritional therapist. The nutritional supplement can be medicinal herbs, vitamins, minerals, amino acids, protein, green foods or fish oil. (*See* Recommended for Ref. No. 3).

COMPLICATIONS

- Orthostatic hypotension occurred more often when the retrocrural (50%) or splanchnic (52%) technique was used than when the anterocrural approach (10%) was used.
- Transient diarrhea—due to irritation of peritoneum.
- The incidence of dysesthesia, interscapular back pain, reactive pleurisy, hiccups, or hematuria was not statistically different.
- Temporary paraplegia.[9]

CONCLUSION

The role of multimodal for chronic upper abdominal pain of any origin affects patients and his family in many ways such as increase in psychological, financial issues and decrease in quality of life. These neurolytic blocks proved to be a safe, cost-effective in such patients. The benefits include improved analgesia, reduced opioid consumption, superior clinical effects due to the deleterious properties of high-dose chronic opioid therapy and favorable economic implications

REFERENCES

1. Kangv JY, Ho KY, Yeoh KG, Guan R. Chronic upper abdominal pain due to duodenal ulcer and other structural and functional causes: its localization and nocturnal occurrence. Journal of Gastroenterology and Hepatology. 1996;11(6):515-9.
2. Jones RR. A technique of injection of the splanchnic nerves with alcohol. Anesth Analg. 1957;36:75.
3. Jain S. The role of celiac plexus block in intractable upper abdominal pain. In: Racz GB (Ed). Technique of Neurolysis. Boston, Kluwer Academic, 1989.p.161.
4. Plancarte, Ricardo, et al. Management of chronic upper abdominal pain in cancer: transdiscal blockade of the splanchnic nerves. Regional Anesthesia & Pain Medicine. 2010;35(6):500-6.

5. Singler RC. An improved technique for alcohol neurolysis of the celiac plexus block. Anesthesiology. 1982;56:137-41.
6. Ischia S, Luzzani A, Ischia A, et al. A new approach to the neurolytic block of the coeliac plexus: the transaortic technique. Pain. 1983;16:333-41.
7. Marra V, Debernardi F, Frigerio A, Menna S, Musso L, Di Virgilio MR. Neurolytic block of the celiac plexus and splanchnic nerves with computed tomography. The experience in 150 cases and an optimization of the technique. Radiol Med. 1999;98(3):183-8.
8. Garcea G, Thomasset S, Berry DP, Tordoff S. Percutaneous splanchnic nerve radiofrequency ablation for chronic abdominal pain. ANZ Journal of Surgery. 2005;75(8):640-4.
9. Baheti DK. Neurolytic coeliac plexus block (NCPB): A ten year review of 212 cases. Bombay Hospital Journal. 2001;43(1).

RECOMMENDED FOR REFERENCES

1. *http//www.cimsasia.com*
2. Baheti D, Bakshi S, Gupta S, Gehdoo RP. Interventional Pain Management: A Practical Approach. Jaypee Medical Publishers, 2010.
3. *www.Nutritional-Supplements-Health-Guide.com.*

CHAPTER 31

Malignant Pelvic Pain and Its Management

Subhash Jain

INTRODUCTION

An estimated 1,530,00 million new cancer patients were reported for the year 2010 excluding basal cell, squamous cell carcinoma and carcinoma *in situ*.[1] National Cancer Institute estimate that approximately 11.4 million cancer patients are living with a history of cancer.[2] An estimated 569,000 Americans are expected to die of cancer and there are more than 1,500 cases each day. Cancer is the second most common cause of death in the United States exceeding heart diseases.

In spite of recent understanding regarding the basic mechanisms and understanding of pathophysiology of cancer and therapies, cancer accounts for 1 death out of every 4 deaths in America. The survival of patients due to cancer depends upon various treatments and newer protocols associated with the illness. The biological and behavioral differences of each individual cannot be taken in account in the estimation or relative survival rate. The overall incidence of cancer has reduced within the last decade. Pelvic cancer is caused by chromosome defect and gene mutation that leads to uncontrolled growth of certain types of cells, including the prostate, uterus, ovaries, testis, bladder, cervix, and fallopian tube. Recent newer diagnostic techniques and studies have shown that pain syndrome can be divided according to activation of various structured stimuli verses a neuropathic pain mechanism.

PATHOPHYSIOLOGY OF PELVIC PAIN

Nociceptive pains are produced by somatic pain predominantly due to tissue injuries of somatic structure, i.e. skin, muscle, bone and soft tissue.

Visceral pain is produced predominantly due to tissue damage or distortion of visceral organs, i.e. cardiac, gallbladder, stomach, and liver. Tissue damage or the response of neural tissue either peripherally or centrally due to injuries produce neuropathic pain. The direct invasion of tumor of soft tissue, bone or muscle mass produces a localized somatic pain in specific body regions. Localized tenderness, throbbing or stabbing sensation are typical characterizations of somatic pain. Contrary to somatic pain the pain produced by visceral obstruction or distortion results in producing diffused, localized, intermittent or cramping abdominal pain. Tissue injuries to the viscera or inflammation cause organs to produce a well localized dermatomal site (referred pain) and many produce tenderness or increase sensitivity.[3] The neural basis of this referral may be viscerosomatic convergence on to wide dynamic range (WDR) spinal neuron.[4] Tumor infiltration or compression of neural tissue, i.e. peripheral nerve, nerve root or infiltration of epidural space produces neuropathic pain.[5] At Memorial Sloan Kettering Cancer Center, New York, approximately 30% of inpatient patients with intractable pain had neuropathic pain.[6] A large percentage of patients with neuropathic pain report abnormal sensations, burning and allodynia (pain due to non-noxious stimuli), i.e. wearing or touching soft cloths or air blowing on their skin. With this abnormal sensation there may or may not have motor sensory or automatic dysfunction or the involved peripheral or central nerves. A small percentage of patient's report various pain problems following cancer therapy including surgery, chemotherapy and radiation treatment[7] (Figs 1 and 2).

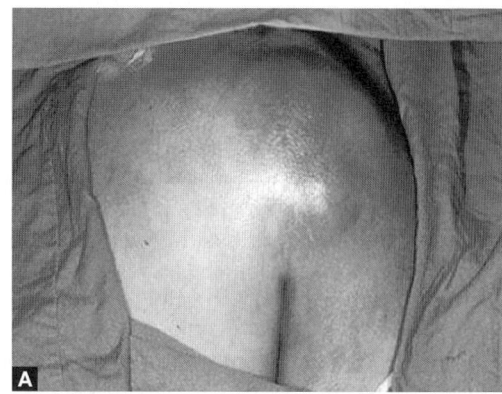

FIG. 2A: Sacral tumor

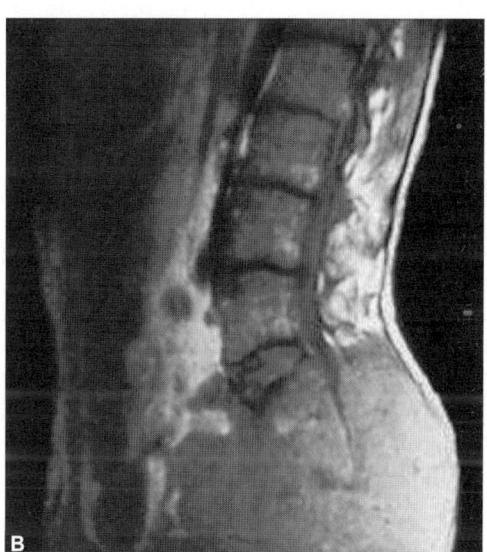

FIG. 2B: MRI sacral tumor

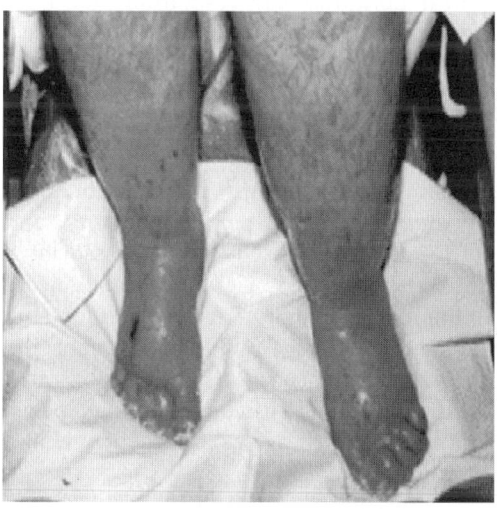

FIG.1: Vincristine legs
(For color version see Plate 10)

ANATOMICAL CONSIDERATION

Chronic pelvic pain may occur in the presence of known or suspected malignant or nonmalignant pathology or in the absence of organic pathology. To understand the various causes and symptoms of pelvic pain due to malignancy of various pelvic organs one must have a clear understanding of the anatomy of various pelvic organs. The intervention of somatic, parasympathetic and sympathetic nerves supplies, are essential to treat these pain syndromes. The parenchyma of various organs is devoid of any pain receptors. The arterial and venous vessels supplying these organs and peritoneum are richly innervated by pain receptors. It is beyond the scope of this chapter to describe the various nerves or fibers responsible for producing visceral and referred pain. Some common pain presentations are described below.[8]

Endometriosis Painful Conditions in Women

An estimated 5 million women are affected by endometriosis. Endometrial tissues, when migrated away from endometrium produce complex situation. The most common location of endometrial tissue outside the uterus is at the ovaries. The migration of endometrial tissue and subsequent lesions are seen throughout the pelvic organs including rectum sigmoid, vaginal, pelvic peritoneum, bladder, round ligament, uterosacral broad ligament, uterus, appendix, vagina, and vulva also including the brain and the lungs, which are far distant from the pelvis region. During menstruation these distant implants show cyclic changes of proliferative and secretor endometrium. Pain may be due to the release prostaglandin.[9] These changes lead to adhesion, scaring and pain. The symptom management includes hormonal therapy, producing pseudomenopause and in extreme cases where the pain is severe, exploratory surgery is indicated to release adhesion or subacute obstruction.[10] For temporary relief a continuous epidural infusion of local anesthetics with opiates alleviates the symptoms.

Adenomyosis

Adenomyosis is most common in patients who are in their late 30s and early 40s. Endometrial tissue invasion of the wall of the uterus produce adenomyosis. An enlarged uterus with a single or multiple nodules are adenomyomas. These tumors are usually benign and are made out of stroma and endometrium. These tumors are associated with other tumors, including endometrial carcinoma, leiomyoma and endometrial hyperplasia. The pain produced by these tumors depends on their location and the way they spread to their surrounding region. These tumors are benign and can be reseated for women of childbearing age. If tumors are large, they require hysterectomy as a curative procedure. The presentation is initially with periodic menstrual pain and increase blood flow during menstruation. In addition to the pain, patients describe a feeling of pressure and a dragging sensation. The sudden sharp pain is usually due to degeneration of a tumor.

Uterine Leiomyoma

These tumors are most common uterine tumors arising from smooth muscles of the myometrium.[11] Estrogen, progesterone and growth hormones are responsible for their growth. The symptoms produced by these tumors depend upon their anatomical location and their relationship to surrounding area[12] and these tumors can be subserosal intramural or submucosal or pedunculated.

Common symptoms include abnormal bleeding, increase pelvic pressure and pelvic pain. Increased pain is associated with tumor necrosis. A rapidly enlarging of abdominal girth and uterus can be due to the transformation of the tumor to malignant. The majority of patients have a history of abnormal uterine bleeding, postcoital spotting, pelvic pain, dysmenorrhea, urinary frequency, and infertility.

Sudden pain and tenderness in a patient with previously stable myoma without any changes indicate a recent vascular compromise and infarction. It is rare that leiomyoma can rapidly grow and become leiomyosarcoma.

The tumors are diagnosed by an ultrasound imaging, saline infusion, sonohysterography, and hysteroscopy. The treatments of the pain produced by these tumors are symptomatic pharmacological management and surgical removal of myomas when they become a larger size.

Endometrium Cancer

These tumors are the most common gynecological cancer in the United States of America. Approximately 43,470 new cases of endometrial cancer are reported each year. It is the eighth leading cause of death for women. An estimated 7,950 deaths are expected from this cancer. The tumor is commonly observed in postmenopausal women. There are two types of endometrial cancer.

Type 1 is the most common cancer which is associated with excessive estrogen while type 2 is rare, but when present, is very aggressive in nature and arises in a atrophic endometrium or a polyp. Global gene expression profile also differs between type 1 and type 2 women treated with tamoxifen, which is used for the treatment of breast cancer, are at risk for developing uterine cancer. These patients usually present with abnormal bleeding. In advanced endometrial cancer, the tumor invades the myometrium and also has pelvic nodal metastasis. Treatment includes surgical therapy, removal of uterus, bilateral salpingoophorectomy, and removal of para-aortic lymph node.[13] During some advance stages, radiation, brachytherapy, chemotherapy with radiation therapy is indicated.[14] Endometrial cancers histological, are different types. They include adenocarcinoma, adenosquamous cell, and mucinous, serous, clear cell, undifferentiated, and mixed carcinoma.

Cervix Cancer

Cervical cancer still remains the cause of mortality second to breast cancer.[15] Overall the incidence and mortality has declined dramatically during the last two decades due to early detection of preinvasive disease. It is estimated that approximately 12,200 new cases are diagnosed with invasive cervical cancer in 2010. Approximately 4,200 deaths are expected due to cervical cancer. The major risk factors include early age indulgence in sexual activity, multiple partners, promiscuous sexual activity, multiple pregnancies, exposure to *Chlamydia*, human papillomavirus, herpes simplex, and close association between HPV and cervical cancer. A reduced risk of cervical cancer is noted in virgins and in women whose sexual partners were circumcised. The most common symptoms include bleeding from the cervix on contact. The squamous cell carcinoma is the most common type of cervical cancer. Cervical cancer commonly spreads to the pelvic wall, parametrial tissue, bladder, and rectum. The uterus and vagina beside local spread, the tumor also spread to lymph nodes at the iliac, inguinal, and aortic regions. There is a small percentage, which spreads as far as the brain, lungs, liver, and the bones. The pain is mostly localized and also depends on the spreading surrounding region. Patient's with larger tumors or locally advanced diseases can be treated with chemotherapy, and radiation. Pain related issues of the patient depends upon the extend of the disease as well as the associated symptoms. It is estimated that approximately 35% of patients with invasive carcinoma of the cervix will have reoccurrence of tumor in spite of earlier chemotherapy, radiation, or surgery.

Condyloma

Vulvar condyloma is produced due to the human papilloma virus type 2 and 6. The pain produced by these lesions depends on the location and invasion of the surrounding structure. These lesions are like warts at the vulvar region, including the labia majora, labia minora, vaginal introitus, and anorectal area. These lesions can be treated by topical application of trichloroacetic acid, 5-fluorouracil and podophyllin. They can also be treated by surgical ablation or laser vaporization. Local application of local anesthesia is helpful in reducing the pain.

Bony Tumors of Pelvis

Chondrosarcoma

It is the second most common bone disease, which develops in the cartilage, pelvis and upper part of the extremity, and it is common in adults over 50 years. These tumors exert great painful pressure on the bony structure and can cause fracture of the bones.

Ewing's Sarcoma

This bone cancer affects children and young adults; it develops in immature nerve tissue in the middle part of the bone. It affects the pelvic bone, legs, ribs, and arms. This cancer can be treated with surgical removal and radiation.

Carcinoma of Urinary Bladder

It is the 5th most common cause of cancer in the United States of America.[16] Approximately 70,530 new cases of bladder tumors were diagnosed in 2010. The incidence of this tumor has increased in the female population by approximately 2% each year. Bladder cancer is predominately present in men and has a higher incidence in white males. In 2010, the number of death reported from bladder cancer was a total of 14,680. The smoking is the most prominent risk factor. A 48% of patients with bladder cancer have a history of smoking. Besides patients who have a history of smoking, the use of cyclophosphamide (Cytoxan) has up to a ninefold risk of developing bladder cancer due to acrotein a metabolite of Cytoxan. More than 90% are transitional cell cancer of the bladder.[17] A gross painless hematuria is the most common symptom. Patients are treated with transurethral resection of tumors. A small percentage of patients require mitomycin, adriamycin and Bacillus Calmette Guerin (BCG) treatment.

Other bladder tumors include adenocarcinoma and squamous cell carcinoma. Advanced bladder cancer patients require radical cystectomy with ileal conduit.

Prostate Cancer

It is the most common malignancy in men and the leading cause of male mortality due to cancer.[18] It is estimated that approximately 23,300 new cases were reported in 2010. Also, more than 30,500 deaths occur from this dreadful disease. The long survival of the male population will further increase the number of new patients. There is a high incidence of prostate cancer in the African American male population. Prostate cancer is most treatable if diagnosed early for patients of 50 years of age or younger. A percentage of patients will present wit urinary symptoms including difficult and painful voiding, increase frequency, hematuria, weight loss, poor appetite, back and pelvic pain.

Prostatic-specific Antigen or PSA Test

These are both diagnostic and used for monitoring tumor activity. Majority of prostatic cancers are prostatic adenoma. The treatment includes radical prostatectomy radiation therapy, hormonal ablation and cryotherapy. The treatment is generally offered to men with at least ten years of life expectancy.

TESTICULAR TUMORS

In the United States of America, approximately 8,000 new cases of testicular tumors are reported each year.[19] These types of tumors are most common among males between the ages of 15 and 40 years. A 95% of these tumors are germ cell tumors and the remaining 5% are sex cord gonadal stromal tumors derived from Leydig cells or Sertoli cells. A large percentage of patients present with a lump in one testis which may or may not be painful. The patient might describe the feeling of heaviness in the scrotum. Besides testicular symptoms patients also report a history of lower back pain when patients have a metastatic spread. Dyspnea, hemoptysis, or a mass in the lungs are reported at a later stage of the tumor due to metastatic spread. A small percentage of patients develop gynecomastia due to the hormonal effects of patient beta-hCG. Most testicular germ cell tumors have too many chromosomes which are triploid, or tetraploid. The management depends upon staging and the type of tumor. Treatment includes surgery, radiation and chemotherapy.

COCCYDYNIA

Patients with a history of anal or rectal cancer, or patients with a history of these tumors treated with chemotherapy, surgery, physical trauma caused by falling backwards, i.e. anterior perineal resection or status postradiation develops coccygeal pain. The pain mostly presents in the coccygeal region, and it becomes worst following sitting or with local pressure due to rectal fullness, i.e. constipation. The pain is relieved by standing or changing posture. Thiel has reported that a high percentage of patients with coccygeal pain has levator ani muscle spasms and other perineal muscle spasms. These painful spasms can be treated by local anesthetic injections or Botox injections to relieve spasms of various rectal muscles. Patients treated with local brachytherapy or radiation therapy occasionally develop post-radiation neuritis, necrosis of tissue, or a chronic nonhealing ulcer.

Pain Description of Pelvic Pain Patients

A large percentage of pelvic tumor patients usually do not present with a history of pain. It is often confusing for patients to describe the characteristics of their pain as the majority of their pain can be a combination of visceral with somatic or somatic with neuropathic pain, or all three together. In advanced stages when tumors become too bulky or invaded surrounding structures, i.e. lymph node, blood vessels, femora sacral plexus or peritoneal invasion produces pain. Patients usually describe the pain as feeling of a hot poker placement, feeling of heavy object pressing or coming out of an organ or burning sensation at the introitus.

MANAGEMENT OF PELVIC PAIN

It is beyond the scope of this chapter to describe all the treatment. The pharmacological management of cancer pain described in other chapters can be well applied to manage pelvic pain; however, there are various interventional treatments that requires a reader's attention. At times a diagnostic neural blockade might not be helpful to pain physicians.[20] In order to prescribe an interventional therapy, a physician must be familiar with pathophysiology of the tumor, tumor locations; histopathology and prior therapy given to the patient including chemotherapy, types of therapy agents used, radiation therapy, and surgery.

Neural Blockade for Relief of Pelvic Pain

It is beyond the scope of this chapter to discuss and describe all appropriate neural blockade techniques and their outcome, risk benefit and complications (Table 1).[21] A few routines procedures will be discussed in this chapter.

Sympathetic Nerve Block

Lumbar Sympathetic Block

The role of a lumbar sympathetic nerve block is limited to manage pelvic pain. However, there are some indirect indications for managing the pain of urogenital and uterine tumors origin. Besides these tumors, there are some selective patients who develop herpetic neuralgia in the distribution of the lumbosacral plexus and selective dermatome peripheral nerve and lumbar sympathetic blocking is helpful.

Superior Hypogastric Plexus Block

For the last 5 decades surgeons were keened to performed presacral neurectomies[22] to relieve various types of pelvic pain for patient

TABLE 1: Neural blockade for management of pelvic pain

• Sympathetic blocks	• Epidural nerve block
○ Lumbar sympathetic block	○ Local anesthetic
– Diagnostic	○ Neurolysis
– Therapeutic	• Intrathecal or epidural drug delivery system
– Neurolytic	○ Opiates
– Chemical neurolysis	○ Local anesthetics
– Radiofrequency	○ Clonidine
– Cryoablation	○ Neostigmine
○ Superior hypogastric plexus block	• Subarachnoid block
– Diagnostic	○ Neurolysis—chemical, alcohol, phenol
– Therapeutic	– Hypobaric
– Neurolytic chemical	– Hyperbaric
○ Ganglion of impar or ganglion of Walther	– Saddle block
• Somatic nerve block	• Plexus nerve block
○ Peripheral nerve block	○ Lumbar plexus
– Diagnostic selective nerve root block	○ Sacral plexus
– Therapeutic nerve root block	○ Coccygeal plexus
– Neurolytic	• Neurosurgical neuroablation
~ Chemical	○ Cordotomy
~ Cryoablation	○ Rhizotomy
~ Radiofrequency	
○ Sacral foraminal nerve block	
– Diagnostic local anesthetic	
– Therapeutic local anesthetic	
– Neurolytic chemical	
○ Pudendal nerve block	
– Diagnostic local anesthetic	
– Therapeutic local anesthetic	
– Neurolytic chemical	

with coccydynia, dysmenorrhea, vulvar pain and dyspareunia in non-cancer pelvic pain patients. The failures and complications related to this procedure causes a very careful selection of patients and result in less frequent surgeries. The role of blocking the superior hypogastric plexus was initially reported by Plancarte[23] and Jain.[24] Following these publication various authors have published two needles versus one needle techniques, a CT-guided notification, and an ultrasound used to perform this block.

The common indication remains for cancer of the cervix, bladder, endometrial, uterus, prostate and rectosigmoid cancers related to pelvic pain. The diagnostic and therapeutic local anesthetic block followed by an injection of 10% phenol in water in a small volume, i.e. 2–3 mL in one injection is a safer way to prevent complications where one can call back the patient in 2–3 weeks for a repeat block. The suspected complications include failure of treatment, intravascular, retroperitoneal hematoma or the impact of an agent on inferior hypogastric plexus can impair sphincter of rectum can produce incontinence (Figs 3 and 4).

Ganglion of Impar

The termination portion of the sympathetic chain at the junction of the sacral coccygeal junction is where the presence of the ganglion is sought. The blocking of the ganglion reduces the burning pain of the sympathetic origin[25] involving various pelvic organs including genitals, rectum, colon, bladder and the cervix. The ganglion lies at the retroperitoneal space like the superior hypogastric plexus and blocking the ganglion is very effective in reducing perineal pain caused by malignancy of the pelvic organs. The original paper

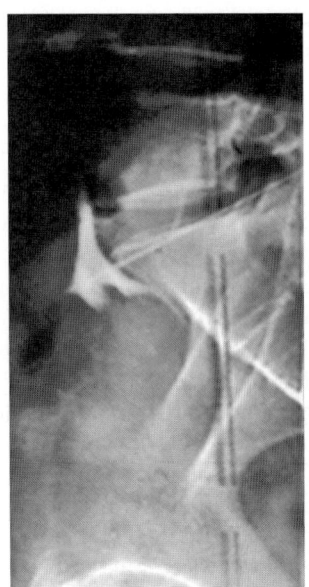

FIG. 4: Hypogastric plexus block—Lateral view

described by Plancarte for newer treatment for malignancy related perineal pain states that a block is very easy to perform and safer without too many complications. Both diagnostic and neurolytic are appropriate for cancer patients.

Sacral Nerve Root Block

Selective blockades of the sacral never root via their dorsal foramina is a useful alternative to subarachnoid or caudal block in patients with pelvic pain due to rectal or uterine cancer with intact bowel and bladder function. Performing a diagnostic local anesthetic block will result in the patient having possible relief.[26,27] A unilateral block with a small of 1–2 cc volume of 4 to 5% phenol will preserve the sphincter function. The second and third sacral roots are most commonly implicated in maintenance of bladder function. One must avoid blocking bilateral S2-3 block to avoid weakness of the detrusor muscle which is responsible for bladder function. A long-term relief of averaging in[26] 5 months was reported in patients with bladder pain where 10 patients had a neurolytic block using 6% phenol was done.

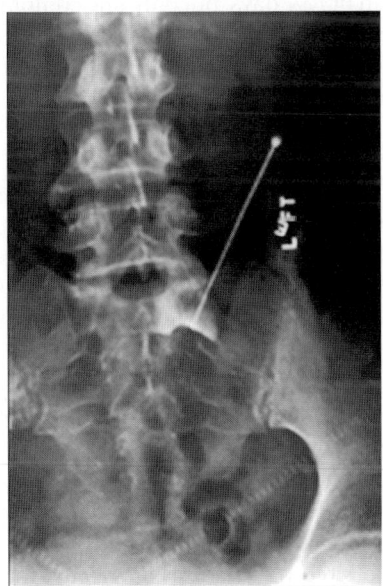

FIG. 3: Hypogastric plexus block—AP view

Subarachnoid and Epidural Neurolytic Block

Classic publications describe the techniques of these and other nerve block procedures in detail,[28,29] and the reader is encouraged to consult them to review technical aspects.[30]

Neuraxial neurolysis—advantages are:
1. Good results in select patients
2. Can perform with minimum equipments
3. Hospitalization for few hours
4. Good pain relief for adequate duration in terminal ill patients.
5. Can be repeated and suitable in debilitated patients
6. Minimum rate of complications.

The chemical rhizotomy is one of lytic neuraxial block procedures pain relief.

The earlier it was thought that phenol was capable of producing selective blockage of small sensory fiber however the pathologic studies have shown that, regardless of size, nervous fibers are affected indiscriminately by both alcohol and phenol.

The concentration and quantity of neurolytic agent decides the degree of sensory loss of type of nerve fiber than number of number of fibers destroyed. Rather than fiber type, which is, in turn, determined by the concentration and quantity of the neurolytic agent. This is supported by recent reports of higher success rates in patients with pelvic malignant neoplasms who were treated with 10% and 15% subarachnoid phenol versus a 7.5% preparation[31] and in patients with a variety of neoplasms treated with 15% versus 10% subarachnoid phenol.[32]

It is agrees that neither agent offers a clear advantage, except insofar as variation in baricity facilitate positioning or the patient in selected cases.[33]

Swerdlow has analyzed the results of 13 series in over 2,500 patients and reported that in 58% of patients, "good" relief was obtained, "fair" pain relief was achieved in an additional 21%, and in 20% of patients "little or no" relief.

The average duration of relief is to be 3–4 months, with a wide range of distribution in one report of analgesia persisting in excess of 1 or even 2 years are not infrequent.[34]

Saddle Block

Perineal and pelvic pain are best managed by neuroaxial lytic blockade. For unilateral pain the approach is placing the patient in a lateral position (dependency dictated by choice of agent) and injecting the neurolytic agent through a low lumbar puncture.

If pain is bilateral, repeat the procedure after a few days. At times bilateral pain can be treated with a unilateral block, so repeat procedure[35] is not required.

A saddle block can be done for pain that crosses the midline. A hyperbaric phenol is injected via a low lumbar puncture, with keeping patient in the sitting position modified by a 45° posterior tilt for 15–30 minutes.

The small volumes of dilute phenol via the caudal route injected in a series of 26 patients with perianal pain due to malignant neoplasm.[36] The pain relief was persisted for a mean of 12.7 days, but only one complication (transient urinary retention). These procedure should be reserved for bedridden patients with risk of addition deficit.

Subarachnoid vs Epidural Neurolysis

It offers the following advantages over epidural techniques:
1. Flow of cerebrospinal fluid confirms subarachnoid needle placement, as compare to localization of the epidural space with epidurograms and/or text doses of local anesthetic.
2. The profound analgesia is seen in subarachnoid neurolysis and reinjection is not required.
3. Subarachnoid injection can be done on an outpatient basis or at the bedside. The epidural neurolysis needs repeated

injection of phenol through an indwelling catheter and a mandatory hospitalization.
4. The gravity and position can be partially relied on to control the effect of epidural block with hyperbaric phenol[37] these factors can be utilized in the case of subarachnoid injection.
5. The excessive viscosity of pure phenol glycerin preparation prevents injections through small caliber tubing.

If epidural block is planned with the phenol-glycerin mixture must be diluted with water, saline, or dye, reducing baricity and introducing the potential for reduced control of spread. A newly designed epidural catheter made from spiral stainless steel coils coated with fluoropolymers has recently been introduced with intention of facilitation radiologic localization, aspiration, and repositioning.[38] No controlled studies have been conducted comparing epidural and subarachnoid neurolysis. The main advantage of phenol epidural neurolysis is its applicability for pain that occupies a wide distribution or is bilateral. Despite the considerations noted above, the main disadvantages cited for classic epidural neurolysis are impressions of a shorter duration of action and inferior intensity of analgesia when compared with subarachnoid techniques. Recent studies suggest that these shortcomings may be overcome by repeated administration over time through an indwelling catheter.[39-41]

It is postulated that epidural injection limits the spread to dorsal nerve roots to reduce motor dysfunction. Using an *in vitro* model, Racz et al. have demonstrated those sections of canine dura opposed to reservoirs of cerebrospinal fluid are relatively impermeable to 2.75% and 5.5% phenol in saline. The risk of meningeal irritation, postdural puncture headache and intracranial spread is less with epidural than subarachnoid neurolysis. The most commonly recommended neurolytic agent for epidural use is still phenol. Although there are of favorable results utilizing alcohol,[42] but its injection causes severe pain in awake patients, this pain can be reduced by injection of local anesthetic following alcohol. The neuropathy and neuralgia have been observed after epidural alcohol.

CONCLUSION

Patient with chronic pelvic pain often are challenging. A broad understanding of tumors, their pathophysiology, outcome and natural history is essential for their management. Both pharmacological and neural blockade management are essential for patients to effectively manage their dreadful pain and proved a better quality of life.

ACKNOWLEDGMENT

I am very thankful to my office manager Ms. Jazmin Garcia for her help and typing this manuscript.

REFERENCES

1. Cancer Facts and Figures. American Cancer Society, Atlanta, Georgia, 2010.
2. National Cancer Institute (NCI). Current Survival of Cancer Patient.
3. Cope, et al. The Early Diagnosis of the Acute Abdomen. Oxford University Press. London.pp.1957-58.
4. Zimmerman M. Central Nervous System Mechanism Modulating Pain Related Inflammation After Lesion of Peripheral or Central Nervous System.
5. Casey Kl. Pain and the Central Nervous System Disease: The Central Pain System. Raven Press, New York, NY; 1991.pp.183-99.
6. Gonzales GR, Elliot KJ, et al. The impact of a comprehensive valuation in the management of cancer pain. Pain 1991;47:141-4.
7. Foley KM. Pain syndrome in patients with cancer. Med Clin North American. 1987;71:169-84.
8. Guzinski GM, Bonica JJ, McDonald, JS. In: Gynecologic Pain Bonica JJ (Ed.). Management of Pain. Philadelphia: Lea and Febriger 1990.
9. Olive DL, Pritts EA. Treatment of endometriosis. N Eng J Med. 2001;345:266-75.
10. Moghissi KS, Schalaff WD, et al. Zoladex with or without hormone replacement therapy for the treatment of endometriosis. Fertile Sterile. 1998;69:1056-62.

11. But tram VC, Reiter RC. Uterine leiomyomata: Etiology, symptomatology and management. Fertile Sterile. 1981;36:433-45.
12. Straughn JM, Huh WK, Kelly FL, et al. Conservative management of stage I endometrial carcinoma after surgical staging. Gynecol Oncol. 2001.pp.191-3.
13. Keys H, Roberts J, Brunetto V, et al. A phase III trial of surgery with or without adjuvant external pelvic radiation therapy in intermediate risk endometrial adeno carcinoma. A gynecology group study. Gynecol Oncol. 2004;92:744-51.
14. Delgado G, Bundy B, Zaino R, et al. Prospective surgical pathological study free interval in patients with stage 1B squamous cell carcinoma of the cervix. Gynecol Oncol. 1900;38:352-7.
15. Steed H, Rosen B, Murphy J, et al. A comparison of laparoscopic. Assisted radical vaginal hysterectomy and radical abdominal hysterectomy in the treatment of cervical cancer. Gynecol Oncol. 2004;93:588-93.
16. Lamm DL, Torti FM. Bladder Cancer. 1996;46(2):93-112.
17. Stein JP, Lieskovsky, et al. Radical cystectomy in the treatment of invasive bladder cancer. Long term results in 1054 patient. J Clinical Oncology. 2001;19: 666.
18. Coopenberg MR, Moul JW, Carrol PR. The changing face of prostate cancer. J Clinical Oncology. 2005;23:8146.
19. Carver BS, Sheinfield J. Germ cell tumors of the testis. Ann Surg Oncology. 2005;12:871.
20. Maher RM. Relief of pain in incurable cancer. Lancet. 1955;1:18.
21. Bonica JJ. Management if pain. Philadelphia: Lea and Febiger; 1954.pp.672-701.
22. Lee RB, et al. Presacral neurectomy in gynecology. Obstetric Gynecol. 1968;68:517-21.
23. Plancarte R, Amescua C, Patt RB, et al. Superior hypogastric plexus block for pelvic cancer pain. Anesthesiology. 1990;73:236.
24. Jain S, Kestenbaum A, Shah N, Khan Y. Hypogastric plexus block: An new technique for treatment of perineal pain. Anesth Analg. 1990;70:S175.
25. Plancarte R, et al. Presacral blockade of ganglion of impar (ganglion of Waltzer). Anesthesiology. 1990;73: A 751.
26. Robertson DH. Transsacral neurolytic nerve block. Br J Anaesth. 1983;55:873-5.
27. Simon DL, Carron H, Rowlingson JC. Treatment of bladder pain with transsacral nerve block. Anesth Analg. 1983;61:46-8.
28. Bonica JJ. The management of pain of malignant disease with nerve blocks. Anesthesiology. 1954;15:280-301.
29. Swerdlow M. Intrathecal neurolysis. Anaesthesia. 1978;33:733-40.
30. Peyton WT, Semansky EJ, Baker AB. Subarachnoid injections of alcohol for relief of intractable pain with discussion of cord changes found at autopsy. Am J Cancer. 1937;30:709.
31. Ischia S, Luzzani A, Ischia A, et al. Subarachnoid neurolytic block (L5-T) and unilateral percutaneous cervical cordotomy in the treatment of pain secondary to pelvic malignant disease. Pain. 1984;20:139-49.
32. Takagi Y, Koyama T, Yamamoto Y. Subarachnoid neurolytic block with 15% phenol glycerine in the treatment of cancer pain. Pain. 1987; S4 :T33.
33. Katz J. Current role of neurolytic agents. Adv Nuerol. 1974;4:471-6.
34. Swerdlow M. Subarachnoid and extradural blocks. Adv Pain Res Ther. 1979;2:325-37.
35. Watson CPN, Evans RJ. Intractable pain with cancer of the rectum. Pain Clin. 1986;1:29-34.
36. Rohde J, Hankemeier U. Neurolytic caudal blocks for the relief of perianal cancer pain. Pain. 1987;S4:T32.
37. Ferrer-Brechner T. Epidural and intrathecal phenol neurolysis for cancer pain. Anesthesiol Rev .1981;8:14-9.
38. Racz GB, Sabonghy M, Gintautas J. Intractable pain therapy using a new epidural catheter. JAMA. 1982;24 B :579-81.
39. Jain S, Foley K, Thomas J, et al. Factors influencing efficacy of epidural neurolysis therapy for intractable cancer pain. Pain. 1987;S4:T32.
40. J Shitbutani K, Kizelshteyn G, Allyne L, et al. Low volume intermittent lumbar epidural phenol injection for relief of cancer pain. Pain. 1987;S4:T32.
41. Racz GB, Heavner J, Haynsworth R. Repeat epidural phenol injections in chronic pain and spasticity, In: Lipton S, Miles J (Eds). Persistent Pain. New York, Grune and Stratton. 1985;5:157-79.
42. Korevaar WC, Kline MT, Donnelly CC. Thoracic epidural neurolysis using alcohol. Pain. 1987;S4:T33.

Metastatic Bone Pain Management

Raghbir Singh P Gehdoo, Jasmeen Kaur

INTRODUCTION

Metastases in the bones are the frequent conditions encountered in oncology practice. Bones are the third most common metastatic site after lungs and liver[1] and is also usually affected in multiple myeloma.[2] Tumors leading to bone metastases include breast (50.1%), prostate (16.6%), and lung (11%).[1] Other primaries include bladder, kidney, uterus, melanoma, thyroid tumors, multiple myeloma and unknown primaries.[1,3]

Bone metastases are comparatively less frequent in patients with gastrointestinal tumors, lymphomas and other hematologic malignancies.[4] Median survival of patients with bone metastases is 2–3 years in breast cancer[5], 2 years in prostate cancer[6] and less than 1 year in lung cancer.[7,8]

Pain is the most common symptom in majority of these patients and develops gradually over weeks to months, becoming progressively more severe. However, Schaberg and Gainor[9] reported that 36% of patients with spinal metastases did not complain of bone pain, and also noted that 66% of their patients with back pain who had a history of previous malignancy had bone metastases. In 50-70% patients, pain combined with other complications (e.g. hypercalcemia, pathologic fracture, nerve root compression, spinal cord compression, focal neurologic deficits, and forced immobilization) can lead to a decrease in patients' quality of life. Therefore, treatment must be structured toward the prevention and reduction of these complications. Bone metastases are usually multiple. Solitary metastasis is produced only in <10% of cases. Most commonly affected areas are spine, pelvis, ribs, proximal thigh, and skull,[10] as shown in the Figure 1.

The bone scan may miss lesion without new bone formation as bone scan depends on osteoblastic activity. In case of tumors of prostate or breast being slow progressive disease and has high risk of bone metastasis.

MECHANISMS OF BONE METASTASIS

Bone metastases are classified as osteolytic, osteoblastic, or mixed, according to the primary mechanism of interference with normal bone remodeling. The balanced activity of osteoblasts and osteoclasts is the basis for physiologic bone remodeling. Activated osteoclasts are responsible for the resorption of bone, while osteoblasts form bone at the same site.[11] In many cases, both osteolytic and osteoblastic processes are involved (Fig. 2).

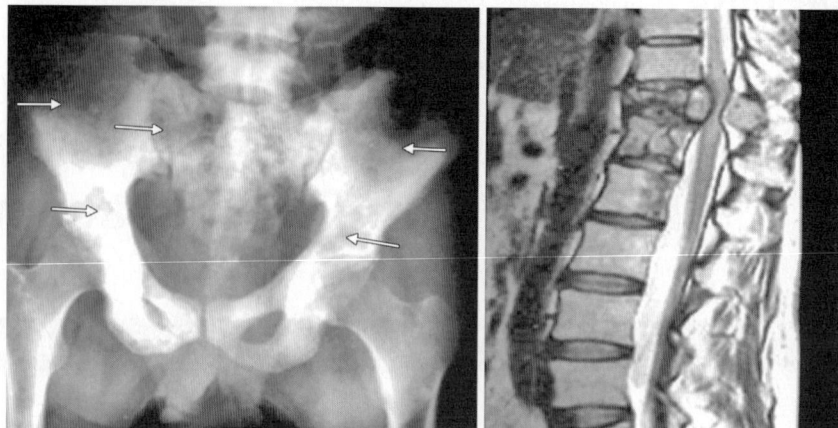

FIG. 1: Multiple metastases in the pelvic bones and spine

The pathogenesis of osteolytic damage is far from elucidated. Osteolysis is mediated by osteoclasts, and does not result from the direct action of tumor cells on bone. Bone-derived transforming growth factor beta (TGFβ) and the tumor-derived parathyroid hormone-related protein (PTHrP) seem to be the major mediators involved in osteolytic metastases.[11] The bone metastases shows ranges of phenotype which can be osteolytic and osteoblastic in breast cancer whereas in prostate cancer it is osteoblastic.[12] The hypocalcemia and bone loss leading to calcium retention can be secondary to hyperparathyroidism. There is increase in bone resorption from osteoblastic metastatic site.[13]

CLINICAL FEATURES

The bone metastatic can be clinically silent some time pain can be a morbidity. Skeletal complications present as pathologic fractures (10–30%), spinal cord compression (5%), or hypercalcemia (10%). The majority of these patients will require palliative radiotherapy.

Pain

Pain is the most common symptom, present in 75% of patients[14] and develops gradually over weeks to months, becoming progressively more severe. Metastatic bone pain is somatic in nature.[15] The pathology of bone pain is poorly understood. The pain associated with bone metastasis could be either of biologic or mechanical origin. The biologic pain is related to the local release of cytokines and chemical mediators like prostaglandins by the tumor cells, periosteal irritation, stimulation of intraosseous nerves, nerve entrapment. It is necessary to control pain to reduce complication such as anxiety and depression to avoid decrease in quality of life.[16]

Bone Fracture

Pathologic fractures most frequently occur in proximal parts of the long bones, and the femur accounting for over half of all cases. The majority of all pathologic fractures registered in solid tumors occur in breast cancer patients (60%),[1] while lung cancer accounts for only 10% of cases. Too much force or stress on a bone will lead to fracture.

Spinal Cord Compression

Spinal cord compression is more commonly seen in breast cancer (20–30% of all cases) and lung cancer (15%) as well as prostate cancer. The development of back pain in a patient

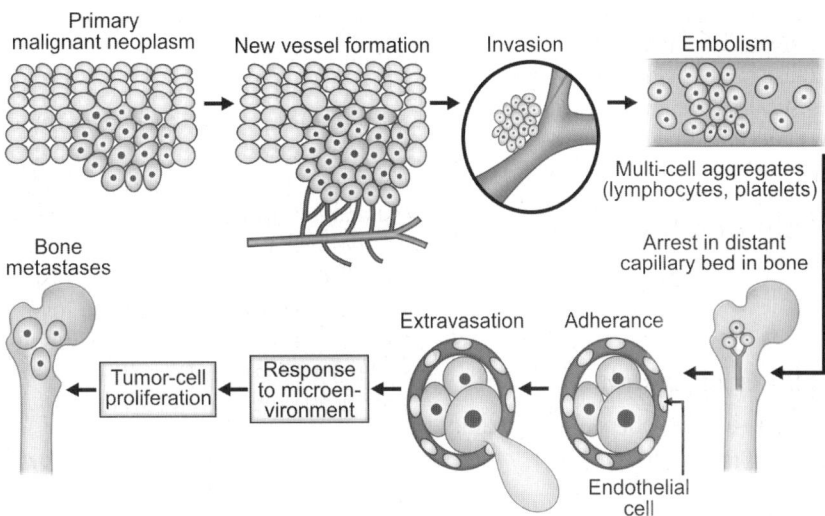

FIG. 2: Putative mechanism by which tumor cells invade the bones

with cancer, associated with an abnormality on a plain spinal radiograph, should serve as a warning for spinal cord compression. It can also clinically present as back ache, tingling and numbness, weakness in both lower limbs, while in severe cases, as paraparesis or paraplegia, with or without bladder and bowel involvement. More than 60% of such patients will have magnetic resonance imaging (MRI) evidence of epidural disease. The key to successful rehabilitation is early diagnosis, high-dose corticosteroid treatment, decompressive surgery, and spinal stabilization or radiotherapy.[17] Neurologic recovery is unlikely if spinal compression is not relieved within the first 24–48 hours.

Other Symptoms

Such patients can experience a number of other symptoms, particularly due to adverse effects associated with chemotherapy and radiotherapy, such as anemia, leucopenia, thrombocytopenia, anorexia, weight loss, weakness and fatigue. Moreover, these patients are also susceptible to infection.

DIAGNOSIS

Laboratory Tests

Apart from at least one of the above mentioned signs and symptoms, the diagnosis of the bone metastases is also based on abnormal serum values of alkaline phosphatase (ALP) and calcium, along with imaging data, such as plain X-ray, bone scans, CT and or MRI scan studies. Altered serum calcium, phosphorus, and ALP levels helps to identify markers of bone turnover and evaluate for hypercalcemia.[18]

Alkaline phosphatase is elevated in most cases, but normal levels do not rule out the presence of bone disease. The sensitivity of this ALP test is questionable. In addition, acid phosphatase and PSA are elevated in the majority of prostate cancer patients with bone metastases, but neither is pathognomonic for bone involvement from cancer.

Hypercalcemia in the serum can also be indicative of bone metastases, unless proved otherwise. Hypercalcemia associated with cancer can be seen in carcinomas of breast, renal, ovary, esophagus, and head and neck, multiple myeloma, lymphomas, etc.[19]

In patients with local osteolytic hypercalcemia, the hypercalcemia results from the marked increase in osteoclastic bone resorption in areas surrounding the malignant cells within the marrow space.[11,20] The condition known as humoral hypercalcemia of malignancy (HHM) is caused by systemic secretion of parathyroid hormone (PTH)–related protein (PTHrP) by malignant tumors.[21,22] PTHrP causes increased bone resorption and enhances renal retention of calcium.[23]

Radiographic Examination

Radiographs are a fast, cheap, and readily available technique for evaluating bone metastases. Radiographs give the best integration of overall bone structure and alignment.

Plain X-ray

Plain X-rays of the affected bone should be the first test in the evaluation of bone pain and it's metastatic lesions. It is highly specific test, but sensitivity is low. Indeed, metastatic lesions may not appear on X-rays for several months.[24] Therefore, plain radiology is less sensitive (44–50%) than bone scan for detecting initial bone metastasis. The radiologic appearance of the lesion depends on the predominance of the osteolytic or osteoblastic process. Lytic lesions are most often detected through plain X-rays. Lesions in trabecular bone (medullary lesions) are more difficult to detect by X-rays than are lesions in cortical bone because of the limited contrast in trabecular bone. Lesions up to 1 cm might go undetected, while more than 50% of trabecular bone must be destroyed before it will be evident on X-ray film.[25]

Computerized Tomography Scan

CT scan or magnetic resonance imaging (MRI) is useful for assessing disease extent and for RT planning. CT scans are generally more sensitive than X-rays. Therefore, the scans can more clearly show the shape of the tumor and its exact location in the body. Rosenthal reported that the sensitivity of CT for the diagnosis of bone metastases ranges from 71% to 100%.[26]

Magnetic Resonance Imaging

Patients who experience bone pain but have normal bone scans may be referred for MRI. MRI can detect changes in the bone marrow caused by tumors or infections. It is helpful for imaging soft tissues such as that of the marrow, but CT scans are better at imaging the bones. An MRI is required to diagnose spinal cord compression, and it can also provide detailed images of the involved bone and bone marrow; the diagnostic sensitivity of skeletal MRI ranges from 82% to 100%, and its specificity ranges from 73% to 100%.[27,28]

Bone Marrow Aspiration and Biopsy

A sample of bone marrow can give the information regarding the spread of cancer and subsequent involvement of the bone marrow. Bone biopsy, however, can explain the detailed pathology behind the bone involvement and probably the primary origin of the metastases.

Bone Scan

Radionuclide bone scanning is highly sensitive but usually has a low specificity, as it relies on the detection of an osteoblastic reaction to suggest the presence of bone damage. In comparison of sensitivity bone scan range from 62% to 89% with false positive rate 40%.[29] Bone scans are more sensitive and specific as compare to plain films while Algra et al. reported MRI is superior while evaluating vertebral metastasis.[30]

Positron Emission Tomography Scans

PET scan detects quantifying metabolic activity and are superior in detection of bone metastases in lung cancer. PET and bone scanning had, respectively, an accuracy of 96 and 66% in the evaluation of osseous involvement in 110 patients with NSCLC.[31]

PET also proved superior in detecting osteolytic bone metastases from breast cancer, with 95% sensitivity and 94% specificity, compared to 93% and 78% with bone scanning.[32]

PET appears to permit earlier diagnosis of bone metastases, especially in multiple myeloma, with imaging of bone resorption sites undetected with conventional diagnostic methods.[33]

TREATMENT OPTIONS

Pain Management Therapy

Pain usually results when a tumor pushes on bones, nerves, or other organs in the body. Many different drugs including non-narcotics and narcotics or drug combinations along with adjuvants like steroids, antidepressants and anticonvulsants, in case of neuropathic involvements can be used to treat bone metastasis pain. Sometimes medications are used along with surgery, radiation, or other treatments to provide relief. The side effects of the different drugs and drug combinations can vary. Some patients experience mild side effects while others have a more intense reaction.

Chemotherapy

Use of tamoxifen, can reduce tumor size, thereby relieving bone pain in most cancer patients. Its major adverse effect being a bone marrow toxicity.[34]

Hormonal Therapy

This is effective only in metastatic bone pain patients with a carcinoma breast, uterus or prostate. However, the pain may become refractory to this kind of treatment as well.[34] Hormones are responsible for growth of some of the cancers. Estrogen, for example stimulates breast and uterus cancer growth. Similarly, testosterone is associated with prostate cancer. The principle of hormonal therapy is to either stop or lower hormone production or to block site of action of hormones thereby affecting growth of cancer cells. However, decreased estrogen level can lead to hot flashes, depression, myalgia and joint pains. Testosterone deficiency results in weight gain, loss of sex drive, anemia and osteoporosis.

Radiation Therapy

Radiation therapy, often called radiotherapy, involves the use of ionizing radiation. The goal of radiotherapy is to destroy cancer cells so that they cannot reproduce and grow. Patients also benefit from radiotherapy because it reduces bone pain and lessens the chance of fractures. In bone metastases radiotherapy indicated for pain, reduce risk of pathologic fracture and neurological complications due to spinal cord compression. The prospective randomized trial showed no difference in effectivity in single fraction regimens (mostly 8 Gy) and fractionated regimen.[35] The single fraction regimen is useful for surgical stabilization for bone to reduce fracture risk to decrease further destruction of bone. In these patients 20–30% there was no pain relief.[36]

Systemic Radioisotope Pharmaceutical Therapy

In patients with advanced cancer in whom both radiotherapy and hormone therapy fail and drug therapy is not sufficiently efficient for palliative care because patients often develop tolerance or adverse effects that are unacceptable, use of the radiopharmaceuticals is an appealing alternative for standard metastatic bone pain treatment modalities. The purpose of this therapy is to deliver radiation to tumor cells without harming normal cells. This type of therapy involves the injection of active metals that give off radiation particles in the patient. Currently, these include the metals Samarium and Strontium. By providing radiation directly to the bone, these metals target and destroy the active cancer cells in the bone. Pain is also decreased or relieved entirely. Radiopharmaceuticals also have a role in the palliation of bone pain. A variety of radioisotopes are available for clinical use.[37] Phosphorous-32 (^{32}P) and strontium-89 (^{89}Sr) have considerably longer half-lives (12 and

50 days, respectively) than samarium-153 (^{153}Sm) or rhenium-186 (^{186}Re) that have half-lives of 2 and 4 days, respectively. Currently, the only Food and Drug Administration (FDA) approved radiopharmaceuticals with an affinity for bone are ^{89}Sr and ^{153}Sm.[38]

- Strontium-89 (^{89}Sr)
  - Strontium-89 (^{89}Sr) is a form of an isotope-based metastatic bone pain management. It is a pure β-emitting isotope based on ^{89}Sr chloride.[43] From a chemical point of view, it is similar to calcium; thereby it fixes on bone areas in which the maximum calcium absorption occurs. Bone uptake is proportional to the bone regenerative activity, so that uptake peaks in the most osteogenic sites. Between 30% and 40% of the administered dose is excreted in the urine within 48 hours, with the remaining dose being taken up by the bone. Biological half-life in metastases is somewhat longer than 50 days, compared to the normal healthy bone (14 days). The use of this isotope is traditionally limited to metastatic bone pain from prostate cancer. The patients can be treated on outpatient basis as there is no radiation risk to others after Sr-89 administration.
- Samarium-153 (^{153}Sm)
  - Samarium-153 (^{153}Sm) is a sodium salt composed of a radioactive complex consisting of samarium bound to lexidronam. The physical half-life is 46.3 hours. It emits β particles. (^{153}Sm) is a combined gamma and beta emitter with a half-life of approximately 2 days. 60% to 75% of treated patients reported an improvement in pain, which usually occurred within the first month of therapy and lasted 2–4 months.[43] It shows a high affinity for bone tissue. It accumulates five times more commonly in metastatic area than normal bone tissue thereby increasing radiation dose to malignant areas. ^{153}Sm, at a dose of 37 MBq/kg, is the most suitable dose. Duration of pain relief is approximately 3–6 months. ^{153}Sm is usually indicated for palliative metastatic bone pain treatment in patients with osteoblastic bone metastases, like those seen in prostate cancer, and in those presenting osteolytic metastases with a osteoblastic component, as is the case in many breast cancer patients.[44]

Furthermore, ^{153}Sm administration-associated adverse effects like thrombocytopenia are mild and reversible.[45]

Indications

Any patient diagnosed to have osteoblastic bone metastasis by bone scintigraphy with associated uncontrolled pain falls into inclusion criteria for palliative pain therapy using radiopharmaceuticals. Practically, it is commonly used for patients suffering from excruciating bone pain due to metastasis not controlled by external radiotherapy.

Contraindications

The absolute contraindication is pregnancy and breastfeeding. A pregnancy test should be done before starting the therapy. It is advisable not to conceive for six months post single therapeutic dose. Breastfeeding needs to be stopped completely before the therapy.[39]

The presence of cytopenia accounts for relative contraindication because bone seeking agents aggravate myelotoxicity further decreasing counts. G-CSF maybe required prior to or following therapy. However, the bone marrow recovers spontaneously. The guidelines used by most centers as cut off for using these agents include Hb (<9 g%), WBC <3500/dL, platelets <1,00,000/dL.[40-42] Born marrow involvement does not account for absolute contraindication. The presence of "superscan" appearance suggests limited reserve but if counts are stable, radiopharmaceuticals can be used at a lower dose or fractionated smaller doses.

In patients with GFR <30 mL/min, it is advisable to avoid using these agents for fear of greater risk of bone marrow toxicity. The total should be decreased if GFR 30–50 mL/min. Sm-153 Lexidronan and RE-186 Etidronate are good options in this category of patients because of the shorter half-life. However, currently there is no data to support the efficacy, safety and side effects.

Radiopharmaceuticals are generally not the option for patients with life expectancy less than 4 weeks.

Precautions

The administration of radiopharmaceuticals requires certain preventive measures to be taken by the patient and the administrator to avoid dangerous effects. The hazards of radiation therapy can be minimized by undertaking following precautions.
- Avoid conceiving for 6–12 months.
- Avoid use of shared toilets (contamination with radioactive urine).
- Flush the toilet twice for a week at least.
- If patient is incontinent, catheterize bladder before injection.
- Avoid sexual contact for one week post therapy.
- Universal safety precautions by administrator.

Medical Therapy

Bisphosphonates are a class of medications shown to be effective in treating bone metastases in both breast cancer and myeloma patients. Specifically, they decrease the risk of fractures and decrease pain from bone metastasis. They also reduce the number of future radiation treatments for these patients.

Bone-targeting Agents (Bisphosphonates)

These drugs help to reset the balance between bone growth and destruction. They are analogs of inorganic pyrophosphate that inhibit osteoclast activity and, consequently, reduce bone resorption in a variety of illnesses.

The apoptosis[46] can occur after bisphosphonates which may bind to hydroxyapatite crystals of bone matrix leads in resorption lacunae which may lead to internalization by osteoclasts.[46]

Many trials reported that there is no variation in toxicity among tumor types as bisphophonates are well tolerated.[47] The uncommon events such as fever; bone, joint and myofascial pain; anemia may occur however these events are of mild-to-moderate nature. The bisphosponates some time raises serum creatinine levels[48] so it is advised to monitor serum creatinine levels.

Pamidronate has been extensively used based on evidence that IV infusion of 90 mg every 3–4 weeks significantly reduced the incidence and delayed the onset of skeletal complications as well as reduction in pain, in the patients of carcinoma breast with bone metastases compared with placebo[49,50,51] and in the patients with bone metastases and multiple myeloma.[52,53] The dose usually recommended is 60–90 mg IV (infused over 2–4 hours) every 3–4 weeks. The reduction of skeletal morbidity (pathological fractures, need for bone radiation or surgery, spinal cord compression, hypercalcemia) described with the administration of pamidronate in multiple myeloma and breast cancer patients is another incentive to use it as an adjuvant. Adverse effects, including hypocalcemia and a flu-like syndrome, are dose related and typically transitory. Nephrotoxicity can occur rarely, usually following a rapid infusion, and typically it is transitory. It is better to keep a note on serum calcium and creatinine levels.

Zoledronic acid (Zometa) is a bisphosphonate that is about 2–3 times more potent than pamidronate. It is safe and easy to administer on an outpatient basis and has an infusion time that is shorter than that of pamidronate. When administered intravenously, it has demonstrated significant benefits like delaying the onset of complications and pain relief, for patients who present with bone metastases from a wide variety of tumors including multiple myeloma, breast, kidney, and prostate cancer.[52-55] Moreover, it also reduces skeletal complications in both osteolytic and osteoblastic bone lesions.[56,57]

In a phase II trial of Berenson et al., it was more potent than pamidronate in the inhibition of bone resorption[53] and also in the treatment of hypercalcemia of malignancy, as noted by Lipton et al.[58]

The recommended dose of zoledronic acid is 4 mg administered IV via 15-min infusion every 3 or 4 weeks. Patients should be adequately hydrated, and calcium plus vitamin D3 oral supplementation is recommended.

The side effects are similar to those encountered with pamidronate, and the dose does not have to be adjusted in patients with mild-to-moderate renal failure.[59]

Ibandronate a highly potent, third-generation aminobis-phosphonate, has been developed in both IV and oral formulations for the management of metastatic bone disease. It has been shown to reduce significantly the risk of skeletal complications, alleviate bone pain, and improve QOL in patients with metastatic breast cancer, in the absence of renal safety concerns.[60] Long-term data have shown that ibandronate is well tolerated either IV or orally, with a renal safety profile similar to placebo and no evidence of cumulative renal damage. It is usually given intravenously in the dose of 6 mg to be infused in 15 minutes approximately every 3-4 weeks. Osteonecrosis of jaws are reported after chemotherapy[61] in some patients with bone metastases and of multiple myeloma.

Clodronate has been shown to be effective in prostate cancer and multiple myeloma[62] The main advantage of clodronate over pamidronate is its good oral bioavailability, which avoids the need for IV administration. An oral dose of 1,600 mg daily seems to be optimal.[62]

In randomized, placebo-controlled multi-centre study conducted by Powel et al.[63] reported benefit in survival. Oral clodronate often causes gastrointestinal disturbances, particularly diarrhea; compliance is often poor because of the large tablet size and multiple daily dosing.

Clinical use—Hillner et al. and American Society of Clinical Oncolgy[64,65] recommended guidelines for treatment of breast cancer patients with bone metastases.

Role of bisphosponates for hypercalcemia of malignancy—Hypercalcemia is a common complication in cancer patients and symptoms such as nausea, vomiting, confusion, anorexia, polyuria, polydipsia are present. Hypercalcemia is seen in about 15% in advanced cancer patients.[66]

Bisphosponates intravenously is administered for patients of hypercalcemia with dehydration.[67] Major et al.[68] reported that pamidronate was more effective that zoledronic acid in patients with hypercalcemia with bone metastases.

Calcitonin

Calcitonin is a peptide composed of 32 amino acids which binds to osteoclasts and inhibits bone resorption.[69] Exact mechanism of analgesic action is not known, but possible mechanisms include, both central and peripheral mechanisms—interaction with serotonergic and catecholaminergic systems, an effect on specific CNS receptors (central), increased endorphin release, inhibition of prostaglandin, and other inflammatory mediator synthesis (peripheral), and calcium flux modulation (central and peripheral).[70,71] Calcitonin has been used in the palliative care for the management of pain from bone metastasis.[72,73] The most frequent routes of administration are subcutaneous and intranasal. If subcutaneous boluses are used, they should be preceded by skin testing with 1 IU to screen for hypersensitivity reactions, especially in patients with a history of reactions to salmon or seafood.[74] Usual dose of subcutaneous calcitonin is 100 IU daily for 5-7 days or 200-400 IU IM 6 hourly for

48 hours. The intranasal formulation can also be used in the dose of 200 IU daily for 7-8 days. It can also be given by rectal route in the dose of 100 IU daily for 21 days.[75] Apart from infrequent hypersensitivity reactions associated with subcutaneous injections, the main side effect is nausea. Periodic monitoring of calcium and phosphorus is prudent during treatment.

Denosumab

Denosumab is a human monoclonal antibody with affinity for Receptor Activator of Nuclear factor-κB Ligand (RANKL), secreted by osteoblasts. It prevents activation of osteoclasts thereby decreases bone resorption and increases bone mass. There are many studies which have shown promising results when comparing Denosumab to Zoledronic acid. In a study, by Fizazi et al. comparing Denosumab to Zoledronic acid in castration resistant prostate cancer showed superiority of Denosumab in increasing the median time to first on study skeletal-related event. (20.7 months vs 17.1 months, P = .0002 for non-inferiority; P = .008 for superiority).[76]

In the study by Stopeck et al. while Denosumab delayed the onset of pain compared to Zoledronic acid, the median time to pain improvement was similar between treatment arms (82 versus 85 days: HR 1.02; p = 0.72) [35].[77]

In a review by Irelli et al. comparing denosumab and bisphosphonates, it depicted that toxicity profile was comparable. However, former is associated with higher rate of fever, bone pain, hypercalcemia and renal failure whereas toothache and hypocalcemia is found with use of denosumab.[78]

Surgical Therapy

In most cases, surgery can restore the function of the original bone. The type of surgery will depend upon the location and size of the bone metastasis tumor. Surgery usually involves removing all or part of the tumor and stabilizing the bone to prevent breakage. With fractures or impending fractures, surgery could include placement of metal plates, rods, screws, wires, nails, and/or pins, or prostheses. The purpose of these tools is to strengthen or provide structure to the bone.

The short-term prognosis of most patients with bone metastases should be taken into account, with intervention limited to cases expected to recover from surgery relatively quickly or when potential fractures could generate major morbidities. Surgery is indicated for fractures of long bones and hip joints, in spinal cord involvement, or peripheral nerve compression. Another option for surgery includes reconstruction of bones or joints. Reconstruction is a procedure where metal, plastic, allografts or a combination of these replaces the damaged bone in the area of the metastasis. A guideline for prophylactic surgical fixation[79] is recommended in some patients.

Percutaneous vertebroplasty and kyphoplasty are also advised for prophylactic spinal fixation[80,81] and can be done on outpatient basis with minimal complications and proved effective.[82] Taylor et al.[83] reported significant pain reduction with vertebroplaty and kyphoplasty in verterbral body fractures due to osteoporosis and in osteoporotic compression fractures.[84-86]

The complications reported with these procedures are cement in epidural space, paralysis due to involvement of spinal cord[87] or radiculopathy.[88] The less vascular and transcortical extra vacation reported with kyphoplasty than vertebroplasty.[83,89]

Other Interventions

Some patients experience inadequate pain control despite pharmacological and all other forms of therapies or may not tolerate an opioid titration program because of side effects. The epidural, intrathecal, plexus blocks; disk procedures; neurostimulations reduces pain significantly and also drug requirements.[90] In patients with somnolence and/or confusion, intrathecal opioid is another option.[90]

In patients unresponsive to radiation but still has pelvic pain then hypogastric plexus block and in localizes bony lesion paravertebral or dorsal root blocks are considered. One needs to explain the side effects of these blocks.

Nonpharmacologic Management

Cutaneous Therapy

It comprises of thermotherapy (application of superficial heat) and cryotherapy. Thermotherapy can be given using hot water bottles, hot packs, electric pads and by immersion in warm water whereas ice packs, cold towels and gel packs are used in cryotherapy. Care needs to be taken that tissues destroyed with radiation therapy should not undergo this form of therapy. In patients with active cancer, one should be vigilant while using deep heat therapy and to avoid direct use over cancer site.[91]

Transcutaneous Electrical Nerve Stimulation

In this technique, low voltage electrical stimulation is applied to large, myelinated nerve fibers. It relieves pain by keeping pain gates closed. The transmission of pain by unmyelinated C and delta fibers is inhibited. Currently, there is not much evidence to prove efficacy of transcutaneous electrical nerve stimulation (TENS) in cancer related pain and further research in this area is warranted.[92,93]

Massage Therapy

Massage therapy reduces generalized bodyache particularly in bedridden patients. In a study by Jane et al. it was found that it had immediate benefit in terms of pain and anxiety. There were no adverse effects noted.[94]

Exercise

Generally, all patients should be encouraged to do physical activity to improve musculoskeletal endurance and to decrease psychosocial regress.

Psychotherapeutic Management

This includes relaxation techniques, mindfulness based stress reduction, hypnosis and psychotherapy.

CONCLUSION

The presence of bone metastases is an ominous sign of a disseminated disease and portends a short-term prognosis in cancer patients. The assessment of bone pain in patients with cancer requires frequent evaluation, treatment, documentation, and reevaluation of the quality, severity, sites, accompanying neurological symptoms, and effectiveness of pain relief with prescribed interventions.[95] Palliation of symptoms, especially pain and quality of life, remains the first aim of any therapeutic approach in the management of bone metastases. It is very important that a patient's analgesic therapy is optimized before initiating more intensive therapies. In most cases, the use of a single treatment method is insufficient in relieving and maintaining sufficient relief from bone pain; a combination of both local and systemic therapies may be necessary.[96] Clinicians caring for patients with bone metastases should be well versed in all available options to maximize care and comfort for the patient. A multidisciplinary team comprising of medical oncologist, radiotherapist, pain physician, interventional radiologist, orthopedician must all be involved at different steps, without forgetting the favorable impact of psychological aid.

Finally, studies at the basic research level continue to elucidate the interactions that occur between tumor cells and the bone microenvironment, and thus are identifying potential novel targets for future therapeutic interventions.

REFERENCES

1. Coleman RE. Metastatic bone disease: clinical features, pathophysiology and treatment strategies. Cancer Treat Rev. 2001;27:165-76.
2. Oxford textbook of oncology. Oxford; 2002.pp.995-1006.
3. Acrageli G, Micheli A, Tollis A, et al. The responsiveness of bone metastases to radiotherapy: The effect of site, histology and radiation dose on pain relief. Radiother Oncol. 1989;14:95-101.
4. Mundy GR. Myeloma bone disease. Eur J Cancer. 1998;34:246-51.
5. Paterson AHG. Bone metastases in breast cancer, prostate cancer and myeloma. Bone. 1987;8:17-22.
6. Crawford D, Faulkner J, Thompson IM, et al. Ten-year survival in patients with metastatic (M+) prostate cancer: analysis of South-West Oncology Group (SWOG) 8894. J Urol. 2002;167:304 (abstr 1202).
7. Schiller JH, Harrington D, Belani CP, et al. Comparison of four chemotherapy regimens for advanced non-small-cell lung cancer. N Engl J Med. 2002;346:92-8.
8. Noda K, Nishiwaki Y, et al. Irinotecan plus cisplatin compared with etoposide plus cisplatin for extensive small-cell lung cancer. N Eng J Med. 2002;346:85-91.
9. Schaberg J, Gainor BJ. A profile of metastatic carcinoma of the spine. Spine. 1985;10:19-20.
10. Falkmer U, Jarhult J, Wersall P, Cavallinstahl E. A systemic overview of radiation therapy effects in skeletal metastases. ActaOncologica. 2003;42:620-33.
11. Roodman GD. Mechanisms of bone metastasis. N Engl J Med. 2004;350:1655-64.
12. Hortobagyi GN. Bone metastases in breast cancer patients. SeminOncol. 1991;18:11-15.
13. Guise TA, Yin JJ, Mohammed KS. Role of endothelin-1 in osteoblastic bone metastases. Cancer. 2003;97:779-84.
14. Powers WE, Ratanatharathorn V. Palliation of bone metastases. In: Perez CA, Brady LW (Eds). Principles and practice of radiation oncology, 3rd ed.Lippincott-Raven Publishers, Philadelphia. 1997.pp.2199-217.
15. Goltzman, D. (1997), Mechanism of the Development of Osteoblastic Metastases. Magazine supplement: Skeletal complications of Malignancy. Cancer. 1997;80:1581-7.
16. Spiegel D, Sands S, Koopman C. Pain and depression in patients with cancer. Cancer. 1994;74:2570-8.
17. Marta Penas-Prado, Monica Loghin. Spinal cord compression in cancer patients: review of diagnosis and treatment. Current Oncology Reports. 2008;10(1):78-85.
18. Demers LM, Costa L, Chinchilli VM, Gaydos L, Curley E, Lipton A. Biochemical markers of bone turnover in patients with metastatic bone disease. Clin Chem. 1995;41:1489-94.
19. Stewart AF, Broadus AE. Malignancy associated hypercalcemia. In: DeGroot L, Jameson LJ, eds. Endocrinology. 5th ed.Philadelphia: Saunders (in press). Washington DC: American Society for Bone and Mineral Research; 2003.pp.251-6.
20. Guise TA, Yin JJ, Taylor SD, et al. Evidence for a causal role of parathyroid hormone-related protein in he pathogenesis of human breast cancer-mediated osteolysis. J Clin Invest. 1996;98:1544-9.
21. Horwitz MJ, Stewart AF. Humoralhypercalcemia of malignancy. In: Favus MF (Ed). Primer on the Metabolic Bone Diseases and Disorders of Mineral Metabolism, 5th ed. Washington DC.: American Society for Bone and Mineral Research; 2003.pp.246-50.
22. Nakayama K, Fukumoto S, Takeda S, et al. Differences in bone and vitamin D metabolism between primary hyperparathyroidism and malignancy-associated hypercalcemia. J Clin Endocrinol Metab. 1996;81:607-11.
23. Bonjour J-P, Philippe J, Guelpa G, et al. Bone and renal components in hypercalcemia of malignancy and response to a single infusion of clodronate. Bone. 1988;9:123-30.
24. Vinholes J, Coleman R, Eastell R. Effects of bone metastases on bone metabolism: implications for diagnosis, imaging and assessment of response to cancer treatment. Cancer Treat Rev. 1996;22:289-331.
25. Adams JE, Isherwood I. Conventional techniques in radiological diagnosis. In: Stoll BA, Parbhoo S (Eds). Bone metastases: monitoring and treatment. New York, NY: Raven; 1983.pp.107-48.
26. Rosenthal DI. Radiologic diagnosis of bone metastases. Cancer. 1997;80:1595-607.
27. Evans AJ, Robertson JF. Magnetic resonance imaging versus radionuclide scintigraphy for screening in bone metastases. Clin Radiol. 2000;55:653.
28. Godersky JC, Smoker WR, Knutzon R. Use of magnetic resonance imaging in the evaluation of metastatic spinal disease. Neurosurgery. 1987;21:676-80.
29. Quinn DL, Ostrow LB, Poerter DK, et al. Staging of non-small cell bronchogenic carcinoma: relationship of the clinical evaluation to organ scans. Chest. 1986;89:270-5.
30. Algra PR, Bloem JL, Tissing H, et al. Detection of vertebral metastases: comparison between MRI and bone scintigraphy. Radiographics. 1991;11:219-32.
31. Bury T, Barreto A, Rigo P. Fluorine-18 deoxyglucose positron emission tomography for the detection of bone metastases in patients with non-small cell lung cancer. Eur J Nucl Med. 1998;25:1244-7.

32. Yang J, Liang JA, Lin FJ, et al. Comparing whole-body 18FDG PET and technetium-99m methylene diphosphonate bone scan to detect bone metastases in patients with breast cancer. J Cancer Res Clin Oncol. 2002;128:325-8.
33. Schirrmeister H, Guhlmann A, Elsner K, et al. Sensitivity in detecting osseous lesions depends on anatomic localization: planar bone scintigraphy versus 18F PET. J Nucl Med. 1999;40:1623-9.
34. Krishnamurthy G and Krishnamurthy S. Radionuclides for metastatic bone pain palliation: a need for rational re-evaluation in the new millennium. Journal of Nuclear Medicine. 2000;41:688-91.
35. Nielsen OS. Palliative radiotherapy of bone metastases: there is now evidence for the use of single fractions. Radiother Oncol. 1999;52:95-6.
36. Steenland E, Leer JW, van Houwelingen H, et al. The effect of a single fraction compared to multiple fractions on painful bone metastases: a global analysis of the Dutch Bone Metastasis Study. Radiother Oncol. 1999;52:101-9.
37. McEwan AJ. Use of radionuclides for the palliation of bone metastases. Semin Radiat Oncol. 2000;10:103-14.
38. Maini CL, Bergomi S, Romano L, Sciuto R. 153Sm-EDTMP for bone pain palliation in skeletal metastases. Eur J Nucl Med Mol Imaging. 2004;31:S171-8.
39. Bodei L, Lam M, Chiesa C, et al. EANM procedure guideline for treatment of refractorymetastatic bone pain. Eur J Nucl Med Mollmaging. 2008;35(10):1934-40.
40. Paes FM, Serafini AN. Systemic metabolic radiopharmaceutical therapy in the treatment of metastatic bone pain. Semin Nucl Med. 2010;40(2):89104.
41. IG, Mason MD, Shelley M. Radioisotopes for the palliation of metastatic bone cancer: asystematic review. Lancet Oncol. 2005;6(6):392-400.
42. Farhanghi M, Holmes RA, Volkert WA, et al. Samarium-153-EDTMP: pharmacokinetic, toxicity and pain response using an escalating dose schedule in treatment of metastatic bone cancer. J Nucl Med. 1992;33(8):1451-8.
43. Resche I, Chatal J F, Pecking A and Wilkins D. A dose-controlled study of 153Sm-(EDTMP) in the treatment of patiens with painful bone metastases. Eur J Cancer. 1997;33(10):1583-91.
44. Tian J H, Zhang J M, Hou Q & T and He I & J et al, Multicentre trial on the efficacy and toxicity of single-dose samarium-153 as a palliative treatment for painful skeletal metastases in China. Eur J Nucl Med. 1999;26:2-7.
45. Serafini AN. Systemic metabolic radiotherapy with samarium-153 EDTMP for the treatment of painful bone metastasis. Quart J Nucl Med. 2001;45:91-9.
46. Rogers MJ, Frith JC, Luckman SP, et al. Molecular mechanisms of action of bisphosphonates. Bone. 1999;24(S5):73-9.
47. Body JJ, Diel I, Bell R. Profiling the safety and tolerability of bisphosphonates. SeminOncol. 2004;31(S10):73-8.
48. Green JR, Rogers MJ. Pharmacologic profile of zoledronic acid: a highly potent inhibitor of bone resorption. Drug Dev Res. 2002;55:210-24.
49. Theriault RL, Lipton A, Hortobágyi GN, et al. Pamidronate reduces skeletal morbidity in women with advanced breast cancer and lytic bone lesions: a randomized, placebo-controlled trial. Protocol 18 Aredia Breast Cancer Study Group. J Clin Oncol. 1999;17:846-54.
50. Hortobagyi GN, Theriault RL, Porter L, et al. Efficacy of pamidronate in reducing skeletal complications in patients with breast cancer and lytic bone metastases. N Engl J Med. 1996;335:1785-91.
51. Glover D, Lipton A, Keller A et al. Intravenous pamidronate disodium treatment of bone metastases in patients with breast cancer. A dose-seeking study. Cancer. 1994;74:2949-55.
52. Rosen LS, Gordon D, Kaminski M et al. Zoledronic acid versus pamidronate in the treatment of skeletal metastases in patients with breast cancer or osteolytic lesions of multiple myeloma: a phase III, double-blind, comparative trial. Cancer J. 2001;7:377-87.
53. Berenson JR, Lichtenstein A, Porter L, et al. Long-term pamidronate treatment of advanced multiple myeloma patients reduces skeletal events. Myeloma Aredia Study Group. J Clin Oncol. 1998;16:593-602.
54. Berenson JR. Recommendations for zoledronic acid treatment of patients with bone metastases. Oncologist. 2005;10:52-62.
55. Rosen LS, Gordon D, Tchekmedyian S, et al. Zoledronic acid versus placebo in the treatment of skeletal metastases in patients with lung cancer and other solid tumors: a phase III, double-blind, randomized trial—The Zoledronic Acid Lung Cancer and Other Solid Tumors Study Group. J Clin Oncol. 2003;21:3150-7.
56. Lipton A, Small E, Saad F, et al. The new bisphosphonate, Zometa (zoledronic acid), decreases skeletal complications in both osteolytic and osteoblastic lesions: a comparison to pamidronate. Cancer Invest. 2002; 20(Suppl 2):45-54.
57. Berenson JR, Rosen LS, Howell A, et al. Zoledronic acid reduces skeletal-related events in patients with osteolytic metastases. Cancer. 2001;91:1191-1200.
58. Lipton A, Demers L, Curley E, et al. Markers of bone resorption in patients treated with pamidronate. Eur J Cancer. 1998;34:2021-6.
59. Skerjanec A, Berenson J, Hsu C et al. The pharmacokinetics and pharmacodynamics of zoledronic acid in

cancer patients with varying degrees of renal function. J ClinPharmacol. 2003;43:154-62.
60. Body JJ, Diel IJ, Lichinitser MR, et al. On behalf of the MF 4265 Study Group. Intravenous ibandronate reduces the incidence of skeletal complications in patients with breast cancer and bone metastases. Ann Oncol. 2003;14:1399-405.
61. Bagan JV, Murillo J, Jimenez YJ, et al. Avascular jaw osteonecrosis in association with cancer chemotherapy: series of 10 cases. Oral Pathol Med. 2005;34:120-3.
62. Fulfaro F, Casuccio A, Ticozzi C, et al. The role of bisphosphonates in the treatment of painful metastatic bone disease: a review of phase III trials. Pain. 1998;78:157-169.
63. Powles T, Paterson S, Kanis JA, et al. Randomized, placebo controlled trial of clodronate in patients with primary operable breast cancer. J Clin Oncol. 2002;20:3219-24.
64. Hillner BE, Ingle JN, Berenson JR, et al. American Society of Clinical Oncology guideline on the role of bisphosphonates in breast cancer. J Clin Oncol. 2000;18:1378-91.
65. Hillner BE, Ingle JN, Chlebowski RT, et al. American Society of Clinical Oncology 2003 update on the role of bisphosphonates and bone health issues in women with breast cancer. J Clin Oncol. 2003;21(21):4042-57.
66. Coleman RE. Bisphosphonates: clinical experience. Oncologist. 2004;9 (Suppl 4):14-27.
67. Saunders Y, Ross JR, Broadley KE, Edmonds PM, Patel S. Systematic review of bisphosphonates for hypercalcaemia of malignancy. Palliat Med. 2004;18(5):418-31.
68. Major P, Lortholary A, Hon J, et al. Zoledronic acid is superior to pamidronate in the treatment of hypercalcemia of malignancy: a pooled analysis of two randomized, controlled clinical trials. J Clin Oncol. 2001;19:558-67.
69. Carstens JH, Jr, Feinblatt, JD. Future horizons for calcitonin: a U.S. perspective. Calcif Tissue Int 1991; 49 Suppl 2:S2.Eastell, R. Treatment of postmenopausal osteoporosis. N Engl J Med. 1998;338:736.
70. Braga PC. Calcitonin and it's antinociceptive activity: animal and human investigations, 1975-1992, Agents Actions. 1994;41:121-31.
71. Azria M. Possible mechanisms of the analgesic action of calcitonin : Bone. 2002;30(5):805-35.
72. Szanto J, Ady N, Jozsef S. Pain killing with calcitonin nasal spray in patients with malignant tumors. Oncology. 1992;49:180-2.
73. Roth A, Kolaric K. Analgesic activity of calcitonin in patient with painful osteolytic metastases of breast cancer: results of a controlled randomized study. Oncology. 1986;43:283-7.

74. Lussier D, Huskey A, Portenoy R. Adjuvant analgesics in cancer pain management. The Oncologist. 2004; 9(5):571-91
75. Mannarini M, Fincato G et al. Analgesic effects of salmon calcitonin suppositories in patients with bone pain; Current Therapeutic Research. 1994;56(9):1079-83.
76. Fizazi K, Carducci M, Smith M, et al. Denosumab versus zoledronic acid for treatment of bone metastases in men with castration resistant prostate cancer: a randomized, double-blind study. Lancet. 2011;377(9768):813-22.
77. Stopeck AT, Lipton A, Body JJ, Steger GG, Tonkin K, de Boer, RH, Lichinitser M, Fujiwara Y, Yardley DA, Viniegra M, et al. Denosumab compared with zoledronic acid for the treatment of bone metastases in patients with advanced breast cancer: A randomized, double-blind study. J Clin Oncol. 2010;28:5132-9.
78. Irelli A, Cocciolone V, Cannita K, Zugaro L, Di Staso M, Baldi PL, et al. Bone targeted therapy for preventing skeletal-related events in metastatic breast cancer. Bone, 2016.
79. Mirels H. Metastatic disease in long bones. A proposed scoring system for diagnosing impending pathological fracture. Clin Orthop. 1989;249:256-64.
80. Harrington KD, Sim FU, Enis JE, Johnston JO, Dick HM, Gristina AG. Methylmethacrylate as an adjunct in internal fixation of pathological fractures: experience with three hundred and seventy-five cases. J Bone Joint Surg. 1976;58:1047-55.
81. Fourney DR, Schomer DF, Nader R, et al. Percutaneous vertebroplasty and kyphoplasty for painful vertebral body fractures in cancer patients. J Neurosurg. 2003;98(1):21-30.
82. Gaitanis IN, Hadjipavlou AG, Katonis PG, Patwardhan AG. Balloon kyphoplasty for the treatment of pathological vertebral compressive fractures. Eur Spine J, 2004.
83. Taylor RS, Taylor RJ, Fritzell P. Balloon kyphoplasty and vertebroplastyfor vertebral compression fractures: a comparative systematic review of efficacy and safety. Spine. 2006;31:2747-55.
84. Weill A, Chiras J, Simon JM, et al. Spinal metastases: indications for and results of percutaneous injection of acrylic surgical cement. Radiology. 1996;199:241-7.
85. Jensen ME, Evans AJ, Mathis JM, et al. Percutaneous polymethylmethacrylatevertebroplasty in the treatment of osteoporotic vertebral body compression fractures: technical aspects. Am J Neuroradiol. 1997;18:1897-904.
86. Mathis JM, Barr JD, Belkoff SM, et al. Percutaneous vertebroplasty: a developing standard of care for vertebral compression fractures. Am J Neuroradiol. 2001;22:373-81.

87. Lee BJ, Lee SR, Yoo TY. Paraplegia as a complication of percutaneous vertebroplasty with polymethylmethacrylate: a case report. Spine. 2002;27:E419-22.
88. Ratliff J, Nguyen T, Heiss J. Root and spinal cord compression from methylmethacrylatevertebroplasty. Spine. 2001;26:E300-2.
89. Phillips FM, Todd Wetzel F, Lieberman I, et al. An in vivo comparison of the potential for extravertebral cement leak after vertebroplasty and kyphoplasty. Spine. 2002;27:2173-9.
90. National Comprehensive Cancer Network. Clinical Practice Guidelines in Oncology, 2005.
91. Jacox AK, Carr DB, Payne R, et al. Management of cancer pain. Clinical practice guideline no. 9. Rockville, MD: Agency for Health CarePolicy and Research. AHCPR Publication no. 94-0592;1994.
92. Robb K, Oxberry SG, Bennett MI, et al. A cochrane systematic review of transcutaneous electrical nerve stimulation for cancer pain. JPain Symptom Manage. 2009;37(4):746-53.
93. Carroll D, Moore RA, McQuay HJ, et al. Transcutaneous electrical nerve stimulation (TENS) for chronic pain. Cochrane Database Syst Rev.2001;(3):CD003222.
94. Jane SW, Wilkie DJ, Gallucci BB, et al. Effects of a full-body massage on pain intensity, anxiety, and physiological relaxation in Taiwanese patients with metastatic bone pain: a pilot study. J Pain Symptom Manage. 2009;37(4):754-63.
95. Campa JA 3rd, Payne R. The management of intractable bone pain: a clinician's perspective. Semin Nucl Med. 1992;22(1):3-10.
96. Serafini AN. Current status of systemic intravenous radiopharmaceuticals for the treatment of painful metastatic bone disease. Int J Radiat Oncol Biol Phys. 1994;30(5):1187-94.

SECTION 8

Neuropathic Pain

8

CHAPTER 33

Neuropathic Pain: Approach, Pathophysiology, and Management

Satish V Khadilkar, Abhinay M Huchche, Nahush P Dilip, Madhu B Singla

INTRODUCTION

The International Association for Study of Pain (IASP) has defined pain as "an unpleasant sensory and emotional experience associated with actual or potential tissue damage, or described in terms of such damage".[1] Traditionally, pain has been classified into nociceptive and neuropathic pain. Neuropathic pain is pain arising primarily from lesion or disease of the somatosensory nervous system. Neuropathic pain differs from nociceptive pain in terms of chronicity and refractoriness to conventional analgesics [nonsteroidal anti-inflammatory drugs (NSAIDs)]. This explains the high prevalence of neuropathic pain in the population. Studies from the West have shown that one in three people are affected by chronic pain.[2] Limited studies available from India corroborate with the West, diabetic neuropathy being the most common cause of neuropathic pain.[3,4] Thus, neuropathic pain poses a formidable challenge for diagnosis and management.

Over the last few years, revisions have been made in the definition and the therapeutic algorithm. Also, a new grading system has been proposed to categorize chronic neuropathic pain as "possible", "probable" and "definite". More and more research is being made to understand the pathophysiology of neuropathic pain so as to develop treatment modalities directed at these mechanisms.

DEFINITION

The definition of neuropathic pain has undergone changes in the recent past. The Neuropathic Pain Special Interest Group (NeuPSIG) has revised the definition in 2008 as "pain arising as a direct consequence of a lesion or disease of the somatosensory system".[5] Lesion refers to macro-or microscopically identifiable damage. Disease refers to an identifiable process like infection, inflammation, channelopathy, etc. The new definition excludes the relatively nonspecific term "dysfunction" and includes the term "somatosensory". Thus, it serves the purpose of defining a more specific entity (e.g. pain arising from spasticity/spasms would not be labeled as neuropathic pain as it results from lesion of the motor system).

ETIOLOGY

Neuropathic pain actually comprises of positive and negative sensory symptoms caused by different etiologies. The somatosensory nervous system begins from the peripheral

> **Box 1: Peripheral and central causes of neuropathic pain**
>
> **Peripheral neuropathic pain:**
> - Mononeuropathies and multiple mononeuropathies:
>   - Entrapment (Carpal tunnel syndrome)
>   - Diabetic mononeuropathy
>   - Postherpetic neuralgia
>   - Cervical and lumbosacral radiculopathy due to disk disease
>   - Traumatic and metastatic plexopathy
>   - Trigeminal neuralgia
> - Polyneuropathy
>   - *Metabolic/Nutritional*: Diabetes, vitamin deficiencies
>   - *Toxic*: Chemotherapy related, ART, isoniazid
>   - *Immune*: Sjögren's syndrome, CIDP
>   - *Hereditary*: Fabry's disease
>
> Central neuropathic pain:
> - Traumatic spinal cord injury
> - Thalamic stroke
>
> ART, antiretroviral therapy; CIDP, chronic inflammatory demyelinating polyneuropathy

nerve endings (first order neurons) which travel rostrally to the spinal cord (second order neurons) and then ascends the spinal cord to synapse in the thalamus (third order neurons). From the thalamus, it projects to the somatosensory cortex. Thus, pain can arise from a lesion anywhere along the system. For simplifying things, it is divided into peripheral neuropathic pain and central neuropathic pain (Box 1).

PATHOPHYSIOLOGY

Injury to the somatosensory system leads to changes not only at the level of injury but also rostral to it. Thus, each level of the somatosensory system plays a role in sustaining neuropathic pain. The changes occurring at each level have been mentioned here. These mechanisms help understanding the symptoms of neuropathic pain (hypersensitivity/allodynia) and also the ways by which medicines and other modalities act on the pain.

Peripheral Mechanisms

Sensitization

This occurs at the level of pain receptor endings. The inflammatory mediators released after nerve injury contribute to the sensitization. The inflammatory cascade has been shown in Figure 1.

Glutamate acts on metabotropic glutamate (metGlu) receptors), protons act on vanilloid receptor [transient receptor potential vanilloid 1 (TRPV1)] and acid sensitive ion channels (ASIC), adenosine triphosphate (ATP) acts on purine (P2X3) receptor, prostaglandins act on (EP) receptors and bradykinin on B1 and 2 receptors. When these receptors are activated, kinases are activated which lead to phosphorylation of sodium (NaV1.8) and vanilloid receptor. Phosphorylated channels are hyperexcitable and open in response to lower threshold.

The final common pathway is change in the intracellular signaling leading to phosphorylation of ion channels [sodium and vanilloid receptor [transient receptor potential vanilloid 1 (TRPV1)] which become more excitable and respond to lower thresholds. The resultant outcome is increased pain (hyperalgesia) even to lower thresholds.

Central Sensitization

This occurs at the level of the dorsal horn in the spinal cord. The changes occur in terms of neurotransmitter receptors especially glutamate receptors [N-methyl-D-aspartic acid (NMDA) and α-amino-3-hydroxy-5-methyl-4-isoxazolepropionic acid (AMPA)]. This modification in the NMDA-receptor allows prolonged depolarization and thus

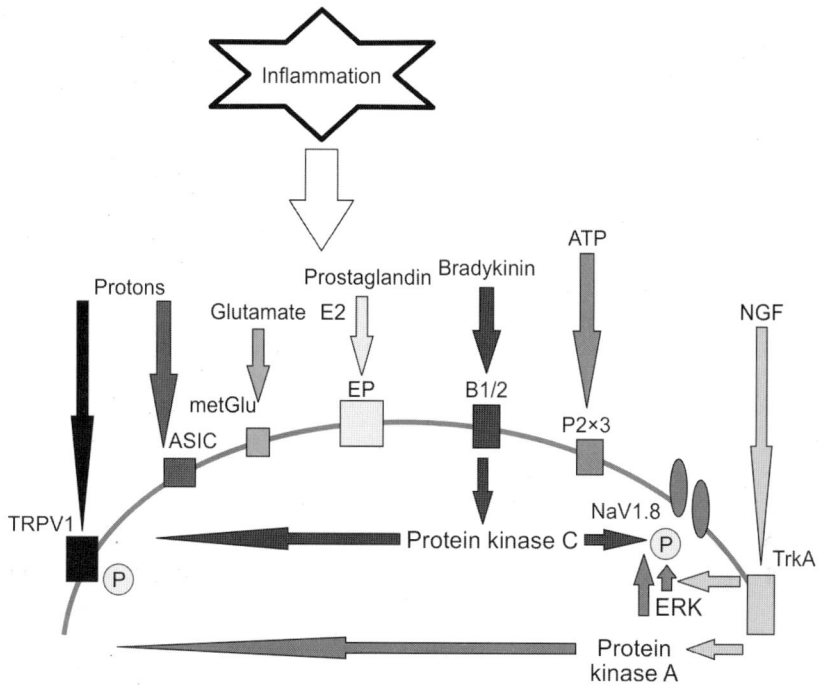

ERK; TrkA; NGF; metGlu, metabatropic glutamate receptors; E2

FIG. 1: Role of inflammatory mediators in peripheral sensitization

constant firing of dorsal horn neurons and pain transmission. Also, increased excitability of neurons explains the activation of pain pathways in response to touch (due to decrease in threshold) thus explaining tactile allodynia. These pathways are illustrated in Figure 2.

Central Modulation of Pain

The spinal dorsal horn output can be modulated by descending pathways originating in the brainstem. These centers include the periaqueductal gray (PAG), locus coeruleus and the raphe magnus. Neurotransmitters released from these sites help modulate pain at the level of dorsal horn also explaining the mechanism of action of certain antidepressants in the treatment of neuropathic pain (Table 1).

TABLE 1: Neurotransmitters involved in descending pathways for pain modulation

Transmitter	Released from	Project to
Norepinephrine	Locus coeruleus	Spinal cord
Serotonin	Raphe magnus	Spinal cord
Endogenous opioids	PAG	Spinal cord

PAG, periaqueductal gray

CLINICAL APPROACH

History

Most patients with neuropathic pain would have paid visits to "n" number of doctors before coming to the pain specialist. Also, they frequently feel that their symptoms are under-appreciated by their physicians as well as family members. Thus, listening to the self-spoken

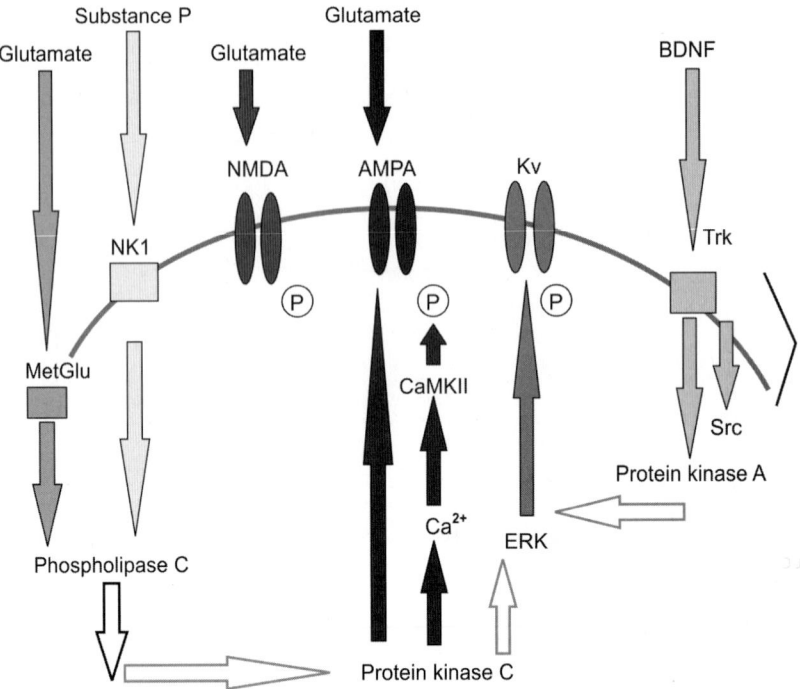

metGLU, metabotropic glutamate receptors; NK1----;Trk-------;SrC ------;ERK,-----;CaMKII---;extracellular signal-regulated kinase

FIG. 2: Mechanisms of central sensitization. In the spinal cord, the pain pathway synapses in the dorsal horn. Thus, neurotransmitters such as glutamate, substance P and brain-derived neurotropic factor (BDNF) are released. These act on their respective postsynaptic receptors resulting in activation of various kinases. These in turn phosphorylate the N-methyl-D-aspartic acid (NMDA) and α-amino-3-hydroxy-5-methyl-4-isoxazolepropionic acid (AMPA) receptors and potassium channels (Kv). The phosphorylation of these receptors and channels leads to constant firing of the postsynaptic neurons irrespective of the stimulus leading to central sensitization

story of his/her pain forms the beginning of a good interaction. Once the patient is done with his description, some active questioning has to be done so as to get a grip of the possible inciting event, perpetuating factors and the impact on QoL. The list of essential questions to be asked in every patient is summarized in Table 2.

Various screening tools (questionnaires) are available for assessment of patients with chronic pain which aid in the diagnosis of pain as neuropathic or non-neuropathic. The neuropathic pain [Douleur Neuropathique (DN4)] is available free for use on the website *http://dn4.ca/en/splash/*.

EXAMINATION

Body sketch for mapping: A diagram for mapping of pain gives a good idea of the possible localization in the somatosensory system. Illustrations of some conditions have been given in Figures 3A to C.

The somatosensory system consists of neurons and axons carrying two broad types of sensations; (1) exteroceptive (pain/temperature) and (2) interoceptive (light touch/vibration/joint position). Sensory abnormalities are characterized by decrease, absence or perversion of sensation. The role of sensory examination is to delineate these

TABLE 2: History taking in neuropathic pain

History of pain (Mnemonic: NOPQRSTU)	*Negative symptoms*: Numbness, emptiness
	Onset: Gradual or sudden
	Progress: Plateau, better or worse
	Precipitating factors: Cough/sneeze (radicular), bedsheet/fan air
	Quality: Sharp or dull, shock like, burning, pins and needles, etc.
	Region/Radiation: Localized or widespread; any radiation
	Relieving factors: If any
	Severity: On a pain scale (e.g. Visual analog scale)
	Time/Trophic changes: Duration of pain/color change, swelling, hair and ulcer
Past medical/surgical history	*Example*: Trauma/fracture, diabetes, shingles and stroke
Sleep	Sleep latency, awakenings cause of pain and duration
Diet habits	Vegan diet, weight loss/gain and oral ulcers
Coping mechanisms	*Negative*: Substance abuse, dissociation, etc.
	Positive: Exercise, support group, etc.

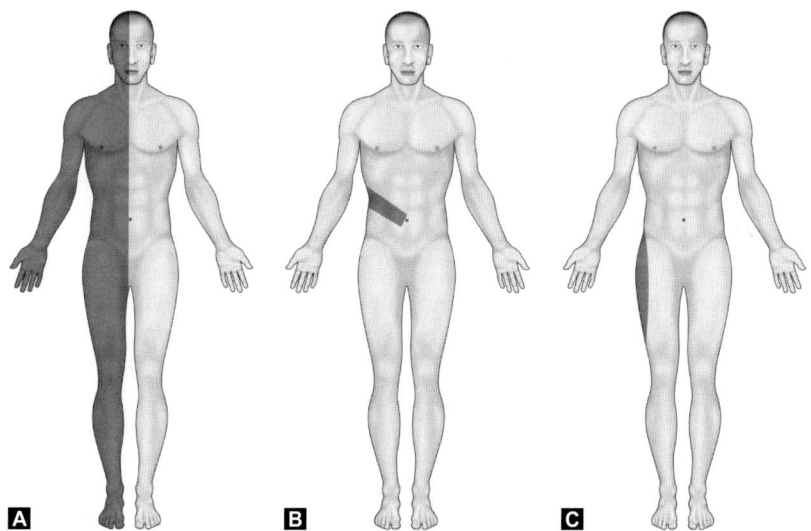

FIGS 3A to C: Mapping of pain in different conditions. (A) Distribution of pain and analgesia in a patient with left thalamic infarct; (B) Pain mapping in a patient with postherpetic neuralgia in the D9 dermatome; (C) An obese patient with meralgia paresthetica in the right lateral cutaneous of thigh distribution

areas of decreased, absent, exaggerated and perverted sensation; the degree of abnormality; type of sensation involved and distribution.

There are two patterns of testing: Side to side and distal to proximal. Pain is usually tested with a pin; temperature with a hot and cold test-tubes. Light touch is tested

TABLE 3: Definitions of different terminologies

Term	Definition
Allodynia	Painful response to a normally innocuous stimulus
Analgesia	Absent pain perception (nociception)
Anesthesia	Complete absence of skin sensation to all stimuli
Dysesthesia	All types of abnormal sensations, including painful ones, regardless of whether a stimulus is evident
Hypoalgesia	Reduced pain perception (nociception),
Hyperalgesia	Denotes severe pain in response to a mildly noxious stimulus
Hyperpathia	A broad term which encompasses all the phenomena described by hyperesthesia, allodynia, and hyperalgesia
Paresthesia	Abnormal sensations of tingling or pins-and-needles except pain

with a brush. A 128 Hz tuning fork is used for testing vibration. Joint position sense is tested using small degree movements at distal joints. A body sketch can be drawn to show the distribution of abnormality with different designs/colors indicating various modalities. These sketches can help us in follow-up and also other physicians for comparison. This part of neurological examination is the most difficult one to perform and interpret.

After examination, we may like to use various terms to describe the sensory abnormalities which have been provided in Table 3. Also, at the end of history and examination, one should be possible to judge the level of surety of neuropathic pain as per the new grading system (Box 2).

> **Box 2: Grading of neuropathic pain[5]**
> - Pain distribution fits into a plausible neuroanatomical site
> - History of a relevant lesion affecting the peripheral or central somatosensory system
> - Demonstration of the distribution in the neuroaxis by at least one confirmatory test
> - Demonstration of the lesion or disease by at least one confirmatory test
> - Definite: From 1 to 4
> - Probable: 1 and 2 plus either 3 or 4
> - Possible: 1 and 2 but no evidence from 3 to 4

INVESTIGATIONS

In order to categorize the pain as "probable" or "definite" additional tests are needed. The European Federation of Neurological Societies (EFNS) provides guidelines which were revised in 2009[6] (Table 4).

Investigations only help to support the diagnosis. Thus, they should be used judiciously and guided by history and examination.

MANAGEMENT

Active participation of the patient is a must for successful management of chronic neuropathic pain. Maintaining a pain diary will give a good understanding of their pain, how it affects their lives and the coping strategies for them. Thus, he/she will know as to what works and what does not and they can make appropriate choices in future. The use of the "visual analog scale" makes it simple to report pain.[7] Team management is preferred. The team leader should be the patient himself being supported by family members, friends and health professionals (family doctor, pain specialist and physiotherapist, etc.). Also, a list of desired coping strategies should be given to the patient. This list could be fed into his electronic gadget and then he/she will know what they are following (Box 3).

TABLE 4: European Federation of Neurological Societies (EFNS) guidelines for assessment of neuropathic pain[6]

Test	Recommended
History and clinical examination for diagnosis	Good practice point
Screening and assessment tools	
• Screening tools for diagnosis	Grade A for nonspecialist
○ LANSS, DN4, NPQ, Pain DETECT, ID Pain, StEP	
• Pain quality assessments to evaluate treatment	Grade A
○ NPS, NPSI	
Quantitative sensory testing (QST)	
• QST for diagnosis not sufficient	Good practice point
• Used in combination with bedside examination	
• Use simple tests—brush and pinprick	Grade A
• QST to quantify effects of treatment on allodynia	
Neurophysiology	
• Nerve conduction studies	Grade A
• Trigeminal reflexes for A beta fibers	To distinguish classical from symptomatic trigeminal neuralgia
• Laser evoked potentials for A delta fibers	
Functional neuroimaging	
• Functional neuroimaging—all technique	Encouraged-expert opinion
Skin biopsy	
IENFD for diagnosis of painful or burning feet	Grade B

Abbreviations: LANSS, leeds assessment of neuropathic symptoms and signs; DN4, neuropathic pain [Douleur Neuropathique 4 (DN4)]; NPQ, neuropathic pain questionnaire; ID, identification; StEP, standard evaluation of pain; NPS, neuropathic pain scale; NPSI, neuropathic pain symptom inventory; IENFD, intraepidermal nerve fiber density; pain DETECT,—

Box 3: Desired list of coping strategies
- *Nutrition*: Healthy meals, multivitamins, reduce caffeine and sugar
- *Exercise*: A walk in the morning or evening
- *Sleep*: Proper sleep hygiene with fixed timings
- *Hobbies*: Pursue your hobbies and do something you like everyday
- *Stress*: Take up only that much that you could tolerate
- Prioritize your tasks
- Plan outings which will give you enough rest
- Meditation

PHARMACOTHERAPY

Neuropathic pain, in general, is difficult to treat. The pain does not respond to over-the-counter analgesics. Even with neuropathic pain medications, the relief is incomplete and individuals usually require a combination of drugs. Thus, for research purpose, individuals with 50% pain relief are regarded as "responders", whereas 30% pain relief is considered "clinically relevant."[8] Therapy for neuropathic pain needs to be individualized. Before initiating treatment, some factors need to be considered. These have been given in Box 4.

Box 4: Factors to be considered before initiating treatment

- Age (Elderly more prone to adverse effects)
- Comorbid conditions (Drug interactions)
- Previous abuse/suicidal history
- Previous tried medications (start with a different one)
- Cost concerns

Box 5: Differences between recent and previous Neuropathic Pain Special Interest Group (NeuPSIG) therapeutic algorithm

- Duloxetine has been proposed as first-line therapy
- Lidocaine patches are no more first-line and are included in second-line therapy for peripheral NP
- Strong opioids which were first/second-line have been pushed to third-line because of the abuse potential and mortality with high doses
- Recommendation has been made against use of cannabinoids because of potential misuse and mental health risks

Clinical practice guidelines (CPGs) are recommendations made on the basis of systematic review of evidence so as to optimize patient care. Worldwide, many organizations have published their guidelines; but they vary a lot in terms of quality. Recently, a systematic review of all the published CPGs for neuropathic pain has been published.[9] Also, a recent revision of the NeuPSIG recommendations is available.[10] The differences between the recent and previous NeuPSIG recommendations have been elucidated in Box 5. Making use of these recent guidelines, we discuss the pharmacologic treatment of neuropathic pain.

Principles of Therapy

- "Start low and go slow" has to be kept in mind while starting these medicines. Starting with a higher dose may lead to dizziness and excess sedation which may lead to discontinuation of therapy and create fear for the agent. Thus, that particular medicine has to be excluded from the list.
- Assess the patient at periodic intervals for pain relief and adverse effects.
- Titration of dosages should be at 2-4 weeks intervals.
- Take precautions especially in the elderly and women of child bearing age.

The "first-line agents" fall into two broad categories: (1) antidepressants and (2) gabapentinoids[9] (Table 5). Amongst antidepressants, tricyclic antidepressants (TCAs) and serotonin-norepinephrine reuptake inhibitors (SNRIs) are used as first-line drugs. Surprisingly, the doses used for analgesia are much lower than for depression. Also, the efficacy of selective serotonin reuptake inhibitors (SSRIs) for pain relief is limited. These antidepressants act by inhibiting uptake of serotonin and norepinephrine. Both these neurotransmitters are involved in the descending pathways for pain modulation. The gabapentinoids (gabapentin and pregabalin) attach to the alpha 2-delta ligand of calcium channel. Thus, they reduce calcium influx in an excited neuron inhibiting neurotransmitter release. Compared to traditional anticonvulsants, this group has no hepatic enzyme induction and minimal drug interactions.

Adverse effects of the first-line agents and their monitoring is arranged in Table 6.

TABLE 5: First-line medications for neuropathic pain[9]

Molecule	Dose and regimen
SNRI (Duloxetine)	30–60 mg once a day
Gabapentin	300–900 mg in three divided doses
Pregabalin	150–450 mg in two divided doses
TCA (Amitriptyline)	25–150 mg once a day

TCA, tricyclic antidepressant

TABLE 6: Adverse effects and monitoring of first-line drugs

Molecule	Contraindication	Caution	Monitor	Interactions
Amitriptyline (TCAs)	Cardiac conduction	Prostate hypertrophy Narrow angle Glaucoma	ECG screen Heart rate IOP Weight	Tramadol (serotonin syndrome) Warfarin
Duloxetine	Uncontrolled hypertension, liver disease			SSRIs and tramadol (serotonin syndrome)
Pregabalin		Renal disease	Creatinine clearance Peripheral edema	Not significant
Gabapentin		Renal disease	Renal clearance	Not significant

ECG, electrocardiogram; IOP, intraocular pressure; SSRIs, selective serotonin reuptake inhibitor; TCAs, tricyclic antidepressants

TABLE 7: Second-line and third-line recommendations[9]

Molecule	Recommendation	Dose and regimen
Tramadol	Second-line	200–400 mg in two or three divided doses
Lidocaine patch	Second-line*	One to three patches once a day for 12 hours
Capsaicin 8% patch	Second-line*	One to four patches every 30–60 minutes
Botox A (subcutaneous)	Third-line*	50–200 units
Strong opioids	Third-line	Individual titration

*Only for peripheral neuropathic pain

Opioids have been used for their analgesic properties since ages. The World Health Organization (WHO) has divided them into weak and strong opioids. Weak include tramadol, codeine, dextropropoxyphene; whereas strong ones include morphine, oxycodone, and tapentadol, etc. Most of the randomized controlled trials (RCTs) have been in peripheral neuropathic pain (diabetic neuropathy) and maximum studies are with oxycodone and morphine. Though the evidence for efficacy has been moderate, the low level of safety precludes their use. The second-and third-line agents with their dosages are enumerated in Table 7.

Trigeminal Neuralgia

This condition needs special mention as the choice of medicines differs as compared to other conditions. Carbamazepine has been the first choice since a long time and most of the patients respond. Eventually, as months and years pass, these patients require a combination of medicines for effective pain relief. Baclofen, lamotrigine and pregabalin have shown benefit in trials over placebo. Those refractory to the combination will have to be subjected to minimally invasive procedures (stereotactic radiosurgery).[11]

INTERVENTIONAL PAIN MANAGEMENT

The need for interventional therapy arises as neuropathic pain relief is often incomplete with drugs. Interventional treatment is defined as "invasive procedures involving delivery of drugs into targeted areas, or ablation/

modulation of targeted nerves" for the treatment of pain.[12] There is paucity of high quality clinical trials in this field. Thus weak recommendations have been made by the NeuPSIG.[13] Having said that, interventions carry their own potential risks (e.g. procedural risks and infection). The various modalities that have been tried include nerve blocks, epidural steroids, intrathecal drugs and neuromodulation (spinal cord stimulation and deep brain stimulation).

The NeuPSIG has made weak recommendations for use in the following conditions: (a) steroid injections for radiculopathy; (b) spinal cord stimulation for failed back surgery syndrome and (c) spinal cord stimulation for chronic regional pain syndrome type 1. Interventional treatment should ideally be offered in clinical and research settings. Readers are requested to refer to the above guidelines for details of different modalities in different pain conditions.

CONCLUSION

Neuropathic pain is a common complex pain syndrome of varied etiologies with pathologic changes occurring at more than one level of the somatosensory system. A detailed history and examination making use of suitable questionnaires is essential to guide investigations and treatment. A multidisciplinary stepwise approach starting with counseling and coping strategies, pharmacologic therapy and if needed appropriate interventions should help majority of patients with pain relief.

REFERENCES

1. Bonica JJ. The need of a taxonomy. Pain. 1979;6(3):247.
2. Simon LS. Relieving pain in America: A blueprint for Transforming Prevention, Care, Education, and Research. J Pain Palliat Care Pharmacother. 2012;26(2):197-8.
3. IndlNeP Study Group. Burden of neuropathic pain in Indian patients attending urban, specialty clinics: results from a cross sectional study. Pain Pract. 2008;8(5):362-78.
4. Jain PN, Chatterjee A, Choudhary AH, Sareen R. Prevalence, etiology, and management of neuropathic pain in an Indian cancer hospital. J Pain Palliat Care Pharmacother. 2009;23(2):114-9.
5. Treede RD, Jensen TS, Campbell JN, Cruccu G, Dostrovsky JO, Griffin JW, et al. Neuropathic pain redefinition and a grading system for clinical and research purposes. Neurology. 2008;70(18):1630-5.
6. Cruccu G, Sommer C, Anand P, Attal N, Baron R, Garcia Larrea L, et al. EFNS guidelines on neuropathic pain assessment: revised 2009. Eur J Neurol. 2010;17(8):1010-8.
7. McCormack HM, David JD, Sheather S. Clinical applications of visual analogue scales: a critical review. Psychol Med. 1988;18(4):1007-19.
8. Farrar JT, Young JP, LaMoreaux L, Werth JL, Poole RM. Clinical importance of changes in chronic pain intensity measured on an 11-point numerical pain rating scale. Pain. 2001;94(2):149-58.
9. Deng Y, Luo L, Hu Y, Fang K, Liu J. Clinical practice guidelines for the management of neuropathic pain: a systematic review. BMC Anesthesiol. 2015;16:12.
10. Finnerup NB, Attal N, Haroutounian S, McNicol E, Baron R, Dworkin RH, et al. Pharmacotherapy for neuropathic pain in adults: a systematic review and meta-analysis. Lancet Neurology. 2015;14(2):162-73.
11. Zahra H, Teh BS, Paulino AC, Yoshor D, Trask T, Baskin D, et al. Stereotactic radiosurgery for trigeminal neuralgia utilizing the BrainLAB Novalis system. Technol Cancer Res Treat. 2009;8(6):407-12.
12. Accident Compensation Corporation. (2012) Interventional guidelines for pain management. [online] Available from http://www.acc.co.nz/for-providers/clinical-best-practice/interventional-pain-management/interventions/intervention-index/WCM1_034233 [Accessed December, 2016].
13. Dworkin RH, O'Connor AB, Kent J, Mackey SC, Raja SN, Stacey BR, et al. Interventional management of neuropathic pain: NeuPSIG recommendations. Pain. 2013;154(11):2249-61.

SECTION 9

Ischemic Pain

CHAPTER 34

Peripheral Vascular Disease: Causes and Pain Management

Kailash M Kothari

INTRODUCTION

Each year 1-2% of patients with peripheral arterial occlusive disease (pAOD) develops critical limb ischemia (CLI), characterized by rest pain and peripheral ulcer or gangrene. This aggravation of the disease is accompanied by an increase of the 1-year mortality rate up to 25% and a similarly increased frequency of major amputation.[1] Peripheral vascular disease (PVD) includes a range of arterial syndromes that are caused by the altered structure and function of the noncoronary arteries. Peripheral vascular disease (PVD) is a nearly pandemic condition that has the potential to cause loss of limb or even loss of life. Peripheral vascular disease manifests as insufficient tissue perfusion caused by existing atherosclerosis that may be acutely compounded by either emboli or thrombi. In some patients, PVD can become life-threatening because of acute limb ischemia, and they require emergency intervention to minimize morbidity and mortality. The pain associated with PVD can be ranging from mild to very severe.

ETIOPATHOPHYSIOLOGY

Peripheral vascular disease, also known as arteriosclerosis obliterans, is primarily the result of atherosclerosis, this process gradually occlude medium and large arteries and ultimately results in to vascular disease.

Thromboses are often of an atheromatous nature and occur in the lower extremities more frequently than in the upper extremities. Multiple factors predispose patients for thrombosis.

The predisposing factors which may lead to thrombosis are sepsis, hypotension, low cardiac output, aneurysms, aortic dissection, bypass grafts, and underlying atherosclerotic narrowing of the arterial lumen.

Etiology

The primary and most common cause is Atherosclerosis.[2]

Some other less common causes are:
- Aortic coarctation
- Arterial fibrodysplasia
- Arterial tumors
- Arterial dissection
- Arterial embolism/thrombosis
- Vasospasm
- Trauma
- Takayasu arteritis
- Temporal arteritis
- Thoracic outlet obstruction
- Burger's disease
- Adventitial cystic disease

- Occluded limb aneurysms
- Popliteal artery entrapment
- Iliac endofibrosis
- Ergot toxicity
- Radiation fibrosis
- Retroperitoneal fibrosis.

Pathophysiology

The pathophysiology of PVD is as diverse as the diseases it encompasses, but it centers on damage, inflammation, and structural defects of blood vessels. It includes atherosclerosis, degenerative diseases, dysplastic disorders, vascular inflammation, and thrombosis as well as thromboembolism.[2] However, the pathophysiology, of intermittent claudication is most likely due to hemodynamic compromise. The other factors include reconditioning, metabolic changes, such as accumulation of acylcarnitines and ADP, impaired synthesis of phosphocreatine, and skeletal muscle injury characterized by muscle fiber loss.

CLASSIFICATION

Fontaine Stages

The four increasing stages of severity:
- Stage I: Asymptomatic
- Stage IIa: Mild claudication
- Stage IIb: Moderate-to-severe claudication
- Stage III: Ischemia rest pain
- Stage IV: Ulceration or gangrene.

Rutherford Categories

There are a total of seven increasing categories of severity:
- Grade 0, category 0: Asymptomatic
- Grade I, category 1: Mild claudication
- Grade I, category 2: Moderate claudication
- Grade I, category 3: Severe claudication
- Grade II, category 4: Ischemia rest pain
- Grade III, category 5: Minor tissue loss
- Grade IV, category 6: Major tissue loss.

Asymptomatic/Claudication/Critical Limb Ischemia/Acute Limb Ischemia

The American College of Cardiology/American Heart Association (ACC/AHA) Practice Guidelines use the following divisions:
- Asymptomatic: Absence of leg claudication symptoms
- Claudication: Inadequate blood flow during exercise, causing fatigue, discomfort, or pain
- Critical limb ischemia: Compromise of blood flow to extremity, causing limb pain at rest. Patients often have ulcers or gangrene
- Acute limb ischemia: A sudden decrease in limb perfusion that threatens limb viability
- Associated with the "5 Ps": Pain, paralysis, paresthesias, pulselessness, and pallor.

HISTORY

Peripheral vascular disease rarely exhibits an acute onset; it instead manifests a more chronic progression of symptoms. Patients with acute emboli causing limb ischemia may have new or chronic atrial fibrillation, valvular disease, or recent MI, whereas a history of claudication, rest pain, or ulceration suggests thrombosis of existing PVD. Radiation-induced PAD is becoming more common, perhaps due to the efficacy of current antineoplastic treatment and increased survival.

Look for associated diseases
- Coronary artery disease (CAD)
- Myocardial infarction (MI)
- Arial fibrillation
- Transient ischemic attack
- Stroke
- Renal disease

Studies have suggested that even asymptomatic peripheral arterial disease (PAD) is associated with increased CAD mortality.

Risk factors
- Smoking
- Hyperlipidemia
- Diabetes mellitus

- Old age
- Hyperviscosity.

Symptoms

- Intermittent claudications relieved by rest.
- Collateral circulation may develop, reducing the symptoms of intermittent claudication.
- The ischemic at rest pain is more worrisome and reference suggest of PVD and inadequate perfusion.
- Ischemic rest pain often is exacerbated by poor cardiac output, it is relieved by effects of gravity.
- Many patients with chronic painful diabetes mellitus have coexisting small fiber damage and PVD.

In these patients, neuropathic pain tends to improve with time and can resolve completely inspite of continuing deterioration of small-fiber function, indicating that these peripheral measures do not predict the evolution of painful symptoms. The presence or absence of PVD does not appear to affect the natural history of neuropathic pain or its symptomatology.[3] Leriche syndrome is a clinical syndrome described by intermittent claudication, impotence, and significantly decreased or absent femoral pulses. This syndrome indicates chronic peripheral arterial insufficiency due to narrowing of the distal aorta.

Other Symptoms and Signs

Further symptoms and signs may lead to a diagnosis of PVD in the presence of risk factors:
- Calf or foot cramping with walking that is relieved with rest
- Thigh or buttock pain with walking that is relieved with rest
- Erectile dysfunction
- Pain worse in one leg
- Diminished pulse.

Critical limb ischemia should be suspected with the following:
- Leg pain at rest
- Gangrene
- Nonhealing wound
- Muscle atrophy
- Dependent rubor
- Pallor when the leg is elevated
- Loss of hair over the dorsum of the foot
- Thickened toe nails
- Shiny/scaly skin.

Acute limb ischemia should be suspected with the following:
- Peripheral signs of peripheral vascular disease with acute ischemic limbs are the classic "5 P's":
  - Pulselessness
  - Paralysis
  - Paresthesia
  - Pain
  - Pallor
- No pulse in lower extremity
- Pale extremity
- Nerve loss.

CLINICAL EXAMINATION

1. *Cardiac*: Assess the heart for murmurs or other abnormalities. Investigate all peripheral vessels, including carotid, abdominal, and femoral, for pulse quality and bruit. Note that the dorsalis pedis artery is absent in 5–8% of normal subjects, but the posterior tibial artery usually is present. Both pulses are absent in only about 0.5% of patients. Exercise may cause the obliteration of these pulses.
2. *Neurological examination*: Paralysis and paresthesia suggest limb-threatening ischemia and mandate prompt evaluation and consultation.
3. Allen test to know information about radial and ulnar arteries.
4. Skin may have an atrophic, shiny appearance including alopecia; dry, scaly, or erythematous skin; chronic pigmentation changes; and brittle nails.
5. In advanced PVD, there may be pulselessness; numbness; cyanosis; paralysis leading to coldness followed by gangrene.

6. Semiquantitative assessment for the degree of pallor. If pallor manifests when the extremity is level, the pallor is classified as level.[4]

LABORATORY STUDIES

- Routine blood tests such as CBC, BUN, creatinine, and electrolytes studies help evaluate factors that might lead to worsening of peripheral perfusion. Risk factors for the development of vascular disease (lipid profile, coagulation tests) can also be evaluated, although not necessarily in the ED setting.
- An ECG for evidence of dysrhythmia, chamber enlargement, or MI.
- The levels of inflammatory blood markers for example D dimer, C-reactive protein, interleukin 6, and homocysteine are decreased lower extremity tolerance of exercise,[4] and higher levels of activity in daily life have been shown to decrease these levels.

IMAGING STUDIES

- Doppler ultrasonographic studies are useful to know flow status (Tables 1 and 2).
- Magnetic resonance imaging (MRI) (Table 3) for presence of plaques.

TABLE 1: First tests to order

Test	Result
Ankle brachial index (ABI) Segmental pressure examination	ABI <0.90 gradient of >20 mmHg between adjacent segments
Duplex ultrasound Pulse volume recording (PVR)	Peak systolic velocity ratio >2.0 any qualitative sequential decrease in pulsatility of the waveform
Continuous wave Doppler Ultrasound	Pulsatility index decrease between adjacent proximal and distal anatomic seoments
Exercise ABI Angiography	Postexercise ABI < pre-exercise ABI stenosis

TABLE 2: Other tests to consider

Test	Result
CT angiogram	Presence of significant stenosis

TABLE 3: Emerging test

Test	Result
MR angiography (MRA)	Stenosis

The benefits of angiography to provide even higher detail and can replace traditional arteriography. The utility of MRI is limited in the emergency setting, often due to location of the device and the technical skill required to interpret, the highly detailed images.

- Computerized tomography (CT)—The noncontrast studies may show image calcification and arteriosclerosis, and contrast studies are useful to image arterial insufficiency.

OTHER TESTS

- The ankle-brachial index (ABI) is a useful test to compare pressures in the lower extremity to the upper extremity (Fig. 1).
- The ABI this test can be influenced by arteriosclerosis and small vessel disease (e.g. diabetes), reducing reliability. Progressive PAD, indicated by ABI decline of greater than 0.15, has been associated with increased cardiovascular disease risk.
- Transcutaneous oximetry affords assessment of impaired flow secondary to both microvascular and macrovascular disruption.
- Stiffening and thickening of arterial wall are two important components of atherosclerosis. Femoral artery intima-media thickness (FA-IMT) and stiffness parameter beta (FA-stiffness beta) can be measured by ultrasound methods. The symptomatic patient's shows greater FA-stiffness beta values than the asymptomatic subjects. Stiffening of arterial wall has a significant impact on PVD manifestations,

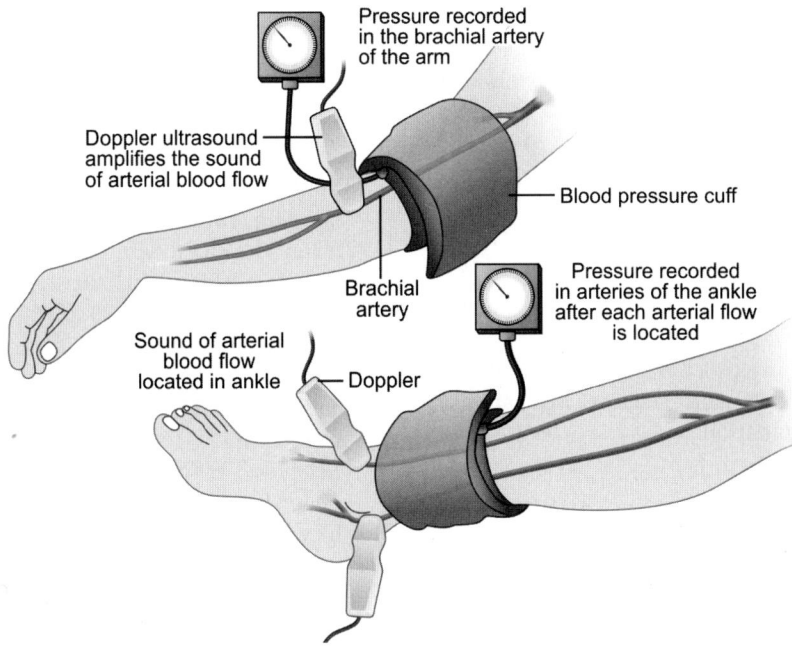

FIG. 1: How to measure ABI?

particularly on the leg symptoms, especially in patients with type 2 diabetes.[5]

TREATMENT

All patients regardless of their symptoms should have aggressive risk factor modification. Control of blood pressure (diabetic patients <130/80 mmHg, nondiabetic <140/90 mmHg), lipid control (LDL <100 mg/dL).

Smoking cessation (level of evidence C), diabetes control (HgA1c <7.0), and antiplatelet therapy are recommended[2] (level of evidence A).

Immediate Management

This involves the basics control ABCs, obtain intravenous access, and administer oxygen
- Generally, do not elevate the affected limbs
- Thorough neurological, cardiovascular including peripheral vascular and skin examination should be performed and findings should be recorded for future references.

In Hospital Management
- Check vitals, obtain good intravenous access, and obtaining baseline laboratory
- Take an ECG and chest radiograph
- As a routine empirical protocol initiate a heparin infusion with the goal of increasing activated partial thromboplastin (aPTT) time to 1.5 time's normal levels
- Identify emergency surgical need
  - Acute leg pain
  - A cool distal extremity
  - Diminished or absent distal pulses
  - An ankle blood pressure less than 50 mmHg.

ACUTE LIMB ISCHEMIA

Patients who have sudden decrease in limb perfusion with threatened tissue viability require urgent history and physical examination to determine symptom onset.
- Emergency vascular study assessment should be performed with ankle brachial index (ABI) or duplex ultrasound

- If there is severe PVD, then patient should immediately be treated with anticoagulation and assessed for etiology of acute limb ischemia.[2,6] Etiologies of acute limb ischemia are embolic, progressive PVD with *in situ* thrombosis, bypass graft thrombosis, arterial trauma, popliteal cyst, or entrapment, hypercoagulable state or phlegmasia cerulea dolens.

Nonviable Limb

These patients will have signs of tissue loss, nerve damage, and sensory loss and will require amputation.

Viable Limb

These patients will have no significant tissue loss, nerve damage, or significant sensory loss. Patients should have arterial anatomy defined and undergo revascularization.
- Localized intra-arterial infusion of thrombolytic with or without the concomitant use of mechanical thrombectomy device has been successful.
- Randomized controlled trials and case series suggest that intra-arterial thrombolytic therapy is as effective as surgery, and it has become the modality of choice.
- Systemic infusion of thrombolytic therapy is no longer used due to poor efficacy and increased bleeding complication.
- Urokinase is the most widely studied thrombolytic in acute limb ischemia, although there are emerging data about alteplase, reteplase, and tenecteplase.
- Although there are number of comparative studies, no single thrombolytic has emerged as the drug of choice. Streptokinase is no longer used due to lower efficacy, increased bleeding rate, and antigenicity issues.
- There have been small studies with thrombolytics and glycoprotein IIb/IIIa inhibitors showing increased lysis effectiveness but increased bleeding time and they are currently not recommended.

Anticoagulants

- *Urokinase:* Complete lysis rates are (64–79%).[7] The range of incidence of major bleeding is 0–16.7%
- *Alteplase:* The efficacy ranges from 61 to 86% in nonweight-based continuous infusion protocol. The efficacy ranges from 75 to 88% with continuous weight-based infusion. In small studies, the efficacy ranged from 70 to 100% for bolus and infusion studies. In a large registry of thrombolytics, tissue plasminogen activator major bleeding complications were 11.9%[7]
- *Reteplase*: Efficacies in small trials have been shown to be over 85% However, the bleeding complications have ranged from 6 to 19%.
- *Tenecteplase:* Efficacy in one study of 24 patients was 87%. There was one major bleeding complication during that trial (1.8%).
- *Heparin:* The optimal dosing is unclear since there has been no uniform reporting. As a consequence, the role of concomitant heparin is unclear.
- It augments activity of antithrombin III and prevents conversion of fibrinogen to fibrin and does not actively lyse but is able to inhibit further thrombogenesis also prevents reaccumulation of clot after spontaneous fibrinolysis.
- *Adult:* 80 U/kg IV bolus, followed by infusion of 18 U/kg/h.
- *Pediatric:* Administer as in adults.

For patients who continue to have symptoms, revascularization is recommended.[8]

Claudication (Not lifestyle-limiting)

For patients with claudication and established PVD who have no significant functional disability, no additional treatment is required.

Follow-up visits, at least annually, are required to monitor development of coronary, cerebrovascular or leg ischemic symptoms.

Claudication (Lifestyle-limiting)

Patients with lifestyle-limiting symptoms should undergo both a supervised exercise program and pharmacological therapy for symptom relief for 3 months (level of evidence C).

Exercise therapy has been shown in multiple studies (but of limited quality) to improve walking time and relieve symptoms. A supervised exercise training program consists of 30–45 minutes per session, 3 times a week for 12 weeks.

Symptom relief can be achieved with cilostazol or pentoxifylline. Cilostazol may improve pain-free walking distance in patients with intermittent claudication.[9] However, cilostazol is contraindicated in patients with congestive heart failure and ejection fraction <40%.

Pentoxifylline is also widely used; however, it is no more effective than placebo in randomized controlled trials and is contraindicated in patients with recent cerebral and/or retinal hemorrhage and in patients with intolerance of methylxanthines (theophylline).

Patients with intermittent claudication may improve their walking distance with naftidrofuryl therapy.[10]

If there is clinical improvement with an exercise program and medication, follow-up visits are recommended. However, if there is no improvement, patients should be referred to a vascular specialist and have their anatomy defined and assessed for revascularization. Some patients choose to take an herbal supplement (L-arginine, propionyl L-carnitine, ginkgo biloba). However, the clinical benefit of these supplements is not well established.

CHRONIC SEVERE LIMB ISCHEMIA (CRITICAL LIMB ISCHEMIA)

These patients have chronic ischemic leg symptoms, such as ischemic rest pain, gangrene, and nonhealing wounds.

For these patients, ischemic etiology must be established urgently by physical examination and vascular studies. If patients have documented PVD, they should be immediately referred to a vascular specialist for revascularization. The patients who have been able to walk before the episode of critical limb ischemia, have a life expectancy of more than 1 year and are able to withstand surgery may be candidates for revascularization.

If the patient is not a candidate for revascularization, the patient should be assessed for amputation where necessary and be on appropriate risk factor reduction medication.

Revascularization Referral

The following patients should be referred to a vascular specialist to have their anatomy defined and assessed:

- Patients with lifestyle-limiting claudication who have had no improvement with exercise and symptom relief
- Patients with critical limb ischemia symptoms (ischemic rest pain, gangrene, nonhealing wounds)
- Patients with acute limb ischemia (sudden decrease in limb perfusion with threatened tissue viability).

Revascularization is recommended if patients have lifestyle-limiting claudication, and have failed to achieve benefit from medications combined with an exercise program.

Procedures (Endovascular or Surgical Revascularization)

Endovascular techniques include percutaneous transluminal angioplasty (PTA) with balloon dilation, stents, atherectomy, laser, cutting balloons, and thermal angioplasty.

- For aortoiliac disease, endovascular revascularization is recommended for stenosis that is <10 cm in length and chronic occlusions that are <5 cm
- For other lesions with stenosis >10 cm, chronic occlusions >5 cm, heavily calcified

lesions, and lesions associated with aortic aneurysm, surgery is recommended
- Surgery should not be offered to patients with a large amount of tissue loss or extensive infection
- For femoropopliteal artery stenosis, endovascular therapy is recommended if there is a discrete stenosis <10 cm or calcified stenosis <5 cm
- Surgical revascularization is recommended for lesions involving the common femoral artery, lesions >10 cm, heavily calcified lesions >5 cm, lesions involving the ostium of superficial femoral artery, and lesions involving the popliteal artery
- For infrapopliteal artery lesions, endovascular treatment has been limited to threatened limb loss only. Unlike femoropopliteal lesions or aortoiliac lesions, failed endovascular intervention can preclude surgical revascularization. Therefore, careful selection is essential. Surgical revascularization patency rate for infrapopliteal artery is poor but may be slightly better with in situ technique. Regardless of the procedure selected, all patients undergoing surgical or endovascular revascularization should receive lifelong aspirin treatment (75–100 mg/day).

CONTINUED INTERVENTIONAL MANAGEMENT

- Depending on the case, the surgeon may involve interventional radiology or proceed operatively
- Emboli may be treated successfully by an intravascular catheter with a balloon at the tip known as Fogarty catheter. The balloon is passed distal to the lesion; the balloon is inflated, and the catheter is withdrawn along with the embolus. This technique most commonly is used for iliac, femoral, or popliteal emboli.

Surgical Management
- Definitive treatment is aortobifemoral bypass (Fig. 2)
- Its 5-year patency rate is approximately 90%
- Remember these patients have associated comorbid medical conditions, such as cardiovascular disease, diabetes, and chronic obstructive pulmonary disease, which increase procedural morbidity and mortality
- Axillobifemoral bypass and femoral-femoral bypass are alternatives, both of which have lower 5-year patencies but have lower procedural mortality
- Some areas of arteriostenosis can be revascularized with percutaneous transluminal coronary angioplasty (PTCA)
- If the occlusion is complete, a laser may be useful in making a small hole through which to pass the balloon
- Restenosis is a concern with PTCA, particularly for larger lesions. Stents and lasers are still considered experimental.

Improving health-related quality of life (HRQL) is the main goal of surgery to treat peripheral vascular disease (PVD); however, HRQL is rarely measured directly. Rather, most surgeons use other measures, such as patient symptoms and ankle-brachial index (ABI) to determine the need for intervention in PVD. The accuracy of these surrogates in representing HRQL has been untested. Multivariate analysis demonstrated that quality of life questionnaire short form-36 (SF-36) and walking impairment questionnaire (WIQ) physical summary scores are better predicted by symptoms than by ABI (P <0.01). Data suggest that sole reliance on these surrogates may not accurately reflect the effect of PVD on HRQL, or the potential benefit of vascular surgery in improving HRQL.

An initial study shows promise in relieving the pain of PAD with topically applied lidocaine

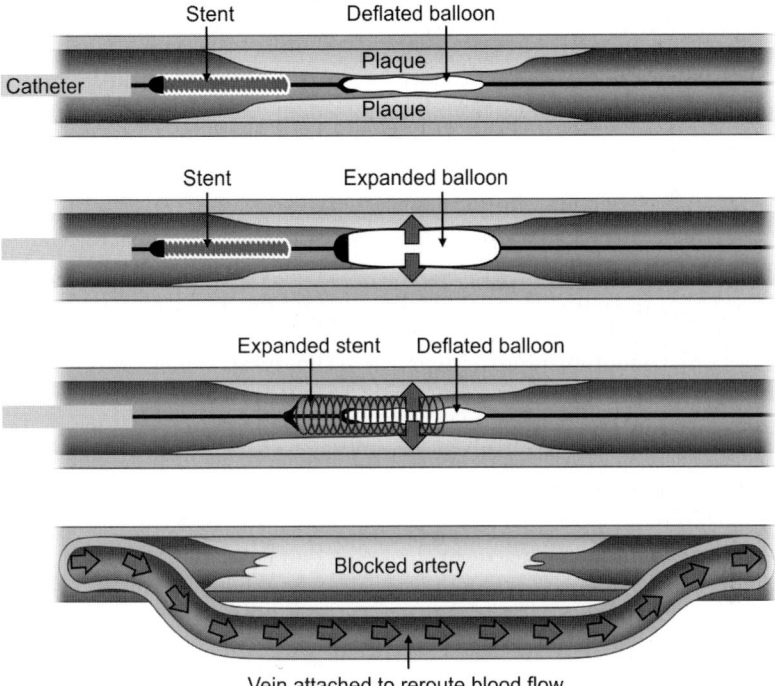

FIG. 2: Diagrammatic representation of bypass surgery for the blocked segment

spray. Suzuki and colleagues studied 24 subjects with PAD and noted a significant drop in pain associated with PAD by applying an 8% lidocaine metered dose spray to the affected areas. Blood levels of lidocaine were minimal, and this technique may show promise for those affected with focal PAD pain.[6]

Amputation

Preservation of the knee joint has enormous advantages for wearing artificial limbs and subsequent mobility. Similarly, a patient with good prospects of wearing an artificial limb will fare better with an above-the-knee amputation, if below-the-knee amputation seems unachievable. Local amputation of ulcerated or gangrenous toes will not heal without revascularization.

Pain Relief

The limb ischemia causes severe pain needs a slow-release opiate, such as morphine is good to start with and can be supplemented by nonsteroidal anti-inflammatory drugs.

The lumbar sympathectomy (surgical or chemical) or spinal cord stimulation are another options.

The phantom limb pain may complicate major amputation.

In addition amitriptyline hydrochloride, carbamazepine, transcutaneous nerve stimulation, and acupuncture are of great help.

Role of Interventional Pain Procedures

- Sympathetic blocks: (Stellate Ganglion, Lumbar and Thoracic). This can be helpful in rest pain and in pregangrene stages. Lumbar sympathectomy is a minimally invasive procedure with a low complication rate. Sympathectomy is proposed to act primarily via its vasodilator effects on the collateral circulation secondary to decreased sympathetic tone, improve tissue oxygenation and ulcer healing, and decrease tissue damage and pain. Pain is also decreased by interrupting sympathetic–nociceptive coupling and by a direct neurolytic action on nociceptive fibers.

Randomized controlled trials have failed to identify any objective benefits for lumbar sympathectomy, but subjective improvements in symptoms for patients with highly symptomatic critical leg ischemia have been consistently demonstrated in multiple cohort studies with sustained symptom improvements in approximately 60% of patients. Lumbar sympathectomy should be considered for symptomatic patients with critical leg ischemia as an alternative to amputation in patients with otherwise viable limbs.

Cohort Studies on Sympathetic Blocks in PVD

- Kim et al. in 1976, 61 lumbar sympathectomies on 58 patients with PVD, overall improvement rate (defined as disappearance of rest pain, healing of tissue and a generally nonpainful useful limb for at least 6 months postoperative) was 60% while early amputation rate was 40%. The immediate postoperative death was 6.5% from cardiac causes.
- Van Driel et al. in 1988, 60 consecutive patients, surgical lumbar sympathectomy in critical leg ischemia, good results (defined as absence of rest pain, healing of ischemic lesions and no major amputation) in 48% of limbs at six months, limb survival at 6 months and 2 years were 65% and 59%, respectively.
- Norman et al. in 1988 performed 174 surgical lumbar sympathectomies on 153 patients, 67% of the claudicant and 54% of the rest pain patients avoided further surgery after 5 years.
- Alexander et al. in 1994, 544 chemical lumbar sympathectomies on 489 patients, improvement in symptoms in 72% of the patients immediately and 35% at 8 months follow-up. The amputation rate was 24% at 2 years.
- Perez-Burkhardt et al. in 1999, 100 surgical lumbar sympathectomies on 93 patients for invalidant claudication, ischemic rest pain and trophic lesions; good results (judged by absent rest pain, healed ischemic ulcers no major amputation at 6 months) were seen in 58.5% of patients with claudication or rest pain and 61.7% of patients with trophic lesions. Amputation rate was 18.3% at 30 days postoperatively.
- Spinal cord stimulator implantation: Epidural spinal cord stimulation (SCS) has been used as a method to improve microcirculatory blood flow, relieve ischemic pain and reduce amputation rate in patients with severe peripheral arterial occlusive disease (PAOD).[11]
- Randomized controlled trials, mostly from Europe, have evaluated clinical and physiologic aspects of spinal cord stimulation in the treatment of PVD.

A systematic review and meta-analysis published in 2004 from nine European trials of spinal cord stimulation and critical leg ischemia encompassing 444 patients[12] received controlled treatments.

And two studies showed significantly increased the number of patients whose clinical picture improved from stage III or IV to stage II. Number to treat with SCS is 3 patients for 1 patient to reach stage II. There were no differences in wound healing or in patients with diabetes compared with no diabetes. Ankle-brachial index data were inconclusive.

- Raynaud's phenomenon and Buerger's disease is promising field for spinal cord stimulation. Many patients are successfully treated. The assessment of the efficacy via randomized controlled trials is extremely challenging due to relatively small patient population. To date, only a few case reports or case series have been published, all reported high success and minimal complication rates with this modality.

- The report was published in 2009 which addressed the question 'What is the clinical and cost-effectiveness of spinal cord stimulation (SCS) in the management of chronic neuropathic or ischemic pain?'[13]
- Thirteen electronic databases [including MEDLINE (1950-2007), EMBASE (1980-2007) and the Cochrane library (1991-2007)] were searched.[10]
- 6000 citations, 11 RCTs–3 of neuropathic pain–SCS was more effective than conventional medical management (CMM) or reoperation in reducing pain, 8 of ischemic pain–small sample sizes—failed to demonstrate that pain relief in critical limb ischemia (CLI) was better for SCS than for Conservative Medical Management.[13]
- The evidence suggested that SCS was effective in reducing the chronic neuropathic pain of FBSS and CRPS type I, vasospastic diseases like Raynaud's disease; collagen vascular disease and diabetic arteriopathy and in claudication with rest and/or night pain, life expectance of at least 3-6 months with no significant tissue involvement. Especially for ischemic pain, there may need to be selection criteria developed for CLI, and SCS may have clinical benefit for refractory angina short-term.[13, 14]
- Addition of the SCS to the standard conservative treatment improves limb salvage, ischemic pain and general clinical condition in patients with inoperable chronic critical limb ischemia. Patients with extensive gangrene with Fontaine 4b stage should not be treated with SCS. These patients usually do not respond to conservative management and are inoperable. They should be treated with amputation.[15]

CONCLUSION

Peripheral vascular disease is multifactorial and pain relief in these patients can be challenging. The multimodal approach is mandatory such as pharmacological, interventional modalities and rehabilitation to achieve pain relief and improve quality of life.

Refer following for details of interventional pain techniques

1. Interventional Pain Management-Practical Approach 2nd edition (2016) by Baheti, et.al, Jaypee.
2. Radiological Imaging for regional Anaesthesia and Pain Management by P Prithviraj, et al. Churchill Livingstone.

REFERENCES

1. Treitl M, Ruppert V, Mayer AK, Degenhart C, Reiser M, Rieger J. Chronic critical ischemia of the lower leg: Pretherapeutic imaging and methods for revascularization. Radiology. 2006; 46(11):962-72.
2. Hirsch, AT, Haskal, ZJ, Hertzer, NR, et al. ACC/AHA 2005 Practice guidelines for the management of patients with peripheral arterial disease (lower extremity, renal, mesenteric, and abdominal aortic). Circulation. 2006; 113:e463-4.
3. Benbow SJ, Chan AW, Bowsher D, MacFarlane IA, Williams G. A prospective study of painful symptoms, small-fibre function and peripheral vascular disease in chronic painful diabetic neuropathy. Department of Medicine, University of Liverpool, UK. Diabet Med. 1994; 11(1):17-21.
4. Long J, Modrall JG, Parker BJ, Swann A, Welborn MB 3rd, Anthony T. Department of Surgery, University of Texas Southwestern Medical Center, USA. Correlation between ankle-brachial index, symptoms, and health-related quality of life in patients with peripheral vascular disease. J Vasc Surg. 2004; 39(4):723-7.
5. Taniwaki H, Shoji T, Emoto M, Kawagishi T, Ishimura E, Inaba M, Okuno Y, Nishizawa Y. Femoral artery wall thickness and stiffness in evaluation of peripheral vascular disease in type 2 diabetes mellitus. Second Department of Internal Medicine, Osaka City University Medical School, 1-4-3, Asahi-machi, Abeno-ku, Osaka 545-8585, Japan. Atherosclerosis Sep. 2001; 158(1):207-14.
6. Dagher NN, Modrall JG. Pharmacotherapy before and after revascularization: Anticoagulation, antiplatelet agents, and statins. Semin Vasc Surg. 2007; 20:10-4.
7. Razavi MK, Lee DS, Hofmann LV. Catheter-directed thrombolytic therapy for limb ischemia: Current status and controversies. J Vasc Interv Radiol. 2004; 15:13-23.

8. Rajagopalan S. Approach to and management of intermittent claudication. In: Rajagopalan S, Mukherjee D, Mohler ER (Eds). Manual of Vascular Diseases. Philadelphia, PA: Lippincott, Williams and Wilkins; 2005; pp70-87.
9. Robless P, Mikhailidis DP, Stansby GP. Cilostazol for peripheral arterial disease. Cochrane Database Syst Rev. 2008 ;(1):CD00374.
10. De Backer T, Vander Stichele R, et al. Naftidrofuryl for intermittent claudication: Meta-analysis based on individual patient data. BMJ. 2009; 338:b603.
11. Sciacca Vincenzo and T Kyventidis. Epidural spinal cord stimulation in lower limb ischemia. Operative Neuromodulation Acta Neurochirurgica Supplementum, 2007 Volume 97/1, Part 4, 253-8, DOI: 10.1007/978-3-211-33079-1_34.
12. Ubbink DT, Vermeulen H, Spincemaille HJJ, et al. Systematic review and meta-analysis of controlled trials assessing spinal cord stimulation for inoperable critical leg ischemia. Br J Surg. 2004;91:948-55.
13. Simpson EL, Duenas A, Holmes MW, Papaioannou D, Chilcott J. Spinal cord stimulation for chronic pain of neuropathic or ischaemic origin: Systematic review and economic evaluation. Health Technol Assess Mar 2009; 13(17): iii, ix-x, 1-154, School of Health and Related Research. The University of Sheffield, UK.
14. Breast Chronic lower limb ischemia. Department of Vascular Surgery, Sheffield Vascular Institute, Northern General Hospital, Sheffield, UK. West J Med. 2000; 173(1):60-3.
15. Smith HS, Deer TR, Staats PS, et al. Intrathecal drug delivery. Pain Physician 2008; 11 (2 Suppl) S89-104. Current Therapy in Pain, Howard S. Smith, 2008.

SECTION 10

Myofascial Pain

CHAPTER 35

Management of Myofascial Pain

Kritika M Doshi

INTRODUCTION

The anatomic frame of the human body is made up of the bony skeleton covered by muscles and fascia. Despite the fact that skeletal muscles account for nearly half the body weight, there is no medical specialty linked to it. Also research and development of muscle specific ailments, pathophysiology, diagnosis and therapeutic options have only recently gained attention.[1] Every movement requires coordinated activity of skeletal and muscular tissues. This means that muscle pain is very common but due to the lack of data, there is controversy about the nature and relevance of muscle pain.

Some of the explanations for muscles being painful include:

- According to Cooper G, Bailey B, and Bogduk N,[2] muscle pain is secondary to underlying tendonitis, muscle strain, inflammation or degeneration or injuries to joints and nerves.
- Kirmayer LJ, Looper KJ consider persistent muscle pain as a manifestation of a somatoform disorder[3]
- Chan Gunn has proposed a model based on Cannon and Rosenblueth's law of Denervation—that myofascial pain is a manifestation of peripheral neuropathy.[4]

The term "Myofascial pain" was coined by Janet Travell who observed that referral pain from fascia was similar to that of the contractile muscle element.[5] Pain originating from muscles and/or its covering fascia is labeled as myofascial pain. Muscle pain is a natural accompaniment to physical activity—hence, its meaning is not always negative.[6] However, muscle pain is also a common manifestation of many chronic pain conditions and is described as diffuse, aching pain that may refer to deep somatic structures.[7]

RELEVANT ANATOMY

Skeletal muscles are made up of contractile elements. The basic unit of these muscles is called a sarcomere.

Skeletal muscles cells are made up of groups of fascicles containing tubular myofibrils. Each myofibril is separated from surrounding fibrils by mitochondria, sarcoplasmic reticulum and the transverse tubules (T-tubules). The T-tubules lie perpendicular to the long-axis of the muscle fiber and conduct impulses from the exterior to the interior of the muscle with release of Ca+ from the sarcoplasmic reticulum.

The sarcomere is made up of alternate thick (myosin) and thin (actin) fibrous proteins filaments (Fig. 1) that slide past each other when a muscle contracts or relaxes. Myofibrils are composed of repeating sections of sarcomeres which appear under the microscope as dark and light bands. The Z-lines separate sarcomeres. The area of only thin bands is called I-band and H-zone has only thick filaments. A-band is area of overlapping. During a contraction, the I-band and H-zone decrease while A-band remains same length.

Motor endplate is the synapse between terminal ends of motor neurons and skeletal muscle. Neuromuscular junction is the functional area of the motor endplate where the impulse from motor neuron reaches the nerve terminal. This causes depolarization with opening of voltage-gated Ca+ channels and influx of Ca+ and release of acetylcholine (Ach). This Ach binds to the postsynaptic membrane and depolarizes it causing a miniature endplate potential (MEPP).

Trigger point is defined as an exquisitely tender spot in discrete taut bands of hardened muscle that produce local and referred pain, among other symptoms. An individual contraction-knot appears as a segment of a muscle fiber with extremely contracted sarcomeres and an increased diameter. Most research has shown the presence of "trigger" points in muscle and its association with almost all reported musculoskeletal problems[8] (migraine, tension type headache, lateral epicondylitis, low back pain, etc.).

The integrated trigger point hypothesis postulates that in myofascial pain motor endplates release excessive acetylcholine, which is evidenced histopathologically by the presence of sarcomere shortening.[9] These areas of intense focal sarcomere contraction have been described in animals and humans.

CLINICAL FEATURES

According to the integrated trigger point hypothesis, myofascial pain is characterized by the presence of trigger points (Fig. 2) with characteristic referred pain areas (Fig. 2). It is not possible to enumerate various muscles and their painful syndromes. However, some salient features are mentioned here.

- The patient can present with:
  ○ Spontaneous pain or
  ○ Pain with tenderness in the muscle on applying pressure, characteristic referred pain, muscle tension, and restriction of motion.
- Myofascial pain syndrome (MPS) can be acute or chronic; primary or secondary. Secondary MPS can be seen in the presence of acquired or congenital abnormalities and skeletal conditions like scoliosis, limb-length discrepancies, etc. The skeletal changes lead to asymmetrical and disproportionate loading of muscles and hence development of trigger points.
- Myofascial trigger points (MTrPs) can be seen in coincidental pathologic states like radiculopathies, nerve entrapments, bone or joint in the stage of healing, and congenital musculoskeletal abnormalities, metabolic disorders, nutritional imbalances, and regional biomechanical imbalances.[10]
- Psychosocial factors can contribute to chronicity, along with metabolic disorders, nutritional imbalances, and regional biomechanical imbalances.[11]

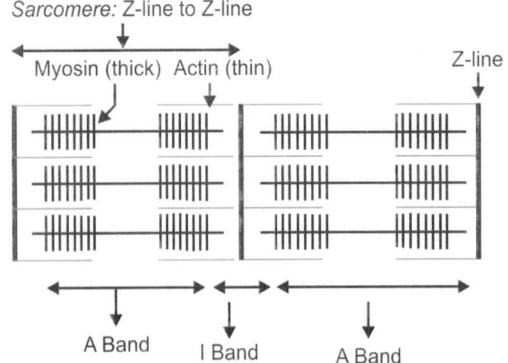

FIG. 1: Muscle structure—line diagram

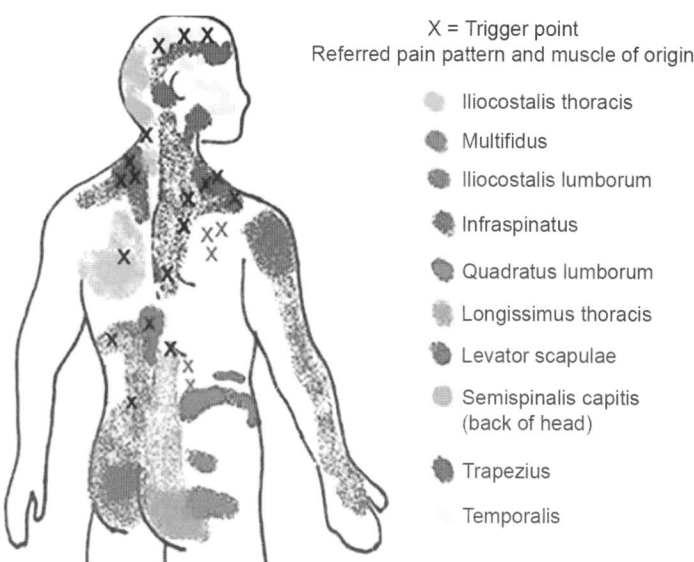

FIG. 2: Various tender points with the areas of referred pain *(For color version, see Plate 10)*

- Patients with MPS have higher scores for anxiety and depression.[12]
- Referred-pain from MTrPs can mimic visceral pain syndromes, visceral pain syndromes can induce trigger point development and MPS, and referred pain syndrome can outlast the initial event, making diagnosis difficult.[13]

This means that almost all chronic pain patients will have some contribution from myofascial component. These trigger points can exist in active or latent states.

DIAGNOSING MYOFASCIAL PAIN

History

This is the most important aspect while dealing with patients presenting with vague pains. A good history will help elicit subtle indicators of myofascial pain. The pain is described as deep, aching and poorly circumscribed. There may be numbness, stiffness, "shifting" of pain, erythema or swelling.[14] Pain can be perpetuated by depression, mental stress, cold-damp weather, sleep disturbance and fatigue.[15] Pain is also felt when muscle is used after a period of inactivity. Pain is aggravated by physical stress on the muscle containing the trigger points. This includes posture, workplace ergonomics, etc.

Examination

A regular physical examination is done. In addition, look for trigger point by palpation, joint dysfunction, posture is examined and restriction of range of motion (ROM) at affected joint is noted. Autonomic features (vasoconstriction, vasodilatation, lacrimation, piloerection) may accompany trigger point. Figures 3A and B shows "swelling" accompanying the trigger point of cervical muscles as well as piloerection.

Jinkins JR, Whittemore AR, and Bradley WG have described a mechanism to explain the autonomic features seen in painful muscles.[16]

All patients should be examined thoroughly to identify underlying serious medical conditions. A good neurological examination, evaluation of posture and biomechanical assessment of joint motion is essential.

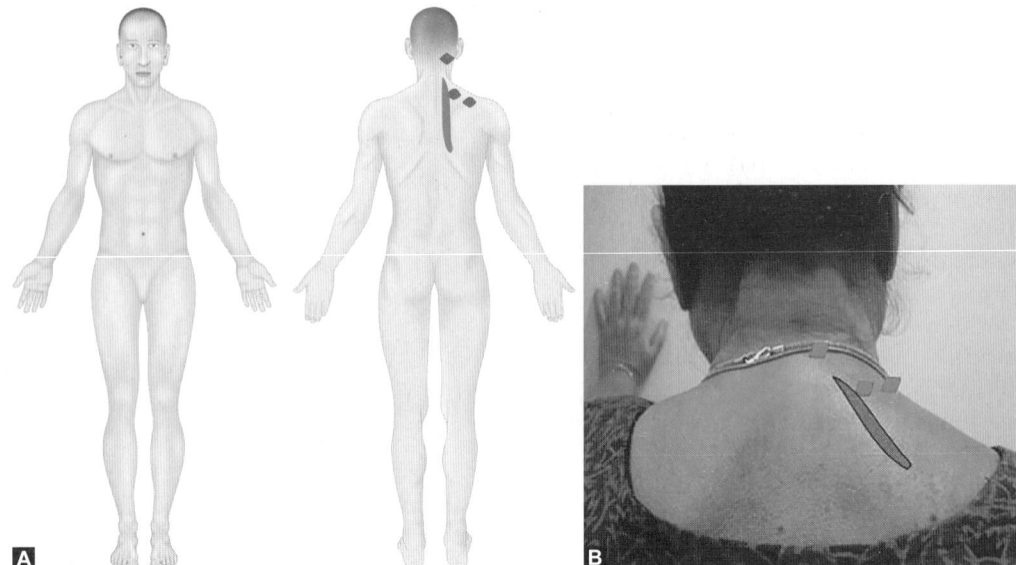

FIGS 3A and B: (A) Line diagram showing Red: Trapezius trigger ares, Blue: levator scapulae trigger point; (B) Patient with visible taut, levator scapulae, trigger point; Taut muscle band visible. referred pain to head, weakness restricted ROM *(For color version, see Plate 11)*

Palpation of trigger points manually is mainly used to arrive at a diagnosis. *Magnetic resonance enterography* (MRE) and ultrasound (USG) may be helpful routine investigations in the future. The muscle is palpated with the flat-palm or by using the "pincer" technique. Prolonged pressure on the trigger will elicit the "jump-sign" where the patient recoils in response to the painful stimulus.

"Red-flags" include[6]
- Central distribution of pain close to the body in neck or shoulder or pelvic areas
- Diffuse spread of muscle pain
- Lack of precipitating factor

Some trigger points may mimic radicular symptoms, e.g. Teres minor trigger may resemble C8 radicular pain, Gluteus minimus trigger may appear like L5 radicular pain, etc.

To give examples of some medical diseases where muscle pain may be seen:
- Diaphragmatic disease like gallstones may present with neck or shoulder pain
- Intra-abdominal diseases like duodenal ulceration, pancreatic cancer (CA-pancreas), etc. may present with low thoracic or lumbar pain
- Heart disease may present with neck or shoulder or arm pain.

Investigations

The diagnosis of myofascial pain is difficult because it is difficult to identify muscle as the primary pain generator with present diagnostic tools. However, now high-resolution USG imaging called US elastography can pick-up trigger point in muscle. Myofascial trigger points are hypoechoic on two dimensional (2D) USG and appear stiffer than the surrounding muscle on vibration sonoelastography. The patients with symptomatic myofascial trigger points have increased tissue heterogeneity at the trigger point site and the surrounding muscle tissue.[17]

A new modality of magnetic resonance imaging (MRI) called magnetic resonance elastography (MRE) can confirm presence of taut bands and decreased elasticity of muscles and can be useful to pick-up trigger point.

DIFFERENTIAL DIAGNOSIS

Initially, myofascial pain with trigger points and fibromyalgia (both present with pain in muscles) were considered to be similar; however, now myofascial pain with trigger points is considered a peripheral pain conditions with wide range of symptoms and hence called a "syndrome".

Fibromyalgia is characterized by widespread pain and tenderness and is described as a central augmentation of nociception giving rise to deep tissue tenderness that includes muscles.

MANAGEMENT

As the cause of MPS is difficult to pin point, there are numerous options and there is no evidence of effect of any one therapy over other for muscle pain.

However, if the patient and physician define their goals of treatment needed and possible respectively, the patient can be helped to a great extent. Patient education about the complex nature of myofascial pain is helpful. This helps reduce disability, guides patient to make correct choice of activities of daily living (ADL) and increase physical activity.[18,19]

The principles of treatment should be:
- Improve functioning
- Avoid precipitating factors
- Cognitive behavior therapy
- Invasive interventional treatment when conservative therapy fails (Dry needling, trigger point injection)
- Preventive measures.

Physical therapy requires a therapist used to deal with chronic pain patients. They can help in trigger point release (myofascial release), breathing exercises, relaxation exercises, electrotherapeutic modality, posture training and physical conditioning[20,21] (Fig. 4).

Available Therapeutic Options[6] (Evidence and Recommendations)

Pharmacologic Treatment of Myofascial Pain

- *Nonsteroidal anti-inflammatory drugs (NSAIDs)*: Though NSAIDs are the most commonly used drugs, there is a lack of strong evidence for the role of an anti-inflammatory in MPS. However, there is clear evidence that the analgesic properties of NSAIDs relieve pain in acute musculoskeletal (MSK) disorders.[22-25]
- *Tramadol:* Though it is effective and well-tolerated in low back pain, some chronic pain syndromes, and osteoarthritis; it is useful in myofascial pain patients due its multimodal analgesic effects and low-abuse potential.[25]
- *Muscle relaxants*
  - Tizanidine is useful for decreasing pain intensity, disability and also improves sleep. Malanga G et al. suggest that tizanidine should be considered as a first-line agent for the treatment of MPS[26]
  - Benzodiazepines cause muscle relaxant effect via the gamma-aminobutyric acid (GABA) inhibitory pathways. But, due to the associated adverse effects, they should be used with caution.[23]
- *Anticonvulsants* are useful in fibromyalgia syndrome (FMS) but, there is no evidence that they are effective for MPS and should be withheld until other interventions have been attempted.[27]

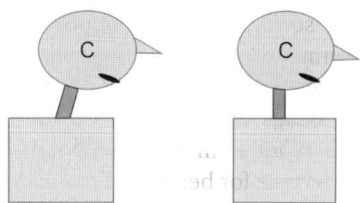

FIG. 4: Posture correction of crane neck

- *Antidepressants* are useful in many painful syndromes. Their pain-mitigating effects are not clear, but it is postulated that tricyclic antidepressants (TCAs) work on central serotonergic and noradrenergic signals, which affect central pain pathways.[28] Currently, there is no indication for the use of these medications in the treatment of MPS; however, the growing body of evidence for their efficacy in chronic pain syndromes suggests an increased role in MPS when conventional treatments fail.[29]
- *Others*:
    - *Botulinum toxin (BoNT)* is a neurotoxin which produces analgesia by decreasing the production of substance P and glutamate. The evidence suggests that BoNT-A injection is a promising therapy to alleviate MPS, especially when it persists despite conservative treatment[30] due to the short-life of its adverse effects.
    - *Ketamine* has insufficient evidence to support its role in MPS.

Nonpharmacologic Treatment Options

- Dry needling (Fig. 5) is an effective treatment and equal in efficacy to trigger point injections, and should be used as the mainstay of acute treatment, despite complaints of postinjection soreness[31,32]
- Manual therapy for local muscle pain
    - Norregaard et al. found that eccentric exercise was helpful for patients presenting with achillodynia or heel pain. This also gave long-term results as seen by marked improvement in symptoms and findings during the 1-year follow-up period.
    - Massage is being favored by patients for relief from myofascial pain. Some evidence for benefits of massage are as follows:

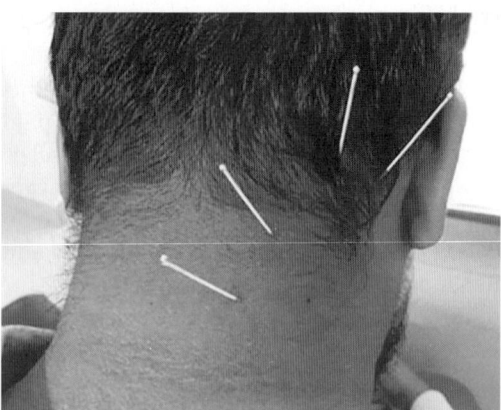

FIG. 5: Dry needling for upper trapezium trigger *(For color version, see Plate 11)*

- Dryden and Moyer immediate and "long-term benefits" have been observed from a series of massage therapy treatments
- "Therapeutic massage can decrease pain, tenderness, and improve range of motion for subacute and chronic neck pain".[33]
- Massage therapy provided by trained massage therapists for chronic, subacute and nonspecific low back pain will alleviate pain, reduce swelling and increase function.[34]
- There is no evidence of effect of electrotherapy, short-wave, USG, laser, injections of steroids or NSAIDs.[35]
- Accupuncture is used by many clinicians but there is contradictory evidence of acupuncture, which should not be used for long-term therapy.[36]
- Transcutaneous electrical nerve stimulation (TENS) is useful as an adjunct therapy to give short-term relief from pain.
- Magnetic stimulation is a newer treatment that is being investigated for MSK pain and MPS.

CONCLUSION

Myofascial pain is a chronic pain that erodes the quality of life and causes a lot of suffering to the patient. Patient education about the condition and helping the patient cope with the condition need an understanding physician and physical therapist trained in chronic pain.

The diverse treatment options are an indicator of the complex pathology of MPS with its underlying central and peripheral neural mechanisms. The goal of the clinician in treating a patient with myofascial pain should focus primarily on identifying and correcting the underlying cause of the symptoms. Medications help to reduce the intensity of pain and physical therapy is essential to rehabilitate and retrain muscles.

ADDENDUM

The author[37] has presented a new observation as a poster presentation at the International Association for the Study of Pain (IASP)-16th World Congress on Pain held at Yokohama in September 2016.

The author has observed that patients presenting with "nonspecific pain", have small discrete, 1–4 mm in diameter, hypo- or depigmented spots (KD-spots 1,2), (KD-spot 3 with corresponding dermatome-MRI) present on the skin surface (Figs 6 to 8). Though these are obviously visible, the patients' themselves were not aware of their existence or the time of origin of the spots. This is not an isolated finding but a recurring observation seen in patients presenting to the pain clinic many of whom responded to physical therapy.

The author has proposed a hypothesis that is yet to be proved based on various reports that have described the morphology and receptive fields of C-polymodal afferent fibers. According to the hypothesis, KD-spots indicate an objective sign of disk pathology which causes sensitization of the somatic nerve with distal effects on the myotome seen as hyperexcitable myofibrils progressing to obvious myofascial trigger points on sustained immunologic or inflammatory stimulation of the *dorsal root ganglion* (DRG) cells with predictable referred pain-patterns.

(If proved, detection of myofascial pain could be possible clinically with a probable diagnosis of somatic origin pain).

The reports of the receptive field of polymodal C-afferent fibers and morphology of nociceptors appear to have features similar to the observations seen:

1. Christenson and Perl in 1970 and Schouenborg and Sjolund in 1983 have reported that many neurons, driven by C-fibers in laminae I and II have small receptive fields on the skin.

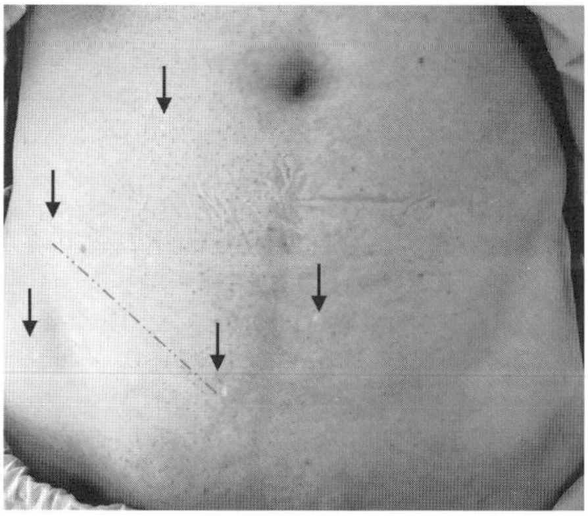

FIG. 6: KD Spots on abdominal dermatomes *(For color version, see Plate 11)*

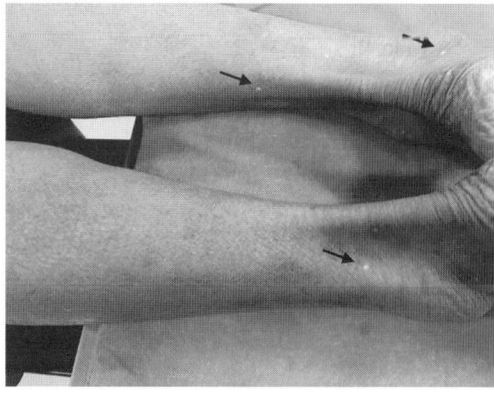

FIG. 7: KD spots *(For color version, see Plate 12)*

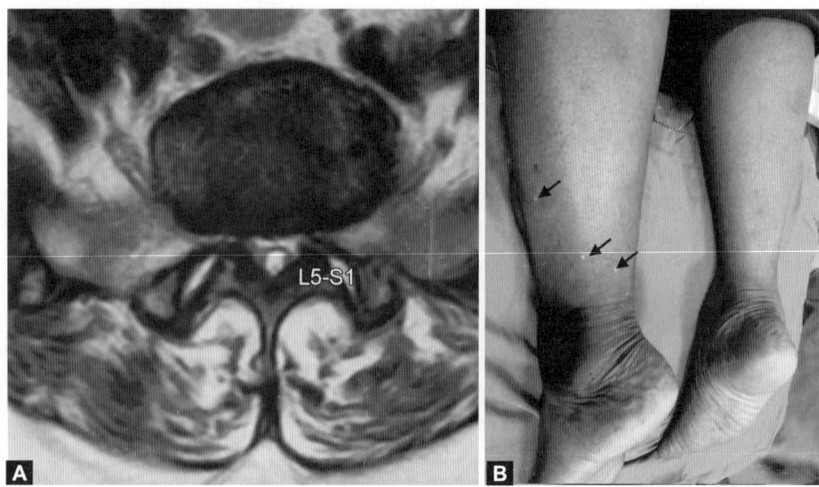

FIGS 8A and B: KD Spots, MRI of L5-S1 *(For color version, see Plate 12)*

2. Other studies have defined the receptive field properties of unmyelinated tactile afferents in the human skin[38,39] and the morphological features of Nociceptive C-afferents from muscle.[37-41]

REFERENCES

1. Simons DG. Orphan organ. J Musculoskel Pain. 2007;15(2):7-9.
2. Cooper G, Bailey B, Bogduk N. Cervical ZA joint pain maps. Pain Med. 2007;8(4):344-53.
3. Kirmayer LJ, Looper KJ. Abnormal illness behavior: physiological, psychological and social dimensions of coping with distress. Curr Opin Psychiatry. 2006;19(1): 54-60.
4. Gunn CC. Radiculopathic pain: Diagnosis and treatment of segmental irritation or sensitization. J Musculoskel Pain. 1997;5(4):119-34.
5. Travell JG, Rinzler SH. The myofascial genesis of Pain. Postgrad Med. 1952;11(5):425-34.
6. Bliddal H. Fundamentals of Musculoskeletal Pain. In: Graven-Nielsen T, Arendt-Nielsen T, Mense S (Eds). Seattle: IASP Press; 2008; Table VII; pp. 342.
7. Chaiamnuay P, Darmawan J, Muirden KD, Assawatanabodee P. Epidemiology of rheumatic disease in rural Thailand: a WHO-ILAR COPCORD study. Community oriented program for the control of Rheumatic Disease. J Rheumatol. 1998;25(7):1382-7.
8. Dommerholt J, Bron C, Franssen JL. Myofascial trigger points: an evidence informed review. J Man Manip Ther. 2006;14(4):203-21.
9. Simons D. Review of enigmatic MTrPs as a common cause of enigmatic musculoskeletal pain and dysfunction. J Electromyogr Kinesiol. 2004;14:95-107.
10. Manolopoulos L, Vlastarakos PV, Georgiou L, Giotakis I, Loizos A. Nikolopoulos TP. Myofascial pain syndromes in the maxillofacial area: a common but underdiagnosed cause of head and neck pain. Int J Oral Maxillofac Surg. 2008;37:975-84.
11. Gerwin RD. A review of myofascial pain and fibromyalgia—factors that promote their persistence. Acupunct Med. 2005;23:121-34.
12. Lavelle ED, Lavelle W, Smith HS. Myofascial trigger points. Med Clin North Am. 2007;91:229-39.
13. Bladry P. Superficial versus deep needling. Acupunct Med. 2002;20:78-81.
14. IASP Subcommittee on taxonomy: Classification of chronic pain, descriptions of chronic pain syndromes and definitions of pain terms. Pain. 1986;3:S1-S225.
15. Simons DG: Muscle Pain syndromes, Part I and II, Am J Phy Med. 1975;54(6);289-311 and part II 1976;55:(1)15-42.
16. Jinkins JR, Whittemore AR, Bradley WG. The anatomic basis of vertebrogenic pain and the autonomic syndrome associated with lumbar disk extrusion. AJR Am J Roentgenol. 1989;152(6):1277-89.
17. Ballyns JJ, Turo D, Otto P, Shah JP, Hammond J, Sikdar S, et al. Office-Based Elastographic Technique for Quantifying Mechanical Properties of Skeletal Muscle
18. J Ultrasound Med. 2012;31(8):1209-19.

19. Bandura A. Self efficacy mechanism in physiological activation and health promoting behavior. In: Madden Jl, Matthysse S, Barchas S (Eds). Adaptation, learning and Affect. New York: Raven Press;1986.
20. Wittink H, Hoskins Michel T. Chronic Pain Management for Physical Therapists. Boston: Butterworth Heinemann; 2002.
21. Banks SL, Jacobs DW, Gevirtz R, Hubbard D. Effects of autogenic relaxation training on electromyographic activity in active myofascial trigger points. J Muscoloskel Pain. 1998;6(4):23-32.
22. Chaitow L. Breathing pattern disorders, motor control, and low back pain. J Osteop Med. 2004;7(1):33-40.
23. Lacey P, Dodd G, Shannon D. A double blind, placebo controlled study of piroxicam in the management of acute musculoskeletal disorders. Eur J Rheumatol inflamm. 1984;7:95-104.
24. Van Tulder M, Koes B, Bouter L. Conservative treatment of acute and chronic nonspecific low back pain: a systematic review of randomized controlled trials of the most common interventions. Spine. 1997;22:2128-56.
25. Amlie E, Weber H, Holme I. Treatment of acute low-back pain with piroxicam: results of a double-blind placebo-controlled trial. Spine. 1987;12:473-6.
26. Borg-Stein J, Simons D. Focused review: Myofascial pain. Arch Phys Med Rehabil. 2002;83(1):540-7.
27. Malanga G, Gwynn M, Smith R, Miller D. Tizanidine is effective in the treatment of myofascial pain syndrome. Pain Physician. 2002;5:422-32.
28. Wiffen P, Collins S, McQuay H, Carrol D, Jadad A, Moore A. Anticonvulsant drugs for acute and chronic pain. Cochrane Database Syst Rev. 2005;20(3):CD001133.
29. Botney M, Fields H. Amitriptyline potentiates morphine analgesia by a direct action on the central nervous system. Ann Neurol. 1983;13:160-4.
30. Desai MJ, Saini V, Saini S. Myofascial Pain Syndrome: A Treatment Review. Pain and Therapy. 2013;2(1):21-36.
31. Sławek J, Madali ski M, Maciag-Tymecka I, Duzynski W. Frequency of side effects after botulinum toxin A injections in neurology, rehabilitation and gastroenterology. Pol Merkur Lekarski. 2005;18:298-302.
32. Borg-Stein J. Treatment of fibromyalgia, myofascial pain, and related disorders. Phys Med Rehabil Clin N Am. 2006;17:491-510.
33. Edwards J, Knowles N. Superficial dry needling and active stretching in the treatment of myofascial pain: a randomised control trial. Acupunct Med. 2003;21:80-6.
34. Brosseau L, Wells G, Tugwell P, Casimiro L, Novikov, M, Loew L, et al. Ottawa panel evidence-based clinical practice guidelines on therapeutic massage for neck pain. J Bodyw Mov Ther. 16(3),300-25.
35. Gam A, Johanssen F. Ultrasound therapy in muscoloskeletal disorders: a meta-analysis. Pain. 1995;63: 85-91.
36. Furlan AD, et al. Spine. 2005;30(8):pp. 944-63.
37. PAIN Reports: November/December 2016 - Volume 1 - Issue 5 - p e581.
38. Moyer C, Rounds J, Hannum J. A meta-analysis of massage therapy research. Psychol Bull. 2004;130:3-18.
39. Liljencrantz J, Olausson H. Tactile C fibers and their contributions to pleasant sensations and to tactile allodynia. Frontiers in Behavioral Neuroscience. 2014;8: 37.
40. Wessberg J, Olausson H, Fernström KW, Vallbo AB. Receptive field properties of unmyelinated tactile afferents in the human skin. J Neurophysiol. 2003;89(3):1567-75.
41. Bessou P, Perl ER. Response of cutaneous sensory units with unmyelinated fibers to noxious stimuli. J Neurophysiol. 1969;32:1025-43.

CHAPTER 36

Fibromyalgia: Causes and Pain Management

Muralidhar Joshi

INTRODUCTION

Fibromyalgia is a chronic clinical condition of unknown etiology which represents with generalized pain with fatigue and sleep disturbances. The condition is known to affect 2% of general population. Up to 70% of patients with fibromyalgia meet the criteria for a depressive or anxiety disorder. People often report high disability levels and poor health-related quality of life.

HISTORY

In 1904, the British neurologist Gowers coined the term fibrositis to describe a persistent form of lumbago. Later, in 1976, Hench introduced the term fibromyalgia to emphasize soft tissue pain as the main clinical feature. Smythe is recognized for his emphasis on tender points in discrete locations as aids to the diagnosis of fibromyalgia. Each of these tender points was locally tender with pressure but did not refer pain as did the trigger points of the myofascial syndrome. In 1990, a multicenter study of patients with fibromyalgia, supervised by the American College of Rheumatology (ACR), resulted in the statistical development of research criteria for the classification of fibromyalgia based on widespread pain and multiple soft tissue tender points.[1-5]

EPIDEMIOLOGY

This disorder has been found in both developed and developing countries. It has a prevalence of 2-12% in the general population.[6] Its prevalence increases with age, most dramatically in women, with a peak in seventh decade. The risk factors for its development include physical trauma, a febrile illness or a family history of fibromyalgia.

Diagnosis is made between the ages of 20 years and 50 years (Stefano Coaccioli et al. 2008).[7] High incidence is seen in female sex and being divorced. Failing to complete high school and low income are also associated with the demographic and social profile.

Psychological factors associated with this syndrome include somatization disorder, anxiety, and personal or family history of depression. 80% of these patients also fulfill the criteria for chronic fatigue syndrome. 70% of these patients have headaches, 75% temporomandibular joint disorders and 60% irritable bowel symptoms.[8] Fibromyalgia is also more common in relatives of patients with fibromyalgia, suggesting that there is contribution of both genetic and environmental factors.[9]

PATHOLOGY

The cause of fibromyalgia is unknown. It is not a form of arthritis nor is it associated with inflammation.[3] It is a form of soft tissue rheumatism, a broad term including a group of disorders that cause pain and stiffness around the joints, and in muscles and bones. Of late certain evidences are available to suggest that fibromyalgia is a disorder of abnormal processing of sensory information within the central nervous system, and it exhibits a limited array of recognized objective physiological and biological abnormalities. Functional brain mapping techniques have supported this conclusion.[10] One of the most commonly noted abnormalities is elevated level of substance P in the cerebrospinal fluid (CSF) of affected individuals.[11] About one-third of fibromyalgia patients report that one of the family members was suffering from similar disorder. There are many studies talking about neuroendocrine, neurotransmitter and neurosensory dysfunctions in fibromyalgia. A lot of them need validation in the long run.

CLINICAL FEATURES

It presents with varied symptoms like headache, anxiety, depression, paresthesia and various complaints which do not fit into any particular systems.

SYMPTOMS

The region-wise[2] generalized body pain is main symptom which is in form of fatigue; disturbances of sleep, feeling tired,[3] mood alteration[4] exhaustion may be associated with flu,[4] headache and abdominal pain.

SIGNS

The result of a general physical examination is usually normal and individual may look healthy; a specific examination of the muscles of people with fibromyalgia reveals tender areas at locations known as tender points.[12] The presence of these characteristic tender points separates fibromyalgia from other conditions.

A tender point on one side of the body usually has a matching tender point in the same place on the opposite side of the body. Although the tender points are common, many other muscles and areas of soft tissue can be sites of pain as well. People often will not be aware of the exact location or even the presence of these tender points until doctor performs a tender point examination.

In 1990, the ACR gave criteria to diagnose fibromyalgia. A person has fibromyalgia if he or she has a history of widespread pain of at least 3 months' duration and pain in at least 11 of 18 specific tender point sites to a standard force of 4 kg of digital palpation. That amount of pressure can be standardized against an algometer, but a reasonably accurate clinical estimate of the correct amount of pressure can be obtained by pressing the examining thumb against a surface until the blood flow to the mid-portion of the thumb nail blanches.

LIMITATIONS

There are certain limitations to ACR definition for fibromyalgia which are as mentioned here:
- If a patient is having a good day or bad day, variation is not considered. No objective measurements exist.
- Can the pain be regional, as in complex regional pain syndrome (CRPS)? The guidelines do not address associated symptoms or severity of the symptoms other than pain may be present.

MANAGEMENT

Most often the diagnosis is clinical[13] as no laboratory tests or X-ray that can help the diagnosis. But laboratory tests can help to rule it out. For example, hypothyroidism can cause many symptoms of fibromyalgia; one can always get a thyroid profile to rule out the problem. Because the complaints of fibromyalgia are so general and often bring to mind other medical disorders, many people undergo complicated and often repeated evaluations before they are diagnosed with fibromyalgia.[14] It is difficult to achieve complete resolution of symptoms, but always should be aimed at controlling symptoms.

INVESTIGATIONS

All investigations like biochemical, hematological, radiological and components might be normal if there are no comorbid conditions. As of now, there are no specific genetic markers for fibromyalgia.

TREATMENT

By now we know fibromyalgia is characterized by persistent, widespread pain and tenderness, sleep problems and fatigue. Common pain-relieving medicines such as paracetamol and ibuprofen are not usually considered effective, though they can be used as rescue analgesics. Medicines used to treat epilepsy or depression can be effective in some people with fibromyalgia and other forms of chronic (persistent, long-lasting) pain where there may be nerve damage. We are yet to arrive at a standardization to manage fibromyalgia. Currently we are working on general guidelines for treatment.

Nonpharmacological Treatment

Counseling

Patient has to be counseled about the problem and the preventive measures to be taken. Education about fibromyalgia and coping strategies are very important.

Exercises

Low-impact exercises to start with like walking, cycling, swimming and physical exercises every other day. In the beginning, start with about 5 minutes three times a day, to get a total of 15 minutes for that day. Over a period of time, try to extend the endurance part of exercise program to get a total of 30 minutes each day for exercise. Lot of these aerobics, strength, flexibility and endurance has been evaluated.

Relaxation Techniques

It is to ease muscle tension and anxiety. Stress management techniques such as alternating periods of activity with periods of rest and breathing exercises will help control the feelings of anger, sadness and panic. The variety of functions, such as pain, tenderness and muscle strength in female patients the evidence is moderate to high intensity resistance training, where to aerobic exercises for 8 weeks the evidence was superior.[15] In comparison to usual care the psychological interventions improves physical functioning but it has low quality evidence and needs further research.

Mind and Body Therapy

Posture and body alignment work goes a long way in improving things. The psychological interventions therapies may be effective in improving physical functioning, pain and low mood for adults with fibromyalgia in comparison to usual care controls but the quality of the evidence is low. Further research on the outcomes of therapies is needed to determine if positive effects identified post-intervention are sustained. The effectiveness of biofeedback, mindfulness, movement therapies and relaxation based therapies remains unclear as the quality of the evidence was very low or low. The small number of trials and inconsistency in the use of outcome measures across the trials restricted the analysis.[16]

Aquatic Exercise Training for Fibromyalgia

Low-to-moderate quality evidence relative to control suggests that aquatic training is beneficial for improving wellness, symptoms and fitness in adults with fibromyalgia. Lowest quality evidence suggests that there are benefits of aquatic and land-based exercise, except in muscle strength (very low quality evidence favoring land). No serious adverse effects were reported.[17]

Cognitive Behavioral Therapy

Cognitive behavioral therapies (CBTs) provided a small incremental benefit over control interventions in reducing pain, negative mood and disability at the end of treatment and at long-term follow-up. The dropout rates due to any reason did not differ between CBTs and controls.[18]

Tips to Get Sound Sleep

- Do not sleep during daytime. Avoid exercise, alcohol, caffeine and tobacco at least 3 hours before going to bed
- Do not watch TV, read or work in bed
- Sleep at same time each night and get up at same time in the morning
- Sleep only in a bed
- Relax during weekend period.

Pharmacological Treatment

Medications to Diminish Pain

- Nonsteroidal anti-inflammatory drugs (NSAIDs), paracetamol, tramadol 50 mg BID/TID
- *Cannabinoids for fibromyalgia*: We found no convincing, unbiased, high quality evidence suggesting that nabilone is of value in treating people with fibromyalgia. The tolerability of nabilone was low in people with fibromyalgia.[19]
- *Oxycodone for fibromyalgia*: There is no randomized trial evidence to support or refute the suggestion that oxycodone, alone or in combination with naloxone, reduces pain in fibromyalgia.[20]

Other Medications Used

- *Anxiolytics*: Tablet alprazolam 0.25–0.5 mg HS or clonazepam 1.0 mg HS (this Cochrane review of 2012 uncovered no evidence of sufficient quality to support the use of clonazepam in chronic neuropathic pain or fibromyalgia).[21]
- *Antidepressants*: Tablet amitriptyline 10–25 mg HS (amitriptyline has been a first-line treatment for fibromyalgia for many years. The fact that there is no supportive unbiased evidence for a beneficial effect is disappointing, but has to be balanced against years of successful treatment in many patients with fibromyalgia. There is no good evidence of a lack of effect; rather our concern should be of overestimation of treatment effect. Amitriptyline will be one option in the treatment of fibromyalgia, while recognizing that only a minority of patients will achieve satisfactory pain relief. It is unlikely that any large randomized trials of amitriptyline will be conducted in fibromyalgia to establish efficacy statistically or measure the size of the effect).[22]
- *Selective serotonin reuptake inhibitors (SSRIs)*: Fluoxetine (10–20 mg/day), paroxetine, citalopram, escitalopram and sertraline (there is no unbiased evidence that SSRIs are superior to placebo in treating the key symptoms of fibromyalgia, namely pain, fatigue and sleep problems. Selective serotonin reuptake inhibitors (SSRIs) might be considered for treating depression in people with fibromyalgia. The black box warning for increased suicidal tendency in young adults aged 18–24 years, with major depressive disorder, who have taken SSRIs, should be considered when appropriate).[23]
- *Balanced serotonin and noradrenaline reuptake inhibitors*: Duloxetine 20–30 mg/day [approved by Food and Drug Administration (FDA) in 2008]. Some studies show that duloxetine dose of 60 mg and 120 mg is effective for pain relief in diabetic neuropathy with minor side effects.[24] The combination of duloxetine 20 mg with pregabalin is effective in neuropathic pain.

- *Noradrenalin-enhanced and serotonin reuptake inhibitors*: Milnacipran (approved by FDA in 2009). Milnacipran 100–200 mg is effective for relief of pain as compared to placebo. In higher doses, milnacipran has more adverse events and withdrawals.[25]

The duloxetine and milnacipran has some benefit to placebo in relief of pain where as it did not help in reducing fatigue and improvement in quality of life. The post withdrawal symptoms includes nausea, dry mouth, constipation, headache and insomnia. Rarely suicidal tendency, liver damage, abnormal bleeding, high blood pressure and urinary hesitation are reported.[26]

- *Serotonin receptor antagonists*: Tropisetron
- *Alpha-2 adrenergic agonists*: Tizanidine
- 5-hydroxytryptophan
- *Anticonvulsants*: Gabapentin (900–3,600 mg), pregabalin (75–600 mg).

The gabapentin in 1200 mg was effective in some neuropathic pain and in 50% cases it reduced sleep disturbance, fatigue and depression.

It also improved quality of life, function and work and it is observed that gabapentin is effective in postherpetic neuralgia and diabetic neuropathy.[27]

In some neuropathic pain conditions, gabapentin and pregabalin only help in pain relief. In some patients, antiepileptics other than gabapentin and pregabalin is beneficial. These strategies rather than interventions produce pain relief for short duration and are cost-effective.[28]

[The anticonvulsant, pregabalin (approved by FDA in 2007), demonstrated a small benefit over placebo in reducing pain and sleep problems. Pregabalin use was shown not to substantially reduce fatigue compared with placebo. Study dropout rates due to adverse events were higher with pregabalin use compared with placebo. Dizziness was a particularly frequent adverse event seen with pregabalin use. At the time of writing this review, pregabalin is the only anticonvulsant drug approved for treating fibromyalgia in the US and in 25 other non-European countries. However, pregabalin has not been approved for treating fibromyalgia in Europe. The amount and quality of evidence were insufficient to draw definite conclusions on the efficacy and safety of gabapentin, lacosamide and levetiracetam in fibromyalgia].[29]

- *Muscle relaxants*: Benzodiazepines, methocarbamol and baclofen
- *NMDA receptor antagonists*: Ketamine and dextromethorphan
- Local anesthetics as trigger point injections
- *Lignocaine infusion*: About 5 mg/kg over 60 minutes. It can be repeated 3–4 times.
- *Acupuncture*: This technique is debated for years together to establish its role in fibromyalgia.

When compared with no treatment, standard therapy, acupuncture for improvement in pain and stiffness the level of evidence is low to moderate.

To reduce pain, stiffness and fatigue and for improvement in global well-being, sleep the electrical acupuncture is probably better than mechanical evidence. The larger studies are warranted.[30]

Some of the refractory trigger points, which are widespread, might respond to injection of botulinum toxin type A. This toxin is derived from Clostridium botulinum. It is a di-chain polypeptide, which reduces muscle tone when injected into spastic and hypertrophic muscle. Usually, 5–10 units are injected at each trigger point and maximum up to 300 units. Each trigger part injected with 1 mL solution containing 10 units of toxin. The drug should not be repeated before 3–6 months for fear of antibodies formation.

Sometimes the tender points themselves become trigger points for pain.[31] The impulse arising from these points bombard the central nervous system to produce local or referred pain or both and the associated effects in the area of reference or activation. Trigger point injection gives many people good relief from pain for very long duration. If necessary, the trigger point injection can be done at weekly intervals. The injections usually consist of depot Medrol 40–80 mg with 0.5% bupivacaine. During the post injection period, patient might complain of slight discomfort at the site of injection. Reassurance is sufficient. As soon as the trigger point is reached with the needle, many patients complain of relief from pain. Sometimes daily needling also gives relief from trigger point pain.

Recent thinking has been about infusion of lignocaine 5 mg/kg over 60 minutes for three consecutive days. This is supposed to suppress both injury-induced nociception and secondary wind-up sensitization of wide dynamic range neurons in the dorsal column of the spinal cord. There has been suggestion about use of N-Methyl-D-aspartate (NMDA) receptor antagonists like dextromethorphan and ketamine; other drugs like alpha-2 adrenergic agonists (tizanidine) can be used for spasmolysis in fibromyalgia.

Fortunately, fibromyalgia is not a life-threatening problem and does not lead to deformity. Although symptoms may vary in intensity, the overall condition rarely worsens over time.

Newer Strategies

There are many studies which are going through protocols to establish or re-establish certain hypothesis which might have long-term implications in proving or disproving certain hypotheses. Some of them are as follows:
- Transcutaneous electrical nerve stimulation (TENS) for fibromyalgia[32]
- Gabapentin for fibromyalgia in adults[33]
- Combination pharmacotherapy for the treatment of fibromyalgia[34]
- Oral NSAIDs for fibromyalgia[35]
- Probiotics for fibromyalgia.[36]

CONCLUSION

The evidence for any particular treatment of fibromyalgia syndrome is difficult to assess. The diversity of symptoms and the number of potential outcome measurements that could be made mean that it is difficult to interpret the data from randomized controlled trials. Formal psychosocial and functional assessment with appropriate cognitive/behavioral approaches may be required for patients who do not respond to the measures outlined above.

REFERENCES

1. Wolfe F, Smythe HA, Yunus MB, Bennett RM, Bombardier C, Goldenberg DL, et al. The American College of Rheumatology 1990 Criteria for the Classification of Fibromyalgia. Report of the Multicenter Criteria Committee. Arthritis Rheum. 1990;33:160-172.
2. Reynolds MD. The development of the concept of fibrositis. J Hist Med Allied Sci. 1983;38:5-35.
3. Simons DG. Muscle pain syndromes—Part 2. Am J Phys Med. 1976;55;15-42.
4. Smythe H. Fibrositis syndrome: a historical perspective. J Rheumatol Suppl. 1989;19:2-6.
5. Wallace DJ. Fibromyalgia: unusual historical aspects and new pathogenic insights. Mt Sinai J Med. 1984;51:124-31.
6. Wolfe F, Ross K, Anderson J, Russell IJ, Hebert L. The prevalence and characteristics of fibromyalgia in the general population. Arthritis Rheum. 1995;38;19-28.
7. White KP, Speechley M, Hart M, Ostbye T. The London Fibromyalgia Epidemiology Study: the prevalence of fibromyalgia syndrome in London, Ontario. J Rheumatol.1999;26:1570-6.
8. Aaron LA, Burke MM, Buchwald D. Overlapping conditions among patients with chronic fatigue syndrome, fibromyalgia and temporomandibular disorders. Arch Intern Med. 2000;160:221-7.
9. Neumann L, Buskila D. Epidemiology of fibromyalgia. Curr Pain Headache Rep. 2003;7:362-8.
10. Mountz JM, Bradley LA, Modell JG, Alexander RW, Triana-Alexander M, Aaron LA, et al. Fibromyalgia in women. Abnormalities of regional cerebral blood flow in the thalamus and the caudate nucleus are associated with low pain threshold levels. Arthritis Rheum. 1995;38;926-38.

11. Russell IJ. Advances in fibromyalgia: possible role for central neurochemicals. Am J Med Sci. 1998;315: 377-84.
12. Fam AG, Smythe HA. Musculoskeletal chest wall pain. Can Med Assoc J. 1985;133:379-89.
13. Calabro JJ, Jeghers H, Miller KA, et al. Classification of anterior chest wall syndromes. JAMA. 1980;243:1420-1.
14. Kraft GH, Johnson EW, LaBan MM. The fibrositis syndrome. Arch Phys Med Rehabil. 1968;49:155-62.
15. Busch AJ, Webber SC, Richards RS, Bidonde J, Schachter CL, Schafer LA, et al. Resistance exercise training for fibromyalgia. Cochrane Database Syst Rev. 2013;12:CD010884.
16. Theadom A, Cropley M, Smith HE, Feigin VL, McPherson K. Mind and body therapy for fibromyalgia. Cochrane Database Syst Rev. 2015;4:CD001980.
17. Bidonde J, Busch AJ, Webber SC, Schachter CL, Danyliw A, Overend TJ, et al. Aquatic exercise training for fibromyalgia. Cochrane Database Syst Rev. 2014; 10:CD011336.
18. Bernardy K, Klose P, Busch AJ, Choy EHS, Häuser W. Cognitive behavioural therapies for fibromyalgia. Cochrane Database Syst Rev. 2013;9:CD009796.
19. Walitt B, Klose P, Fitzcharles MA, Phillips T, Häuser W. Cannabinoids for fibromyalgia. Cochrane Database Syst Rev. 2016;7:CD011694.
20. Gaskell H, Moore RA, Derry S, Stannard C. Oxycodone for pain in fibromyalgia in adults. Cochrane Database Syst Rev. 2016;9:CD012329.
21. Corrigan R, Derry S, Wiffen PJ, Moore RA. Clonazepam for neuropathic pain and fibromyalgia in adults. Cochrane Database Syst Rev. 2012;5:CD009486.
22. Moore RA, Derry S, Aldington D, Cole P, Wiffen PJ. Amitriptyline for fibromyalgia in adults. Cochrane Database Syst Rev. 2015;7:CD011824.
23. Walitt B, Urrútia G, Nishishinya MB, Cantrell SE, Häuser W. Selective serotonin reuptake inhibitors for fibromyalgia syndrome. Cochrane Database Syst Rev. 2015;6:CD011735.
24. Lunn MP, Hughes RA, Wiffen PJ. Duloxetine for treating painful neuropathy, chronic pain or fibromyalgia. Cochrane Database Syst Rev. 2014;1:CD007115.
25. Cording M, Derry S, Phillips T, Moore RA, Wiffen PJ. Milnacipran for pain in fibromyalgia in adults. Cochrane Database Syst Rev. 2015;10:CD008244.
26. Häuser W, Urrútia G, Tort S, Üçeyler N, Walitt B. Serotonin and noradrenaline reuptake inhibitors (SNRIs) for fibromyalgia syndrome. Cochrane Database Syst Rev. 2013;1:CD010292.
27. Moore RA, Wiffen PJ, Derry S, Toelle T, Rice ASC. Gabapentin for chronic neuropathic pain and fibromyalgia in adults. Cochrane Database Syst Rev. 2014;4: CD007938.
28. Wiffen PJ, Derry S, Moore RA, Aldington D, Cole P, Rice AS, et al. Antiepileptic drugs for neuropathic pain and fibromyalgia—an overview of Cochrane reviews. Cochrane Database Syst Rev. 2013;11:CD010567.
29. Üçeyler N, Sommer C, Walitt B, Häuser W. Anticonvulsants for fibromyalgia. Cochrane Database Syst Rev. 2013;10: CD010782.
30. Deare JC, Zheng Z, Xue CC, Liu JP, Shang J, Scott SW, et al. Acupuncture for treating fibromyalgia. Cochrane Database Syst Rev. 2013;5:CD007070.
31. Smythe HA. Non-articular rheumatism and the fibrositis syndrome. In: Hollander JL, Mc Carty DJ (Eds). Arthritis and Allied Conditions, 8th edition. Philadelphia: Lea and Febiger; 1972.
32. Johnson MI, Claydon LS, Herbison GP, Paley CA, Jones G. Transcutaneous Electrical Nerve Stimulation (TENS) for fibromyalgia in adults (Protocol). Cochrane Database Syst Rev. 2016;4:CD012172.
33. Cooper TE, Moore RA, Derry S, Wiffen PJ. Gabapentin for fibromyalgia pain in adults (Protocol). Cochrane Database Syst Rev. 2016;5:CD012188.
34. Gilron I, Shum B, Moore RA, Wiffen PJ. Combination pharmacotherapy for the treatment of fibromyalgia (Protocol). Cochrane Database Syst Rev. 2013;6: CD010585.
35. Derry S, Wiffen PJ, Häuser W, Mücke M, Tölle TR, Bell RF, et al. Oral nonsteroidal anti-inflammatory drugs for fibromyalgia in adults (Protocol). Cochrane Database Syst Rev. 2016;8:CD012332.
36. Supraha V, Francis DK, Utrobicic A, Choy EH, Tenzera D, Kordic A. Probiotics for fibromyalgia (Protocol). Cochrane Database Syst Rev. 2013;3:CD010451.

SECTION 11

Scar Pain

Post-herniorrhaphy Pain and Its Management

Lakshmi C Vas

INTRODUCTION

Hernia is common anatomical problem that has the potential to lead to serious complications. Surgical repair provides a definitive solution irrespective of the type of hernia or its anatomical origin.[1] Hernia repair forms about 10–15% of all planned general surgical procedures.[2] The annual number of hernia repairs is over 20 million across the world.[3] Inguinal hernias occur in about 15% of adult men and hernioplasty is the most common procedure performed by general surgeons. Females have a lesser incidence of inguinal hernia probably because of a stronger inguinal anatomy.[4]

A serious long term problem of hernia surgery appears to be chronic post surgical pain (CPSP) known as chronic postoperative inguinal pain (CPIP) syndrome.[5-7] An incidence of 0–54% up to 63% has been reported for CPIP 1 year after hernia repair[8-11] and with a cumulative prevalence of 30% at 3 years postoperatively. About 2–25 % of patients report that the pain is severe enough to interfere with activities of daily life.[12] Certain risk factors for CPSP have been reported in young patients, women, patients perceiving intense preoperative pain, patients with postoperative infection or hematoma, patients with tendency to develop anxiety and depression, and patients with previous history of high sensibility to nociceptive pain. Recurrent hernia repair, day care surgery, delayed onset of symptoms and high pain scores in the first week of surgery were also identified to be risk factors for the development of chronic pain.[13]

Chronic postoperative inguinal pain is characterized by persistent pain in and around the surgical incision (Fig. 1), of at least 2–3 months duration after surgery. There are

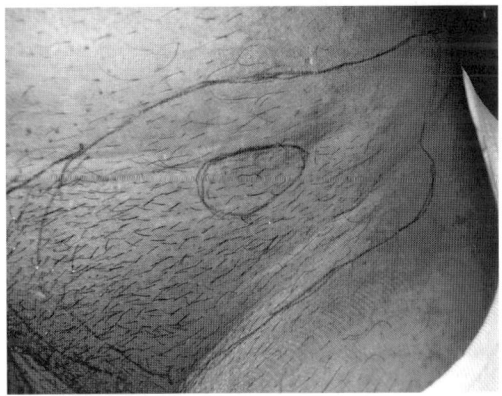

FIG. 1: Pain distribution in a patient with post-hernioplasty pain (laparoscopic). He had maximum pain (8–9/10 NRS) and allodynia in the small circular area marked next to the surgical scar. The surrounding areas including the root of penis and scrotum had pain of 6–7/10 NRS *(For color version, see Plate 12)*

few studies that have explored the natural course of CPSP which may progress as well as regress with time.

The acute postoperative pain following herniorrhaphy is a physiological reaction to tissue trauma and comprises nociceptive or inflammatory pain due to visceral or somatic tissue irritation/damage from surgical dissection, sutures, or application of meshes. Pains caused by mechanical compression or tension that follow the acute phase may gradually decrease with time as a result of tissue rearrangement. Thus nociceptive pain is expected to be self limiting.

Nerve lesions causing neuropathy play a major role in the development of persistent pain following hernia repair. Approximately 30% of post-herniorrhaphy pain is neuropathic[14,15] and overall, 1% of patients who undergo hernia repair will need to be referred to a chronic pain specialist for management.[7]

Neuropathic pain is a type of pain that results from a disturbance in the nerve, including injury to the nerves with later nerve regeneration. Inflammatory reaction of the healing tissues around the nerve causing nerve entrapment or an entrapment within surgical sutures, chronic inflammation, tension or local compression from a dislocated mesh ("meshoma") can all cause neuropathic pain.[16] Neuropathic pain is typically located in the distribution of ilioinguinal (II), iliohypogastric (IH), genital branch of the genitofemoral (GF) nerve (Fig. 1), and, rarely, the lateral femoral cutaneous nerve distributions.[17]

Standardized tools for assessment of post-operative pain include the Brief Pain Inventory and Short Form McGill Pain Questionnaire. There are also instruments specifically aimed at assessing post-herniorrhaphy pain, including the Carolina Comfort Scale[18] and Inguinal Pain Questionnaire.[19]

To understand the pathogenesis of CPIP in its entirety it is necessary to understand the anatomical as well as and neuroanatomical implications of hernia surgery, the implications of the altered pathophysiology leading to peripheral and central sensitization.

ANATOMY OF INGUINAL CANAL

The canal is simply the medial half of the thickened lower free edge of the external oblique aponeurosis (also known as the inguinal ligament), which curls back on itself to form a gutter that is U-shaped in cross-section. The inguinal gutter contains the round ligament in females and spermatic cord, its fascial coverings in males. The spermatic cord contents include ductus (vas) deferens and its artery, testicular artery and pampiniform plexus, genital branch of genitofemoral (GF) nerve, lymphatic vessels and sympathetic nerve fibers, fat and connective tissue. The II nerve runs along the front of the cord.

Conceptually, the fascial arrangements in the region reflect the passage of the testis, spermatic cord (or round ligament), and neurovascular structures through the muscular and fascial layers of the anterior abdominal wall during fetal life. These structures pass through the deep inguinal ring (which lies about halfway along the posterior wall of the ligament, lateral to the inferior epigastric artery), traverse the canal, and emerge through the superficial inguinal ring (superior and medial to the pubic tubercle). The fascial coverings are extensions of external oblique aponeurosis (external spermatic fascia), internal oblique (cremasteric muscle and fascia), and transverses abdominis and transversalis fascia (internal spermatic fascia).

NEUROANATOMY OF ILIOINGUI-NAL NERVE

It is the inferior branch of anterior division of L1 after it receives branches from T12 (subcostal nerve). It emerges from the lateral border of the psoas major, and passes obliquely across the quadratus lumborum and iliacus. The II nerve then perforates the transversus abdominis near the anterior part of the iliac crest, and

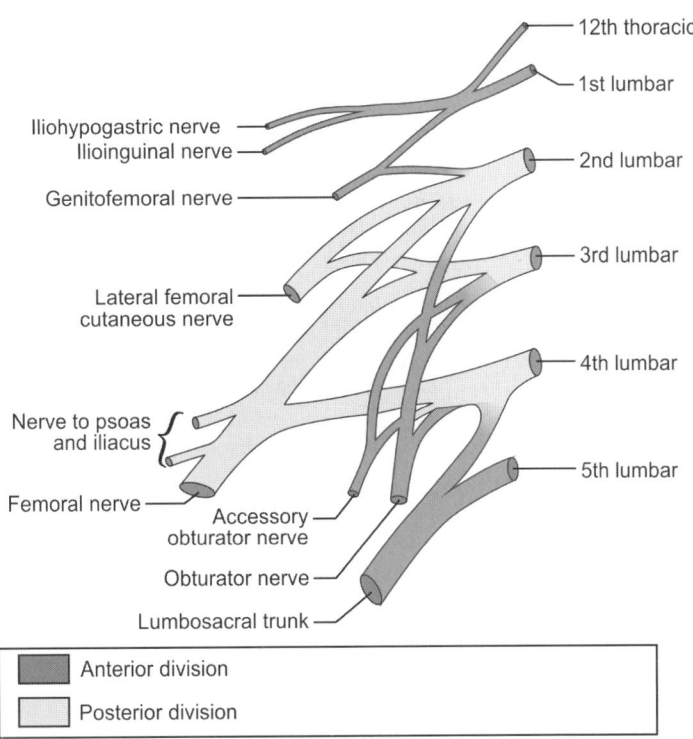

FIG. 2: Illustrates the nerves of the lumbar plexus. Both ilioinguinal and Iliohypogastric nerves arise from T12 and L1 and the genitofemoral from the L1-2 nerve roots
(*Courtesy:* Figs 3 and 4 drawing by Dr KS Waghmare, postgraduate fellow in chronic pain medicine at Ashirvad Institute for Pain Management and Research)

communicates with the iliohypogastric (IH) nerve between the transversus and the obliquus internus. It then pierces the obliquus internus, distributing filaments to it, and then accompanies the spermatic cord through the superficial inguinal ring. Its fibers are then distributed to the skin of the upper and medial part of the thigh, and to the following locations in the male and female (which corresponds to the pain distribution of CPIP (Fig. 1).
- *In the male (anterior scrotal nerve)*: To the skin over the root of the penis and upper part of the scrotum.
- *In the female (anterior labial nerve)*: To the skin covering the mons pubis and labium majus.
- Variations.

The II nerve may not pass through the deep inguinal ring, only travelling through part of the inguinal canal. The size of this nerve is in inverse proportion to that of the IH nerve. occasionally it nerve may be altogether absent or be very small, and ends by joining the IH; in such cases, a branch from the IH takes the place of the II.

NEUROANATOMY OF ILIOHYPO-GASTRIC NERVE (FIG. 2)

The IH nerve is the superior branch of the anterior ramus of spinal nerve L1 which also receives fibers from T12 (subcostal nerve). It emerges from the upper part of the lateral border of the psoas major, and crosses

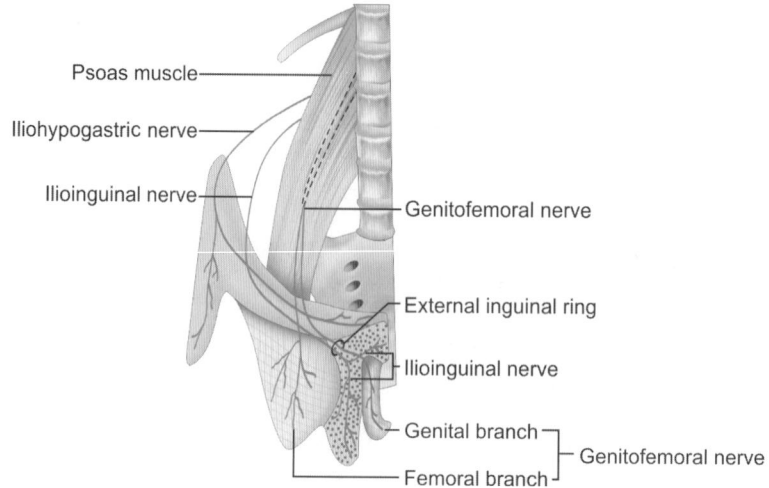

FIG. 3: Illustrations of the inguinal nerves and their dermatomal distribution which is also likely to be the area of pain referral in postherniplasty pain. The GFN arising from L1 and L2 roots, pierces the psoas muscle, and divides into the genital and femoral branches. The genital branch travels along with the ilioinguinal nerve in the inguinal canal and there is an overlap sensory distribution along the medial aspect of the thigh and scrotum. The femoral branch travels more laterally, piercing the fascia lata to travel within the femoral sheath, and supply cutaneous sensation to the anterior aspect of the upper thigh, over the femoral triangle. There is an overlap of sensory distribution with the iliohypogastric nerve also in the inguinal region but the area over the gluteus medius is supplied solely by the iliohypogastric nerve. [Copied with permission from Wiley Publishers.][35]

obliquely in front of the quadratus lumborum to the iliac crest. Running posterior to the kidneys, it then perforates the posterior part of the transversus abdominis, near the crest of the ilium, and divides between that muscle and the obliquus internus abdominis into a lateral and an anterior cutaneous branch. It provides sensory innervation to the skin over the lateral gluteal region and above the pubis. Its motor fibers supply the internal and transverse abdominal muscles (Fig. 3).

GENITOFEMORAL NERVE

This nerve originates in the first and second lumbar nerves, passing over the psoas major before splitting into two branches which innervate 2 different areas. One branch, the femoral branch, heads to the femoral triangle in the upper inner thigh. The genital branch innervates the genital area. The area of innervation is the same as the name genito- femoral suggests (Fig. 3).[20]

Chronic postsurgical pain is marked by hypersensitivity to painful stimuli around a localized site, and also is felt in noninjured areas nearby. When a patient undergoes surgery, tissues and nerve endings are traumatized, resulting in incision pain. Neuropathic pain may involve actual anatomical injury to the nervous system as in axonal damage, local neuritis, atrophy, altered Schwann cell activity, etc. or as a physiological insult which initiates an alteration of the plasticity of the nervous system. After the initial injury, C-fibers have 1–2% spontaneous activity in the first week increasing to 4–6% by one month.[21] This afferent bombardment of the spinal cord sets up a central neuroplasticity phenomenon which keeps the pain cycle going on which contributes to chronicity with overloading of messages to the spinal cord, which becomes over stimulated. The resultant central sensitization is a type of post-traumatic stress to the spinal cord, which interprets any stimulation, painful or otherwise as unpleasant. In addition, the central neuronal plasticity recruits the adjacent areas of the spinal cord which provides neurons for the surrounding nerves in the incision area.[22] That is why a patient may feel pain on physical touch in locations far from the surgical site.

Mild neural insult might spontaneously recover during the usual postoperative period. Persistent postsurgical pain beyond the natural tissue healing process is most likely neuropathic in nature. The two nerves most commonly injured during and after an inguinal hernia repair are the II and IH. Mild pain due to injury to these nerves is usually responsive to pharmacological management with "analgesic ladder" ranging from nonsteroidal anti-inflammatory drugs, like ibuprofen (diclofenac is more commonly used in Indian practice) and membrane stabilizers, like gabapentin,[23] to opioids, reoperation and interventions.[24] Interventions include peripheral nerve blocks which can be diagnostic as well as being therapeutic, radiofrequency treatment, cryoanalgesia ablation, transcutaneous electrical nerve stimulation, mesh/staple removal, peripheral nerve stimulation,[25-28] spinal cord stimulation[29,30] and finally therapeutic neurectomy.[31] Intraoperative neurectomy has also been described as a preventive/pre-emptive measure.[32,33] Ultrasound-guided interventions are preferred for accuracy.[34-36] Adjunctive therapies like mental preparation of the patient, meditation, deep breathing, and hypnosis, physical modalities like transcutaneous electrical nerve stimulation (TENS), ultrasound and physical stretches have also been utilized.

TREATMENT MODALITIES FOR CHRONIC POSTSURGICAL INGUINAL PAIN

Preventive Approach

Laparoscopic surgery instead of open hernioplasty has been claimed to be better (less acute post operative pain and lesser incidence of chronic pain). However, the literature seems to be equivocal about the benefit of laparoscopic over open surgery.

Mesh can be a cause of chronic pain by probably being a source of irritation. Infection, mesh migration, adhesion formation, erosion into intraperitoneal organs, entrapment of nerves, vessels or the vas deferens, obstruction of vas deferens as a result of fibroblastic reaction to mesh (can present at times as long lasting pain during copulation), attachment of suture to the periosteum of pubic tubercle, to muscles or due to electrocoagulation can induce pain reaction. Mesh fixation by glue (tissucol) might overcome the effects of suturing, though expensive.

The review by Aasvang and Kehlet [37] suggests that in hernia surgeries, chronic pain is to be considered a more important outcome variable (since it is resistant to treatments and has greater socioeconomic impact) rather than recurrent hernia (since this is amenable to cure by re-do surgery). Inguinal hernia repair is the most common elective procedure in general surgery. Therefore, patient number having complications (1% of all hernia surgeries require referral for pain management) is relatively large.[7]

International guidelines for the prevention of CPIP recommended identification and preservation of all three inguinal nerves during surgery to reduce the risk of CPIP. Elective resection of a suspected injured nerve was also recommended. There was no recommendation for using glue during hernia repair.[33]

Therapeutic Approach

The pain complex syndrome of inguinodynia includes pain (neuralgia), burning sensation (paresthesias), hypoesthesia, hyperesthesia, with radiation of the pain to the skin of the corresponding hemiscrotum/labium majus, and Scarpa's triangle. The symptoms are frequently triggered or at least aggravated by walking, stooping, or hyperextension of the hip and can be reduced in supine position with thigh flexion. The neuropathic pain can also be reproduced by tapping the skin medial to the anterior superior iliac spine or over an area of localized tenderness (Tinel's test). It

is extremely difficult to pinpoint the involved nerve because.
- Innervation field of the 3 nerves overlap.
- Peripheral communications developing between II, IH and genital branch of genitofemoral nerve resulting in an overlap of their sensory innervations.
- Both II and IH nerves derive from T12, L1, and both GF and II run in relation to the spermatic cord with its autonomic nerve supply.

A 2015 international consensus algorithm for CPIP recommends a multidisciplinary approach with a consultation from a pain management team. Pharmacologic, behavioral, and interventional modalities including nerve blocks are essential. If conservative measures fail and surgery is considered, triple neurectomy, correction for recurrence with or without neurectomy, and meshoma removal if indicated should be performed.[38]

Multimodal treatment strategies including pharmacotherapy, physical therapy, and biofeedback techniques should be the first choices in the chronic pain management. Pharmacologically, gabapentin has been shown to be beneficial in some cases, and it may have a protective effect against chronic nerve pain if used preoperatively II/IH nerve block can provide clinical evidence for nociceptor pathways. However, pain responses to nerve blocks should be cautiously interpreted.

The neural involvement is diagnosed by assessing response to local infiltration and then doing repeated infiltration with anesthetic and cortisone. Using this as algorithm for assessment and treatment of CPIP has been suggested.[39]

A 2016 review concluded that paucity of data, heterogeneity and lack of appropriate control groups in the contemporary literature precluded firm conclusions on the efficacy and safety of perineural steroids for CPIP.[17]

If the pain relief by perineural injections is inadequate, Interventional treatment options for post-herniorrhaphy pain vary greatly. They are, transcutaneous electrical nerve stimulation, peripheral nerve stimulation[40] repeated ilioinguinal blocks using a catheter technique[41] cryoanalgesia ablation,[42] pulsed radiofrequency,[43,44] spinal cord stimulation[29,30] and combined spinal cord and peripheral nerve field stimulation.[45] If all these fail, surgical measures like mesh/staple removal and triple neurectomy have to be undertaken.

In one case report, repetitive infusion of local anesthetic and clonidine for 3 weeks was successful for a year in a patient with recalcitrant ilioinguinal neuralgia. In a case series, cryoanalgesia ablation of the II and GF nerves resulted in decreased pain scores and medication use. Pulsed radiofrequency (PRF) treatment of these nerves has been reported to be successful in one case report and another case series. Five studies (3 case series and two case reports) reported peripheral nerve stimulation for CPIP with follow-up of 6 weeks to 11 months. Pre-implant pain scores of 8–10/10 decreased to postimplant scores of 0–1/10. However, 3 reports mentioned several technical drawbacks. First, electrodes of the stimulator were placed either immediately next to the targeted nerve through surgical exploration or empirically on the incisional scars. Both techniques required repetitive testing and awake intraoperative assessment. Second, a period of trial stimulation is often required before the efficacy of the stimulator could be reliably determined. Therefore, surgical manipulation was always needed as part of the diagnostic process.

A small case control study using peripheral nerve field stimulation (PNFS) showed reduction in mean pain intensity from 7.2/10 to 4.7/10 ($P < 0.001$). Once spinal cord stimulation (SCS) was added to PNFS the pain inventory and SF36 scores reduced at 12 months follow-ups ($p < 0.05$).

Placement of a percutaneous lead of electrical nerve stimulation relies on ultrasound guidance to accurately position the device around the II, IH nerves. The II usually enters the abdominal wall 2.8 ± 1.1 cm medial and 4.

6 ± 1.2 cm inferior to the anterior superior iliac spine (ASIS) and terminates 3.6 ± 0.5 cm lateral to the midline. The IH enters the abdominal wall 2.8 ± 1.3 cm medial and 1.4 ± 1.2 cm inferior to the ASIS and terminates 4 ± 1.3 cm lateral to the midline.[46] Once stimulation of the II and IH nerves has been confirmed with significant pain control during the 4-day trial stimulation, permanent leads are implanted in the same manner. Peripheral nerve stimulation device is expensive should be reserved for highly selected cases with chronic intractable pain. Psychological consultation for ensuring a well-motivated and psychologically stable patient is a definite prerequisite.

Studies with SCS show that it is difficult to consistently cover the groin/perineum; with paresthesias.[47-49] The groin and lower abdomen are predominantly innervated by the L1-2 while the perineum is innervated by S2-4. Other normal areas, particularly the posterior leg get targeted by the stimulation. The nerves corresponding to the groin contain both fewer fibers and fibers of smaller diameter which is inversely proportional to the amplitude required for activation. Several studies have been published examining the treatment of groin pain using SCS dorsal root ganglion stimulation (DRGS), sacral nerve root stimulation,[50] and combined SCS and PNFS. These studies have obtained excellent pain relief in some patients (but at the cost of 2 separate stimulator sets, more than ₹10 lakhs in the Indian scenario), however there remain difficulties with consistently treating these pain areas. SCS can result in unwanted stimulation of the lower limb and other body areas, while PNS has issues with erosion and migration.[51]

In one study of 32 patients with SCS and/or dorsal nerve root stimulation (DNRS) for neuropathic groin, pelvic, and abdominal pain, a total of 42 trial operations were required, 3 had a superficial skin infection, 5 had a lead migration, and one had a cerebrospinal fluid (CSF) leak headache. During the follow-up period, 8 patients required a total of 15 revision operations. Reasons for revision were lead migration in 9, lead fracture in 1, increase of paresthesias in 3, and device removal in 2. There were 4 CSF leaks during the permanent implant and revision operations. A small number of patients with good trial results were ultimately long-term failures but the authors concluded that overall, their patients had sustained pain reduction, opioid reduction, and improved quality of life at 12 months follow-up after DNRS.

Thus to summarize, most of the evidence on posthernioplasty pain is from case reports and case series.

Triple neurectomy is not commonly preferred but has been suggested as a last resort in severe CPIP since a 90% success has been claimed.[52] Several publications have concluded that either open or laparoscopic triple neurectomy may produce immediate, profound, and consistent positive effects across multiple mechanical, pressure, and thermal QST variables, and marked improvements of clinical outcomes in selected CPIP patients. However, large, high powered studies are warranted to determine whether preoperative or repeated longitudinal QST may guide patient selection and predict effectiveness of neurectomy. Late postneurectomy complications like anesthesia dolorosa have not been investigated. Orchidectomy and triple neurectomy has also been suggested as a treatment for severe orchialgia after hernia surgery.[53] Severe testicular pain, testicular atrophy, azoospermia have all been reported after hernia surgery, but it is fortunately much less common than inguinal pain. The orchialgia could be secondary to ischemic orchitis, epididymitis, edema, infection, cord fibrosis and scarring, varicocele or hydrocele formation, torsion, referred pain from radiculitis or ureteral pathology, and entrapment or disruption of the genital branch of GF, II nerves, paravasal nerve fibers, or autonomic plexus within the cord. Nociceptive orchialgia secondary to intraoperative testicular tissue injury, including ischemia, edema, and infection. Typically, a dull aching pain is elicited by pressure and the testis may be enlarged or atrophic. These patients can get pain relief by means of orchiectomy. However in one study, 24% of these patients continued to have severe orchialgia after orchiectomy indicating that it might be neuropathic.[54] Neuropathic orchialgia manifests with burning, hyper/hypoesthesia, and radiation of the pain to the skin of the corresponding scrotum which is triggered or aggravated by walking, stooping, or hyperextension of the hip and can be decreased by supine posture and thigh flexion.[55] Neuropathic pain might benefit from triple neurectomy.[55,56] There is no established treatment for this fortunately rare complication.

The great variety of techniques developed to treat CPIP is a clear indication that no treatment modality (even advanced and very expensive) has been uniformly satisfactory. It has been suggested that this failure is because of the development of peripheral and central sensitization of both primary small fiber afferents and second-order spinal neurons. Pain management after involvement of the central nervous system has traditionally been difficult.

At Ashirvad Institute of Pain Management and Research (AIPMR), we initially used to address the issue of spinal sensitization by a pharmacological deafferentation of the involved nerves with a continuous catheter technique targeting the lumbar plexus to break the pain cycle developing secondary to chronic plasticity. A nerve stimulating catheter was placed under aseptic conditions with antibiotic coverage in 2 patients of severe crippling pain from CPIP. The catheter for continuous infusion of local anesthetic from an elastomeric pump was kept *in situ* for about 20 days in one patient (with CPIP of 2 months duration) but another patient with CPIP of 2 years duration required the infusion for 40 days to overcome the pain. Both patients returned to their prior professions with no residual issues from CPIP.[57] The continuous catheter technique overcomes the pain from plasticity but, it takes very long time for physiotherapy alone to overcome stiffness like discomfort from "tightness, band round the abdomen, a dragging discomfort in lower abdomen" that worsens on standing walking movements, etc. In some later patients we found that the patients continued to have stiffness related complaints even after 4–5 weeks of continuous infusion. There is also concern regarding the complications from an indwelling catheter like infection, accidental extrusion, etc. As we treated more patients of CPIP, we have come to understand the pathogenesis of postsurgical pains better. In the past 8 years; we have come to realize a very important factor; that all neuropathic pains have a neuro-myopathic component. In CPIP and orchialgia, we believe that it is not just the sensory fibers in II, IH and GF nerves that are affected by neuropathy. The motor fibers from these 3 nerves that supply the muscles of the abdominal wall are equally (or even primarily) involved. The muscle abnormalities on USG seem to be consistently present. Figure 4 shows the decrease in size, and hyperechogenecity (indicative of fibrosis) in the abdominal muscles on the operated side after hernioplasty in comparison with the unoperated side. It is our constant finding that unless this motor nerve involvement affecting muscles is addressed, the patients will not get satisfactory relief of CPIP. We have described similar motor neuropathy in other visceral neuromyopathic conditions.[58,59]

Increased firing from the II, IH and GF nerves rendered irritable by the post-hernioplasty motor neuropathy leads to development of myofascial trigger points (MTrPs) in the rectus abdominis, the internal, external obliquus and transversus abdominis muscles. These MTrPs are exquisitely painful accounting for symptoms like severe pain, hyperalgesia, allodynia, and hyperesthesia. We believe it is pain from these MTrPs that cause

Chapter 37: Post-herniorrhaphy Pain and Its Management

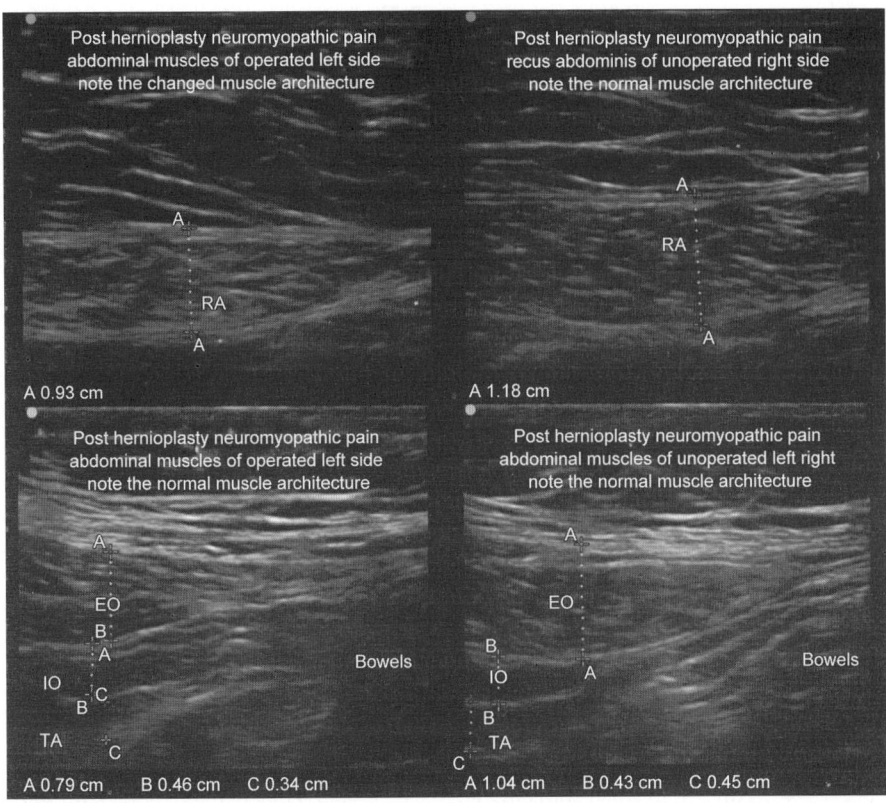

FIG. 4: The musculoskeletal ultrasonography of the abdominal muscles of the operated left side with the unoperated right side shows more hyperechogenecity as well as a reduction in the size of rectus abdominis, the internal and external oblique's as well as transversus abdominis

the movement difficulties reported by CPIP patients. The pain from these MTrPs sets up a parallel stream of spinal sensitization that is independent of the original spinal sensitization from the hernioplasty induced injury to the II, IH and GF nerves. It is the pain from these MTrPs that persists even after interventions addressing nerves like nerve blocks, cryoablation, RF procedures and peripheral and spinal nerve stimulator procedures. It is this recalcitrant myofascial pain that has made CPIP and orchialgia treatment so difficult as reported in the hernioplasty literature. It is because hitherto, the contribution from the MTrPs in CPIP has been largely ignored. There is only one publication of a randomized clinical trial of 2013 that mentions trigger point infiltration with lidocaine to diagnose anterior cutaneous nerve entrapment syndrome.[60]

We have developed a protocol where we address the neural component of neuro myopathy with USG guided PRF of II, IH and GF nerves followed by a systematic ultrasound guided dry needling (USGDN) of the abdominal wall muscles (Figs 5A to C) to address the myopathic component of neuromyopathy. With this combination, we have been able to achieve a routine reversal of CPIP in several patients including some with testicular pain referred to the scrotum. Our CPIP patients go off neuromodulatory and analgesic medications after 6–8 sessions of USGDN and are able to return to their prior lifestyle (manuscript in preparation stage).

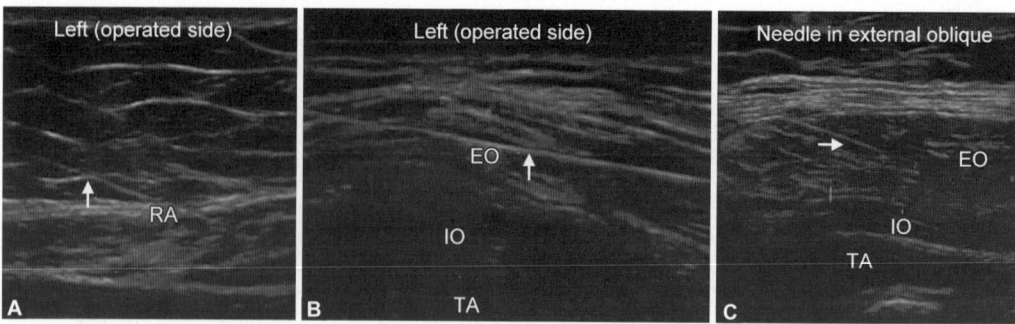

FIGS 5A to C: Illustrates ultrasound guided dry needling of the oblique muscles. The arrow in (B) shows the needle going horizontally through external oblique. The arrow in (C) points to the 50 mm long needle traveling to internal oblique and transversus abdominis through the external oblique muscle

CONCLUSION

In conclusion, hernioplasty could result in a state of chronic post-herniorrhaphy pain which can have serious personal, social and economic impact to the patient and a difficult challenge to the pain physician.

Newer, comprehensive studies keeping post-herniorrhaphy pain as an important variable to assess and quantify its time course are necessary. Equally or more important is to look at novel pathogenetic factors like the myofascial component of CPIP, since the older pathogenetic theories have failed to produce an effective treatment.

REFERENCES

1. Rosenberg J, Bisgaard T, Kehlet H, et al. Danish Hernia Database recommendations for the management of inguinal and femoral hernia in adults. Dan Med Bull. 2011;58:42-3.
2. Rutkow I. Demographic and socioeconomic aspects of hernia repair in the United States in 2003. Surg Clin North Am. 2003;83:1045-51.
3. Bay-Nielsen M, Kehlet H, Strand L, et al. Quality assessment of 26, 304 herniorrhaphies in Denmark: a prospective nationwide study. Lancet. 2001;358:1124-1128. doi:10.1016/S0140-6736(01)06251-1.
4. Jaiswal, LCSS, Chaudhry, BR Agrawal, MA. Chronic groin pain following Lichtenstein mesh hernioplasty for inguinal hernia. Is it a myth? Indian Journal of Surgery. 2009;71(2):84-8.
5. Macrae WA. Chronic post-surgical pain: 10 years on. Br J Anaesth. 2008;101:77-86.
6. Fitzgibbons RJ, Forse RA Groin hernias in adults. N Engl J Med. 2015;372:756-63.
7. Hindmarsh AC, Cheong E, Lewis MP, et al. Attendance at a pain clinic with severe chronic pain after open and laparoscopic inguinal hernia repairs. Br J Surg. 2003;90(9):1152-4.
8. Aasvang EK Bay-Nielsen, M Kehlet H. Pain and functional impairment 6 years after inguinal herniorrhaphy. Hernia. 2006;10(4):316-21.
9. Kehlet H, Jensen TS, Woolf CJ. Persistent postsurgical pain: risk factors and prevention. Lancet. 2006;367:1618-25.
10. Poobalan AS, Bruce J, Smith WCS, et al. A review of chronic pain after inguinal herniorrhaphy. Clin J Pain. 2003;19:48-54.
11. Poobalan AS, Bruce J, King PM, et al. Chronic pain and quality of life following open inguinal hernia repair. Br J Surgery. 2001;88:1122-26.
12. Simons, MP Aufenacker, T Bay-Nielsen, M et al. European Hernia Society guidelines on the treatment of inguinal hernia in adult patients. Hernia. 2009;13(4):343-403.
13. Sandblom G. Chronic post-herniorrhaphy pain always chronic? A literature review. Journal of Pain Research. 2015;8;241.
14. Haroutiunian S, Nikolajsen L, Finnerup NB, et al. The neuropathic component in persistent postsurgical pain: A systematic literature review. Pain. 2013;154:95-102.
15. Magnusson N, Heberg M, Osterberg J, et al. Sensory disturbances and neuropathic pain after inguinal hernia surgery. Scand J Pain. 2010;1:108-111.
16. Amid PK. Radiologic images of meshoma: a new phenomenon causing chronic pain after prosthetic repair of abdominal wall hernias. Arch Surg. 2004;139(12): 1297-8

17. Khan JS, Rai A, Rajan RS et al. A scoping review of perineural steroids for the treatment of chronic postoperative inguinal pain. Hernia. 2016;20(3):367-76.
18. Zaborszky A, Gyanti R, Barry JA, et al. Measurement issues when assessing quality of life outcomes for different types of hernia mesh repair. Ann R Coll Surg Engl. 2011;93(4):281-5.
19. Fränneby U, Gunnarsson U, Andersson M, et al. Validation of an inguinal pain questionnaire for assessment of chronic pain after groin hernia repair. Br J Surg. 2008;95(4):488-93.
20. Cesmebasi A, Yadav A, Gielecki, et al. Genitofemoral neuralgia: a review. Clinical Anatomy. 2015;28(1):128-35.
21. Crespi G, Giannetta E, Mariani F, et al. "Imaging of early postoperative complications after polypropylene mesh repair of inguinal hernia". Radiol Med. 2004;108(1-2):107-15.
22. Weyhe D, Belyaev O, Müller C, et al. "Improving outcomes in hernia repair by the use of light meshes—a comparison of different implant constructions based on a critical appraisal of the literature". World J Surg. 2007;31(1):234-44.
23. Sen H, Sizlan A, Yanarate O, et al. The effects of gabapentin on acute and chronic pain after inguinal herniorrhaphy. European Journal of Anesthesiology. 2009;26:772-6.
24. Thomassen I, van Suijlekom H, van der Gaag A, et al. Intervention techniques for chronic post herniorrhaphy pain. European Surgery. 2012;44:132-7.
25. Elahi F, Reddy C. Ultrasound guided peripheral nerve stimulation implant for management of intractable pain after inguinal herniorrhaphy. Pain Physician. 2015;18(1):E31-8.
26. Stinson LW Jr, Roderer GT, Cross NE, et al. Peripheral subcutaneous electrostimulation for control of intractable post-operative inguinal pain: A case report series. Neuromodulation. 2001;4:99-104.
27. Rauchwerger JJ, Giordano J, Rozen D, et al. On the therapeutic viability of peripheral nerve stimulation for ilioinguinal neuralgia: putative mechanisms and possible utility. Pain Pract. 2008;8:138-43.
28. Rosendal F, Moir L, de Pennington N, et al. Successful treatment of testicular pain with peripheral nerve stimulation of the cutaneous branch of the ilioinguinal and genital branch of the genitofemoral nerves. Neuromodulation. 2013;16:121-4.
29. Levine AB, Parrent AG and MacDougall, KW. Stimulation of the Spinal Cord and Dorsal Nerve Roots for Chronic Groin, Pelvic, and Abdominal Pain. Pain Physician. 2016. pp.405-12.
30. Yakovlev AE, Al Tamimi M, Barolat G, et al. Spinal cord stimulation as alternative treatment for chronic post-herniorrhaphy pain. Neuromodulation. 2010;13:288-90.
31. van Assen T, Boelens, O.B, van Eerten, P.V., et al. Long-term success rates after an anterior neurectomy in patients with an abdominal cutaneous nerve entrapment syndrome. Surgery. 2015;157(1):137-43.
32. Johner A, Faulds J, Wiseman SM. Planned ilioinguinal nerve excision for prevention of chronic pain after inguinal hernia repair: a meta-analysis. Surgery. 2011;150(3):534-41.
33. Alfieri S, Amid PK, Campanelli G, et al. International guidelines for prevention and management of post-operative chronic pain following inguinal hernia surgery. Hernia. 2011;15(3):239-49.
34. Gofeld M, Christakis M. Sonographically guided ilioinguinal nerve block. Journal of Ultrasound in Medicine. 2006;25:1571-5.
35. Eichenberger U, Greher M, Kirchmair L, et al. Ultrasound guided blocks of the ilioinguinal and iliohypogastric nerve: Accuracy of a selective new technique confirmed by anatomical dissection. Br J Anaesth. 2006;97:238-43.
36. Thomassen I, van Suijlekom J, van de Gaag A, et al. Ultrasound-guided ilioinguinal/iliohypogastric nerve blocks for chronic pain after inguinal hernia repair. Hernia. 2013;17:329-32.
37. Aasvang E, Kehlet H. Chronic postoperative pain: the case of inguinal herniorrhaphy. British Journal of Anaesthesia. 2005;95(1):69-76.
38. Voorbrood CEH, Burgmans JPJ, Van Dalen T, et al. An algorithm for assessment and treatment of postherniorrhaphy pain. Hernia. 2015;19(4):pp.571-7.
39. Lange JFM, Kaufmann R, Wijsmuller AR et al. An international consensus algorithm for management of chronic postoperative inguinal pain. Hernia. 2015;19(1):33-43.
40. Slavin KV. Peripheral nerve stimulation for neuropathic pain. Neurotherapeutics. 2008;5:100-6.
41. Maaliki H, Naja Z, Zeidan A. Repeated Ilioinguinal block using a catheter technique for pain relief in inguinal neuralgia. Pain Practice. 2008;8:144-6.
42. Fanelli R, DiSiena M, Lui F, et al. Cryoanalgesic ablation for the treatment of chronic post herniorrhaphy neuropathic pain. Surgical Endoscopy and Other Interventional Techniques. 2003;17:196-200.
43. Mitra R, Zeighami A, Mackey S. Pulsed radiofrequency for the treatment of chronic ilioinguinal neuropathy. Hernia. 2007;11:369-71.
44. Cohen SP, Foster A. Pulsed radiofrequency as a treatment for groin pain and orchialgia. Urology. 2003;61:645.
45. Lepski G, Vahedi P, Tatagiba MS, et al. Combined spinal cord and peripheral nerve field stimulation for persistent post-herniorrhaphy pain. Neuromodulation. 2013;16:84-9.
46. Klaassen Z, Marshall E, Tubbs RS, et al. Anatomy of the ilioinguinal and iliohypogastric nerves with observations of their spinal nerve contributions. Clin Anat. 2011;24:454-61.

47. Barolat G, Massaro F, He J, et al. Mapping of sensory responses to epidural stimulation of the intraspinal neural structures in man. J Neurosurg. 1993;78:233-9.
48. Holsheimer J, Barolat G. Spinal geometry and paresthesia coverage in spinal cord stimulation. Neuromodulation. 1998;1:129-36.
49. SchuS, Gulve A, El Dabe S, et al. Spinal cord stimulation of the dorsal root ganglion for groin pain—a retrospective review. Pain Pract. 2015;15:293-9.
50. McJunkin TL, Wuollet AL, Lynch PJ. Sacral nerve stimulation as a treatment modality for intractable neuropathic testicular pain. Pain Physician. 2009;12:991-5.
51. Stuart RM, Winfree CJ. Neurostimulation techniques for painful peripheral nerve disorders. Neurosurg Clin N Am. 2009;20:111-20, vii-viii.
52. MacQueen IT, Chen DC, Amid PK. Open Triple Neurectomy. In The SAGES Manual of Groin Pain. Springer International Publishing; 2016.pp.319-31.
53. Narita M, Moriyoshi K, Hanada K, et al. Successful treatment for patients with chronic orchialgia following inguinal hernia repair by means of meshoma removal, orchiectomy and triple-neurectomy. International journal of surgery case reports. 2015;16:157-61.
54. Ronka K, Vironen J, Kokki T., et al. Role of orchiectomy in severe testicular pain after inguinal hernia surgery: audit of the Finnish Patient Insurance Centre. Hernia. 2015;(1):53-9.
55. Amid PK. A 1-stage surgical treatment for post-herniorrhaphy neuropathic pain: triple neurectomy and proximal end implantation without mobilization of the cord. Arch Surg. 2002;137(1):100-4.
56. D.C. Chen, P.K. Amid. Persistent orchialgia after inguinal hernia repair:diagnosis, neuroanatomy, and surgical management, Hernia. 2015;19(1):61-3.
57. Vas L. Management of 2 patients with post hernioplasty pain. Indian Journal of Pain, 2011.
58. Vas L, Phanse S, Pai R. A new perspective of neuro-myopathy to explain intractable pancreatic cancer pains; dry needling as an effective adjunct to neurolytic blocks. Indian journal of palliative care. 2016;22(1):85-93.
59. Vas L, Pattanik MP, Titarmore V. Interstitial cystitis/painful bladder syndrome treated as a neuropathic pain condition with a combination of caudal epidural analgesia followed by botox injection of the perineal muscles Indian Journal of Urology. 2014;30(3):350-3.
60. Boelens, O.B.A., Scheltinga, M.R., Houterman, S., et al. Randomized clinical trial of trigger point infiltration with lidocaine to diagnose anterior cutaneous nerve entrapment syndrome. British Journal of Surgery. 2013;100(2):217-21.

Post-coronary Artery Bypass Grafting Scar Pain and Its Management

Madhuri A Lokapur

INTRODUCTION

Post-thoracotomy pain syndrome (PTPS) (chronic post-thoracotomy pain or post-thoracotomy neuralgia) is defined by the International Association for the Study of Pain (IASP) as 'pain that recurs or persists along a thoracotomy incision at least two months following the surgical procedure'. In general, it is burning and stabbing pain with dysesthesia and thus shares many features of neuropathic pain. PTPS is increasingly acknowledged by anesthesiologists and surgeons alike.[1]

PREVALENCE OF POST-THORACOTOMY PAIN

Coronary artery bypass grafting (CABG) is one of the most common surgical procedures performed in thorax worldwide. Chronic postoperative pain is a well-recognized problem. Sternotomy causes considerable postoperative pain and patients with chronic poststernotomy pain are often referred to pain clinics. Epidemiological studies on chronic poststernotomy pain are few. In a study done by Kalso E et al. in the CABG group, 28% of the patients still had poststernotomy pain at the end of two to three years, which was moderate-to-severe in 38% of patients. Of the patients who had poststernotomy pain, one-third reported sleep disturbances due to the pain.[2] Morone NE et al. concluded that pain and depression had an impact on recovery after coronary artery bypass grafting.[3] Choinière M et al. found 9.5% of participants experienced persistent postoperative pain at 24 months after CABG surgery.[4] There are several studies done to lessen post-thoracotomy pain in the immediate period and possibly avoid development of chronic pain.

CAUSES [5-7]

The exact mechanism for the pathogenesis of PTPS is still not clear, but cumulative evidence suggests that it is a combination of neuropathic and non-neuropathic (Myofascial) pain. Choinière M et al. identified significant risk factors namely increased anxiety before surgery and acute postoperative pain in the first week after surgery in development of chronic post-CABG pain.[4]

Post-thoracotomy pain may be due to:
- Retraction, resection, or fracture of ribs
- Dislocation of costovertebral joints.
- Injury of intercostal nerves
- Irritation of the pleura by chest tubes
- Sternal malunion

- Sternal wires and retained epicardial pacing-wires, especially when infected.

Signs and Symptoms [7, 8]

A patient may have moderate-to-severe chest wall pain with or without radicular intercostal pain often associated with hypoesthesia, mechanical allodynia, dysesthesia and elevated thermal threshold. The patient may exhibit signs of clinical depression and behavioral changes due to chronic illness.

CLINICAL EXAMINATION

The examination of a patient with PTPS includes inspection of the scar and respiratory excursion movements. Next palpation is done to test scar adherence and local tenderness. Neurological testing for hypoesthesia, allodynia and hyperalgesia should be noted. In case of autonomic dysfunction, symptoms like swelling change in skin color and temperature may be present. Assessment of regional musculature for postoperative disruption, atrophy and myofascial pain should be done. It is important to elicit trigger points in the tissues. Active and passive range of motion of upper limbs must be tested.

INVESTIGATIONS

The patient must be investigated to rule out neoplasm or recurrent cardiac origin pain by doing CT/MRI of thorax and cardiac function tests. CT will also give information about mal union of sternum or rib fractures. Causative factors for neuropathic pain including diabetes and vitamin B_{12} deficiency should be evaluated.

DIFFERENTIAL DIAGNOSIS

It is mandatory to exclude recurrence of disease or malignancy as a cause for the pain prior to initiating treatment.
- Pain of cardiac origin
- Underlying visceral pathology, including neoplasm
- Nerve entrapment syndrome
- Neuroma formation
- Myofascial pain syndrome.

TREATMENT PROTOCOL

At the outset cardiogenic causes of pain after CABG must be ruled out by the cardiothoracic surgeon and cardiologist. Once it is established that the origin of the ongoing pain is most likely to be noncardiogenic, patient should be offered suitable pain relieving therapies.
- The old adage of prevention being the best way to avoid pain is very true in CABG patients. Aggressive management of early postoperative pain may reduce the likelihood of long-term post-thoracotomy pain.[9] By choosing the most appropriate and least traumatic surgical incision, adhering to meticulous surgical techniques and avoiding intercostal nerve injury or rib fractures, surgeons can minimize postoperative pain. Aggressive perioperative and postoperative pain management is best accomplished with use of an epidural anesthetic and covering breakthrough pain with an IV-PCA. Alternatively, an infusion system for continuous administration of local anesthetics directly in the subpleural plane, posterior to the intercostal incision, also provides excellent pain control. Again, use of an IV-PCA as adjuvant therapy is recommended.[10] Thoracic paravertebral block has been tried with success as well.[11,12]
- Physiotherapy and osteopathy techniques may be used. Ligamentous articular release, myofascial release, strain-counter strain, diaphragm balancing can be tried in the acute phase. In patients with chronic pain treatments like rib rising, facilitated positional release, muscle energy, diaphragm redoming may be tried.

- First-line pharmacologic therapies include NSAIDs, tricyclic antidepressants, anticonvulsants and low-dose opioids. At our clinic, we found the combination of tramadol and paracetamol gives good pain relief to majority of patients with minimal side effects. Second line pharmacologic therapy may be prescribed for neuropathic pain including tricyclic antidepressants, SSRI, neurostabilizers.
- Some patients require more sophisticated treatment from multidisciplinary pain-management clinics. This treatment may include trigger point injections, intra muscular stimulation, intercostal nerve blocks, sympathetic ganglion blocks or cryoneurolysis. In properly selected cases, advanced interventional therapies like continuous spinal analgesia or spinal cord stimulation may be offered.[10]
- Sternal wire removal should be offered to patients with persistent anterior chest wall pain after sternotomy, when other serious postoperative complications have been excluded.[7]
- Isolated studies pertaining to use of acupuncture or stellate ganglion block have been published, but more data is required before any conclusions can be drawn.[13-15] As Karmarkar, et al. stated, as pain does not cause disability in the majority of patients, management is usually conservative. If pain is causing disability then multidisciplinary pain management involving the pain specialist, social worker, physical therapist, and a psychologist is required. As with most forms of neuropathic pain, treatment of post-thoracotomy pain syndrome (PTPS) is also difficult and patients might require more than one form of therapy to control pain and reduce disability.

Based on current evidence, it is not possible to draw any firm conclusion regarding whether any form of analgesic or surgical technique can influence the occurrence of PTPS. Pre-emptive analgesia initiated prior to surgery shows promise and might help reduce the incidence of PTPS. Scientific evidence is steadily growing but there is still a need for large, prospective, randomized trials evaluating PTPS. Until more is known about this condition and how to prevent the central and peripheral nervous system changes that produce long-term pain after thoracotomy, patients must be warned preoperatively about the possibility of developing PTPS and how it might affect their quality of life after surgery.

CONCLUSION

Chronic post-CABG pain is a well-known condition following thoracotomy. It needs to be assessed and investigated thoroughly. Multimodal treatment is the best option in most patients.

REFERENCES

1. Koehler RP, Keenan RJ. Management of post thoracotomy pain: Acute and chronic. Thorac Surg Clin. 2006;16(3):287-97.
2. Kalso E, Mennander S, Tasmuth T Nilsson E. Chronic post-sternotomy pain. Acta Anaesthesiologica Scandinavica. 2001;45:935-9.
3. Morone NE, Weiner DK, Belnap BH, Karp JF, Mazumdar S, Houck PR, He F, Rollman BL. The impact of pain and depression on recovery after coronary artery bypass grafting. Psychosom Med. 2010;72(7):620-5.
4. Choinière M, Watt-Watson J, Victor JC, et al. Prevalence of and risk factors for persistent postoperative nonanginal pain after cardiac surgery: a 2-year prospective multicentre study. CMAJ : Canadian Medical Association Journal. 2014;186(7):E213-E23. doi:10.1503/cmaj.131012.
5. Gerner P. Post-thoracotomy pain management problems. Anesthesiol Clin. 2008;26(2):355–vii. Doi: 10.1016/j.anclin.2008.01.007.
6. Karmakar MK. Post-thoracotomy pain syndrome. Thorac Surg Clin. 2004;14(3):345-52.
7. Nørgaard MA, Andersen TC, Lavrsen MJ, Borgeskov S. The outcome of sternal wire removal on persistent anterior chest wall pain after median sternotomy. Eur J Cardiothorac Surg. 2006;29:920-4.
8. Eisenberga E, Pultoraka Y, Pudab D, Bar-Elc Y. Prevalence and characteristics of post coronary artery bypass graft surgery pain (PCP). Pain. 2001;92(1):11-7.

9. Obata H, et al. Epidural block with mepivacaine before surgery reduces longterm post-thoracotomy pain. Can J Anesth. 1999;46(12):1127-32.
10. D'Amours RH, Riegler FX, Little AG. Pathogenesis and management of persistent postthoracotomy pain. Chest Surg Clin N Am. 1998;8(3):703-22.
11. De Cosmo G, Aceto P, Gualtieri E, Congedo E. Analgesia in thoracic surgery: Review. Minerva Anestesiol. 2009;75(6):393-400.
12. Savage C, McQuitty C, Wang D, Zwischenberger JB. Postthoracotomy pain management. Chest Surg Clin N Am. 2002;12(2):251-63.
13. Vickers AJ, Rusch VW, Malhotra VT, Downey RJ, Cassileth BR. Acupuncture is a feasible treatment for post-thoracotomy pain: Results of a prospective pilot trial. BMC Anesthesiol. 2006;3(6):5.
14. Khan MU, Ahmed I. Role of Stellate ganglion block in post CABG sympathetically mediated chest pain. J Pak Med Assoc. 2007;57(9):470-2.
15. Kwon S-Y, Joo J-D, Kim JH, Jeong J-T. Sympathetically mediated upper back pain after coronary artery bypass graft surgery. Korean Journal of Anesthesiology. 2013; 65(6 Suppl):S135-S6. doi:10.4097/kjae.2013.65.6S.S135.

SECTION 12

Challenging Pain

CHAPTER 39

Complex Regional Pain Syndrome: Where We Stand?

Samyadev Datta

INTRODUCTION

Complex regional pain syndrome (CRPS) is a painful condition that is usually regional, but may be widespread. It is manifested by symptoms that may be intermittent or continuous. Symptoms could be provoked by tissue damage and/or nerve damage as seen in CRPS (II) and only tissue damage in CRPS (I). The injury may be trivial and remote. CRPS may lead to aberrant sensory, motor, and trophic changes.[1,2]

The syndrome shows variable progression over time. CRPS may occur at any age and affects both men and women, but is more common in women. The intensity and extent of symptoms and signs are not related to the magnitude of initial trauma. In addition, course of the diseases is unpredictable. Patients may have various periods of reduced symptoms and various factors may precipitate recurrence of symptoms.

CAUSES

The causes of CRPS are unknown. CRPS likely has multiple causes.

The sympathetic nervous system plays an important role in sustaining pain. Theories suggest that pain receptors in the effected part of body become responsive to catecholamines. Animal studies indicate that norepinephrine can activate pain pathways after injury. The incidence of sympathetically mediated pain in CRPS is unknown.[1]

Another theory suggests that CRPS is a result of the triggering of the immune response, which results in inflammatory symptoms of redness, warmth and swelling in the affected areas.

Physiological windup and central sensitization are key neurologic processes involved in the conduction and maintenance of CRPS. There is evidence of NMDA receptors involved in central nervous system (CNS) sensitization. Elevated CNS glutamate levels may promote physiological windup and central sensitization. There is clear evidence to indicate that there are very high levels of glutamate in the white matter of the brain. This is area of the brain with highest density of glia cells. The immune process may contribute to peripheral and central sensitization.[1]

GENETICS IN COMPLEX REGIONAL PAIN SYNDROME

Involuntary, sustained muscle contractions or dystonia are seen in 25% of CRPS patient. Cause of dystonia remains unclear. There is some evidence associating genetics and CRPS.

This is more evident in patients with CRPS and dystonia.[3]

CRPS with dystonia has an onset time of about 11 years earlier than CRPS without dystonia. To date no causative gene has been identified.[3] The same group in Netherlands studied association of HLA subtypes in CRPS patient's without dystonia. Analysis of the data suggests that CRPS with and without dystonia may be genetically different but overlapping.

Maternally inherited mitochondrial disease may also play a role in development of CRPS in children. Researchers in a tertiary care pediatric genetic practice suggest that mitochondrial DNA sequence variants may predispose children to development of CRPS. Their recommendations are that children complaining of unexplained pain be investigated for mitochondrial diseases.[4]

Role of Glia

Watkins and her group have done some pioneering work on the role of glia both in pathological and protective roles. Astrocytes and microglia have been known to modulate neuronal function at the synaptic level, and play a major role in pain facilitation. Various neuropathic states including diabetic neuropathy, chemotherapy-induced neuropathy and peripheral neuropathies appear to have a common mechanism in which the spinal glia play an important role. This results in pathological pain.[5]

Activated glial cells may produce pathological pain by various mechanisms. The release of inflammatory cytokines, tumor necrosis factor, etc. may cause release of various neuromodulators include glutamate that may result in pain. Glial cell activation is associated with increase glutamate receptor density.[5]

Activated glia may also play a protective role by the release of anti-inflammatory factors that help to clear tissue debris. They also reduce the release of proinflammatory proteins.

Research shows that glia plays an important role in pain, and there is interesting research targeting the glial cells for pain control. Animal research has shown the role of glia in neuropathic pain, CRPS is a classic example of neuropathic pain. Tumor necrosis factor and interleukins play a very important role in the initiation and maintenance of neuropathic pain. These chemicals may oppose opioids and lead to reduced pain suppression by opioids. Another study showed that administration of naloxone results in antagonism of TLR4 receptors, an important glial receptor. Naloxone was shown to reverse neuropathic pain induced by microglial activation.[5] These findings will help us decide on various approaches in the management of CRPS.

SYMPTOMS AND SIGNS

Symptoms of CRPS are usually neuropathic in nature. They usually manifest near the site of injury but it is well documented that symptoms can spread and be widely manifest. Patients describe symptoms as being burning with shooting sensation. They also report sensitivity to touch and report that even light breeze can precipitate symptoms. These are described as allodynia and hyperalgesia. Depending on the severity of the disease process, patient's may have muscle spasm, dystonia, changes in skin color, stretching and thinning of skin, dryness of skin, with associated swelling and changes in skin temperature, trophic changes. These may be different in intensity based on the stage of the diseases. In addition, there may be changes in growth of hair and nails. As the disease progresses, patients may have joint stiffness with restriction of movement. Dystonia or muscle contractures are seen in about 25% of patients.[6,7]

The pain in CRPS pain is continuous and results in emotional physical stress. Moving or touching the area is often intolerable. Symptoms may vary in severity and duration. Various stages of CRPS have been identified.

Stage I is characterized by severe burning pain at the site of injury, muscle spasm, joint stiffness, reduced mobility and change in hair and nail growth. In addition, vasospasm with change in color and temperature is also noted.

Stage II is characterized by more severe pain. There is an extension of swelling, decreased hair growth, loss of integrity of the nails, osteoporosis, thickening of joints and muscle atrophy.

Stage III is characterized by irreversible changes in skin and bones and pain is unyielding and affects an extensive area. Bone resorption may be noted on bone scan at this stage. Muscle atrophy is severe and contractures are extensive. Often the pain spreads to an entire arm or leg and sometimes to the opposite extremity.[6,7] At this stage of the diseases, the patients have a very poor quality of life. In the occasional patient, the signs and symptoms of CRPS may burn out and leave the patient with no pain. There is a significant decrease in functional status and recovery is very unlikely.

DIAGNOSTIC CRITERIA

The CRPS is diagnosed primarily through observation of signs and symptoms but other conditions have similar symptoms. This makes it difficult to make a firm diagnosis of CRPS in the early stages of the disease. Simple nerve entrapment may cause severe pain and mimic CRPS. Further, some patients will improve gradually over a period of time without treatment, making the diagnosis complicated.

Diagnostic criteria used in CRPS (I) and (II) are the same. These include allodynia, pain evoked with normal touch, pain that non-dermatomal in distribution and associated with hyperesthesia, an excessive response to painful stimuli. Other additional symptoms include vasomotor changes including abnormal and excessive sweating, changes in blood flow associated with color changes and temperature changes.[7,8]

The International Association for the Study of Pain (IASP) list diagnostic criteria for CRPS as follows:
- Presence of an initiating noxious event or a cause of immobilization.
- Allodynia or hyperalgesia disproportionate to the inciting event.
- Evidence of edema, change in skin blood flow, or abnormal sudomotor activity in the area of pain.
- The diagnosis is excluded by the existence of any condition that would otherwise account for the degree of pain and dysfunction.

The IASP criteria for CRPS diagnoses have sensitivity ranging from 98 to 100% specificity ranging from 36 to 55%.

No specific test is available to diagnose CRPS. However, thermography, sweat testing, X-rays, electrodiagnostics and sympathetic block can be used to help diagnose the condition. A delay in diagnosis and treatment can result in severe physical and physiological problems. Early recognition and prompt treatment provide the greatest opportunity for recovery.[7,8]

Harden et al. in a 2010 publication have been able to validate the Budapest criteria for confirming the diagnosis of CRPS. They report that the Budapest criteria maintain the exceptional sensitivity for diagnosis, but increase the specificity to 0.79.

It is recommended that Budapest criteria be the preferred criteria used for diagnosis of CRPS. It is included below:

Budapest clinical diagnostic criteria for CRPS:
- Continuing pain, which is disproportionate to any inciting event
- Must report at least one symptom in three of the four following categories:
  - *Sensory:* Reports of hyperesthesia and/or allodynia
  - *Vasomotor:* Reports of temperature asymmetry and/or skin color changes and/or skin color asymmetry

- *Sudomotor/edema:* Reports of edema and/or sweating changes and/or sweating asymmetry
- *Motor/trophic:* Reports of decreased range of motion and/or motor dysfunction (weakness, tremor, dystonia) and/or trophic changes (hair, nail, skin)
- Must display at least one sign at time of evaluation in *two or more* of the following categories:
  - *Sensory:* Evidence of hyperalgesia (to pinprick) and/or allodynia (to light touch and/or deep somatic pressure and/or joint movement)
  - *Vasomotor:* Evidence of temperature asymmetry and/or skin color changes and/or asymmetry
  - *Sudomotor/edema:* Evidence of edema and/or sweating changes and/or sweating asymmetry
  - *Motor/trophic:* Evidence of decreased range of motion and/or motor dysfunction (weakness, tremor, dystonia) and/or trophic changes (hair, nail, skin)
- There is no other diagnosis that better explains the signs and symptoms.

INVESTIGATIONS SUGGESTED

It is extremely important to remember that there is no investigation that will help to diagnose CRPS.

Thermography

It is a diagnostic test used to measure the heat emitted by the body. Use of a color coded thermogram gives a visual indication of variations of blood flow in various parts of the body of the subject. In thermography, temperature is measured in symmetrical parts of the body. A temperature difference of greater than 1°C is considered significant.[7,8]

Radiography

Complex regional pain syndrome (CRPS) may lead to disuse of the extremity. Changes in bone density maybe noted as early as 2 weeks after onset of symptoms. A plain X-ray may show patchy osteoporosis. A bone scan would confirm changes in bone density. This may take a few months before it is manifest.

Bone Scintigraphy

Al Sharif et al. reported on a retrospective analysis of CRPS patient's, they divided the patient's into four groups. After analysis of specific symptoms and bone scintigraphy, they report bone scintigraphy changes are more likely to be associated with vasomotor symptoms and seen in patients with motor and trophic changes. They postulated that this may explain some of the variability of results seen in CRPS patients.[9]

Electrodiagnostic Testing

Nerve injury that characterizes CRPS cannot be detected by EMG in contrast to peripheral mono neuropathy.

Neuropsychological Testing

In a very extensive investigation on the neuropsychological deficits associated with CRPS, Schwartzmann and his colleagues administered various neuropsychological tests. Based on the group, they noted significant neuropsychological deficits present in 65% of patients, with many patients presenting with elements of a dysexecutive syndrome and some patients presenting with global cognitive impairment.[10]

CRPS in Children

Sherry and his team at the Children's Hospital of Philadelphia, USA, have been working with children with CRPS for many years. Their approach has been a combination of intense inpatient physical therapy and psychotherapy. They have avoided the use of medications and interventions in their patients. Published findings and results validate their approach.[11]

Exercises therapy was continued for about 14 days. More recently the duration of exercise therapy was 6 days. The majority of the children

(92%) were symptom free at the end of therapy. A 2 year follow-up showed 88% of the children were free of symptoms, 10% maintained full function but did have some continued pain. The group's recommendation is that intense exercise therapy is highly effective in childhood CRPS and results in less long-term symptoms and dysfunction.[11]

In a more recent paper, the group from the Children's Hospital in Boston report on a Day-hospital Approach to treatment of Pediatric Complex Regional Pain Syndrome. The results indicate using an interdisciplinary day-hospital treatment for pediatric CRPS, seems effective in reducing disability and improving physical function. The emotional functionality and occupational performance also improved in patients after they had failed to improve with outpatient treatment.[12]

TREATMENT PROTOCOL

Because there is no cure for CRPS, treatment is aimed at relieving painful symptoms so that patient can maintain function and attempt to resume a normal life as best possible.

Control of pain and maintenance of function are the corner stones of therapy. It is highly recommended that treatment be started early and be aggressive to be able to get the best results.

One of the stumbling blocks has been the lack of medical education of CRPS among medical and nursing professional. In addition as it is a rare disease, it has been designated the same by NIH recently, signs and symptoms are not consistent, there is real reluctance to believe patients. In addition, there may be no external manifestations, and no diagnostic test to confirm the condition. This results in patients being labeled as malingers and these results in further reluctance to provide treatment.

Medications

Many different classes of medications are used to treat CRPS including topical analgesic drugs that act on the painful nerves, skin and muscles, antiepileptics, antidepressants, corticosteroids, and opioids. No single drug or combination has produced consistent long-term improvement in symptoms.

Gabapentin is available in an extended release form using gastro retentive technology. It allows the side effect of sedation to be used effectively to improve the sleep patterns for patients. Sleep disturbance is a common complaint in CRPS patients. During the day time, patients experience pain relief with reduced sedation. Pregabalin, duloxetine, milnacipran are some of the other choices.

Neuropathic pain symptoms are commonly seen in complex regional pain syndrome patients. Use of calcitonin to treat neuropathic pain symptoms is well documented. Ito et al. in experiments on rats concluded that normalization of sodium channel expression may affect the peripheral nerve tissue and not the DRG neurons. Activation of calcitonin receptors may result in antihyperalgesic effect.[13]

Use of opioids in the management of CRPS is not recommended. They may be used to control symptoms during the acute phase and use of short-acting medications can be recommended. Long-acting opioids are not recommended. Use of opioids can cause activation of glial cells. That results in central sensitization. A common finding in CRPS.

Low Dose Naltrexone

Since the approval of naltrexone in the 1980's, Bihari has been investigating the potential benefits of naltrexone in low dose. Naltrexone is now approved for opioid and alcohol dependency. The daily dose of naltrexone 50 mg tab is about 100 mg. It is also available in a depot preparation and is administered as a monthly injection of 350 mg. At the higher doses of naltrexone, there is suppression of immune system

The administration of low dose naltrexone (LDN) in doses of 1.5-4.5 mg, results in a temporary inhibition of endorphin production, followed by a reactive increase in production of endorphins, resulting in reduction of pain and increased well-being.[14,15]

Increased levels of endorphins stimulate the immune system, promoting an increase in number of T lymphocytes. This may be to the tune of 300%. This was documented by Bihari. Increase T cells results in apparent restoration of normal balance of T cells and helps to reduce symptoms in various diseases states.[14-16]

Low dose naltrexone also results in suppression of production of a proinflammatory cytokine, resulting in decrease glial inflammation, a core finding in CRPS.

The LDN has now been used in pain management and especially in chronic neuropathic pain states. Its use for treatment of symptoms in CRPS is now being reported. Chopra et al. have published a case series and have reviewed the literature. The LDN is administered orally as an immediate release capsule, tablet or liquid. The medication must not be administered in the presence of opioids, as it will precipitate opioid withdrawal, other immune suppressants and high dose steroids. Prednisone above 20 mg/day would be a contraindication. The medication is usually administered at night on an empty stomach, and it is recommended that patient be NPO for at least 1 hour after taking the medication. It may be necessary to start the medication in the morning and then switch to a night time dose.[14] Occasionally patients have a surge of energy after ingesting LDN and so have difficulty with sleep. This resolves in about 7-10 days.

The starting dose for LDN is about 1.5 mg and the maximum suggested dose is 4.5 mg daily. It is recommended that the medication be titrated slowly every 10-15 days. As the medication is not available as a pill, it needs to be compounded by a compounding pharmacist. It is important that medication be available as an immediate release formulation and not a sustained released medication. As patients are not able to use opioids along with LDN, breakthrough pain can be managed using oral ketamine. Ketamine troche at 5-10 mg 2-3 times daily is usually adequate.[14]

The adverse effects of the medication are minimal including temporary increase in symptoms including, change in sensation, muscle spasm, fatigue and weakness and wakefulness. These symptoms are thought to be related to increase in brain levels of endorphins and may also result in disturbed sleep. These symptoms usually resolve in about 2-3 weeks. Patients may also complain of headaches. Gastritis has been noted possibly as medications have to be taken on an empty stomach. If gastritis is problem, use of a topical paste is a very simple alternative.

Toxicity of the drug is mainly to do with reversible effects on the liver. This was noted at very high doses. It is recommended that LDN be used very cautiously in patient with significant liver and renal impairment. No reports of effects on liver or kidney have been reported at low doses.

The author has used LDN on about 400 patients with an approximate 70% response rate. Patients on long-term opioids have been weaned and started on LDN with very good results.

Following therapies have been used:

Physical Therapy

In a systematic review published recently, it was noted that physical therapy and occupational therapy are central in the management of complex regional pain syndrome. The main purpose of physical therapy is to restore and maintain functional status. In addition, physical therapy attempts to desensitize the affected body.[17] There is some evidence to indicate that introduction of efforts to desensitize early in the process may prevent development of hyperesthesia. Although it should be noted that, some patients at certain stages of the disease are incapable of participating in physical therapy, due to touch intolerance. The graded motor imagery in combination with mirror therapy can be used to reduce symptoms of complex regional pain syndrome. A recent review does validate this method of treatment.[18]

Psychotherapy

Chronic pain syndromes are associated with profound psychological changes. The psychological effect, are not limited to the patient but includes the family. CRPS patients will also manifest similar psychological effects. This may be more manifest as the patient population is usually younger and occasionally there are no obvious signs of distress. This results in depression, anxiety and occasionally post-traumatic stress disorder. As a result, rehabilitation in this patient population can be very difficult. Using a multidisciplinary approach including psychologists trained in pain management have been extremely beneficial and should be recommended early in the process. Sherry and his coworkers have been very successful in their approach with children.[11] Patient may be reluctant to see a psychologist, but it is the responsibility of the treating clinician in educating patient on the profound benefits of working with a psychologist.[8]

Sympathetic Nerve Block

Some patients attain significant relief from sympathetic nerve block. Intravenous administration of phentolamine into the affected limb as a Bier block has been beneficial. Application of the tourniquet can be extremely painful. Sympathetic plexus block at various levels has been used. Stellate ganglion nerve block is conducted with placement of the needle over the C6 transverse process. Spread of dye is confirmed under fluoroscopy (Figs 1 to 3). Lumbar sympathetic plexus block is conducted with either one or two needles. There should be an adequate spread of dye as confirmed under fluoroscopy (Figs 4 to 7). Initially it is recommended that they be conducted with local anesthetic and be repeated twice weekly. This can be continued for about 3–4 weeks. Recently the use of long acting lisosyme based bupivacaine (Exparel) has been very effective. The block lasts about 72 hours and patients can participate in physical therapy Ideally physical therapy should follow the block.[8] Use of sympathetic plexus block in chronic CRPS has very limited value and not recommended.

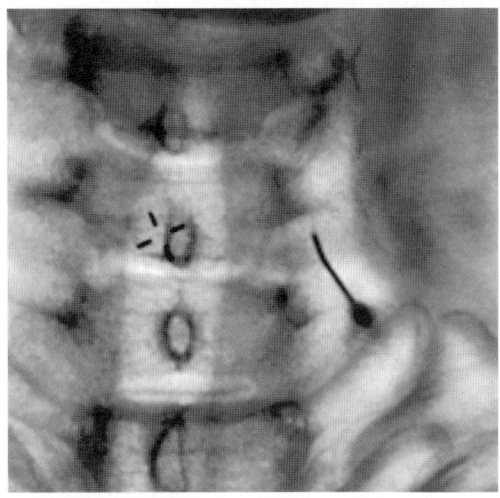

FIG. 1: Stellate ganglion block needle position—Anteroposterior view

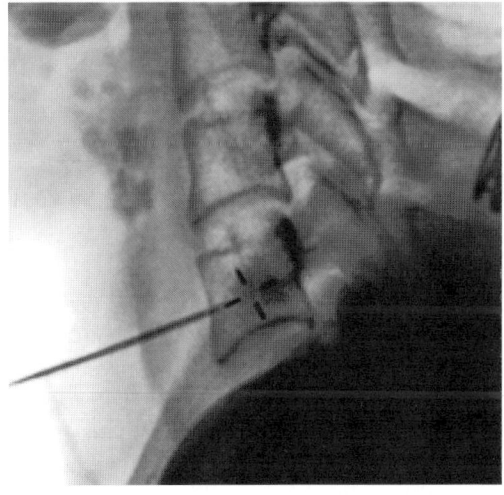

FIG. 2: Needle—Lateral view

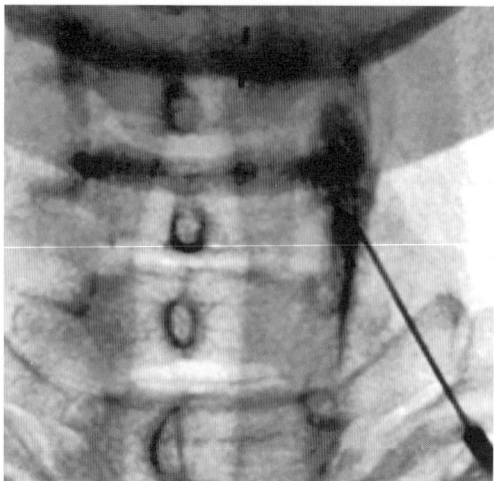

FIG. 3: Stellate ganglion block spread of dye—anteroposterior view

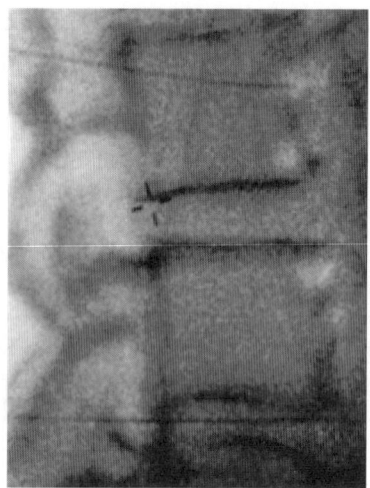

FIG. 5: Lumbar plexus spread of dye—anteroposterior view

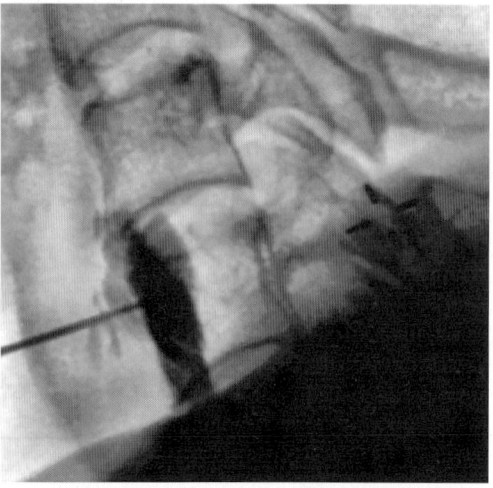

FIG. 4: Stellate ganglion block spread of dye—Lateral view

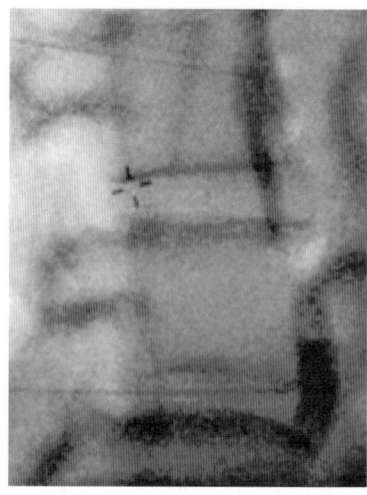

FIG. 6: Lumbar plexus spread of dye—Lateral view

In some patients, early in their diseases process the situation may convert from sympathetically mediated pain to sympathetically independent pain. This may be considered in situations where after a sympathetic block the patients have all the signs of a successful sympathetic block, including vasodilatation and temperature changes, but have none to minimal pain relief. Continued sympathetic blocks are not recommended in these settings.

Neurolytic sympathetic nerve block can also be considered. Lidocaine is the preferred local anesthetic while performing stellate ganglion block because of the proximity to blood vessels. 4% phenol dissolved in water is recommended for neurolytic nerve blocks. Neurolytic lumbar

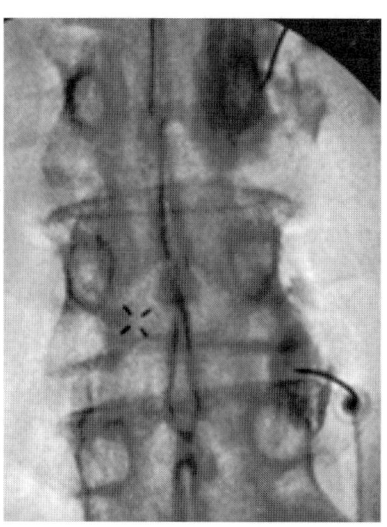

FIG. 7: Lumbar plexus needle position

sympathetic plexus block should be conducted using three needles placed at the L2, L3, and L4 level. Correct spread of dye needs to be confirmed before administration of neurolytic agents. Needles may need to be repositioned if the dye is noted to be spreading into the muscles. Reverse Trendelenburg's position maybe helpful during stellate ganglion block. It is recommended that neurolytic agents be injected incrementally, under fluoroscopic or CT guidance.

Straube et al. in review of neurolytic sympathetic plexus blocks concluded that the high quality evidence to perform chemical or surgical sympathectomy in CRPS patient's is limited. Their recommendations are that neurolytic sympathetic plexus block be used in CRPS patient's only when other modalities have failed.[19] It is very important to inform patients about the potential complications of neurolytic sympathetic plexus blocks either in the cervical or lumbar area. It is of critical importance that while performing these procedures, the practitioners be very aware of the anatomy. All necessary measure for resuscitation must be immediately available when performing these procedures.

MC5-A Calamare Device

The MC5-A Calmare© delivers patient-specific cutaneous electrostimulation, resulting in 'scrambling' pain information with 'no pain' information. The goal is to reduce the perception of pain intensity. Researchers from Italy recently published there findings and concluded that cutaneous electrostimulation with the MC5-A Calmare© can be part of a multimodality approach to the treatment of chronic pain.[20,21] They also recommended larger trial with a sham arm.

HYPERBARIC OXYGEN THERAPY

There has been a lot of interest in the use of hyperbaric oxygen therapy (HBOT) for treatment of chronic CRPS. Katznelson et al. in a recent publication mention the case of 40-year-old male with chronic CRPS responding very well to HBOT.

The therapeutic effects of HBOT are based on a supraphysiologic increase in the mount of dissolved oxygen carried by the blood. This increase allows oxygenation of ischemic areas with compromised circulation. HBOT activates oxidant-antioxidant mechanisms via an endothelial nitric oxide (NO) pathway, which plays a key role[6] in stimulating secretion of growth factors such as vascular endothelial growth factor, hypoxia inducible factor-1, and stem cells. By activating signal transduction cascades, HBOT has been shown to mediate tissue healing and improve postischemic and inflammatory injuries.[7] Furthermore, HBOT may cause an immediate and prolonged analgesic effect which is initiated and maintained by NO and NO dependent release of endogenous opioids.[8-10]

It has been suggested that CRPS is related to dysfunction of the central and autonomic nervous systems,[23-25] inflammation,[26] immune system dysfunction[27,28] and microvascular pathology leading to tissue hypoxia and ischemia.[3,29]

Amputation

Bodde et al. discusses the merits of amputation in CRPS. They report that the primary reason for amputation was pain followed by a dysfunctional limb. They also report that there is a significant recurrence of CRPS in the stump. In addition, only a small percentage of patient's were able to return to work after amputation. They concluded that amputation as a well-defined modality for treatment of symptoms related to CRPS cannot be recommended.[22]

Spinal Cord Stimulator

The use of spinal cord stimulator in the treatment of CRPS is well-documented. It is very important that a well monitored trial be conducted before placement of a permanent spinal cord stimulator. A systematic review concluded that spinal cord stimulation appears to be an effective therapy in the management of patients with CRPS I and II; however, the study did not find clinically significant improvement in functional status (Figs 8 and 9).[23,24]

The recent improvement is SCS technology has given us more choices. Nevro is a company manufacturing a high frequency device, where the patient does not feel any paresthesia. This is a common complaint among CRPS patients

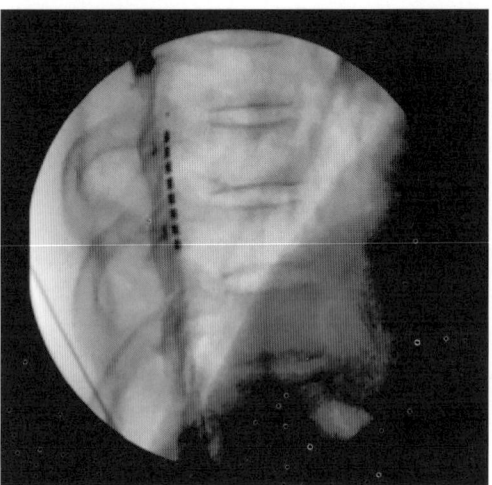

FIG. 9: Lead Position-Lateral View

and may be useful. St Jude's has also introduced a dorsal root ganglion (DRG) stimulator that allows more targeted approach to therapy. These new technologies need more time to evaluate efficacy and patient acceptance.[30]

Intrathecal Pumps

Intrathecal pumps are used to treat resistant CRPS when the patients have either significant side effects of medications, or are requiring large doses of medications. The choices of medications available to administer via intrathecal pump include: opioids, local anesthetic, clonidine, baclofen, and ziconotide.[25]

In a consensus statement from a panel of experts in 2007, it was recommended that ziconotide be in the first line of medications along with morphine and hydromorphone. ziconotide is a nonopioid analgesic and a voltage sensitive, N-type calcium channel blocker, isolated from a marine snail. It may be used in combination or as mono therapy. It appears that in neuropathic pain states, and in difficult to control pain situations, ziconotide may be very effective. The medication does have many side effects that need to be considered before use, but if the benefits outweigh the risks, it may be an effective drug.[26]

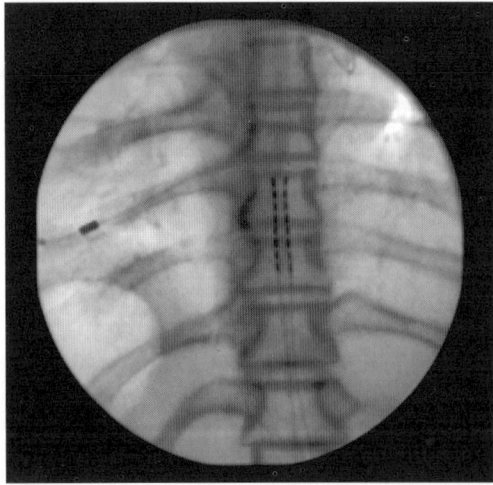

FIG. 8: Lead Position-Anteroposterior View

Earlier trials with ziconotide were conducted with significantly higher doses. Presently the recommendation is for test dose with 2–4 µg given as a single dose intrathecally. If that dose is effective than the expected daily dose it is likely to be about the same as the test dose.

It is recommended that a well-conducted trial showing significant improvement in function be performed before placement of permanent intrathecal pump. In addition, all patients must have a psychological evaluation. It is very important that patients understand the nature of the treatment option and that it is an invasive procedure. Also the final decision for placement of the intrathecal pump must come from the patient. Pumps need to be managed by trained physicians and nurses.

Ketamine

The use of ketamine to treat CRPS remains controversial and has been advanced by Schwartzman. Correll from Australia was the first to use ketamine for treatment of CRPS. Hubbard introduced the same in USA in 1999. The exact mechanism by which the ketamine works is not clear. It is postulated that ketamine is able to manipulate the NMDA receptor. It is also possible that there are multiple other mechanisms by which ketamine works. In CRPS patients, there is excessive release of glutamate in the peripheral receptors. This is a possible mechanism resulting in central sensitization and windup phenomena. Ketamine is a potent NMDA receptor blocker. This is the possible basis on which ketamine has been helpful in the treatment of symptoms of CRPS patients.[27]

There are two treatment modalities: the first consists of a low dose sub-anesthetic ketamine infusion of between 10 and 40 mg per hour for 5 days. This is performed in an inpatients setting. The risks are quite high and must be supervised by trained, competent physicians. It is mandatory that patients be monitored in an ICU type setting. It is also recommended that LFT be monitored daily. Various scales have been used to monitor depth of sedation with ketamine. The second treatment consists of putting the patient into a medically induced coma and administrating an extremely high dose of ketamine typically between 600–900 mg.[27] This is not approved in USA and is associated with very high risk and is not recommended.

The outpatient protocol is conducted in a softly lit, quiet infusion suite over a 10-day period. The infusion is conducted Monday through Friday on 2 consecutive weeks and infused for 4 hours each day. Dose starts at 80 mg and is gradually increased up to 200 mg. It may be necessary to increase the dose gradually due to side effects. Also, all patients receive the same dose as per the protocol. There may be some merit in considering the need to modify the dose based on the weight of the patient.

Before starting the protocol, all patients are evaluated by a cardiologist and psychologist. There is a small cardiac risk. In addition, ketamine is known to cause hallucinations. Hallucinations are one of the side effects of ketamine and may occur during the infusion. Hallucinations are usually self-limiting, but if needed ketamine infusion may be stopped or the rate reduced to stop the hallucinations. Use of midazolam, before and during helps to reduce hallucinations. Premedication with lorazepam also help.

Patients are given midazolam 2 mg at the start of the infusion and 2 mg 2 hours into the infusion. This helps to reduce the hallucinations related to ketamine. Addition of transdermal scopolamine patch to reduce incidence of nausea and vomiting significantly. In addition, clonidine 0.1 mg tablet is given before the infusion. Clonidine helps to potentiate the pain relieving effects of ketamine. In some patients, the blood pressure may be low and administration of clonidine may be withheld. Some practitioners have used dexmidomidine to help alpha-2 effects. In addition lorezepam 1 mg tablet, can be prescribed for anxiety. This is administered the night before and the day of the infusion.[27]

A set of 4 booster infusions follow at the end of ketamine protocol. Each booster is schedule for 2 days. Two weeks after the end of treatment phase, one month after end of treatment phase, 2 months after end of treatment phase, 3 months after end of treatment phase. Booster doses may be scheduled for 2 days every 3-6 months as needed.

Data from our office presented recently on about 100 patients, 2000 infusion sessions over 6 years indicates that this is a very safe modality of treatment. Most patients have stopped use of opioids and are now using low dose naltrexone (LDN) very effectively. Side effects were mainly nausea and vomiting, dizziness, hallucinations were also noted. There were no major side effects noted.

REFERENCES

1. http://www.ninds.nih.gov/disorders/reflex_sympathetic_dystrophy
2. http://en.wikipedia.org/wiki/Complex_regional_pain_syndrome
3. van Rooijen DE, Roelen DL, Verduijn W, Haasnoot GW, Huygen FJ, Perez RS, Claas FH, Marinus J, van Hilten JJ, van den Maagdenberg AM..Genetic HLA Associations in Complex Regional Pain Syndrome With and Without Dystonia. J Pain. 2012;13(8):784-9.
4. Higashimoto T, Baldwin EE, Gold JI, Boles RG. Reflex sympathetic dystrophy: complex regional pain syndrome type I in children with mitochondrial disease and maternal inheritance. Arch Dis Child. 2008;93(5):390-7.
5. Milligan ED, Watkins LR, Pathological and protective roles of glia in chronic pain. Nature Reviews Neuroscience. 2009;10:23-36 (January 2009) doi: 10.1038/nrn2533.
6. Veldman PH, Reynen HM, Arntz IE, Goris RJ. Signs and symptoms of reflex sympathetic dystrophy: prospective study of 829 patients. Lancet. 1993;342(8878):1012-6.
7. Harden RN, Bruehl S, Perez RS, Birklein F, Marinus J, Maihofner C, Lubenow T, Buvanendran A, Mackey S, Graciosa J, Mogilevski M, Ramsden C, Chont M, Vatine JJ. Validation of proposed diagnostic criteria (the "Budapest Criteria") for Complex Regional Pain Syndrome. Pain. 2010;150(2):268-74.
8. Stanton-Hicks MD, Burton AW, Bruehl SP, Carr DB, Harden RN, Hassenbusch SJ, Lubenow TR, Oakley JC, Racz GB, Raj PP, Rauck RL, Rezai AR. An updated interdisciplinary clinical pathway for CRPS: report of an expert panel. Pain Pract. 2002;2(1):1-16.
9. Alsharif A, Akel AY, Sheikh-Ali RF, Juweid ME, Hawamdeh ZM, Ajlouni JM, Abdulsahib AS, Alhadidi FA, Elhadidy ST. Is there a correlation between symptoms and bone scintigraphic findings in patients with complex regional pain syndrome? Ann Nucl Med 2012 (Epub ahead of print).
10. Libon DJ, Schwartzman RJ, Eppig J, Wambach D, Brahin E, Lee Peterlin B, Alexander G, Kalanuria A. Neuropsychological deficits associated with Complex Regional Pain Syndrome J Int Neuropsychol Soc. 2010;16(3):566-73.
11. Sherry, David D.M.D.; Wallace, Carol A.M.D.; Kelley, Claudia O.T.*; Kidder, Monica P.T.*; Sapp, Lyn R.N.,Short- and Long-term Outcomes of Children with Complex Regional Pain Syndrome Type I Treated with Exercise Therapy. Clinical Journal of Pain. 1999;15(3):218-23.
12. Logan DE, Carpino EA, Chiang G, Condon M, Firn E, Gaughan VJ, Hogan M, Leslie DS, Olson K, Sager S, Sethna N, Simons LE, Zurakowski D, Berde CB.. A Day-hospital Approach to Treatment of Pediatric Complex Regional Pain Syndrome: Initial Functional Outcomes. Clin J Pain, 2012 [Epub ahead of print].
13. Ito A, Takeda M, Yoshimura T, Komatsu T, Ohno T, Kuriyama H, Matsuda A, Yoshimura M. Anti-hyperalgesic effects of calcitonin on neuropathic pain interacting with its peripheral receptors. Mol Pain. 2012;8(1):42.
14. http://www.lowdosenaltrexone.org/.
15. Bihari B. Efficacy of low dose naltrexone as an immune stabilizing agent for the treatment of HIV/AIDS [letter]. AIDS Patient Care. 1995;9(1):3.
16. Brown N, Panksepp J. Low-dose naltrexone for disease prevention and quality of life. Med Hypotheses. 2009;72(3):333-7.
17. Daly AE, Bialocerkowski AE. Does evidence support physiotherapy management of adult Complex Regional Pain Syndrome Type One? A systematic review. Eur J Pain. 2009;13(4):339-53.
18. Ezendam D, Bongers RM, Jannink MJ. Systematic review of the effectiveness of mirror therapy in upper extremity function. Disabil Rehabil. 2009;31(26):2135-49.
19. Straube S, Derry S, Moore RA, McQuay HJ. Cervico-thoracic or lumbar sympathectomy for neuropathic pain and complex regional pain syndrome. Cochrane Database Syst Rev. 2010;(7):CD002918.
20. Marineo G, Iorno V, Gandini C, Moschini V, Smith TJ. Scrambler therapy may relieve chronic neuropathic pain more effectively than guideline-based drug management: results of a pilot, randomized, controlled trial. J Pain Symptom Manage. 2012;43(1):87-95.

21. Ricci M, Pirotti S, Scarpi E, Burgio M, Maltoni M, Sansoni E, Amadori D. Support. Managing chronic pain: results from an open-label study using MC5-A Calmare® device. Care Cancer. 2012;20(2):405-12.
22. Bodde MI, Dijkstra PU, den Dunnen WF, Geertzen JH... Therapy-resistant complex regional pain syndrome type I: to amputate or not? J Bone Joint Surg Am. 2011; 93(19):1799-805.
23. Taylor RS, Van Buyten JP, Buchser E. Spinal cord stimulation for complex regional pain syndrome: a systematic review of the clinical and cost-effectiveness literature and assessment of prognostic factors. Eur J Pain. 2006;10(2):91-101.
24. Kemler MA, de Vet HC, Barendse GA, van den Wildenberg FA, van Kleef M. Effect of spinal cord stimulation for chronic complex regional pain syndrome Type I: five-year final follow-up of patients in a randomized controlled trial. J Neurosurg. 2008;108(2):292-8.
25. Koulousakis A, Kuchta J, Bayarassou A, Sturm V. Intrathecal opioids for intractable pain syndromes. Acta Neurochir Suppl. 2007;97(Pt 1):43-8
26. Deer T, Krames ES, Hassenbusch SJ, PhD, et al. Neuromodulation: .Polyanalgesic Consensus Conference 2007: Recommendations for the Management of Pain by Intrathecal (Intraspinal) Drug Delivery: Report of an Interdisciplinary Expert Panel. Technology at the Neural Interface; 2007.pp.300-280.
27. Schwartzman RJ, Alexander GM, Grothusen JR, Paylor T, Reichenberger E, Perreault M. study. Pain. 2009; 147(1-3):107-15.
28. Rita Katznelson, Shira C. Segal, and Hance Clarke, "Successful Treatment of Lower Limb Complex Regional Pain Syndrome following Three Weeks of Hyperbaric Oxygen Therapy," Pain Research and Management, vol. 2016.
29. Thom, Stephen R. "Oxidative stress is fundamental to hyperbaric oxygen therapy. J Applied Physiol. 2009; 106(3):988-995.
30. Verrills, Paul, Chantelle Sinclair, and Adele Barnard. "A review of spinal cord stimulation systems for chronic pain. J Pain Research.2016;9:481.

Phantom Limb Pain: Causes and Pain Management

JD Hoppenfeld

INTRODUCTION

After amputation, patients may experience both phantom sensation and phantom limb pain. Phantom sensation is any nonpainful sensation of an absent limb. Phantom limb pain is the sensation of pain in an amputated limb. Dr. Mitchell, a famous American civil war surgeon in the nineteenth century coined the term "phantom limb pain" and provided a comprehensive description of the condition.

Postoperative studies have shown that 85–90% of patients experience phantom limb pain in the first month postamputation.[1] At one-year follow-up, 60% of patients continue to have pain. However, only 5–10% of those 60% have severe pain at one year.[2] Phantom limb pain is often undiagnosed, and therefore undertreated. When diagnosed the severity of pain is often underestimated and treatment not offered. In one study, 61% of amputees with phantom pain discussed the problem with their doctors and only 17% were offered treatment.[3]

Severe preamputation pain may be a risk factor for phantom limb pain. Chronic pain in the amputated body part was a risk factor for phantom limb pain in some but not all surveys. It is hypothesized that high preoperative pain levels may sensitize the nervous system. However, phantom limb pain has been seen in amputations secondary to trauma when the patient had no history of preamputation pain. Conversely, some patients with a history of severe chronic pain in an extremity before surgery never develop phantom limb pain.

SIGNS AND SYMPTOMS

Phantom limb pain is equally frequent in men and women. It is not influenced by level or side of amputation. Phantom sensations and pain have been reported following of different body parents including the teeth, eyes, tongue breast and bladder but the most common occurrence is following limb amputation. Phantom limb pain usually presents within the first week after amputation.[2] However, there has been anecdotal evidence of presentation being delayed for months and even years. Patients often describe their pain as burning, crushing, or feeling like they have been stabbed with needles in the missing limb (Figs 1A to D).[2] Phantom limb pain is more commonly described as more episodic than constant.

Phantom pain is primarily located in the distal part of the limb. Patients often describe pain in the lower missing extremity as if their toes were tightly flexed and in the upper extremities as if their fingers were

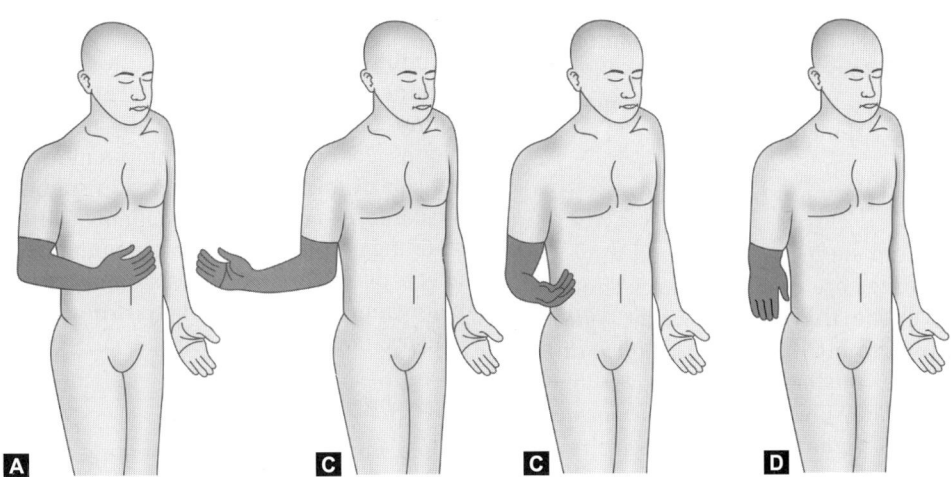

FIGS 1A to D: Types of missing limbs

tightly clenched.[4] It has been theorized that the large cortical representation of the hand and foot may contribute to the sensitivity of the distal part of the extremity as being more susceptible to phantom limb pain. The gradual improvement of phantom limb pain occurs proximal to distal with the toes and fingers being the last pain to dissipate. This is known as telescoping. The patient feels as if the toes are located at the stump as the more proximal pain dissipates. As the proximal pain improves further, the toes or fingers of the phantom limb may even be experienced at or in the stump.

CAUSES

The pathophysiology of phantom limb pain is not fully understood. It may be due to a single mechanism or the combination of multiple mechanisms. There are three primary theorized mechanisms; they include peripheral, spinal plasticity and cerebral reorganization. The peripheral mechanism holds that there is a neuroma that forms after amputation that triggers the sympathetic nervous system. Tap-induced exacerbations of phantom limb pain have been shown to temporarily abate after local anesthetic injection. The spinal plasticity mechanism holds that following amputation the wide dynamic range neurons in the spinal cord go unchecked causing a self-sustained neuronal activity.[5] Reorganization at the level of the spinal cord may lead to the development of referral areas in the dermatome surrounding the injured region. Where stimulation at these sites was previously neutral, it may generate phantom limb pain in the missing limb.

However there has been a lack of response to treatment following complete cordectomy.[6] The cerebral reorganization mechanism holds that neural reorganization takes place in cortical and subcortical structures. Within the somatosensory cortex, distinct processing center exist: One for the processing of sensory input and one for the delivery of motor output. When sensory input is lost, cortical reorganization takes place. It has been shown that the hand area invades the face area after hand amputation.[7] Ramachandran et al showed that when the face was stimulated patients felt phantom limb pain in the missing hand. In this example, the detail of information transmitted was shown to be thermal specific. When warm touch on the face was felt, warmth on the missing hand was also felt. Cerebral reorganization has been observed to occur in a linear relationship between pain and degree of reorganization.[8] It has been suggested that there needs to be maturity of the central nervous system to develop phantom limb pain. Phantom limb pain is exceedingly rare in congenital amputees or children who lose their limb before the age of six.

CLINICAL EXAMINATION

The stump should be examined fully. Often the findings are nonsignificant. There may, however, be trigger points that reproduce the phantom limb pain. Signs of skin abrasions, blisters or breakdown may be present. They are often due to a poor fitting prosthesis. Signs of local infection should be investigated.

DIAGNOSTIC CRITERIA

There are no specific diagnostic criteria for phantom limb pain.

INVESTIGATIONS

Imaging, lab work or electrodiagnostic studies are not typically indicated in the work-up of phantom limb pain. Diagnosis remains clinical.

Differential Diagnosis

It is of importance to rule out stump pain in any patients where the diagnosis of phantom limb pain in being entertained. Stump pain, unlike phantom limb pain, occurs in the part of the body that actually exists. Stump pain can exist after post-surgical healing has occurred. Persistent stump pain has been shown to exist in roughly 14% of patients.[9] Stump pain and phantom limb pain is commonly seen together. Sherman and Sherman reported that stump pain is as present in 61% of amputees with phantom pain but in only 39% of those without phantom pain.[10]

Local trauma may exist at the stump of the amputated limb. This is most often due to a poor fitting prosthesis.

TREATMENT PROTOCOL

Phantom limb pain is typically resilient to treatment. Research has focused on preventing stump pain with regional anesthetic techniques for pre-planned amputations. The efficacy of this has been mixed in studies but a favorable trend exists. In patients with long-standing chronic pain before amputation, the effects of epidural anesthesia one to two days before amputation most likely do not present a true pre-emptive approach.

Mirror Box Manipulation

It is a novel approach to treating phantom limb pain and has shown significant promise (Fig. 2). Patients often report that the missing limb feels as if it is fixed in a painful position: A tightly clenched hand in the upper extremity or tightly curled toes in the lower extremity. With a loss of sensory input from the limb to the somatosensory cortex, motor output is altered. It is hypothesized that patients developed learned paralysis. The motor system needs sensory input to make the limb move and without it, the missing limb

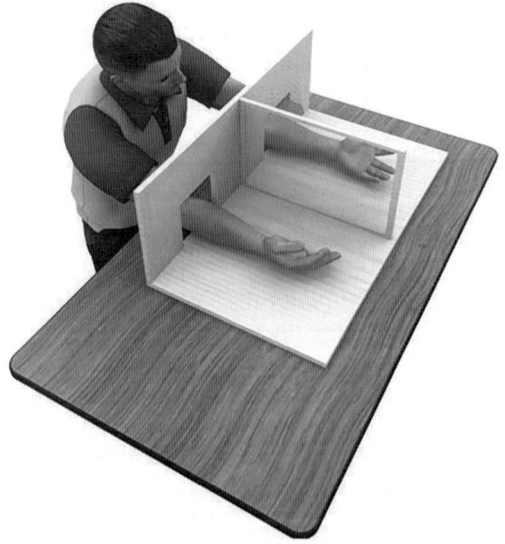

FIG. 2: Mirror image *(For color version, see Plate 12)*

is paralyzed and contracted. The premise of mirror box manipulation is that afferent sensory input must be provided to the brain so that the missing limb can be moved and pain relieved. A mirror is held on side of the intact limb. The patient is asked to move the intact limb. The phantom limb is viewed as moving in the mirror providing the missing sensory input. Preemptive use of analgesics and anesthetics during the preoperative period is believed to prevent noxious stimulus from the amputated site from triggering hyperplastic changes and central neural sensitization which may prevent amplification of future impulses from the amputation site. Small studies have shown this to be a successful treatment of phantom limb pain, but it is unclear whether mirror therapy is better than motor imagery alone. Studies have shown that 20–60% of amputees may be clinically depressed, between three and five times greater than that of the general population.[10] The loss of a limb has social, economical, and psychological implications. Phantom limb pain, like other painful conditions, has been shown to be further exacerbated with depression and anxiety.

A multi-modal approach to the patient's pain, including psychological care should be evaluated. Multiple medications have been used for the treatment of phantom limb pain. At this point, no medication has been shown to be superior. Phantom limb pain is thought to be of a neuropathic pain origin, i.e. pain originating from the peripheral or central nervous system. Commonly, antidepressants and anticonvulsants used to treat neuropathic pain are used to treat phantom limb pain. With severe levels of pain, narcotic therapy has been used as well.

Transcutaneous Electrical Nerve Stimulations

It has been shown in anecdotal evidence that transcutaneous electrical nerve stimulations (TENS) could possibly be helpful for phantom limb pain. The TENS has an inherent safety to it, which adds to its value as a treatment modality. A large limitation to the use of TENS is combining electrode placement and the use of the prosthesis. Spinal cord stimulation has been successfully used for the treatment of phantom limb pain. Its method of pain relief is not fully understood and studies are limited.

Stump Neuromas

The stump neuromas have been shown to trigger phantom limb pain. Injections of local anesthetic to stump trigger points may provide benefit.

Sympathetic Nerve Blocks

Sympathetic nerve blocks may provide pain relief. If helpful, sympathetic nerve blocks are usually transitory however some patients experience long-term benefit.

Surgical Treatment

It is typically only performed when it is apparent that the stump has not healed properly. Proximal extension is not indicated for amputation pain.

Invasive Procedures

The invasive procedures such as cordotomy, dorsal root entry lesions, and sympathetectomy have not produced encouraging results.

CONCLUSION

Phantom limb pain is treated with multi-disciplinary approach to achieve maximum pain relief

REFERENCES

1. Parker CM. Factors determining the persistence of phantom pain in the amputee. J Psychosom Res. 1973;17:97.
2. Nikolajsen L, Ilkjaer S, Kroner K, et al. The influence of preamputation pain on post amputation stump and phantom pain. Pain. 1997b;72:393-405.

3. Sherman RA, Glenda GM. Concurrent variation of burning phantom limb and stump pain with near surface blood flow in the stump. Orthopedics. 1987;10:1395-402.
4. Wilkins KL, McGrath PJ, Finley GA, Katz J. Phantom limb sensations and phantom limb pain in child and adolescent amputees. Pain. 1998;78:7-12.
5. Omer GE. Jr Nerve, neuroma, and pain problems related to upper limb amputations. Orthop Clin North Am. 1981;12:751.
6. Melzack R, Loeser JD. Phantom body pain in paraplegics: Evidence for a central "Pattern generating mechanism" for pain. Pain. 1978;4:195.
7. Pons TP, Garraghty PE, Ommaya AK, et al. Massive cortical reorganization after sensory deafferentation in adult macaques. Science. 1991;252(5014):1857-60.
8. Grüsser SM, Winter C, Mühlnickel W, et al. The relationship of perceptual phenomena and cortical reorganization in upper extremity amputees. Neuroscience. 2001; 102(2):263-72.
9. Pezzin LE, Dillingham TR, Mackenzie EJ. Rehabilitation and the long-term outcomes of persons with trauma-related amputations. Arch Phys Med Rehabil. 2000;81:292-300.
10. Ephraim PL, Wegener ST, MacKenzie EJ, Dillingham TR, Pezzin LE. Phantom pain, residual limb pain, and back pain in amputees: Results of a national survey. Arch Phys Med Rehabil. 2005;86:1910-9.

CHAPTER 41

Postherpetic Neuralgia: Causes and Pain Management

Charles Daknis

INTRODUCTION

Postherpetic neuralgia (PHN) occurs when after an acute infection of herpes zoster (HZ) the afflicted individual develops pain along the affected dermatome. It affects approximately 800,000 people each year; and, most of these patients are elderly or are immunosuppressed in some fashion. The role of stress in the suppression of the immune system can not be underestimated, especially in the younger population. The pain appears a 3 months after the degumming and of the rash has been used as a definition of postherpetic neuralgia. Accordingly, between 25–50% of adults >50 years, develop postherpetic neuralgia, and, in greater than 50 is a large risk factor for herpes zoster. The risk of herpes zoster doubles each decade beyond the 5th, starting with a population-wide incidence of approximately 20%.

Herpes zoster results from the reactivation of varicella-zoster virus (chickenpox). The cell-mediated immunity, which decreases with age, is thought to be the mechanism behind the direct link to increased incidence of zoster with increasing age. Other infections such as HIV-AIDS or even certain malignancies, can increase the risk of zoster outbreaks. In case of malignancies such as Hodgkin's lymphoma, the race contributes to the development of herpes zoster and Caucasians are four times as likely to develop zoster as are darker skinned individuals.

SIGNS AND SYMPTOMS

Classically, the rash of HZ develops after the pain presents in the dermatome of the affected nerve. The rash is characterized by blistering and close groups of red bumps and the affected area appear reddened and new waves of blisters occur for several days as old lesions crust over. The most common is shown in Figure 1.

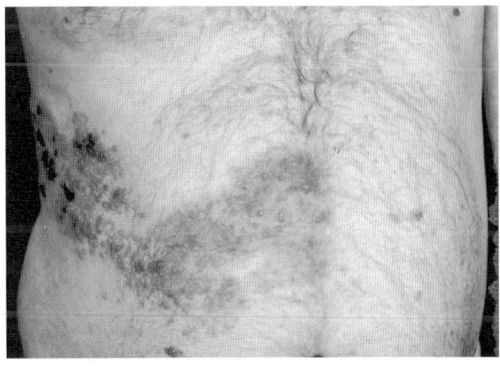

FIG. 1: Thoracic dermatome *(For color version, see Plate 13)*
Source: Mayo Clin Proc. 2009; 84(3):274–80.

The rash is associated with viral manifestations, such as fever, lethargy, as well as lymph adenopathy. Usually within 1–5 days, there is the onset of a rash in the area of pain. After about 4 weeks in the 'typical' patient the lesions will fade and the infection is over; rarely, there will be no cutaneous eruption and only pain along the dermatome 'zoster sine herpete'. This may present some diagnostic challenge!

It is important to remember that the older the patient at the onset of the disease, the more likely they are to have a severe case of the shingles. This includes deeper blisters, motor involvement, including facial nerve paralysis. Motor loss usually improves with time but not always. Pain is usually the primary complaint! As discussed, the most common manifestation is the mid-thoracic dermatomes but there can also be involvement of the trigeminal nerve in—all divisions.

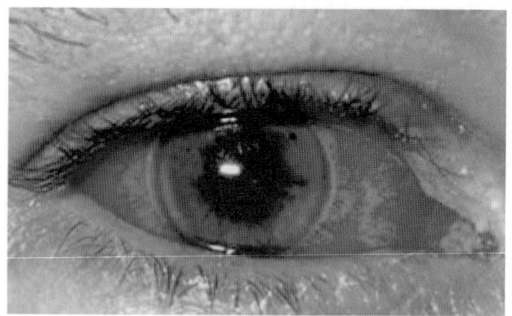

FIG. 2: Anterior uveitis inflammation of the middle layer of the eye, including the iris *(For color version, see Plate 13)*

CLINICAL EXAMINATION

The examination for PHN is to evaluate the skin at the site of pain; and, many times, there can be residual of the lesion of active shingles, and many patients may present with active shingles for management of the pain. Typically, these lesions are distributed along the dermatome of the affected nerve root, including the trigeminal nerve.

In case of trigeminal nerve involvement one must look for the possibility of ocular involvement. If the ophthalmic division of the trigeminal nerve is affected, there is approximately a 50% chance that the patient will manifest ocular symptoms. Ocular symptoms are shown in Figures 2 to 5.

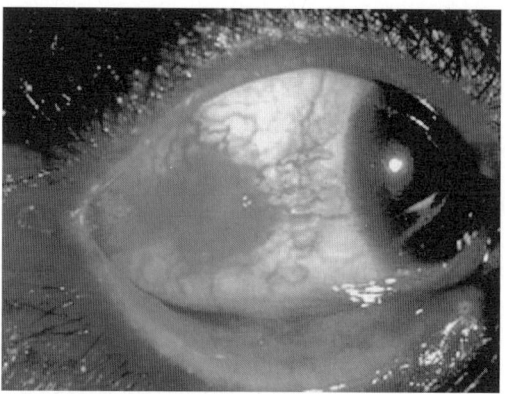

FIG. 3: Episcleritis inflammation of the sclera *(For color version, see Plate 13)*

TREATMENT OPTIONS

Antiviral Treatments

Antiviral treatments of herpes zoster includes treatment of the acute infection. The common ones are as follows:

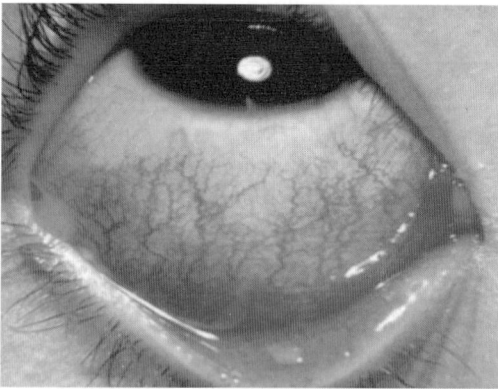

FIG. 4: Mucopurulent conjunctivitis *(For color version, see Plate 13)*

Chapter 41: Post Herpetic Neuralgia: Causes and Pain Management

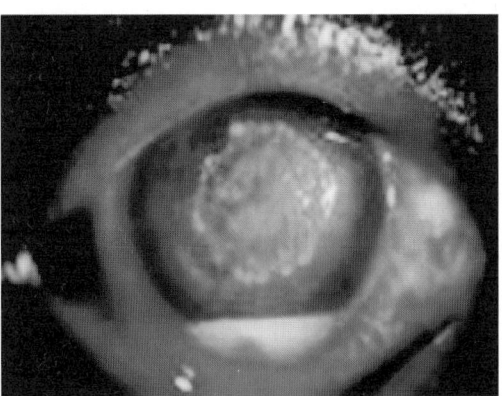

FIG. 5: Keratitis inflammation of the cornea *(For color version, see Plate 13)*

- *Acyclovir*: It is a DNA polymerase inhibitor. It is readily available and relatively inexpensive, has reduced bioavailability as well as being less effective reduc the pain of PHN. The dose is 800 mg orally 5 times per day for 7–10 days.
- *Famcyclovir*: It is also a polymerase inhibitor, has better bioavailability than acyclovir, also an easier dosing schedule only 3 times per day instead of 5 times per day with acyclovir. The dose of famciclovir 500 mg orally 3 times per day for 7 days.
- *Valacyclovir*: It a prodrug to acyclovir, also dosed 3 times per day and dose is 1000 mg orally 3 times per day for 7 days.

The incidence on PHN was noted to be up to 50% 3–6 months after the active infection. This effect was most profound in patients over 50 years of age. Valacyclovir reduces the duration of pain for 51 days and acyclovir for 38 days. At 6th month, pain reduction is 18% with valacyclovir and 26% with acyclovir. The valacyclovir and famcyclovir are very similar in their efficacy but PHN resolves two times faster with famcyclovir than with valacyclovir.[1-4]

In addition to antiviral therapy, corticosteroids have been used in treatment. There is some controversy regarding the use of steroids in the acute phase of the disease.

Chemical Neuromodulatory Therapies

It includes tricyclic antidepressants and the serotonin reuptake inhibitors and they have been used successfully to reduce the incidence and intensity of postherpetic neuralgia. The mechanism of action with these medications has been shown to be inhibition of reuptake of seretonin and norepinephrine, blockade of N-methyl-D-aspartate (NMDA) receptors as well as sodium and calcium channel receptors.[5-7]

Tapentadol has a unique mechanism of action on the mu receptor as well as inhibition of reuptake of norepinephrine. Based on available mechanistic data, it should provide fairly good relief in cases of PHN. As tapentadol is a stronger μ-opioid agonist than tramadol, it is more likely to be associated with typical opioid-induced side effects. Therefore, tramadol may be a more conservative approach before resorting to tapentadol. In addition tramadol also has a dual mechanism of action resulting in inhibition of norepinephrine and serotonin. There has been some data to suggest this medication is helpful in the treatment of PHN.[8]

Narcotic medications: These are used extensively in the treatment of PHN but it has some concerns of side effects, reduction in renal clearance and respiratory depression especially in elderly population of >50 years, These side effects include but are not limited to sedation, constipation, confusion, pruritus, nausea, vomiting, respiratory depression, and addiction.

The discontinuation of narcotic medications must also be done in an appropriate manner, especially if the use of narcotics has been prolonged, i.e. more than 1 month. The appropriate weaning of the narcotic dose with psychological as well as pharmacological support is recommended.

At the end of the day, however, nearly all patients a practitioner will see with the diagnosis of PHN will use these medications.

Topical agents: There is a host of topical agents, which are prepared outside the jurisdiction of the Food and Drug Administration (FDA). It has compounds, which may contain a local anesthetic as well as neuropathic medication such as gabapentin or ketamine. In theory, these agents 'should' work, but there is no data to present at this juncture. The topical agents with data to support their use include lidoderm patches as well as topical capsaicin. The topical capsaicin has been shown to be an agonist on the vanillin 1 receptor present in primary nociceptive receptors. Initially with application, there is severe burning and stinging which reduces after the first several weeks.[9,10]

It is the brave practitioner that uses this agent in an already suffering patient! Lidocaine patches have been shown to be effective in reducing the severity of PHN and up to 3 patches may be used at a time and can be cut to follow the distribution of the pain. The blood levels of lidocaine must remain within acceptable limits with the patch use. The levels of lidocaine can be elevated in hepatic failure.[11]

Interventional Techniques

Postherpetic neuralgia can be treated with interventional pain management techniques. The common ones are epidural steroid administration; sympathetic blockade and spinal cord stimulation. The potential for peripheral stimulation also will be explored.

The epidural steroid administration has been demonstrated to help to reduce the cerebrospinal fluid (CSF) levels of interleukin-8.[12] In some cases, intrathecal administration of steroid methylprednisolone may be useful. However, there has been significant data linking this medication to arachnoiditis when delivered intrathecally.[13-15]

Postherpetic neuralgia has also been treated with sympathetic blockade such as stellate ganglion blockade for facial zoster; chest lesions and upper extremity lesions. In case of lower extremity, pain can be treated with epidural steroid and lumbar sympathetic block. The low dose local anesthetic will provide dermatomal sympathetic interruption when instituted through a thoracic epidural catheter.[16]

The downside to the use of sympathetic blockade is that it does not seem to produce long-term efficacy in pain reduction during a course of PHN.[17-19]

Spinal cord stimulation has been described as a successful modality in the treatment of recalcitrant PHN. The practical concerns of placement of the electrodes for successful thoracic dermatomal coverage without activation of motor fibers are real issues. Spinal stimulation has been described to be up to 82% effective in PHN;[20] however, technical difficulties with lead placement make this a treatment option of last resort.

From a mechanistic standpoint spinal cord stimulation efficacy in PHN is not well understood. The stimulation of the dorsal column of the relevant dermatomal segment is thought to prevent transmission of nociceptive signal to the thalamus and subsequently cortical projection.

As of 2016 spinal stimulation remains of questionable efficacy in the treatment of post herpetic neuralgia. With the advent of high frequency and burst stimulation there may be an improved role of spinal stimulation treatment of this disorder.

At this point in time, there is no significant body of literature dedicated to this topic and information from individual practitioners regarding efficacy has been mixed. However, potentially, this technology could benefit those with PHN. At the point of chapter submission, recommendations for this technology must remain guarded.

Other Pharmacologic Options

Gabapentin and pregabalin are common medications used for the reduction in PHN. The gabapentin was shown in several studies at doses ranging from 1800 to 3600 mg/day to significantly reduce PHN pain perception.[16,20]

The side effects were somnolence, dizziness, ataxia, peripheral edema and infections these, side effects seem to be related to the rapidity of dose escalation. In renal insufficiency, slow titration of gabapentin and pregabalin dosage must be done to help to reduce the severity of intolerable side effects.

A suggested dosage regimen for gabapentin is as follows.
The dose of should be calculated according to the age, body weight, and in consideration of metabolic, cardiovascular and renal function status:

1. Tablet gabapentin 100–300 mg at hours of sleep (HS) for 3–5 days
2. Tablet gabapentin 100–300 mg in the afternoon
3. The dose to be titrated up to 900 mg of gabapentin.

The Pregabalin can be titrated in similar fashion. However, dosing is usually done up to twice per day with maximum doses of 600 mg/day. It must be pointed out there are no established guidelines for dosing of either of these drugs for the diagnosis of PHN. But as of how gabapentin, pregabalin and lidoderm are FDA approved for use in PHN

Vaccinations for Shingles

Zostavax is the commercially available vaccine for postherpetic neuralgia and is perhaps the best way to treat this disease. Individuals over 50 years of age may have the vaccine, which reduces the rate of infection by 51% and reduces the rate of developing post herpetic neuralgia by over 60% The vaccine can be administered to patients who have had shingles but should not be administered within approximately four weeks of an active infection. There are no specific recommendations on how soon after an infection the patient should get the vaccine. It is generally accepted that the lesions of active infection should have abated. The Centers for Disease Control and Prevention (CDC) has recommendations for individuals over 60 years of age but FDA approves vaccine for anyone over 50 years.

Contraindications for the Vaccine

Pregnant women should avoid the vaccine and those that are immunocompromised and individuals with HIV/AIDS or immunosuppressant from chemotherapy or other therapy that reduces the immune system's integrity and allergy to any component of the vaccine.

Side Effects from the Vaccine

There are minor side effects. They may include swelling or redness at the injection site or a minor outbreak of varicella like lesions surrounding the injection site. Headache has also been described after the vaccine.

CONCLUSION

Post herpetic neuralgia is a commonly occurring pain disorder especially in the population of individuals greater than 50 years of age. Treatment of this disease lacks significant long-term well designed studies to develop effective paradigms.

Early intervention with antiviral therapy and aggressive pain control during the acute phase of the viral infection remains the mainstay of treatment. Other modalities including interventional treatment for this disorder have been attempted but they lack clear evidence to support efficacy in a long term situation.

Postherpetic neuralgia is an extremely disabling disorder and the temptation to "try anything" will certainly present itself. The wise practitioner would exhaust FDA approved treatments prior to considering off label treatments.

Practitioners are encouraged to familiarize themselves with proper dosing and monitoring of opioid analgesic regimens for PHN prior to using these medications.

REFERENCES

1. Wood MJ, Kay R, Dworkin RH, Soong SJ, Whitley RJ. Oral acyclovir therapy accelerates pain resolution in patients with herpes zoster: A meta-analysis of placebo-controlled trials. Clin Infect Dis. 1996;22:341-7.
2. Beutner KR, Friedman DJ, Forszpaniak C, Andersen PL, Wood MJ. Valaciclovir compared with acyclovir for improved therapy for herpes zoster in immunocompetent adults. Antimicrob Agents Chemother. 1995;39: 1546-53.
3. Tyring SK, Beutner KR, Tucker BA, Anderson WC, Crooks RJ. Antiviral therapy for herpes zoster: Randomized, controlled clinical trial of valacyclovir and famciclovir therapy in immunocompetent patients 50 years and older. Arch Fam Med. 2000;(9):863-9.
4. Tyring SK. Efficacy of famciclovir in the treatment of herpes zoster. Semin Dermatol. 1996;15:27-31.
5. Ishii Y, Sumi T. Amitriptyline inhibits striatal efflux of neurotransmitters via blockade of voltage-dependent Na^+ channels. Eur J Pharmacol. 1992;221:377-80.
6. Deffois A, Fage D, Carter C. Inhibition of synaptosomal veratridine-induced sodium influx by antidepressants and neuroleptics used in chronic pain. Neuroscience Letters. 1996;220:117-20.
7. Lavoie PA, Beauchamp G, Elie R. Tricyclic antidepressants inhibit voltage-dependent calcium channels and Na^+ Ca^{2+} exchange in rat brain cortex synaptosomes. Can J Physiol Pharmacol. 1990;68:1414-8.
8. Boureau F, Legallicier P, Kabir-Ahmadi M. Tramadol in postherpetic neuralgia: A randomized, double-blind, placebo controlled trial. Pain. 2003;104:323-31.
9. Bernstein JE, Korman NJ, Bickers DR, Dahl MV, Millikan LE. Topical capsaicin treatment of chronic postherpetic neuralgia. J Am Acad Dermatol. 1989;21:265-70.
10. Watson CP, Tyler KL, Bickers DR, Millikan LE, Smith S, Coleman E. A randomized vehicle-controlled trial of topical capsaicin in the treatment of postherpetic neuralgia. Clin Ther. 1993;15:510-26.
11. Comer AM, Lamb HM. Lidocaine patch 5%. Drugs. 2000;59:245-9.
12. Kikuchi A, Kotani N, Sato T, Takamura K, Sakai I, Matsuki A. Comparative therapeutic evaluation of intrathecal versus epidural methylprednisolone for long-term analgesia in patients with intractable postherpetic neuralgia. Regional Anesthesia and Pain Medicine. 1999;24:287-93.
13. Kotani N, Kushikata T, Hashimoto H, Kimura F, Muraoka M, Yodono M, Asai M, Matsuki A. Intrathecal methylprednisolone for intractable postherpetic neuralgia. N Engl J Med. 2000;343:1514-9.
14. Nelson DA. Intraspinal therapy using methylprednisolone acetate twenty three years of clinical controversy spine. 1993;18(2):278-86.
15. Wilkinson HA. Intrathecal depo-medrol: A literature review. Clin J Pain. 1992;8:49-56.
16. L Manchikanti, et al. Interventional techniques in chronic nonspinal pain. ASIIP Publishing; 2009.
17. Dworkin RH, Johnson RW. A belt of roses from hell: Pain in herpes zoster and postherpetic neuralgia. In: Block AR, Kremer EF, Fernandez E (eds). Handbook of Pain Syndromes: Biopsychosocial Perspectives; 1999. pp.371-402.
18. Rowbotham MC, Taylor K. Herpes zoster and postherpetic neuralgia. In: Yaksh TL, Lynch C, Zapol WM, Maze M, Biebuyck JF, Saidman LJ (Eds). Anesthesia: Biologic Foundations, Philadelphia: Lippincott-Raven Publishers; 1998.pp.879-88.
19. Wu CL, Marsh A, Dworkin RH. The role of sympathetic nerve blocks in herpes zoster and postherpetic neuralgia. Pain. 2000;87:121-9.
20. Krames E. Implantable devices for pain control: Spinal cord stimulation and intrathecal therapies. Best Pract Res Clin Anaesthesiol. 2002.16:619-49.

CHAPTER 42

Post-laminectomy Pain and Its Management

Preeti P Doshi

INTRODUCTION

Post-laminectomy pain syndrome specifically refers to recurrent or persistent pain and disability following surgical laminectomy. It constitutes an important variant of chronic back pain and disability affecting millions of individuals across the world. However, the term is often used more broadly to describe failure to achieve satisfactory result after any type of surgery on the spine. Although a pain-free outcome is always desirable, it is not always obtained even when an excellent technical result is achieved after lumbosacral spine surgery. It is indeed very disappointing and frustrating to experience resurfacing of pain with the preoperative anticipation of cure of the problem and ability to live a normal life after surgery. Although unpleasant, it is a hard reality and based on the universal high incidence, it is labeled as failed back surgery syndrome (FBSS), which for obvious reasons is not a very popular term with the surgeons. It is estimated to occur in approximately 5–40% of patients after surgical intervention.

It also poses a significant clinical and economic concern. It is a real challenge for the treating clinician, as it is often known to respond poorly to conservative measures as well as repeat surgeries. It is important to learn that the success rate goes down substantially for each successive surgical intervention. No one treatment is effective for all patients with FBSS. Treatment will vary in every individual based on the underlying cause of FBSS. Patients of FBSS often experience pain which is a combination of nociceptive and neuropathic mechanisms. Knowledge about the potential causes of FBSS facilitates more efficient and cost-effective evaluation and management of these patients. It is, however, important to note that precise etiopathology of pain may often be difficult to determine in view of the complex interplay of biological and psychosocial factors in majority of these patients. Interventional pain specialist plays a vital role in diagnosis and therapy of a possible pain generator in this multifactorial enigma.

ETIOLOGY

The common causes of failed back surgery syndrome are:
- Foraminal stenosis (25–29%)
- Painful disk (20–22%)
- Pseudoarthrosis (14%)
- Neuropathic pain (10%)
- Recurrent disk herniation (7–12%)
- Iatrogenic instability (5%)
- Facet joint pain (3%)

- Sacroiliac joint (SIJ) pain
- Arachnoiditis (1%)
- Epidural and perineural fibrosis [Incidence of perineural fibrosis can increase up to (60%) in patients with multiple revision surgeries].

PATHOPHYSIOLOGY

On removal of disk tissue, two major changes occur in the motion segment locally, namely reduction in disk space height and formation of fibrous tissue. The amount of fibrous tissue developing will depend on patient's intrinsic tendency and certain extraneous factors such as degree of trauma and bleeding during surgery and suboptimal postoperative care.

It is generally the interplay between predisposition, mechanical instability and scarring which determines the degree of post-laminectomy and diskectomy pain. The mechanical instability also leads to or aggravates residual lateral recess stenosis, which with or without scarring can result in radicular pain. Scar tissue can either form bands stretching from nerve root up to the surrounding bone, or engulf the nerve root or increase pressure on venous plexus and cause ischemia to the nerve root and this can result in pain at rest (Fig. 1).

Adhesions hinder the normal movement of nerve root in the lateral recess and produce friction and pain during body movements. Although postoperative scarring is a regular phenomenon, every patient does not have pain as it depends on configuration of scar and overall condition of the motion segment. The time of appearance of pain takes few months when the scar gets more consolidated and patient increases the level of activity and movements. But in poorly performed surgeries associated with severe bleeding, dural or nerve root injury the pain can occur soon after surgery.

If patient has extensive spinal decompression, he can develop mechanical

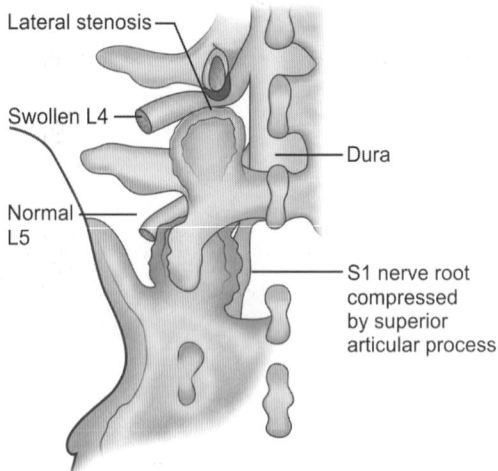

FIG. 1: Mechanism for nerve root inflammation

instability and strain at adjoining level zygapophyseal facet joints resulting in facetogenic pain.

The fusion at the lumbar spine level increases motion and stress at sacroiliac joint (SI joint). This could be a probable reason for low back pain in 20–30% of patients after lumbar spine fusion procedures which is often underdiagnosed.

CLINICAL EVALUATION

It is extremely vital to identify and establish the pain generator in order to institute appropriate treatment algorithm. Detailed history with thorough clinical examination provides very valuable clues pointing to the source of pain. One must remember that some patients may have more than one pain generator.

One needs to broadly figure out a reason for persistent pain like mismatch of surgery performed versus surgery needed, residual pathology, intraoperative complication or a technical failure. The likelihood of postspinal surgery pain is higher in patients suffering from diabetes, peripheral vascular disease (PVD) autoimmune disease and smokers. Hence, it may be useful to note presence of any of these.

HISTORY

Elaborate history about pain can point to a potential generator which can be confirmed with the help of examination and appropriate investigations. It is important to note the following:
- Location of pain
- Comparison with preoperative pain
- Response to mechanical changes in terms of change in intensity of pain. Low back pain or leg pain which worsens with sitting and flexion in standing is likely to be diskogenic or due to instability. If it improves on sitting and stooping, by and large indicates stenosis. Transition from sitting to standing if worsens pain it is likely to arise from the disk or sacroiliac joint and goes against facet joint. If pain worsens on standing and walking it goes in favor of canal stenosis. Localized pain inferior and medial to posterior superior iliac spine (PSIS) points to sacroiliac (SI) joint (Fig. 2)
- *Quality of pain*: Whether sharp, shooting, burning or accompanied by dysesthesia which indicate neuropathic pain.
- *Time course of appearance of pain*: If pain recurs in days to within four weeks, it generally implies inadequacy of the surgery. New leg pain soon after surgery may be due to neural injury, misplaced screw or venous thrombosis. If the patient has initial improvement in pain which recurs within 1-6 months it may be due to residual or recurrent pathology but could also indicate a new pathology. Pain which recurs after 6 months or is different in character generally indicates a new pathology
- Severity of pain
- Aggravating and alleviating factors
- Diurnal variation of pain.

Besides a detailed history about pain, any other significant medical history, ongoing medications, constitutional symptoms, psychosocial history and history of previous therapies including type of surgery and interventions should be elicited. One should be vigilant for presence of any red flags or pre-existing neurological deficits like weakness, bladder and/or bowel disturbances which may warrant immediate intervention. It may be useful in some patients to obtain a baseline detailed disability scoring like Ostwald Disability Index (ODI) to judge the impact of problem on quality of life and to monitor response to therapy. A background of compensation issue may warn the clinician about poor response to an otherwise appropriate line of management.

EXAMINATION

The body language, of the patient right from the time he or she enters the clinic including facial expressions often give a hint of mental status and psychosocial issues. In addition to the general examination a detailed relevant neurological and musculoskeletal evaluation is essential.

On inspection it is important to note the posture, gait, range of movements, deformity or abnormal spinal curves and position of the scar.

Localized tenderness on palpation may help to identify the source of pain such as facet joint, sacroiliac joint, vertebral body or soft tissues. Exacerbation of pain on

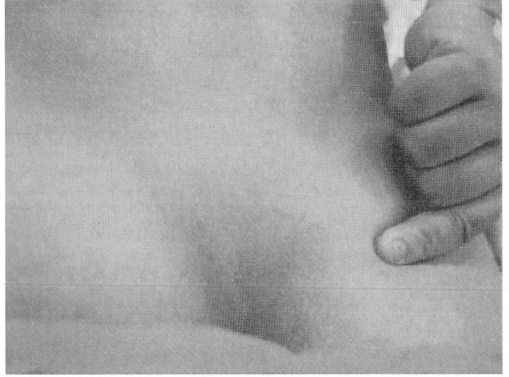

FIG. 2: Fortin finger test for sacroiliac joint mediated pain *(For color version, see Plate 13)*

extension, ipsilateral lateral flexion, rotation of lumbosacral spine indicates lumbar facet joint as the pain generator. One can identify a neuroma by local tenderness over the scar. Any obvious swelling, redness or color change should be noted at the site of incision and in lower extremities for patient with pain in the immediate postoperative period.

It may be worthwhile to feel peripheral pulsations to rule out vascular pathology.

Neurological examination: This includes straight leg raise (SLR), Reverse SLR, deep tendon reflexes, Babinski sign and detailed sensory and motor testing. The SLR test result is considered positive only if the pain radiates to below the knee and not merely in the back or the hamstrings. This is the single best test for determining radiculopathy due to disk herniation with a high sensitivity and moderate specificity.

Analysis of information obtained from sensory, motor and reflexes evaluation helps in dermatomal localization as shown in table 1.

Motor testing of the lower extremity usually provides objective information to identify the location of potential lumbosacral lesions. Joint movement requires 2 opposing movements involving 4 adjacent nerve roots:

1. Hip movement involves L2-L3 for flexion and S1-L5 for extension.
2. Knee movement involves L3-L4 for extension and L5-S1 for flexion.
3. Ankle movement involves L4-L5 for flexion and S1 for extension.

Some foot movements are mediated through a single nerve root:
- Foot inversion is primarily innervated by L4
- Great toe dorsiflexion is supplied by L5
- Foot eversion is predominately S1.

Nonphysiological testing (Waddell signs) should be performed.[1] The presence of 3 or more positive signs out of the 5 may be clinically significant in terms of psychosocial issues yellow flags which may indicate symptom magnification or possible illness behavior and probable nonorganic cause, unlikely to respond to standard therapies. Isolated positive signs are of limited value.

Once a clinical diagnosis is made on the basis of examination, most patients will require investigations mainly in form of imaging to consolidate the same and establish the pain generator.

DIFFERENTIAL DIAGNOSIS

Clinician must rule out the following which might mimic symptoms, before labeling the condition as post laminectomy pain syndrome:
- Peripheral vascular disease
- Drug-seeking behavior
- Osteoporosis
- Seronegative arthritic diseases (e.g., reactive arthritis, ankylosing spondylitis)
- Fractures of the lumbar vertebral body
- Multiple myeloma or metastatic neoplasms
- Aortic aneurysm
- Avascular necrosis of femoral head
- Extra spinal causes (e.g., ovarian cyst, pancreatitis)
- Renal infection/calculi.

INVESTIGATIONS

In patients with chronic persistent pain, it is essential to evaluate the adequacy of the

TABLE 1: Root values for sensory innervation and reflexes

Nerve root	Pin prick sensation	Reflex
L3	Lateral thigh and medial femoral condyle	Patellar tendon reflex
L4	Medial leg and medial ankle	Patellar tendon reflex
L5	Lateral leg and dorsum of foot	Medial hamstring
S1	Sole of foot and lateral ankle	Achilles tendon reflex

surgical result and consider whether persistent symptoms represent an inadequate surgical outcome, a new problem, or an idiopathic pain syndrome. If persistent symptoms are judged on objective imaging studies to be an anatomical problem, such as subsidence or non-union, it will still be necessary to determine whether revision is likely to be beneficial.

Imaging modalities provide immensely useful information to correlate with clinical evaluation although it cannot distinguish symptomatic from asymptomatic radiological findings.

Plain X-rays

Anteroposterior/lateral views will reveal disk space reduction, spondylolisthesis, fractures, loss of lordosis, osteophytes etc. and should be advised if any of these are suspected.

MRI Scan

MRI is superior to CT scanning for detection of many conditions because it presents soft tissue detail and multiple planar points of view. It should be used if infection, cancer or persistent neurologic deficit is strongly suggested. It is also to delineate other soft tissue pathology responsible for pain such as adhesions.

Imaging in the postoperative patients may consist of standard MRI Scan; T1-weighted, T2-weighted, and STIR sequences with the addition of fat-saturated T1-weighted post-gadolinium sequences.

T1-weighted post-gadolinium fat saturated images are critical to identify fibrosis and distinguish it from recurrent disk herniation. It can help to spot other complications which include surgery at the wrong level or inadequate surgery (insufficient decompression), surgical injury to the nerve root (attention of the course of pedicle screws on coronal MRI or coronal CT myelography), lack of mechanical stability or pseudarthrosis (dissectible by CT to dissect bony bridging) versus lucency around the hardware (loosening).

Magnetic resonance imaging (MRI) is useful in demonstrating Modic I changes, which when persisting longer than 6 months post-surgery are suggestive of abnormal-motion/pseudarthrosis.

Axial MRI images are helpful in assessing stenosis and lateral recess narrowing, while parasagittal images are helpful in assessing foraminal stenosis.

MRI scan can also help identify hematoma, abscess, spinal cord injury, infarction or spinal tumor. It can also demonstrate indistinctness of nerve roots within the thecal sac, thickening and clumping of nerve roots pointing to arachnoiditis.

CT Myelography

This is useful when MRI is contraindicated and spinal canal pathology is suspected. It can also be helpful when MRI is equivocal or nondiagnostic.

Bone Scan

This may be indicated if one suspects vertebral fracture, infection or metastasis. Nuclear medicine bone scan utilizes a radiopharmaceutical to demonstrate the abnormal physiology of healing processes in the bony spine such as fracture, infection, tumor, or inflammatory processes (arthritis).

Neurophysiology

Electrodiagnostic studies such as electromyography (EMG) and nerve conduction studies (NCS) can be very helpful in the evaluation of neurologic symptoms and/or neurologic deficits seen during the physical examination in select patients.

EMG/NCS can often help identify which specific nerve root is involved in a given radiculopathy, which can be extremely helpful for correlation with any abnormal lumbosacral imaging study results (especially when the MRI shows multilevel abnormalities, while the nerve root compromise may be occurring in only 1 or 2 specific levels). Identifying the specific nerve root involved can help ensure that any spinal injections or eventual surgery are performed at the appropriate level or site within the lumbar spine.

EMG/NCS findings take a couple of weeks to appear after an acute injury; hence many neurophysiologists wait 2-4 weeks before performing the testing.

Laboratory Studies

If history suggests fever, weight loss, night sweats, one should get a CBC count, erythrocyte sedimentation rate, CRP and urinalysis to rule out cancer or infection. Serum and urine electrophoresis studies may help to rule out multiple myeloma at an early stage when radiographic imaging studies appear negative or inconclusive.

Color Doppler

It may be advised for patients where vascular claudication is suspected.

MANAGEMENT

It is important to reduce the incidence of failed back syndrome by taking precautions right from the time the patient is subjected to the spine surgery. First and foremost is the correct selection of the patient and to plan the most appropriate surgery for an individual patient with preferably a minimally invasive approach wherever possible. Surgery should be based on a sound clinical judgment rather than attempting to correct all radiological features.

Good control of acute post-operative pain is also recommended to reduce the chances of progression to chronic pain or chronic postoperative pain.

Once the diagnosis of post-laminectomy pain is established a multimodal, multidisciplinary approach is advocated to improve chances of success. An individualized plan is made based on clinical evaluation in conjunction with investigations once a potential pain generator is identified.

It is now well accepted that for precision diagnosis, image guided diagnostic blocks can often help the treating practitioner determine the anatomic origin(s) of the patient's pain. These procedures also may facilitate differentiation of a local from a referred somatic pain source, a visceral from a somatic pain source, or a peripheral from a central etiology. Once this is done the decision on further management is made easier. These blocks also may help the practitioner and patient decide whether to proceed with surgery or ablative procedures.

Repeat Surgery

Patient has to be offered repeat surgery when there is a surgically treatable etiology for pain. This requires an accurate diagnosis that demonstrates a structural defect that corresponds with the patient's symptoms and a comprehensive discussion with the patient about the goals of surgery and the risks of failure. The goal of revision surgery will be alleviation of symptoms, but it is important to recognize an inverse relationship between an increasing number of revisions and benefit. Here the patient should recognize that complete alleviation of symptoms is unlikely, but a successful procedure will reduce pain and improve function. The motivation of the patient and his or her ability to express realistic expectations about the outcome may be important variables when considering whether to proceed with a revision.

The main indications are:
- Wrong level of previous surgery
- Recurrent disk herniation
- Residual lateral recess stenosis
- Instability with axial back pain
- Cauda equina syndrome
- Impingement of nerve root by screw.

Waddell et al. documented that, the success of a second operation was only 50%, with an additional 20% considering themselves worse afterwards; with success rate further declining following a third operation to 30%, with 25%

considering themselves worse and, after four operations, 20% success rate, with 45% of the patients considering themselves worse.

Pharmacotherapy

It forms a very useful treatment modality for patients especially in the acute and early phase of postoperative period. No double blind randomized controlled trials have been conducted to prove that any one group of drugs is superior over the other. Detailed analysis of symptoms will enable the practitioner to decide the most appropriate drug. One may consider combining two or more drugs for synergistic effect and also to reduce incidence of dose related side effects.

The commonly used drugs are as follows:

Simple Analgesics and NSAIDs

Acetaminophen (paracetamol) remains one of the safest first-line treatments of acute low back pain (LBP). It is generally well tolerated, has few adverse effects or drug reactions with other medications and is inexpensive. It is also safe in elderly patients. Overdose for long period can result in fatal hepatic injury. The maximum advised dose is 4 g/day.

NSAIDs are the most frequently prescribed analgesic medications for mechanical LBP worldwide for short-term use in acute phase and are proven most effective. Drugs like Diclofenac have been most popular in dose up to 150 mg/day.

There are newer molecules in form of COX II inhibitors like aceclofenac, etoricoxib, and etodolac which are claimed to have a better safety profile for long-term usage especially in the elderly age group.

Muscle Relaxants

Various molecules like chlorzoxazone, caprisoprodol, cyclobenzaprine and thiocolchicoside are used in treating pain due to muscular spasm experienced by many patients.

Antidepressant Drugs (TCAs, SNRI, SSRI)

As already discussed often these patients have psychosocial issues or neuropathic component to the pain for which this group is very useful. Commonly used drugs are amitriptyline (10–50 mg) or nortriptyline (12.5–50 mg) started in small doses and titrated upwards as necessary.

There are newer drugs such as duloxetine which are found to be promising and can be safely used for long-term. It is a potent inhibitor of neuronal serotonin and norepinephrine reuptake. Dose ranges from 20 to 240 mg/day.

Antiepileptic Drugs

The basic mechanism of anticonvulsants is to stabilize neural membranes. This concept has been used to support the use of anticonvulsants for adjunct analgesia suspected to come from neuropathic causes. The drugs most popular from this group are pregabalin (75–300 mg/day), gabapentin (100–3600 mg/day), carbamazepine and topiramate.

Antiarrhythmic Drugs

Such as lignocaine, mexiletine can be offered to patients with neuropathic pain who have not responded to anticonvulsant drugs.

Steroids

These are most useful drugs used by various routes. Centers with lack of expertise of percutaneous interventions advocate use of oral steroids to alleviate inflammatory neuropathy. But the dose required by this route is much higher and may produce undesirable side-effects. In the present scenario it is a regular practice to consider epidural and perineural deposition of steroid to give a targeted delivery for better efficacy. This will also reduce the incidence of steroid related side-effects due to smaller dose.

Tramadol and Codeine

The other popular drugs for pain in failed back syndrome are tramadol and codeine especially in elderly patients who may require them on a regular basis. Both these drugs have a safer side effect profile.

Strong Opioids

Patients with severe intractable pain after exhausting other options may be considered for pure opioids like morphine, oxycodone or Fentanyl. It is said that in patients with genuine pain, the incidence of addiction and drug dependence is much lower than other patients. The only tip here is that the opioid prescription must be given only by a single physician who can monitor the patient for drug abuse.

Pain Interventions

There are a multitude of interventional techniques in the management of chronic pain in failed back patients which include not only neural blockade but also minimally invasive percutaneous to surgical procedures ranging from peripheral nerve blocks, trigger-point injections, epidural injections, facet joint injections, sympathetic blocks, neuroablation techniques, intradiskal thermal therapy, disk decompression, morphine pump implantation and spinal cord stimulation.

The interventions have proven to be cost effective in long-term as compared to the cost of conventional medical management and cost incurred in repeat surgery.

They are used for diagnostic, prognostic and therapeutic purpose. There are some patients where pain generator cannot be established from clinical evaluation and investigations with 100% certainty. For patients where pain can potentially arise from more than one spinal structure a diagnostic block with local anesthetic drug can help to establish the source of pain. It is important to remember when these interventions are for therapeutic purpose that if the source of pain is more than one structure or multiple levels, it is not expected that all the pain will be relieved.

It may be essential to combine, in certain circumstances, more than one block. This may include an epidural and facet-joint block in case of identification of pain generators from both sources; a sympathetic block and facet-joint block if there are two different sources of pain or if two different regions are affected in combination with trigger-point injections. These should ideally be done one at a time to guide the interventionist about contribution of each one to pain.

Transforaminal Epidural Injection

This is the first intervention for a patient with pain in restricted dermatomal distribution. It can also be used to pinpoint the nerve root which is inflamed due to compression by a recurrent disk or vertebral body or adhesions. This may enable surgeon to determine the correct level based on response to this block (Fig. 3).

Facet Blocks

Intra-articular injections, medial branch blocks, and medial branch neurotomy are generally accepted as percutaneous management options for facet joint pain. The use of radiofrequency denervation of the medial branches of the dorsal rami to treat facet joint pain has been employed for over 30 years. Over this time period, the technique and the guidelines have been fine-tuned to improve the outcomes of the procedure and treatment algorithms have been designed to pinpoint specific patients who may benefit. Comparative diagnostic injections, when used

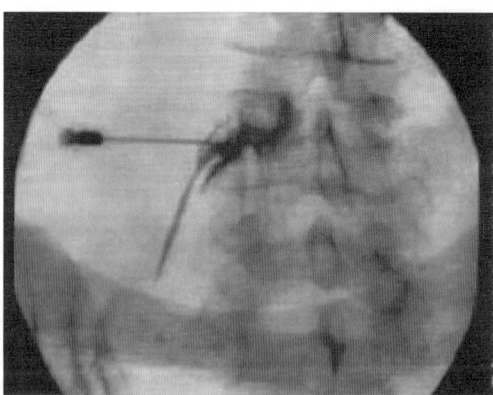

FIG. 3: Transforaminal epidural injection

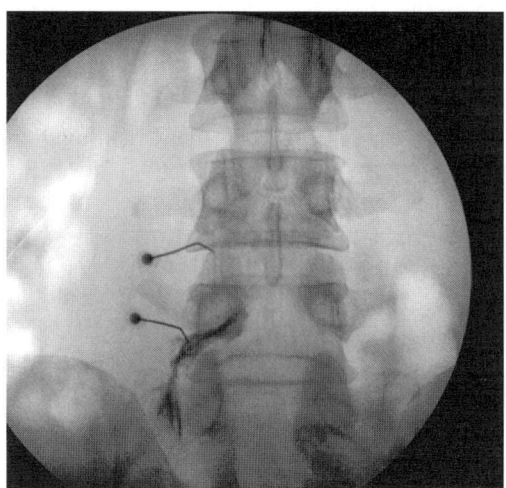

FIG. 4: Medial branch block

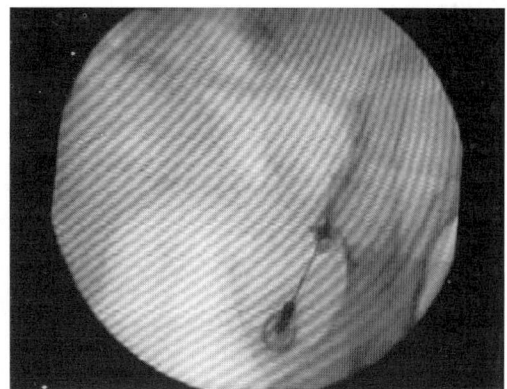

FIG. 5: Sacroiliac joint injection

with the appropriate guidelines, are the best method of diagnosing facet joint pain. Pain relief of more than 80% with medial branch block can establish the diagnosis (Fig. 4).

Medial branch block performed at two adjoining levels for a suspected facet in a comparative controlled manner on two occasions two local anesthetic agents with different duration at least two weeks apart can help to exclude false positive response in 27–47% patients.

Radiofrequency Ablation

It is offered for meaningful long-term attenuation of facetogenic pain with good evidence to support its clinical use. The patients with radicular pain with short-lived but positive response to TFE injection can gain prolonged benefit from a newer modality with unknown mechanism of action called pulsed radiofrequency ablation of dorsal root ganglion (DRG).

Sacroiliac Joint Injection[1]

This is a gold standard to establish SI joint as a pain generator and is offered to patients in whom clinical diagnosis points to this source (Fig. 5).

Caudal Epidural Injection

This is offered by centers where expertise to do TFE injection is not available or when multiple levels are involved. This is an alternative to interlaminar epidural injection which is technically not ideal in presence of a surgical scar which can obscure the entry into the right plane and increase the chances of subdural or subarachnoid needle placement.

Epidural Neuroplasty

The goal of this percutaneous lysis of epidural adhesions is to assure delivery of high concentrations of injected drugs to the target areas. This is performed with special spring loaded navigable catheter designed by Gabor Racz who established a three-day protocol for satisfactory Adhesiolysis. Manchikanti and colleagues modified the Racz protocol from a 3-day procedure to a 1-day procedure.

Epiduroscopy

Epidural lysis of adhesion and direct deposition of corticosteroids on the pathological target in the spinal canal are also achieved with a 3 D view provided by epiduroscopy or spinal endoscopy. Endoscopic adhesiolysis with administration of corticosteroids is a safe and possibly cost-effective technique for relief of chronic intractable pain failing to respond to other modalities of treatments.

Other Interventions

Percutaneous disk decompression at adjacent nonoperated level, sympathetic blocks/ramus communicants block/Trigger point injections, cluneal nerve injections are some other interventions that can be offered in select patients.

Neuromodulation[2]

In patients with severe post-laminectomy pain refractory to all simpler interventions ongoing modulation of nociception may be considered for sustained relief. This requires use of implantable programmable therapies which can be titrated to suit patient requirement for indefinite duration. This modality should be performed only by clinicians with good training and expertise as they are complex and require ongoing titration. The other point to bear in mind is the cost of these systems which are not indigenously made. There are no cost comparative figures available from our country but from many other regions across the globe, the cost analysis clearly indicates that percutaneous, minimally invasive techniques work out less expensive in long-term and their judicious use may prevent the need for more invasive and more expensive techniques and surgery. Two landmark studies published several years ago show that spinal cord stimulation offers better long-term pain relief at lower annualized cost than either repeat spinal surgery or optimized nonsurgical care.[2] It is essential to learn that these therapies also have to be offered at an early stage to have good efficacy. Neuromodulation can be achieved in 2 ways.

Spinal cord stimulation:[3] This is claimed to be very effective for neuropathic variety of radiculopathy pain due to fibrosis, arachnoiditis. There are several proposed mechanisms to explain its efficacy like stimulation of A-β fibers competing with conduction of nociceptive transmission via A-δ and c-fiber activation of central inhibitory pathways, suppressive action on the A-δ fiber and wide dynamic range (WDR) neuron hyperexcitability.

Researchers have found that the costs associated with spinal cord stimulation compare favorably with alternatives, including nonsurgical treatments. The system comprises of two components, configuration varying on a case to case basis. A lead with contact points is placed in dorsal epidural space under fluoroscopic guidance to deliver mild electrical stimulation to dorsal columns (Fig. 6). This is connected to a source of power in form of a compact subcutaneous device (implantable pulse generator (IPG) (Fig. 7).

The best part about the therapy is a testing or trial phase when patient gets an opportunity

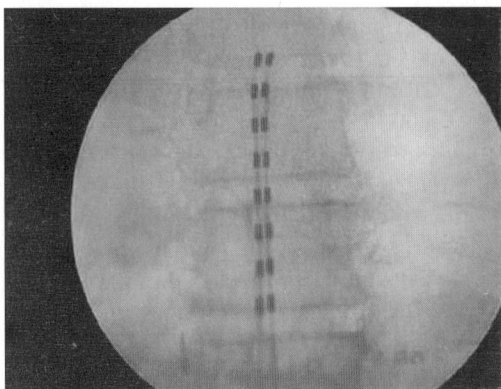

FIG.6: Bilateral octades (anteroposterior view)

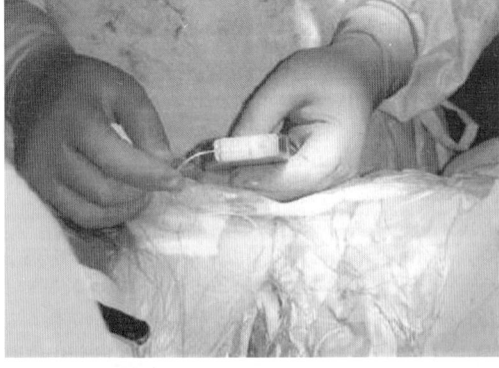

FIG. 7: Subcutaneous implantable pulse generator *(For color version, see Plate 14)*

to feel the therapy briefly and judge the improvement in pain levels.

The success of stimulation therapy depends on the exact pathology, type of pain generator, how much of the pain is neuropathic, patient's motivation and active participation, timely application of the therapy.

Advances are occurring at a rapid pace in the field of neuromodulation and promise much more therapeutic options to come. An innovative system of spinal stimulation has been investigated and proven effective for managing patients with chronic neuropathic pain, including pain associated with failed back surgery syndrome, low back pain and leg pain. In May 2015, the US Food and Drug Administration approved the Senza spinal cord stimulation (SCS) system (Senza System). The Senza System can reduce pain without producing a tingling sensation called paresthesia by providing high frequency stimulation (at 10 KHz) and low stimulation amplitudes[1] and shown better outcomes.

The IPGs can be a nonrechargeable or a newer chargeable variety. Rechargeable generators are often smaller and last longer before they need to be replaced. A potential drawback is that they need to be charged regularly, and the use of high-frequency spinal cord stimulation may require even more frequent charging. Nonrechargeable generators are simpler in terms of day-to-day maintenance, but require a surgical revision to change the battery. This type of generator may be easier for patients who have difficulty with technology.

Spinal cord stimulation is becoming less invasive due to miniaturization of generators and other devices. With smaller generators, the incision needed to insert them has also gotten smaller. For example, one new device offers a generator the size of a matchstick.

A new wireless system takes miniaturization a step further. The leads, electrodes, and a microtransmitter are all implanted in the spinal space with a hollow needle. A small wearable antenna sends signals wirelessly to the electrical contacts in the spinal cavity. This eliminates the need for more extensive surgery to insert the generator as well as the need to eventually replace it. It also avoids potential irritation or infection in the area where the generator is implanted.

There are anecdotal case reports of cases where peripheral nerve field stimulation has been used for localized severe pain such as sacroiliac joint related pain[2] or back pain where all other modalities have failed.

Spinal cord stimulation is considered successful if pain is reduced pain by at least half, but not everyone reaches that goal. With traditional low-frequency therapy, about 50–60% of those using spinal cord stimulation reach that goal, but studies have shown more than 80% experience significant pain relief when using newer, high-frequency therapy.[3]

Intrathecal drug delivery systems[4] (Fig. 8): Intrathecal drug administration by means of an implanted pump has an advantage in that, because the opioids bind directly to the receptors in the dorsal horn, lower dose is required for pain relief. This option is mainly for patient with refractory pain who has significant levels of pain and is on a large dose of opioid like morphine. The system has better efficacy as compared to systemic drug administration and lower chances of adverse effects.

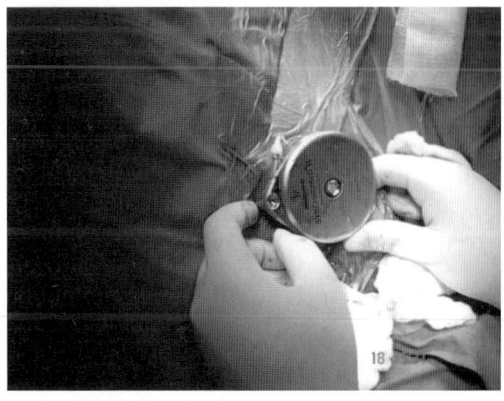

FIG. 8: Intrathecal drug delivery system *(For color version, see Plate 14)*

An implanted hollow intrathecal catheter (made from a biocompatible material) connected to an implanted infusion pump provides continuous intrathecal administration. Permanent implantation is also preceded by a trial period with an external pump. During this trial period, the mode of delivery and the combination and doses of medications are adjusted to achieve optimal pain control. The patient must return regularly to the pain centre for the refilling of the pump with medication which is performed percutaneously on outpatient basis.

The drugs most commonly used with this system for post-laminectomy pain are morphine and the newer one called ziconotide which is claimed to be good for neuropathic variety. There are several other adjuvant drugs used in clinical practice either alone or in combination which are beyond the scope of discussion in this chapter.

Physiotherapy and Rehabilitation

This is extremely useful adjunct therapy with other modalities. An individualized approach will optimize the benefit which may include options like specific workouts for improvement of muscular strength and endurance, restoration of joint ROM and soft tissue extensibility and maintenance exercise programs. It is claimed that some patients may benefit from manipulation or TENS therapy. Hydrotherapy can be recommended for someone with limited ability to perform other exercises.

Psychological Counseling and Cognitive Behavioral Therapy

It may be necessary in many of these patients with dominant psychosocial issues and central sensitization. Biofeedback, relaxation, group therapies, alternative therapies may have a useful role in some select patients.

CONCLUSION

Postspinal surgery pain is a recognized universal problem which may occur even after technically well executed surgery. With an exponential rise in spine surgeries, problem of postsurgery pain is growing!! Detailed clinical evaluation primarily identifies the pain generator. Precision diagnostics have immense value to establish the same. Algorithmic approach permits rational institution of individualized treatment. Timely interventional pain management improves the success rate. Awareness about these available options can help better utilization. Chronic pain specialist can play a vital role as a key person to institute multidisciplinary care to improve quality of life of these unfortunate patients. It is important to realize that these treatments do not take all the pain away but they do make the pain much more bearable in the majority of patients.

REFERENCES

1. Chakrabortty S, Sanjeev Kumar S, Rudraraju S. Intractable sacroiliac joint pain treated with peripheral nerve field stimulation. Anaesthesio Clin. Pharmaco. 2016;32(3).
2. Nagy Mikhail, et al. Clinical Applications of Neurostimulation: Forty Years Later: Pain Practice, 2010;10(2): 103-20.
3. Kapural L, Yu C, Doust MW, et al. Novel 10-kHz High-frequency therapy (HF10 Therapy) is superior to traditional low-frequency spinal cord stimulation for the treatment of chronic back and leg pain: The SENZA-RCT randomized controlled trial. Anesthesiology. 2015;123(4):851-60.
4. Timothy Deer. Intrathecal drug delivery systems: Interventional techniques in chronic spinal pain. ASIPP; 2007.pp.665-80.

Restless Leg Syndrome: Causes and Pain Management

Dwarkadas K Baheti

INTRODUCTION

The exact cause of restless leg syndrome (RLS) is not known and can begin even during childhood. There is a strong genetic link and the risk factor can be iron deficiency. The RLS is thought to be caused by, some type of malfunction of the motor system more specifically of the dopamine pathway. RLS is a sensory cum motor disorder and can be idiopathic or secondary.

Restless leg syndrome can affect people of any age, but susceptible ones are middle-aged and elderly, pregnant women, one with genetic link whose parents had experienced it, one who has sleep disorder called periodic limb movement and people on antidepressants.

The symptoms are characterized by a distressing and uncomfortable urge to move the legs and, sometimes, other parts of the body, such as the arms. It causes a marked sense of discomfort and pain in the legs or other affected parts of body. These symptoms are triggered by rest or inactivity and often relieved by movements of a particular part of the body. This is in contrast to ischemic pain syndrome, where movement causes pain and rest relieves pain. The symptoms are most intense in the evening and night and follow a typical circadian pattern. The restless leg syndrome was first recognized by Wittmaack[1] and clinically studied by Karl Ekbom[2] so it is also known Wittmaack-Ekbom syndrome.

CAUSES

In most cases, there is no definite cause of RLS. It is suspected that genes play a role as a family member may have suffered with this condition. The cause of primary is unknown, however, the secondary RLS can be because either of the following (refer to table 1).

DIAGNOSTIC CRITERIA FOR RESTLESS LEG SYNDROME

These five essential features must be present for a diagnosis of restless legs syndrome:
- You have a strong urge to move your legs (sometimes arms and trunk), usually accompanied or caused by uncomfortable and unpleasant sensations in the legs.
- Your symptoms begin or become worse when you are resting or inactive, such as when lying down or sitting.
- Your symptoms get better when you move, such as when you walk or stretch, at least as long as the activity continues.
- Your symptoms are worse in the evening or night than during the day, or only occur in the evening or nighttime hours.

TABLE 1: Causes of restless leg syndrome

Dysfunction factors	Chronic diseases	Medication Prevention of	Miscellaneous
Dopamine signaling in brain	Parkinson's	Nausea	Alcohol use
Defficient iron metabolism	Kidney failure	Psychotic and depression	Sleep deprivation
Opioid system	Diabetes mellitus	Cold and allergy	Strong genetic basis
	Peripheral neuropathy	Sedation	Pregnancy (usually 3rd trimester)
	Spinocerebellar ataxia types 2 and 3		Axonal neuropathy
	Rheumatoid arthritis		

- Your symptoms are not solely accounted for by another condition such as leg cramps, positional discomfort, leg swelling or arthritis. Willis-Ekbom disease (WED)/RLS often causes difficulty in falling or staying asleep—one of the chief complaints of the syndrome. Many people who have the disease also have periodic limb movements (PLMs)—jerking of the arms or legs that is often associated with sleep disruption.

PREVENTIVE TIPS FOR RESTLESS LEG SYNDROME

Symptoms and Signs

Patient information—aching, creeping, crawling, restless; 'jimmy legs'.

Patients with restless legs syndrome have uncomfortable sensations in their legs (and sometimes arms or other parts of the body) and an irresistible urge to move their legs to relieve the sensations. The condition causes an uncomfortable, 'itchy,' 'pins and needles,' or 'creepy crawly' feeling in the legs. The sensations are usually worse at rest, especially when lying or sitting.

The severity of RLS symptoms ranges from mild to intolerable. Symptoms can come and go and severity can also vary. The symptoms are generally worse in the evening and at night. For some people, symptoms may cause severe night sleep disruption that can significantly impair their quality of life.

- This disease is prevalent in all age groups.
- There is feeling of pulling, cramping, aching, burning, and crawling in legs.
- Irresistible urge to move limbs usually associated with paresthesia/dysesthesia in legs.
- Symptoms worse or exclusively present at rest (lying and sitting).
- Symptoms worse in the evening or at night.
- It is often associated with disturbance in sleep pattern.
- Periodic leg movements during sleep.
- Family history of other member suffering from restless leg syndrome is also present.

Box 1 mentions preventive tips for RLS.

CLINICAL EXAMINATION

Physical Examination

- There will be near-constant leg movement or shifting at rest
- There may be evidence of nerve damage such as paresthesia, allodynia.

Neurological Examination

The patient usually has normal power reflexes of lower limbs (knee and ankle jerk; a flexor plantar response and no obvious sensory deficit to touch and vibration).

Chapter 43: Restless Leg Syndrome: Causes and Pain Management

> **Box 1: Preventive tips for restless leg syndrome**
>
> How to prevent/decrease symptoms of restless leg syndrome
> - Sleep late and sleep longer in the morning
> - Stretch before sleep
> - Decrease or avoid-caffeine, coffee, tea, chocolate, and cola
> - Warm water shower will relax muscles and increase circulation in extremities
> - Warm or chill legs– whatever one is comfortable with
> - Exercise regularly during day in order to have adequate sleep at night
> - Keep mind engaged, i.e. Brain exercise as an empty mind is a devil's paradise,
> - Have calf massage or wear stockings
> - Yoga such as stretching, deep breathing, and relaxation
> - Make your bedroom TV and computer free zone
> - Avoid alcohol and smoking few hours before sleep
> - Take regular iron supplements
> - Avoid antihistaminics, antidepressants, herbal, over-the-counter medicines

INVESTIGATIONS

Blood Investigation
- Vitamin levels (B12, Folate)
- Iron levels (storage level of Ferritin)
- Hormone levels

Sleep Studies
- During periods of wakefulness—can demonstrate excessive muscle activation in the lower extremities through leg leads
- EMG/NCS abnormal in neuropathy with RLS.

DIFFERENTIAL DIAGNOSIS
- Nocturnal leg cramps
- Akathisia (generalized restlessness)
- Periodic leg movement syndrome (PLMD)
- Tardive dyskinesia (extra pyramidal syndrome)
- Insomnia
- Positional discomfort
- Peripheral neuropathy—nutritional or diabetic mellitus.

TREATMENT PROTOCOL
The modal approach is the key, to maximum relief of symptoms of RLS (Table 2).

Medications
- Oxycodone 2.5–25 mg-Painful RLS
- Propoxyphene 100–260 mg-Painful RLS
- Tramadol 50–100 mg-Painful RLS
- Clonazepam 0.5–2 mg-evening dose Drowsiness
- Triazolam 0.125/0.25 mg-Insomnia
- Nitrazepam 2.5–10 mg-Insomnia
- Carbamazepine 100–600 mg-Resistant RLS
- Gabapentin[3,4] 1-4 300–2400 mg-Resistant and painful RLS
- Pregabalin[5] 75–600 mg-Resistant and painful RLS
- Iron sulfate 200 mg TID PO-Iron deficiency
- Dopamine agonists
- Mirapex, Requip 2 mg once daily
- Dopamine-containing medications
- Sinemet 25–100 mg TID.

Nonpharmacologic Therapy
- Sleep improvement
- Mind-distraction activities, e.g. video game, crossword puzzle
- Yoga
- Relaxation exercises
- Music therapy
- Hot bath or soothing massage
- Exercise, e.g. walk in the evening

Interventional
- Botulinum toxin injection
- Nerve block
- Lumbar sympathetic block
- Acupuncture

TABLE 2: Treatment protocol

Medications	Interventional	Miscellaneous	Preventive
Oxycodone 2.5–25 mg		Sleep improvement	To avoid nicotine, caffeine, alcohol, dopamine antagonist, metoclopramide, diphenhydramine, SSRIS, e.g. Prozac
Propoxyphene 100–260 mg	Nerve block	–	–
Tramadol 50–100 mg		Mind-distraction activities, e.g. video game, crossword puzzle	–
Clonazepam 0.5–2 mg evening dose	–	–	–
Triazolam 0.125/0.25 mg	–	–	Watch for tardive dyskinesia
Nitrazepam 2.5–10 mg	Lumbar sympathetic block	Yoga and relaxation exercises, music therapy	Unusual movements which develop after years of therapy
Carbamazepine 100–600 mg	–	–	–
Gabapentin 1–4 300–2400 mg	–	Hot bath or soothing massage	High risk of 'rebound' and 'augmentation'
Pregabalin 5–75–600 mg	Botulinum toxin injection	Exercise, e.g. walk in the evening	Requires alteration in medication dosage
Iron sulfate 200 mg TID PO	–	–	Watch for dizziness and nausea
Dopamine agonists	–	–	Development of augmentation and rebound
Mirapex, requip (ropinirole) 2 mg once daily	Acupuncture	–	–

Preventive/Avoid

- Nicotine, caffeine, alcohol, dopamine antagonist, metoclopramide,
- Diphenhydramine, SSRIS, e.g. Prozac.

Risk Involved to Watch for During the Treatment

- Watch for tardive dyskinesia, dizziness, nausea
- Unusual movements which develop after years of therapy
- High risk of 'rebound' and 'augmentation'
- Require alteration medication dosages
- Development of augmentation and rebound.

CONCLUSION

Restless leg syndrome is very bothersome and psychological disturbing syndrome.

The multimodal approach is mandatory for relief of these symptoms.

REFERENCES

1. Wittmaack T. Lehruch der nervenkrankheiten I. Pahologie und Therapie der Sensibilitat. Neuro-sen; 1861.
2. Ekbom K. Restless legs: A clinical study. Acta Med Scand. 1945:158.
3. Happe, et al. Treatment of idiopathic restless legs syndrome with gabapentin. Neurology. 2001; 57:1717-9.
4. Garcia-Borreguero, et al. Treatment of restless legs syndrome with gabapentin; A double blind, cross over study. Neurology. 2002;59:1573-9.
5. Sommer M, et al. Pregabalin in restless legs syndrome with or without neuropathic pain. Acta Neurol Scand. 2007;115: 347-50.

CHAPTER 44

Calciphylaxis and Its Pain Management

Krishna Poddar

INTRODUCTION

Calciphylaxis or calcemic uremic arteriolopathy (CUA) is a rare and highly morbid syndrome that includes calcification of blood vessels, skin necrosis and thrombosis. It is most commonly associated with end-stage renal disease (ESRD). Calciphylaxis is believed to affect 1-4% of dialysis patients.[1] Other associated disorders may include diabetes mellitus, obesity, hypercalcemia, hyperphosphatemia, secondary hyperparathyroidism and many hypercoagulable conditions. Pathophysiology remains poorly understood; however, current belief is that in ESRD, abnormal calcium and phosphate homeostasis result in the deposition of calcium in the vessels, also known as metastatic calcification. Once the calcium has been deposited, a thrombotic event occurs within the lumen of these vessels, resulting in tissue infarction. It is unknown what the triggers are those because the thrombotic and ischemic event.[2] It is a type of extraskeletal calcification that causes intense pain and cutaneous hyperesthesia. There is no gold standard diagnostic test; it is a clinical diagnosis which can be supported by skin biopsy showing arterial occlusion and calcification in absence of vasculitis. Treatment includes dialysis, wound care, tissue plasminogen activator, hyperbaric oxygen, maggot larva debridement, pain management, urine calcium and phosphate correction and sodium thiosulfate. The cause of mortality and morbidity is fulminant sepsis and severe infection. The prognosis of calciphylaxis remains poor—the overall 1-year survival is 45% and the 5-year survival is 35%, with a relative risk of death of 8.5 compared with other dialysis patients.[3]

BACKGROUND

Calciphylaxis was first reported by Bryant and White in 1898, they associated it with uremia. However, the significance of this relationship became uncertain when vascular calcification was subsequently shown to be prevalent in uremia, yet the syndrome of vascular calcification with cutaneous necrosis remained rare. In 1962, Selye conducted experiments in nephrectomized rats where he observed systemic calcification which was somewhat similar to the clinical features of calciphylaxis.[4] He also coined the term calciphylaxis. It was further explained by Gipstein et al. (1976) who conducted a case series of vascular calcification in 11 patients with chronic renal failure.[5] Hafner et al. in 1995 termed this phenomenon as uremic small artery disease of hands and feet characterize with skin necrosis and acral gangrene due to medial calcification and intimal hyperplasia in arteries of subcutaneous tissue.[6]

EPIDEMIOLOGY

It affects about 1–4% of total patients with ESRD.[7] Widespread use of iron-dextran and parenteral vitamin D has led to increase in incidence in chronic renal failure (stage 5). But, it is extremely rare in patients without chronic kidney disease. More prevalent in whites as compared to blacks, calciphylaxis is seen more in females (female to male ratio 3:1). Mean age of incidence is 48 years (±16 years). Individuals seemingly more predisposed are younger patients who have had a longer duration of renal replacement therapy.

PATHOPHYSIOLOGY

Pathogenesis of calciphylaxis remains obscure and poorly understood. It is a combination of various comorbidities. It is reported to occur from as little as 1 month to as long as 12 years after the onset of ESRD with a median time of 2 years and 9 months.[8] It may be associated with disorders like chronic kidney disease, diabetes, obesity, increased calcium and phosphate concentration, elevated calcium pyrophosphate dihydrate (CPPD) crystal deposition disease, secondary hyperparathyroidism and various hypercoagulable states.

Chronic renal failure, hyperparathyroidism, and a high phosphate diet act as sensitizing agents resulting in a high calcium-phosphate product (Ca x P; normal range 4.2–5.6 $mmol^2/L^2$) with resultant precipitation of Ca-P crystals results in diffuse calcification of the media and internal elastic lamina of small-to-medium-sized arteries and arteriole with intimal proliferation and rarely arterial occlusion causing tissue necrosis. This entity was given the term calcinosis cutis. This results in areas of painful ischemic necrosis in the dermis and subcutaneous fat, mainly involving the abdomen, buttocks and medial aspects of the thighs.

Other triggering events include intravenous iron dextran and albumin infusion, low serum albumin, corticosteroids, immunosuppression, trauma, subcutaneous injections in obese patients, and protein C and S deficiencies causing hypercoagulability and subsequent thrombosis.[9]

There are many cytochemical and molecular mechanisms that are important in bone metabolism. The receptor activator of nuclear factor-kB (RANK), RANK ligand, and osteoprotegerin appear to regulate skeletal and extraskeletal mineralization.[6] Chronic inflammatory conditions reduce serum levels of fetuin-A, an important inhibitor of calcification produced in the liver and thus may predispose to calciphylaxis. Some recent studies show that calciphylaxis occurs as an active form of osteogenesis with upregulation of bone morphogenic protein 2 (BMP-2), Runx2, its target gene and its indirect antagonist sclerostin.[10]

DIAGNOSIS

Early recognition is the key to better treatment outcomes. The diagnosis is most often clinical. The noninvasive tests including plain radiographs, high-resolution computed tomography, bone scans, X-ray and mammography are nonspecific for this condition. In the absence of contraindications, the diagnosis may be confirmed by skin biopsy, which reveals calcifying septal panniculitis and arterial occlusion and calcification in the absence of vasculitic changes.[11]

CLINICAL FEATURES

History

Patients have a long-standing history of chronic renal failure and renal replacement therapy. Very rarely, it may occur in individuals without chronic kidney disease.

Many patients might have a history of renal allograft transplantation. Lesions may have sudden or insidious onset; may be singular or numerous and generally occur on the lower limbs. These lesions are associated with intense burning pain. Patient's history generally reveals hyperphosphatemia with hyperparathyroidism and hypoalbuminemia.

Physical Findings

Early calciphylactic lesions are seen as nonspecific violaceous mottling, as livedo reticularis, or as erythematous papules, plaques or nodules. More developed lesions have a stellate purpuric configuration with central cutaneous necrosis. About 90% of the lesions occur on the lower limbs. Peripheral pulses remain brisk. Other manifestations may include bullae, distinct subcutaneous, erythematous nodules suggestive of erythema nodosum. The lesions begin as painful, symmetrical and evolve into well-demarcated nonhealing ulcers that become necrotic and gangrenous (Figs 1 and 2). The lesions on the upper arm (Fig. 3), trunk, buttocks, and thighs are considered as proximally localized and have a poorer prognosis essentially due to the larger bulk of necrotic and infected tissue. Lesions with distal localization may involve the calves,

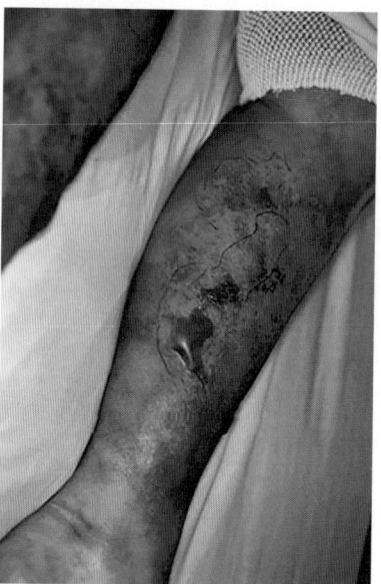

FIG. 2: Calciphylactic lesions at side of leg
(For color version, see Plate 14)

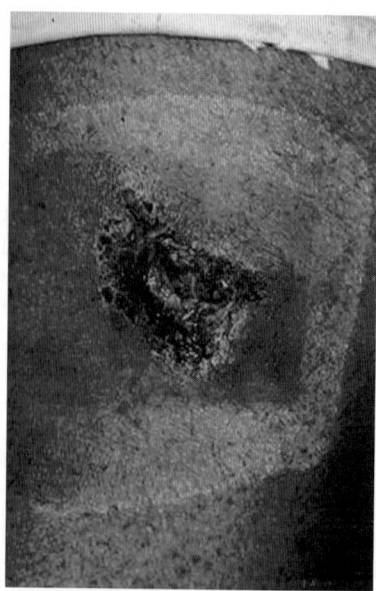

FIG. 1: Nonhealing necrotic ulcer over leg
(For color version, see Plate 14)

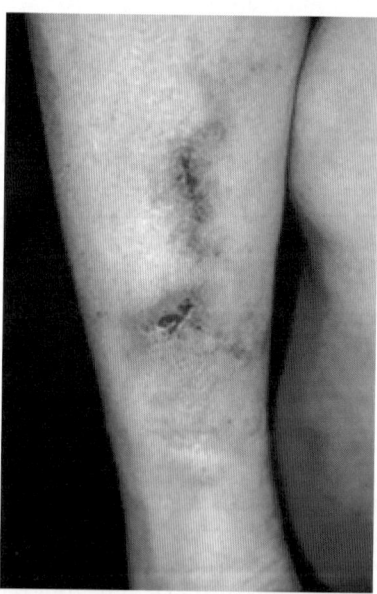

FIG. 3: Calciphylactic lesions at arm
(For color version, see Plate 14)

forearms, acral sites (hands, fingers, feet and toes) and genitalia. Chan et al. in their review of 47 cases reported that 19 of 22 patients with proximal localization died compared with eight of 25 with distal localization.[12] These findings were consistent with Hafner et al.'s review. Thirty-eight of 60 (63%) patients with proximal lesions died as compared with 15/65 (23%) with distal localization or acral gangrene.[13] There is no correlation between age at onset and outcome of the disease. Age at onset ranges from 6 months to 83 years with a mean age of 48 ± 16 years.[10] A female preponderance (61%) is noted due to the tendency to deposit fat in subcutaneous sites, more common in white patients. There is positive correlation with the duration of azotemia, which may alter the internal milieu to an extent to intensify vascular calcification. Vascular insufficiency causing tissue necrosis may coexist due to fibrous obliteration of lumen in response to medial calcification.

CAUSES/ASSOCIATION (TABLE 1)

Differential Diagnosis

- Brown recluse spider envenomation
- Bullous pemphigoid
- Bullous systemic lupus erythematosus (BSLE)
- Cellulitis
- Dermatologic manifestations of necrotizing fasciitis
- Dermatologic manifestations of granulomatosis with polyangiitis (Wegener granulomatosis)
- Erythema nodosum
- Hypersensitivity vasculitis
- Pyoderma gangrenosum
- Venus ulcers
- Vibrio vulnificus infection.

Laboratory Studies

- Creatinine
- Serum proteins and calcium levels
- Liver function test
- Parathyroid hormone level
- Coagulation studies—bleeding, clotting and prothrombin time
- Activated partial thromboplastin time, factor V level
- Triple H
- Erythrocyte sedimentation rate (ESR)
- Rh factor
- Complete blood count (CBC)
- Antineutrophilic antibody (ANA), antineutrophil cytoplasmic antibodies (ANCA) to exclude vasculitis

Imaging Studies

- Plain X-ray of affected area to confirm vascular calcification. Net-like calcification on X-ray is strongly associated with calciphylaxis.
- Bone scintigraphy may be used as a noninvasive diagnostic tool because the bone matrix protein osteopontin has recently been demonstrated in calciphylaxis lesions.

TREATMENT

Nonetheless, the pathogenesis of CUA remains poorly understood and thus there is a lack

TABLE 1: Causes and Association of calciphlaxis

Common association	Speculative association	Others
• Chronic renal failure • Hypercalcemia • Hyperphosphatemia • Hyperparathyroidism • Vascular calcification	• Aluminum toxicity • Coagulation abnormalities • Iron dextran infusion	• Renal transplantation • Immunosuppressive agents • Corticosteroid use • Obesity

of consensus about the optimal treatment. The optimal therapy of calciphylaxis is to prevent its development by rigorous control of phosphate and calcium balance while avoiding or modifying the other risk factors. Treatment includes

- Decreasing parathyroid hormone levels through parathyroidectomy or cinacalcet
- Decreasing serum calcium and phosphate levels through the use of low-calcium dialysis and bisphosphonates.
- Reversing calcium-phosphate deposition through the use of sodium thiosulfate.
- Improving local tissue oxygenation through hyperbaric oxygen and ozone therapy, tissue plasminogen activator and prostacyclin.

A multidisciplinary therapeutic approach is recommended in those with established disease. The utility of parathyroidectomy, corticoid therapy and hyperbaric oxygen therapy remains controversial. However, despite intensive combined treatments, the prognosis of calciphylaxis remains poor. The overall 1-year survival is 45% and the 5-year survival is 35% with a relative risk of death of 8.5 compared with other dialysis patients.

An aggressive *local wound care* program should be initiated to prevent local and systemic infections. This typically involves the use of enzymatic debriding agents, wet to dry dressings, hydrocolloid or hydrogel dressings and systemic antibiotics as needed for infections and avoidance of local tissue trauma including subcutaneous injections. Noncalcium, nonaluminum phosphate binder, such as sevelamer, can be used as an adjunctive therapy. The role of surgical debridement for ulcerations in this condition remains controversial. Improved survival rates have been documented; however, it predisposes the patient to increased risk of sepsis and worsening pain.

Sodium Thiosulfate

Sodium thiosulfate intravenously used as adjunctive for many years as therapeutical.[14] It has relief of pain, reduction in inflammation and healing of ulcers. It is supposed to dissolve insoluble calcium salt embedded in tissues and it reverses endothelial dysfunction and increases vasodilation through its antioxidant properties. Sodium thiosulfate is supposed to be safe and nontoxic drug.[15,16] The suggested dose is 5–25 g intravenously 3–4 times per week for 2–6 years. However, optimum dose and duration is not known yet.

Substitution for sodium thiosulfate intolerance (due to nausea) is deferoxamine.

Bisphosphonates

Bisphosphonates have a powerful inhibitory effect on osteoclast activity and bone resorption. They have also been shown to exert an inhibitory effect on macrophage activity and local proinflammatory cytokine production. Few case reports have shown improvement of calciphylaxis lesions associated with systemic inflammatory response, when treated with intravenous pamidronate and oral etidronate.[17] A dose of 200 mg/day for 14 days has been used with success, effectively lowering the calcium-phosphorus levels.

Hyperbaric Oxygen Therapy

It increases the amount of oxygen in diseased tissue thereby promoting wound healing. The reported schedule hyperbaric oxygen therapy (HBO) is at 2.5 atmospheres absolute has been used for 90 minutes, 5 days per week for 5–7 consecutive weeks. This helps in healing cutaneous ulcers of calciphylaxis. At times there is more pain in some patients ineffective with organ involvement.[18]

Steroids

Its use in calciphylaxis is controversial. Only in one patient its use has resulted in stabilization or improvement in nonulcerating lesions; however, there may be possibility of systemic infection. It is reported that systemic corticosteroids could be a risk factor for calciphylaxis in non-ESRD patients with an autoimmune disorder.

Cinacalcet is a calcimimetic that targets the calcium-sensing receptors of the parathyroid gland chief cells. It is used to lower parathyroid levels as well as improve calcium-phosphorus homeostasis. A dose of 30–60 mg/dL has been shown to be helpful in lowering parathyroid level.[19]

Sterile Maggot Therapy

In some patients, the larvae of the species *Lucilia sericata* have been used for debridement to disinfect skin lesions in patients of calciphylaxis. The mechanism of action is that the maggots have enzymes which liquefy necrotic tissue and secrete phenyl acetic acid and phenyl acetyl aldehyde. This has antibacterial activity that helps to prevent infection.[20] This regime is painless and a promising one. One needs to assess the risks and long-term outcomes.

Anticoagulation therapy: Use of low-dose tissue plasminogen activator and substitution of warfarin with low molecular weight heparin is reported[21] with success in patients with calciphylaxis.

Limb revascularization tried with little success due to presence of progressive gangrene and ischemia.[22,23]

The role of parathyroidectomy in the treatment of calciphylaxis is controversial. It has been reported to be of some help in patients with primary hyperparathyroidism. Hafner et al.[6] noted a survival benefit in patients who underwent parathyroidectomy. Of 58 patients, 38 who underwent parathyroidectomy survived compared with 13 of 37 patients who did not undergo parathyroidectomy. Parathyroidectomy should be avoided in patients without proven primary hyperparathyroidism.

PAIN MANAGEMENT

Pain management is one of the most challenging aspects of calciphylaxis and many patients report severe pain despite administration of potent analgesics. The exact cause of pain is unclear and is thought to be ischemic in origin, but there may be a neuropathic component associated with nerve inflammation.[24] Opioid analgesics are typically required to control severe pain, but morphine, codeine, and hydrocodone should be avoided in dialysis patients due to accumulation of neurotoxic metabolites. Byproducts of morphine can cause hypotension, thereby, slowing the flow in the pannicular arterioles, and thus increasing the risk of thrombosis. Oxycodone and hydromorphone can be used in patients with decreased kidney function but require close monitoring for side effects. Emotional support should be provided to the patient and family. Experience suggests multimodal analgesia combining opioids with nonopioid adjuvants such as neuropathic agents gabapentin and pregabalin. Ketamine may improve symptomatic management of calciphylaxis. Use of nonsteroidal anti-inflammatory drugs may be limited in patients with decreased kidney function. Because of the severity and complexity of pain in this population, pain medicine and palliative care teams play a critical role in calciphylaxis management. Nutritional status of the patient should be well addressed. An increase in dietary protein has been shown to promote wound healing.

The continuous physical examination is to know the response to any therapy. As this disease has high morbidity and mortality in spite of all treatment regimens. The early recognition and use of multimodal therapy is mandatory.

CONCLUSION

Calciphylaxis is a type of metastatic calcification seen in ESRD patients on maintenance hemodialysis. The clinical scenario is in form of ischemic skin ulceration and has high morbidity and mortality. The presence of an abnormal mineral and bone metabolism is the strongest risk factor and use of cortisone for local wound care. The cardinal rule is prevention better though outcome is poor even after best efforts.

REFERENCES

1. Angelis M, Wong LL, Myers SA, Wong LM. Calciphylaxis in patients on hemodialysis: A prevalence study. Surgery. 1997;122:1083-9.
2. Wilmer WA, Magro CM. Calciphylaxis: emerging concepts in prevention, diagnosis, and treatment. Semin Dial. 2002;15(3):172-86.
3. Mazhar AR, Johnson RJ, Gillen D, Stivelman JC, Ryan MJ, Davis CL, et al. Risk factors and mortality associated with calciphylaxis in end-stage renal disease. Kidney Int. 2001;60:324-32.
4. Selye H. Calciphylaxis. Chicago, Ill: University of Chicago Press; 1962.
5. Gipstein RM, Coburn JW, Adams DA, Lee DB, Parsa KP, Sellers A, et al. Calciphylaxis in man. A syndrome of tissue necrosis and vascular calcification in 11 patients with chronic renal failure. Arch Intern Med. 1976;136(11):1273-80.
6. Hafner J, Keusch G, Wahl C, Sauter B, Hürlimann A, von Weizsäcker F, et al. Uremic small-artery diseasewith medial calcification and intimal hyperplasia (so-called calciphylaxis): a complication of chronic renal failure and benefit from parathyroidectomy. J Am Acad Dermatol. 1995;33:954-62.
7. Blumberg A, Weidmann P. Successful treatment of ischaemic ulceration of the skin in azotaemic hyperparathyroidism with parathyroidectomy. Br Med J. 1977;1(6060):552-3.
8. Budisavljevic MN, Cheek D, Ploth DW. Calciphylaxis in chronic renal failure. J Am Soc Nephrol. 1996;7(7):978-82.
9. Rogers NM, Teubner DJ, Coates PT. Calcific uremic arteriolopathy: advances in pathogenesis and treatment. Semin Dial. 2007;20(2):150-7.
10. Kramann R, Brandenburg VM, Schurgers LJ, Ketteler M, Westphal S, Leisten I, et al. Novel insights into osteogenesis and matrix remodelling associated with calcific uraemic arteriolopathy. Nephrol Dial Transplant. 2013;28(4):856-68.
11. Essary LR, Wick MR. Cutaneous calciphylaxis: an underrecognized clinic pathologic entity. Am J Clin Pathol. 2000;113(2):280-7.
12. Chan YL, Mahony JF, Turner JJ, Posen S. The vascular lesions associated with skin necrosis in renal disease. Br J Dermatol. 1983;109:85-95.
13. Hafner J, Keusch G, Wahl C, Burg G. Calciphylaxis: a syndrome of skin necrosis and acral gangrene in chronic renal failure. Vasa. 1998;27:137-43.
14. Schlieper G, Brandenburg V, Ketteler M, Floege J. Sodium thiosulfate in the treatment of calcific uremic arteriolopathy. Nat Rev Nephrol. 2009;5(9):539-43.
15. Meissner M, Kaufmann R, Gille J. Sodium thiosulphate: a new way of treatment for calciphylaxis. Dermatology. 2007;214(4):278-82.
16. Araya CE, Fennell RS, Neiberger RE, Dharnidharka VR. Sodium thiosulfate treatment for calcific uremic arteriolopathy in children and young adults. Clin J Am Soc Nephrol. 2006;1(6):1161-6.
17. Hanafusa T, Yamaguchi Y, Tani M, Umegaki N, Nishimura Y, Katayama I. Intractable wounds caused by calcific uremic arteriolopathy treated with bisphosphonates. J Am Acad Dermatol. 2007;57(6):1021-5.
18. Basile C, Montanaro A, Masi M, Pati G, De Maio P, Gismondi A. Hyperbaric oxygen therapy for calcific uremic arteriolopathy: a case series. J Nephrol. 2002;15(6):676-80.
19. Robinson MR, Augustine JJ, Korman NJ. Cinacalcet for the treatment of calciphylaxis. Arch Dermatol. 2007;143(2):152-4.
20. Tittelbach J, Graefe T, Wollina U. Painful ulcers in calciphylaxis—combined treatment with maggot therapy and oral pentoxyfillin. J Dermatolog Treat. 2001;12(4):211-4.
21. Coates T, Kirkland GS, Dymock RB, Murphy BF, Brealey JK, Mathew TH, et al. Cutaneous necrosis from calcific uremic arteriolopathy. Am J Kidney Dis. 1998;32(3):384-91.
22. Friedman SG. Leg revascularization in patients with calciphylaxis. Am Surg. 2002;68(7):591-2.
23. Weenig RH, Sewell LD, Davis MD, McCarthy JT, Pittelkow MR. Calciphylaxis: natural history, risk factor analysis, and outcome. J Am Acad Dermatol. 2007;56(4):569-79.
24. Polizzotto MN, Bryan T, Ashby MA, Martin P. Symptomatic management of calciphylaxis: a case series and review of the literature. J Pain Symptom Manage. 2006;32(2):186-90.

CHAPTER 45

Regenerative Medicine for Spine and Orthopedic Conditions

Annu Navani, Joshua D Chrystal

INTRODUCTION

The field of regenerative medicine has received great interest in the past decades due to both popularity among patients and physicians alike. The term regenerative medicine is an umbrella-term used to describe the use of biological agents to stimulate a healing response in various tissues throughout the body. Platelet-rich plasma (PRP) has been used with success for decades in various surgical and dermatological settings. There has been a natural progression towards the use of these biologic agents to enhance regeneration and nonsurgical repair of tissue in interventional pain management, sports medicine and orthopedic clinical settings, among others. Proponents consider biologics as the bridge between conservative modalities and invasive surgical interventions. More recently, stem cell therapies have generated great excitement among researchers and clinicians due to promising initial results.

HISTORICAL BACKGROUND

The idea of regenerative medicine is not a new concept. Ancient philosophers such as Aristotle wrote about their observations of various animals such as lizards and worms that had the ability to regenerate tissue and pondered about how this ability could implicate humanity, if it could be harnessed. Applications such as PRP have been described in the literature as early as the 1970s where PRP had been used clinically to help manage various dermatological and oromaxillofacial conditions. Stem cells have been of great interest to scientists for decades. The first methods to isolate and collect stem cells were successfully employed back in 1981. Since then, the clinical applications of this type of medicine have been expanded to include, among others, the fields of interventional pain management, sports medicine and orthopedics.

BIOLOGIC AGENT SOURCES

Biologic agents can be derived from a number of different sources. Each type of source is characterized by where the sample is derived. A tissue-donation sample from a source that is then re-administered to that same source is known as an autologous sample. A prime example is collecting blood, bone marrow or adipose tissue from a patient and after concentrating injecting that solution back into the donor. When graft-versus-host disease (GvHD) and tissue rejection due to immunological incompatibility are concerns, autologous is often the preferred method for these types of procedures. Allogenic samples on the other hand are sourced from donations from a different source, but of the same species. These tissues may need to be processed to "clean and remove" the surface proteins from the donation to reduce the chance of GvHD as the major cause for rejection is human leukocyte antigen (HLA) mismatching. The final category is known as a xenogeneic source. This is when tissue is taken from one species and after processing is transplanted into different species. All tissues donated from nonautologous sources will need to undergo some form of processing before they would be safe (or at least safer) to donate to any other source.

Mesenchymal stem cells (MSCs) possess unique characteristics, which prevent immunological reactions. These cells are young and relatively undifferentiated, therefore lack the surface antigens that may trigger HLA mismatching, they lack major histocompatibility complex-2 expression, as well as having immunological suppression activity mediated by prostaglandin E2.[1] Therefore, theoretically these stem cells can be harvested from a number of different sources and allow compatibility across hosts.

There are, in fact, a number of different sources available. As these types of cells are immature by definition, early sourcing was focused on using embryological samples. Embryonic stem cells represent true pluripotent cells that are capable of differentiating across all cell lines. While this does represent a source of great numbers of these undifferentiated cells, ethical and religious concerns present challenges to research and into the utilization of this sourcing. Fetal stem cells also carry similar concerns among varying groups and represent a more differentiated cell than embryological. Fetal stem cells may be sourced from blood, bone marrow, liver and kidney tissues. On the other hand, umbilical cord stem cells represent an excellent source for multipotent stem cells that have the potential to differentiate into more than one type of cell, but not all cell lines. Cord-blood derived stem cells are rich in hemopoietic stem cells (HSCs) and can differentiate and give rise to all blood cell types, whereas cord tissue is rich in MSCs which can differentiate and give rise to a number of cell lines such as connective tissue, bone, cartilage, muscle, ligament, etc.[2] Placental donations represent another viable source of stem cells. Placental tissue is rich in both HSCs and MSCs. These MSCs can be isolated from placental villous tissue, amniotic fluid and fetal membranes.[3] Finally, scientists have demonstrated the ability to take somatic cell types and "dedifferentiate" them into a type of pluripotent cell known as induced-pluripotent stem cells (iPSCs) through means of transfection in a laboratory setting. Unlike the other viable sources for stem cells, however, this method has been demonstrated to possess oncogenic properties and the possibility to form teratomas and other tumor-types *in vivo*.[4] Research is underway to overcome this limitation.

Clinically, however, all of the above-mentioned sources represent challenges to the practicing physician in both accessibility and point-of-care utilization. In current practice, most physicians are taking advantage of easily accessible methods to harvest and concentrate these cells such as lipo-aspiration and bone marrow-aspiration techniques. While these sources do not contain as high of a ratio of stem cell to fully-differentiated cell sourcing as the above mentioned, these techniques represent a true point-of-care method for collecting and concentrating viable autologous stem cells. In this chapter, we will discuss the clinical applications of commonly used biologics with an emphasis on autologous PRP and autologous MSCs within the context of their use in interventional pain management.

BIOCELLULAR CHEMISTRY

The use of biologics is based on evidence that suggests an increased efficiency and enhancement in wound-healing process.

This process can be divided into three distinct phases: (1) Inflammatory, (2) Proliferative (repair), and (3) Maturation (remodeling) phases. The inflammatory phase begins within the first week. This is typically considered the most painful of the three phases. The inflammatory phase is initiated by the lysis of cells which in-turn release debris and inflammatory mediators such as kinins and prostaglandins. First, platelets aggregate to form a fibrin-matrix. These aggregated platelets then degranulate and release cytokines, signaling and attracting various leukocytes to the area in question. It is the job of neutrophils to kill bacteria and remove extracellular debris. As the platelets are activated, they release a number of growth factors, which attract more cells such as macrophages and fibroblasts. This, along with vasodilation induced by cyclooxygenase-2 (COX-2) helps bring us into the second-stage known as the proliferative phase.

The proliferative phase lasts approximately 2 weeks. During this phase, macrophages perform phagocytosis to further debride the area while fibroblasts begin to form granulation tissue and promote neovascularization.

The final phase that takes place over several months postinjury is known as the remodeling phase. It is during this last phase that the body forms new collagen and scar tissue by replacing the proteoglycan and fibrin networks and forming a new, stronger type-1 collagen matrix. This process continues through remodeling and maturation of new tissue.

Of great interest now is the role and importance of the various growth factors and their role in this symphony of biochemical signaling and healing process. Growth factors stimulate tissue repair and play important roles in cell regulation, differentiation, proliferation, chemotaxis, and matrix synthesis.[5,6] Growth factors released from α-granules within aggregated-platelets help to trigger intracellular signaling pathways. There are many growth factors that have been identified which influence chemotaxis and cell migration via chemical mediators such as: insulin-like growth factor (IGF)-1, transforming growth factor (TGF)-β, platelet-derived growth factor (PDGF), vascular endothelial growth factor (VEGF), basic fibroblast growth factor (b-FGF), hepatocyte growth factor (HGF), and epidermal growth factor. Furthermore, various cytokines, chemokines, and metabolites supplement the action of growth factors[7] (Table 1). These granules contained within the platelets also release calcium, various monoamines and catecholamines such as serotonin, histamine and dopamine, as well as energy providing molecules such as adenosine diphosphate (ADP) and adenosine triphosphate (ATP) to assist in these processes. Additionally, a multitude of other biochemical agents assist and amplify the actions of these growth factors such as cytokines, chemokines and the metabolites formed therein. These agents induce mitosis, contribute to the production of extracellular matrix, and mediate angiogenesis that promotes proliferation, maturation, differentiation, and ultimately repair.[7,8]

Attraction, migration and activation of MSCs also play an integral role in this healing process along with native tissue.[9] This can result in clinical outcome of repair and restoration of injured tissues as is noted in figures 1A and B.

The term "stem cells" represent unspecialized or undifferentiated cells; which at the therapy's basis allows those cells to then differentiate into various target adult cell types.[10] Embryonic stem cells (ESCs), which are formed during the early phases of growth and development within the living source, represent our only source of pluripotent cells that are able to differentiate into any of the three germ layers.[11] However, based on certain ethical perspectives and under current law, the experimentation and research of human-derived ESCs remains controversial.[10]

In 2006, Takahashi and Yamanaka were the first to successfully "dedifferentiate" somatic cell types into an almost ESC pluripotent

TABLE 1: Growth factors involved in wound healing[7]

IGF-1	Early inflammatory phase
IGF-1	Early inflammatory phase
	Anabolic effects
	Protein synthesis, proliferation of myoblasts and fibroblasts
	Enhances collagen and matrix synthesis
	May modulate swelling
TGF-β	Proinflammatory
	Immunosuppressant during inflammatory phase
	Aids cell migration and fibronectin binding
	Augments production of tendon sheath fibroblasts, expression of type I and III collagens
	Improves tendon mechanics during healing
	Controls angiogenesis and fibrosis
PDGF	Early phase of tendon damage
	Facilitates proliferation of other growth factors
	Attracts stem cells and white blood cells
	Stimulates angiogenesis
	Contributes to tissue remodeling
VEGF	Expression peaks after the inflammatory phase
	Promotes angiogenesis-neovascularization
FGF	Appears to stimulate angiogenesis
	Mediates cell migration
	Stimulates proliferation of capillary endothelial cells
	Influences fibroblasts to produce collagenase
	Enhances angiogenesis
	Contributes to production of granulation tissue

IGF-1, insulin-like growth factor; TGF-β, transforming growth factor-Beta; PDGF, platelet-derived growth factor, VEGF, vascular endothelial growth factor, b-FGF, basic fibroblast growth factor.

status by means of transfection using embryonic transcription factors, thus creating "induced-pluripotent stem cells (iPSCs).[12] The applications of these cells in orthopedic medicine have been described well by Schmitt and colleagues.[13] However, dedifferentiated cell types have demonstrated the ability of inducing various tumor types such as teratomas and high rates of other tumor types in mice injected with these (iPSCs) cells.[4] It has been proposed that the mechanism of oncogenesis in regards to the iPSC cell types is due to a suppression of epigenetic remodeling that occurs as a consequence of using known oncogenic retroviuses to direct those transcription factors that induce dedifferentiation. Due to these findings, ethical and safety issues have been underpinned in the concerns of human application utilizing iPSC- and ESC-derived cells.[10,14]

Therefore, much of the application of stem cells in current regenerative medicine focuses on the use of MSCs. These MSCs have been shown to have the ability to migrate from their site of origin by means of chemotaxis after tissue injury and subsequent inflammatory response.[15] Further evidence has demonstrated that like PRP, another mechanism of action is the release of various growth factors such as IGF-1, IGF-2, HGF, VEGF and b-FGF from MSCs, which will promote cell growth, proliferation and angiogenesis.[16,17] Evidence suggests that MSCs have the ability to differentiate and incorporate themselves into tissue matrices and interestingly, there is evidence to suggest that these MSCs even have the ability to differentiate into those tissues of different germ lineages.[18-21] In addition to their direct ability to differentiate, MSCs have been shown to induce both anabolic and anti-inflammatory activity via the release of several cytokines into the surrounding environment.[22] These mechanisms may explain why clinically, patients tend to report earlier-onset of pain relief with this type of therapy versus PRP, as the mechanisms of PRP are more inflammatory in nature. Furthermore, some evidence has

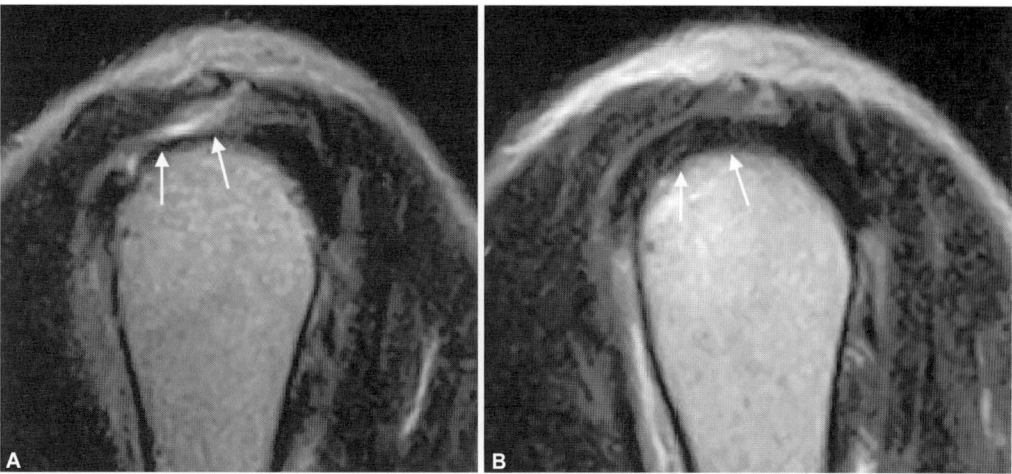

FIGS 1A and B: Pre and post Platelet-rich plasma treatment demonstrating healing of rotator cuff tendinopathy in magnetic resonance imaging

even suggested that the MSCs have such low immunogenic properties that they may be transplanted between different individuals without inducing an immune reaction or rejection of these tissues.[23] The potential of both quickly relieving pain and ultimately restoring function, as well as the potential of unlimited sourcing, makes the use of MSCs very exciting within the field of regenerative medicine.

CLINICAL CONSIDERATIONS

As the popularity of this type of medicine has grown, so as the industry offering a variety of systems and kits used to prepare the biological agents for clinical use. The essential role of these systems is to centrifuge and concentrate the primary biologic agent down to the end-product goal, i.e., concentrated PRP or concentrated MSCs. However, due to the variations in system and preparation techniques, the end-product can be very different from system-to-system. Platelet-rich plasma may need to be prepared differently for different applications such as the concentration and constitution of PRP for an acute injury like a bone fracture should be different from treating a chronic injury such as a tendinopathy or osteoarthritis (OA).[24]

Platelet-rich plasma is defined as a sample of autologous blood with concentrations of platelets above baseline values. In the case of current PRP and MSC concentration systems, most will start with a certain volume of donated whole blood, bone marrow or adipose tissue, ranging on an average from 20 cc to 120 cc. These systems utilize various kits and centrifuges that allow for the separation and concentration of platelets and or stem cells. In PRP and bone marrow aspirate concentrate (BMAC) preparation, an anticoagulant is often used to bind to calcium, thus preventing temporarily the initiation of the clotting cascade by inhibiting the conversion of prothrombin to thrombin.[25] Both PRP and BMAC can be prepared without anticoagulants, however, extra-care and much shorter "draw-to-injection" times must be taken into consideration in preparation and application of the end product. Although several anticoagulants are available, it is proposed that the acid citrate dextrose-A and citrate phosphate dextrose maintain the structural and functional integrity of platelets better than others.[26]

Once the sample has been drawn and is applied to the specific kit, the sample is then prepared in a centrifugation process, most often in at least 2 cycles. The first cycle (soft-spin) separates the sample into 3 distinct fractionated layers: (1) The erythrocyte layer [containing mostly whole red blood cells (RBCs)], (2) The buffy coat layer [containing the leukocytes (white blood cells {WBCs}), platelets and any viable stem cells] and (3) the plasma-protein layer (containing various proteins and growth factors). At this point, during the second cycle, most systems will then either through manual or mechanical means separate out the RBC layer (hard-spin) and allow for concentration of the platelets and stem cells into solution. In the case of PRP, this separation will create both platelet-rich and platelet-poor plasma. The potential beneficial effects of platelet-poor plasma on tissue healing are unknown.

The term PRP was recently expanded to include any combination of concentrated RBCs, WBCs, and any or all of activating factors such as thrombin or calcium chloride.[27-29] Thus, depending on the kit and the centrifuge, the end product may be further categorized leukocyte poor or leukocyte rich PRP. Not all preparations are equivalent. Variations in preparations occur due to everything from the volume of tissue being used, the end concentrations of the cell types, volumes of the concentrated end product, the presence or absence of RBCs or WBCs or both, the pH of the final solution as well as the addition of thrombin or calcium chloride to activate platelets (after preparation and prior to injection) to name a few. At least 40 commercial systems claim to segregate and concentrate various components of whole blood, bone marrow and adipose tissue. Castillo and colleagues investigated this topic by studying several popular automated PRP systems and testing the products against each other utilizing blood samples from a small population. Automated clinical laboratory analyzers were used to count platelet, RBC, WBC and fibrinogen concentrations of the end products. Additionally, enzyme-linked immunosorbent assay (ELISA) was employed to determine growth factor concentrations for $\alpha\beta$ and $\beta\beta$ (PDGF-$\alpha\beta$, PDGF-$\beta\beta$), transforming growth factor β_1 (TGF-β_1), and vascular endothelial growth factor (VEGF). As expected, there were significant differences in end products, most notably in platelet capture efficiency as well as concentrations of WBCs and various growth factors.[30]

It should be noted that unlike prescription drugs and durable medical equipment, which are regulated in the United States by the Food and Drug Administration (FDA), there is little oversight for PRP and MSC concentration systems. This puts the burden of efficacy and application squarely on the practitioner, as an understanding of the end-formulation and its clinical use is paramount for clinical success. Two other studies describe attempts to standardize different PRP systems by classifying them according to activation mechanism, platelet number, and/or cell content.[31,32] The concentrations of platelets and growth factors within solution exhibit a direct proportional relationship to each other.[33] However, although PRP preparations containing higher concentrations of platelets will include higher PDGF concentrations, the relationship is not always directly proportional.[34]

In addition, because TGF-β and VEGF concentrations can vary greatly among individual samples, it makes it difficult to determine the specific differences in these concentrations among different systems. These results may suggest that PDGF concentrations should be used as an indicator when comparing methods for producing PRP.[35] Conversely, some evidence suggests that higher concentration or absolute number of platelets within a particular PRP solution may not, necessarily, lead to an enhanced effect on tissue healing.

For instance, one such study has proposed that the most efficacious platelet concentration for tissue healing is 1.5×10^6

platelets/μL.[36] Additionally, the dose-response curve does not appear linear. Once a high enough concentration of platelets is achieved, a saturation effect occurs that is accompanied by the activation of an inhibitory cascade. As platelets exert the greatest influence on healing during or immediately after the inflammatory phase of healing, some authors have postulated that the timing of the administration of PRP has greater influence on healing than the number of platelet.[33,37]

This has been further demonstrated in a study comparing patellar tendon repair after acute injury using PRP in rat models.[38] During this study, PRP injections were administered to wounded tendons on either 3 days or 7 days following induced-injury. The tendon segments were then harvested 14 days after the initial injury. The tendons injected 7 days after injury showed greater gains in both mechanical properties, including peak loads as well as in the overall maturation of healing, when compared with those injected on day 3. These findings provide further evidence that suggest the optimal time for injecting acute tendon injuries is immediately following the termination of the inflammatory phase, to help augment the initiation and progression of the proliferative phase.

Induced-activation of platelets prior to or during injection of PRP remains a subject of debate. Thrombin, calcium chloride, or both are necessary to catalyze the conversion of fibrinogen to fibrin, and they also induce platelets to secrete growth factors. However, some data suggests that this may not necessarily be beneficial in specific applications, as exogenous thrombin activation of PRP may diminish the ability of PRP to induce bone formation, when compared with non-thrombin-activated PRP. Furthermore, the presence of different cell types such as neutrophils may be included or excluded in PRP and MSC preparations, which may affect both healing as well as the comfort level of these injections for the patient. Depending on preparation techniques and systems, PRP can contain other cell types that potentially benefit, or hinder tissue healing. WBCs such as monocytes and polymorphonuclear neutrophils may trigger localized inflammation, which, while some investigators believe that this inflammatory effect is critical to the repair process, neutrophils have been shown to potentially impede healing, as well as contribute to increased postinjection soreness. Inclusion or exclusion of these different cell types in both PRP and MSC preparation may vary based on clinical indications and goals.

INDICATIONS AND APPLICATIONS

Biologics have been used clinically in a variety of musculoskeletal applications. These techniques have been employed successfully to treat a variety of acute and chronic musculoskeletal and spine injuries such as osteoarthritis, tendinopathy, chondropathy, muscle and ligamentous tears, as well as disks and spinal bony and soft-tissue structures.

Osteoarthritis (OA) is a complicated process involving nearly all of the tissues in the joint. This process is explained in theory by both mechanical and biochemical mechanisms. The interplay of the various tissues throughout the joint, including cartilage, subchondral bone and synovium can become overwhelmed by inflammatory chemicals and decreased cellular functioning, which will perpetuate the degenerative process.[39] There are a multitude of treatment options for OA that have been used in a clinical setting and observed to decrease the symptomatology of OA. Anti-inflammatory treatments have been a mainstay of modern medical treatments used orally, topically and intra-articularly (Figs 2A and B). Oral anti-inflammatories can be effective in pain relief; however, these medications are not without side effects such as the formation of ulcers, liver and kidney damage as well as cardiovascular complications. Topical anti-inflammatories can also address pain however they too carry similar side effect profiles. The most commonly used intra-articular corticosteroid

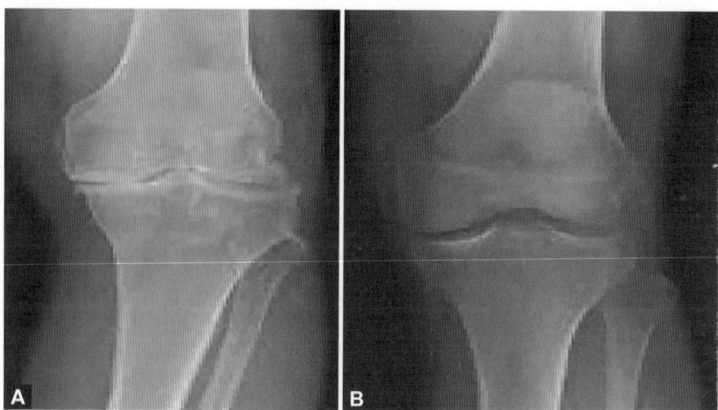

FIGS 2A and B: Radiographs demonstrating pre and post regenerative treatment utilizing mesenchymal stem cells (MSCs) demonstrating reduction in arthritic properties such as subchondral sclerosis and an increase in joint space indicating a correlated increase in the thickness of the intra-articular cartilage

injections can provide significant symptomatic relief; however with increased frequency or higher doses, these too can cause both local and systemic side effects. In higher doses of intraarticular corticosteroid injections, both gross and histological degradation of cartilage and toxicity of chondrocytes has been observed.[40]

There are, of course, risks and contraindications to all injections; however with the use of biologics, we can see marked therapeutic benefit, while demonstrating a greatly reduced side effect profile. In addition, the main difference between regenerative methods and other types of therapies is that with biologic treatments, the aim is to restore cellular integrity and therefore function of the target structures.

As an example, in the case of lateral epicondylitis, local injections of PRP demonstrated clear advantages over corticosteroids achieving significantly greater reduction in visual analog scale (VAS) scores that, unlike corticosteroids, were maintained through 1- and up to 2-year follow-up.[41,42] Similarly, PRP and MSCs have shown positive results in a variety of musculoskeletal conditions (Figs 3A and B).[43]

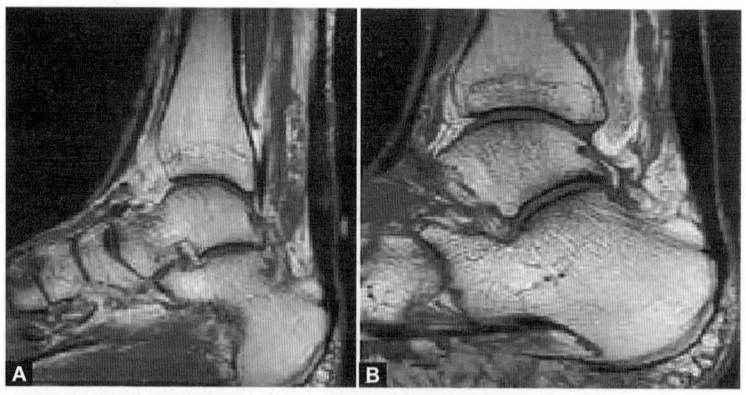

FIGS 3A and B: Pre- and postregenerative treatment images utilizing platelet-rich plasma (PRP) demonstrating healing of a partial thickness intra-substance tear of the Achilles tendon

In terms of spinal pain, conventional therapies have focused on tampering down the inflammatory process to reduce swelling and inflammation. Rest, the use of ice or other cold hydrotherapies, non-steroidal anti-inflammatory drugs (NSAIDs) or corticosteroids and even bracing will fall into this category. Physical and manual therapies have been utilized to rehabilitate muscular functioning and stabilization of skeletal structures. Corticosteroids (as do NSAIDs) work to interfere in the inflammatory process and have been utilized successfully for decades in the treatment of a multitude of musculoskeletal conditions from trigger point or facet injections to epidural injections. The treatment of targeted sensory nerve pain has been advanced by the use of radio-frequency ablation (RFA) techniques. Selective nerve blocks with local anesthetics, such as medial branch blocks (MBB) are utilized to help the practitioner identify the pain generator (or generators) and once identified can help to open up the utilization of more advanced techniques such as radiofrequency ablation.

Intradiskal pathology has been pointed to as a major source and generating factor of back pain and dysfunction. As the intervertebral disk is a cornerstone of biomechanical functioning of the vertebral unit, any disruption in normal functioning will exacerbate the degenerative process, often leading to pain and further disability. Traditional techniques dealing with intervertebral disk pathology had been limited to surgical techniques, however more recently; the use of radiofrequency ablation and other high-energy techniques has been proposed and utilized for various intervertebral disk pathologies. Researchers in the field of regenerative medicine have shown promising results in restoration of disk architecture with the use of biologic agents.[44,45] In the case of intradiskal injections, PRP and platelet lysate have been shown to exert proliferative effects on annulus fibrosus (AF) cells and increase the production of extracellular matrix (ECM) in vitro (Figs 4A and B).[46] Furthermore, biologic agents such as MSCs are capable of altering the microenvironment of the lumbar intervertebral disks and may alter the catabolism within the disk.[46-48] Clinical practitioners have begun to perform intradiskal injections utilizing biologics successfully for therapeutic benefits of pain reduction and restoration of both structure and function.[49-52]

Although the literature is sparse in the use of biologics for nondiskogenic spinal pain recent studies have shed light into its efficacious use (Figs 5A and B).[53,54]

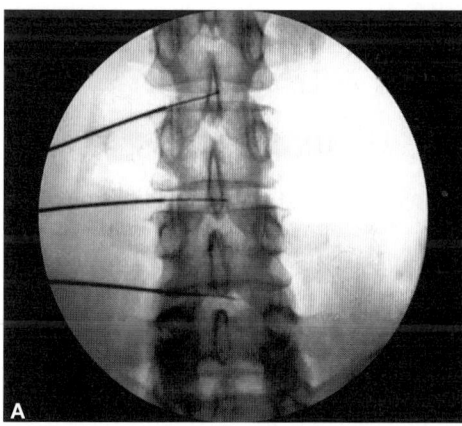 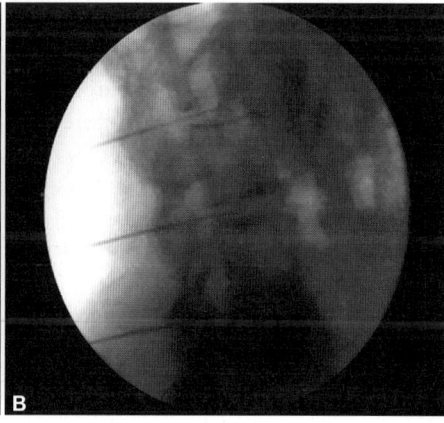

FIGS 4A and B: Anteroposterior and lateral views demonstrating needle placement for intradiskal platelet-rich plasma (PRP) or mesenchymal stem cells (MSCs) injection at L2-3, L3-4, L4-5 levels

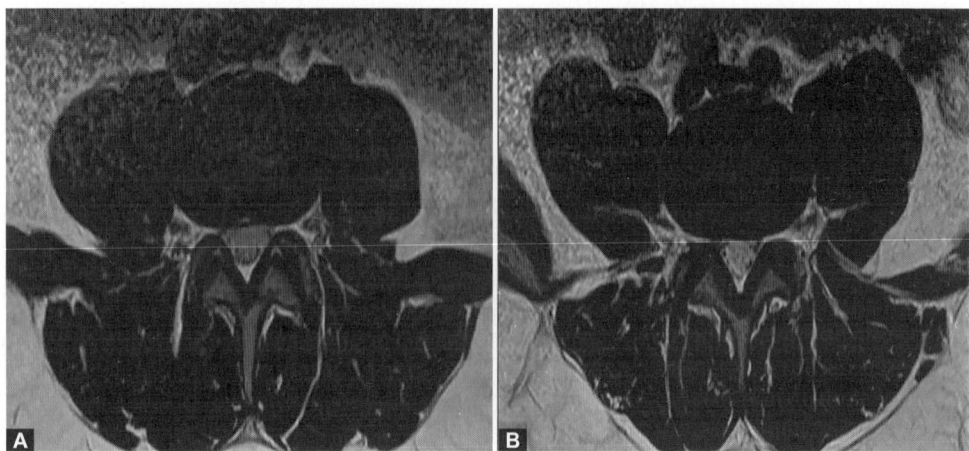

FIGS 5A and B: Axial T2 MRI images identifying resolution of posterior annular tear at L3-4 disk 6 months post-PRP injection

As more studies are performed and techniques refined, early interventions may help to prevent the deterioration of the disks, joints and other orthopedic and spinal structures thereby leading to less pain and disability.

PROCEDURAL PROTOCOLS

There are currently no formal guidelines for the practice of regenerative medicine procedures. One is directed to their regional and national societies for policies and practices related to safe and efficacious use of this therapy in clinical setting. In general, the orthopedic, musculoskeletal and spinal procedures are done in a sterile environment under live visualization of the structures via fluoroscope, ultrasound, computed tomography or magnetic resonance imaging (Fig.).

A clinical center and a practitioner capable of executing the procedure in a manner that meets standard of care in the community and capable of managing complications and providing immediate emergency services are well-suited to perform these procedures (Fig. 6).

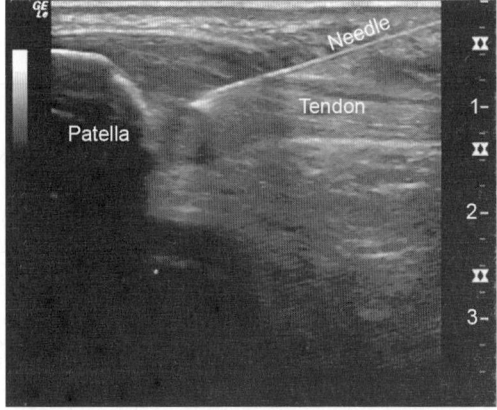

FIG. 6: Demonstration of proper technique utilizing ultrasound guidance to visualize the needle as it approaches the pathological patellar tendon for regenerative injection

CONTRAINDICATIONS

Not all patients are suitable candidates for this type of intervention. As with any therapy, there are several absolute and relative contraindications. Absolute contraindications include local infection or abscess over the site to be injected, septicemia, hemodynamic instability and critical thrombocytopenia. Much like any intervention, typically 100,000 platelets/μL is considered optimal; any values below the standard of 100,000 platelets/μL may affect bleeding times and healing. Additionally, injections about hardware, surgical implants and joint replacements, hematologic and bone marrow cancers, as well as factors that affect healing such as diabetes mellitus and the use of tobacco products are considered relative contraindications.

As a proper inflammatory response is critical in therapeutic benefit from these applications, the use of NSAIDs and corticosteroids around the time of injection is a relative contraindication. For NSAIDs, the last dose is recommended to be taken minimum of 72 hours prior to the treatment and a minimum of 1 week, optimally 21 days after the treatment; oral corticosteroids should be avoided, if possible along the same time frame. As the half-life of injectable corticosteroids are often significantly longer, there should be a minimum of 4-8 weeks since the last corticosteroid injection, especially in the area to be treated, prior to the regenerative treatment. Additionally, therapeutic hydrotherapy techniques should focus on moist heat, as opposed to ice or other cold therapies. As the goals of regenerative therapies are to increase, at least temporarily, inflammation, the use of topical ice or other cold hydrotherapy techniques, postbiologic therapy are discouraged. Furthermore, heat, especially moist heat can help to encourage localized blood-flow and perfusion, bringing cellular nutrients to the area and removal of metabolic waste products; helping to reduce subsequent muscle spasms and discomfort in the treated areas.

LEGISLATIVE AND ETHICAL UPDATE

As the aim of these therapies is to promote and enhance healing, it had in the past been called into question regarding its ethical application and use in professional athletes as a potential performance enhancing substance. In 2010, the World Anti-Doping Agency (WADA) prohibited the administration of intramuscular injections of platelet-derived preparations. Other routes of administration "require a declaration of use in compliance with the International Standard for Therapeutic Use Exemptions." As PRP appears benign, in 2011, WADA removed platelet-derived preparations from the prohibited list, stating that: "after consideration of the lack of current evidence concerning the use of these methods for purposes of performance enhancement, current studies on platelet-derived preparations do not demonstrate a potential for performance enhancement beyond a potential therapeutic effect."

Currently, the FDA, Center for Biologics Evaluation and Research (CBER) and Centers For Disease Control (CDC) are the main regulatory agencies in the United States that hold regulations over the use of biologic therapies and all other blood products. Currently, the FDA names PRP solely for use in operative settings to enhance bone grafts, therefore the use of PRP for any other purpose would be considered "off label".[55] Additionally, sourcing for stem cell treatments are also regulated by these agencies. As with any off-label use, including the use of these agents for techniques mentioned above, the burden falls on the practitioners to be knowledgeable of the product or products they are utilizing, to provide adequate information and obtain informed consent from their patients. It is of the utmost importance that each practitioner research and check in with their regional, state and national regulatory agencies to ensure best practice policies are being followed where ever they are practicing.

CONCLUSION

The changing landscape of health care is rapidly transforming the medical practice. Minimally invasive outpatient procedures are displacing invasive and expensive surgeries associated with prolonged recovery times. Similarly, the focus of treatment in many orthopedic and sports medicine practices have shifted towards a more natural and holistic approach, from traditional medical and surgical treatments. Furthermore, larger studies are required to establish a greater understanding of optimization of the biologic end-products. These studies should aim to help characterize the variability and optimal concentrations in numbers of platelets, WBCs, RBCs, and growth factors and their influence on the biological end product as well as their influence on efficacy and longevity of treatment outcomes. Long-term studies taking into account the timing of these types of interventions and their possible utilization as preventative measures should also be undertaken. Finally, further critical review and rigorous clinical studies are required to formulate a cost-effective and efficacious algorithm for the use of biologics and regenerative medicine in patients with varying spinal and orthopedic conditions.

REFERENCES

1. Lin CS, Lin G, Lue TF. Allogeneic and xenogeneic transplantation of adipose-derived stem cells in immunocompetent recipients without immunosuppressants. Stem Cells and Development. 2012;21(15):2770-8.
2. O'Donoghue K, Fisk NM. Fetal stem cells. Best Pract Res Clin Obstet Gynaecol. 2004;18(6):835-75.
3. Wang Y, Zhao S. Vascular biology of the placenta. Morgan and Claypool Life Sciences; 2010.
4. Rodolfa K, di Giorgio FP, Sullivan S. Defined reprogramming: a vehicle for changing the differentiated state. Differentiation. 2007;75(7):577-9.
5. Anitua E, Andia I, Ardanza B, Nurden P, Nurden AT. Autologous platelets as a source of proteins for healing and tissue regeneration. Thomb Haemost. 2004;91(1):4-15.
6. Anitua E. Plasma rich in growth factors: preliminary results of use in the preparation of future sites for implants. Int J Oral Maxillofac Implant. 1999;14(4):529-53.
7. Nguyen RT, Borg-Stein J, McInnis K. Applications of platelet rich plasma in musculoskeletal and sports medicine. an evidence-based approach. PM R. 2011;3(3):226-50.
8. Hammond JW, Hinton RY, Curl LA, Muriel JM, Lovering RM. Use of autologous platelet-rich plasma to treat muscle injuries. Am J Sports Med. 2009;37(6):1135-42.
9. Saito M, Takahashi KA, Arai Y, Tonomura H, Honjo K, Nakagawa S, et al. Intraarticular administration of platelet-rich plasma with biodegradable gelatin hydrogel microspheres prevents osteoarthritis progression in rabbit knee. Clinical Exp Rheumatol. 2009;27(2):201-7.
10. Wert G, Mummery C. Human embryonic stem cells: research, ethics and policy. Hum. Reprod. 2003;18(4):672-82.
11. Ehnert S, Glanemann M, Schmitt A, Vogt S, Shanny N, Nussler NC, et al. The possible use of stem cells in regenerative medicine: dream or reality? Langenbeck's Archives of Surgery. 2009;394(6):985-97.
12. Takahashi K, Yamanaka S. Induction of pluripotent stem cells from mouse embryonic and adult fibroblast cultures by defined factors. Cell. 2006;126(4):663-76.
13. Schmitt A, van Griensven M, Imhoff AB, Buchmann S. Application of Stem Cells in Orthopedics. Stem Cells International. 2012;2012:394962.
14. Robbins RD, Prasain N, Maier BF, Yoder MC, Mirmira RG. Inducible pluripotent stem cells: not quite ready for prime time? Current Opinion in Organ Transplantation. 2010;15(1):61-7.
15. Wang L, Li Y, Chen X, Chen J, Gautam SC, Xu Y, et al. MCP-1, MIP-1, IL-8 and ischemic cerebral tissue enhance human bone marrow stromal cell migration in interface culture. Hematology. 2002;7(2):113-7.
16. Yu XY, Geng YJ, Li XH, Lin QH, Shan ZX, Lin SG, et al. The effects of mesenchymal stem cells on c-kit up-regulation and cell-cycle re-entry of neonatal cardiomyocytes are mediated by activation of insulin-like growth factor 1 receptor. Molecular and Cellular Biochemistry. 2009;332(1-2):25-32.
17. Chen TS, Lai RC, Lee MM, Choo ABH, Lee CN, Lim SK. Mesenchymal stem cell secretes microparticles enriched in pre-microRNAs. Nucleic Acids Research. 2009;38(1):215-24.
18. Cao Y, Sun Z, Liao L, Meng Y, Han Q, Zhao RC. Human adipose tissue-derived stem cells differentiate into endothelial cells in vitro and improve postnatal neovascularization in vivo. Biochem Biophy Res Comm. 2005;332(2):370-9.
19. Bossolasco P, Cova L, Calzarossa C, Rimoldi SG, Borsotti C, Deliliers GL, et al. Neuro-glial differentiation of human bone marrow stem cells in vitro. Experimental Neurology. 2005;193(2):312-25.
20. Fukuda K. Reprogramming of bone marrow mesenchymal stem cells into cardiomyocytes. Comptes Rendus: Biologies. 2002;325(10):1027-38.
21. Schwartz RE, Reyes M, Koodie L, Jiang Y, Blackstad M, Lund T, et al. Multipotent adult progenitor cells from bone marrow differentiate into functional hepatocyte-like cells. J Clin Inves. 2002;109(10):1291-302.

22. Porada CD, Almeida-Porada G. Mesenchymal stem cells as therapeutics and vehicles for gene and drug delivery. Advanced Drug Delivery Rev. 2010;62(12):1156-66.
23. Devine SM, Bartholomew AM, Mahmud N, Nelson M, Patil S, Hardy W, et al. Mesenchymal stem cells are capable of homing to the bone marrow of non-human primates following systemic infusion. Experimental Hematology. 2001;29(2):244-55.
24. Sánchez M, Filardo G, Yoshioka T. Platelet rich plasma and orthopedics: Why, when, and how. Bio Med Res Int. 2015;2015:949720.
25. Hu X, Wang C, Rui Y. An experimental study on effect of autologous platelet-rich plasma on treatment of early intervertebral disc degeneration. Zhongguo Xiu Fu Chong Jian Wai Ke Za Zhi. 2012;26(8):977-83.
26. Pignatelli P, Pulcinelli FM, Ciatti F, Pesciotti M, Sebastiani S, Ferroni P, et al. Acid citrate dextrose (ACD) formula A as a new anticoagulant in the measurement of in vitro platelet aggregation. J Clin Lab Anal. 1995;9(2):138-40.
27. Lacoste E, Martineau I, Gagnon G. Platelet concentrates: effects of calcium and thrombin on endothelial cell proliferation and growth factor release. J Periondontol. 2003;74(10):1498-507.
28. Martineau I, Lacoste E, Gagnon G. Effects of calcium and thrombin on growth factor release from platelet concentrates: kinetics and regulation of endothelial cell proliferation. Biomaterials. 2004;25(18):4489-502.
29. Wasterlain AS, Braun HJ, Dragoo JL. Contents and formulation of platelet-rich plasma. Operative Tech Orthop. 2012;22(1):33-42.
30. Castillo TN, Pouliot MA, Kim HJ, Dragoo JL. Comparison of growth factor and platelet concentration from commercial platelet-rich plasma separation systems. Am J Sports Med. 2011;39(2):266-71.
31. DeLong JM, Russell RP, Mazzocca AD. Platelet-rich plasma: the PAW classification system. Arthroscopy. 2012;28(7):998-1009.
32. Mishra A, Harmon K, Woodall J, Vieira A. Sports medicine applications of platelet rich plasma. Curr Pharm Biotechnol. 2012;13(7):1185-95.
33. Hsu WK, Mishra A, Rodeo SR, Fu F, Terry MA, Randelli P, et al. Platelet-rich plasma in orthopaedic applications: evidence-based recommendations for treatment. J Am Acad Orthop Surg. 2013;21(12):739-48.
34. Shen W, li Y, Zhu J, Schwendener R, Huard J. Interaction between macrophages, TGF beta 1 and the COX-2 pathway during inflammatory phase of skeletal muscle healing after injury. J Cell Physiol. 2008;214(2):405-12.
35. Kushida S, Kakudo N, Morimoto N, Hara T, Ogawa T, Mitsui T, et al. Platelet and growth factor concentrations in activated platelet-rich plasma: a comparison of seven commercial separation systems. J Artif Organs. 2014;17(2):186-92.
36. Giusti I, Rughetti A, D'Ascenzo S, Millimaggi D, Pavan A, Dell'Orso L, et al. Identification of an optimal concentration of platelet gel for promoting angiogenesis in human endothelial cells. Transfusion. 2009;49(4):771-8.
37. Rodeo SA, Delos D, Williams RJ, Adler RS, Pearle A, Warren RF. The effect of platelet-rich fibrin matrix on rotator cuff tendon healing: a prospective, randomized clinical study. Am J Sports Med. 2012;40(6):1234-41.
38. Chan BP, Fu SC, Qin L, Rolf C, Chan KM. Supplementation-time dependence of growth factors in promoting tendon healing. Clin Orthop Relat Res. 2006;448:240-7.
39. Man G, Mologhianu G. Osteoarthritis pathogenesis: a complex process that involves the entire joint. J Med Life. 2014;7(1):37-41.
40. Wernecke C, Braun HJ, Dragoo JL. The effect of Intra-articular corticosteroids on articular cartilage: a systematic review. Orthop J Sports Med. 2015;3(5):2325967115581163.
41. Peerbooms JC, Sluimer J, Bruijn DJ, Gosens T. Positive effect of an autologous platelet concentrate in lateral epicondylitis in a double-blind randomized controlled trial: platelet-rich plasma versus corticosteroid injection with a 1-year follow-up. Am J Sports Med. 2010;38(2):255-62.
42. Gosens T, Peerbooms JC, van Laar W, den Oudsten BL. Ongoing positive effect of platelet-rich plasma versus corticosteroid injection in lateral epicondylitis: a double-blind randomized controlled trial with 2-year follow-up. Am J Sports Med. 2011;39(6):1200-8.
43. Navani A, Li, G, Chrystal J. Platelet-rich plasma in musculoskeletal pathology: a necessary rescue or a lost cause? Pain Physician accepted for publication August 2016, in Press.
44. Pirvu T, Blanquer S, Li Z, Benneker LM. A combined biomaterial and cellular approach for annulus fibrosus rupture repair. Biomaterials. 2015;42:11-9.
45. Orozco L, Soler R, Morera C, Alberca M, Sanchez A, Garcia-Sancho J. Intervertebral Disc Repair by Autologous Mesenchymal Bone Marrow Cells: A Pilot Study. Transplantation. 2011;92(7):822-8.
46. Chen WH, Lo WC, Lee JJ, Su CH, Lin CT, Liu HY, et al. Tissue engineered intervertebral disc and chondrogenesis using human nucleus pulposus regulated through TGF-beta 1 in PRP. J Cell Physiol. 2006;209(3):744-54.
47. Zeckser J, Wolff M, Tucker J, Goodwin J. Multipotent Mesenchymal Stem Cell Treatment for Discogenic Low Back Pain and Disc Degeneration. Stem Cells Int. 2016;2016:3908389.
48. Monfett M, Harrison J, Boachie-Adjei K, Lutz G. Intradiscal platelet-rich plasma (PRP) injections for discogenic low back pain: an update. Int Orthoped. 2016;40(6):1321-8.

49. Tuakli-Wosornu Y, Terry A, Lutz G, Harrison JR, Gribbin CK, LaSalle EE, et al. Lumbar intradiskal platelet-Rich plasma (PRP) injections: prospective, double-blind, randomized controlled study. PMR. 2016;8:1-10.
50. Levi D, Horn S, Tyszko S, Levin J, Hecht-Leavitt C, Walko E. Intradiscal platelet-rich plasma injection for chronic discogenic low back pain: preliminary results from a prospective trial. Pain Med. 2015;0:1-13.
51. Pettine K, Suzuki R, Sand T, Murphy M. Treatment of discogenic back pain with autologous bone marrow concentrate injection with minimum two year follow-up. International Orthoped. 2016;40(1):135-40.
52. Navani A, Hames A. Platelet-rich plasma injections for lumbar discogenic pain: A preliminary assessment of structural and functional changes. techniques in regional anesthesia and pain management. Published online: November 15, 2016.[In press].
53. Aydin S. Regenerative medicine modalities for nondiscal spinal disorders: techniques in regional anesthesia and pain management. Published online: November 16, 2016.[In press].
54. Navani A, Gupta D. Role of intra-articular platelet-rich plasma in sacroiliac joint pain: techniques in regional anesthesia and pain management. Published online: November 15, 2016.[In press].
55. Beitzel K, Allen D, Apostolakos J, Russell R, McCarthy MB, Gallo G, et al. US definitions: Current Use, and FDA stance on use of platelet-rich plasma in sports medicine. J Knee Surg. 2015;28(01):029-34.

SECTION 13

Physiotherapy

CHAPTER 46

Role of Physiotherapy in Treatment of Patients with Spinal Pain During the Acute/Inflammatory Phase

Rob Naber

INTRODUCTION

The frequency and epidemiology of spinal pain has been well published.[1-3] Acute painful episodes, with or without neurological deficits, frequently force patients to seek medical care from a multitude of healthcare practitioners. At that time, patients receive varied diagnoses related to abnormal anatomy such as degenerative disk disease, degenerative joint disease. However, the pathological anatomy as seen on radiographs does not correlate well with the pain the patient is experiencing at the moment.[4] However, there is sufficient evidence supporting the role of both chemical mediators and mechanical forces playing a significant role in spinal pain.[5] Patients with spinal pain will benefit from medical intervention including medications and injections to address the chemical component of their pain but physical therapy is an underutilized treatment tool that is also available to address the mechanical forces that contribute to patients' symptoms.

Research has identified the cervical, lumbar and sacroiliac joints can all be potential sources of pain.[6-8] The spinal pain can also emanate from muscles, the tendons, joint capsules and ligaments including the innervated portion of the annulus fibrosis. The cause of the patient's pain is very difficult to diagnose partially because the location of the pain is not pathognomonic and how the patient perceives the nociception signal from the periphery.

Once injured, the soft tissues of the spine heal along a fairly predictable pattern which includes the inflammatory phase, reparative phase and remodeling phase. More specific information about soft tissue healing is provided by Woo and Buckwalter.[9] Each phase of healing has implications for the clinician and should result in a tailored intervention to benefit the patient. For example, it would not be surprising that a patient with lateral epicondyle tendinosis may not benefit from anti-inflammatory medication once the condition has entered the remodeling phase of healing.

The patient with an acute episode, or recent onset, of spinal pain should be thought of as being in the inflammatory phase of healing. The role of the inflammatory phase is to eliminate the pathological insult, remove injured tissue, and promote regeneration of normal tissue structure. The strength of the injured tissue is low and related to the strength of the fibrin clot. Therefore, the healing tissue should be protected so as not to delay the recovery process. The typical patient experiences an acute episode of spinal pain superimposed on a chronic history of repeated microtraumas. They present frequently with an insignificant mechanism of injury. However, they do have a long but neglected history of discomfort. They may attribute their antalgic postures, stiffness with sustained flexed positions as age related or the way they slept. Patients may become complacent with their pain because their symptoms progressed slowly, subsides for reasons they do not understand and the pain has repeatedly followed a pattern the patient is familiar with. As one can expect, after consistent abuse of their spine, damage is done, the symptom pattern unexpectedly progresses and now demands the patient's full attention. This concept is well described by Kirkaldy-Wills as the degenerative cascade.[10]

The patient in the inflammatory phase may have a recent mechanism of injury, which may not have been exquisitely painful at that moment. Frequently, the patient awakes from a peaceful night of sleep with low back pain vaguely related to the previous day's activities. Upon careful questioning the patient will recall the mechanism as a sustained flexed posture such as kneeling or a benign slip and fall that at the time did not seem proportional to the amount of pain they are experiencing at your office. The delayed onset of pain can be explained by the accumulation of swelling and the beginning of the inflammatory phase.

The goals of a physical therapy program in the inflammatory phase include the following:

1. Reduce swelling
2. Promote healing if possible but more likely do not impede the healing process.
3. Educate the patient on postures and positions to avoid that may aggravate their condition and further damage the injured tissue
4. Reduce the patient's pain.
5. Maintain the patient's general mobility as needed for basic activities of daily living, while protecting the healing tissue.

We do not recommend aggressive passive range of motion exercise, joint mobilization, neural mobilization or strengthening at this phase. Those treatments are valid but the treatment does not match the phase of healing the patient is in currently. We do emphasize correct body mechanics, alternative movement patterns and trunk muscle activation to protect the injured tissue.

CAUSES OF SPINAL PAIN

The causes of spinal pain are varied and multifactorial and beyond the scope of this chapter but one should appreciate most spinal acute pain does not occur from a macro-trauma. Rather the pains start from benign motions such a bending forward to pick up a pencil superimposed on taxing habitual and sustained flexion postures.[11,12] Nachemson has demonstrated the significant elevated intradiskal pressure associated even with sitting and forward bending.[12]

However, a simplistic pattern of causes does appear based on which plane of motion is most provocative. That is the patient reports their pain is consistently reproduced with flexion activities such as bending, sitting, lifting or they may report extension activities such as standing, walking or reaching overhead are provocative. Patients who are suffering with cervical or lumbar radiculopathies can identify which positions relieve their distal pain by opening or closing the intervertebral foramina.

Asymmetrical postures, such as standing with most of one's weight on one leg will place forces on the spine including tensile loads on the convex side of the spine and compression load on the concave side of the spine (Fig. 1). These convexities influence the lumbar, thoracic and cervical spines. Flexion creates compression forces along the anterior column and tensile forces along the posterior columns. Extension creates tensile forces on the anterior column and compressive forces along the posterior columns. Gait dysfunction due to gluteus medius weakness or knee flexion contractures (Fig. 2) can also lead to asymmetrical forces, resulting in spinal compensations and pain.

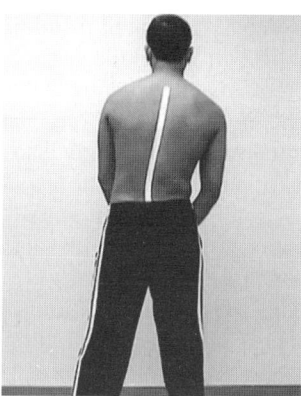

FIG. 1: Asymmetrical stance

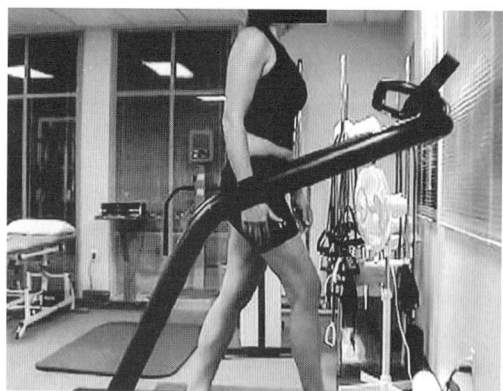

FIG. 2: Patient walking with a right knee flexion contracture at initial contact phase of gait which causes asymmetrical stride length and asymmetrical forces to the spine

Sahrmann postulates that repeated movements and sustained postures can ultimately lead to impairments like these.[13]

This example results (Fig. 1) in tensile forces on the left and compression forces on the right side of the lumbar spine. Scoliotic compensation is seen though the thoracic and cervical spine.

SYMPTOMS

For the subjective portion of the examination the clinician must use excellent communication skills to learn of the patient's mechanism of injury and location(s) of their pain(s). Particular attention is directed to unilateral arm or leg pain versus bilateral extremity pain as its significance to central canal pathology. The behavior of the patient's pain(s) helps define common spinal motions and forces from the aggravating activities. For further reference to subjective examination the reader is referred to Geoffrey Maitland's excellent texts.[14]

To facilitate communication during the history portion of the exam, we use body charts and patient completed function questionnaires such as the Oswestry Low Back Pain Disability Questionnaire (ODI) and the Neck Disability Index (NDI) with a VAS pain intensity scale of zero to ten centimeters. In the acute episode, the patient score frequently is above 50% for the ODI and above 60% for the NDI. Our experience correlates well the original description by Fairbanks[15] of the Oswestry questionnaire and its scoring. Visual analog scale also reveals scores above 6.0 out of 10 centimeters.

In the past decade, research has expanded our understanding of pain. References by Moseley and Butler are suggested.[16] Nociception begins in the periphery, which Moseley refers to as danger receptors, and ascends via multiple neural pathways to the brain. In the brain the different lobes provide meaning and content of the afferent signal. It is here that the patient perceives pain. Their previous experiences influence the meaning of pain and what action the body should take to reduce pain. Sometimes the processing of nociception can be incorrect as in phantom limb pain. It is important for the physical therapist to be attentive during the evaluation for the patient who appears to be anxious about their symptoms or symptoms which are not proportional to the mechanism of injury. Standard tools such the Tampa Scale of Kinesiophobia can assist in identifying patients with biopsychosocial issues which may impair recovery.

CLINICAL EXAMINATION

The objective portion of the examination is next undertaken to determine potential movement faults, the quantity and quantity of spinal AROM, selectively reproduce the patient's pain and obtain specific signs. We begin with observation of the patient's posture and spontaneous movements which may reveal a tendency for how the patient moves outside of the clinic. For example, an increased thoracic kyphosis and increased lumbar lordosis may imply buckling of the spine under vertical load. Compression and perturbations are then applied to the patient in standing or sitting to assess stability of the postural spinal curves (Fig. 3A). Perturbation at the shoulders from anterior to postures may reveal unwanted increased lumbar extension and lack of abdominal muscle reflexive contraction (Fig. 3B)

Spinal active range of motion is next measured best in the clinic with fluid filled inclinometers. Usually painful AROM correlates with the patient's mechanism of injury. Functional motions to also consider examining for pain reproduction is side glides, hip hiking and combined spinal motions (Figs 4A to C). Patients with acute spinal pain demonstrate reduced ranges of motion with recognizable patterns of limitations. We recognize these patterns of limitations as facet closing problems, facet opening problems, diskal presentation and myofascial restrictions (Table 1). In the inflammatory phase, these limited movements are used to identify pain relieving postures.

The examination is continued with appropriate neurological testing even in the absence of radicular pain patterns. This includes upper quadrant, lower quadrant and cranial nerve testing following possible head injuries from

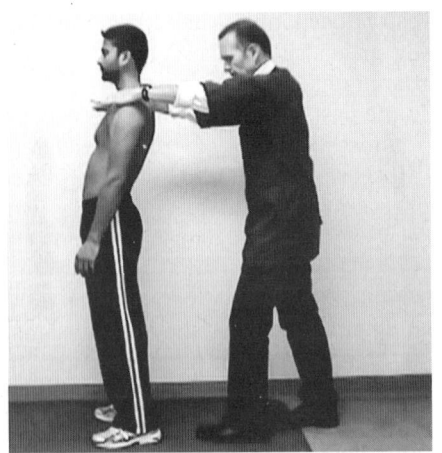

FIG. 3A: Vertical compress to assess stability to postural curves

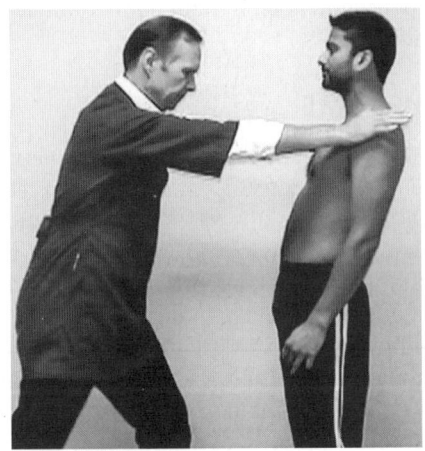

FIG. 3B: Anterior to posterior perturbation to assess abdominal reflexive contraction

TABLE 1: Common patterns of spinal limitations

Facet opening pattern	Limited forward bending, contralateral side bending, contralateral rotation
Facet closing pattern	Limited backward bending, ipsilateral side bending, ipsilateral rotation
Diskal pattern	Proportional limitation of all cardinal plane motions
Myofascial restrictive pattern	Limited bilateral or unilateral side bending

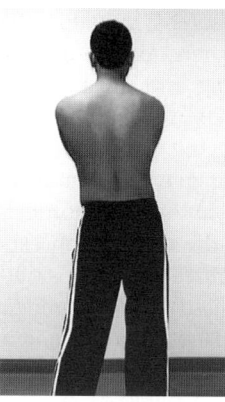

FIG. 4A: Functional motion of the spine—right side glide

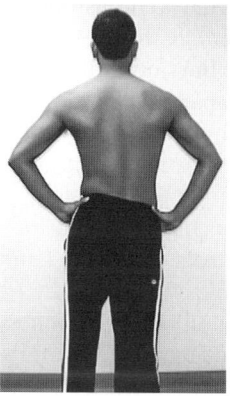

FIG. 4B: Functional motion of the spine—left hip hiking

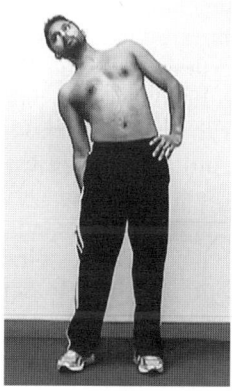

FIG. 4C: Functional motion of the spine—combined motions of backward bending and right side bending

car accidents or falls. Testing includes light touch sensation rather than pinwheel testing, deep tendon reflexes, myotomal strength testing for fatigable weakness, spinal cord reflexes for upper motor lesions and neural mobility testing such as straight leg raise.

Flexibility of specific muscles is next assessed. Hip and pelvic girdle muscles, especially all three gluteals, hamstrings and hip flexors are tested for sufficient length as their tightness will continue to compromise a patient's lumbopelvic posture. Shoulder girdle muscle flexibility, especially pectoral, latissimus dorsi and upper trapezius, and upper thoracic mobility are examined as they too influence a patient's ability to maintain a neutral cervicothoracic posture and obtain positions of comfort.

The clinician now selects special tests to elicit further diagnostic information based on the developing clinical hypothesis. Caution is taken as some special testing such as combined motions and gait analysis may not be appropriate because the patient is in too severe of pain or the results are not valid as the patient assumes antalgic movement patterns. For the patient in the inflammatory phase, their ability to perform actions such as rolling, moving from standing to sitting, moving standing to prone should be examined. It is imperative for the clinician to examine how the patient performs movements that they specifically note as trouble-some. For example, if the patient complains using the sink in the morning to wash their hands is very painful, ask the patient demonstrated how they bend their spine while simulating this activity (Fig. 5). Do not assume how the patient performs their activities of daily livings (ADLs).

TREATMENT

Baring concerns of disease or fracture, and the confirmation the patient is an appropriate candidate for physical therapy, treatment consistent with this phase of healing can

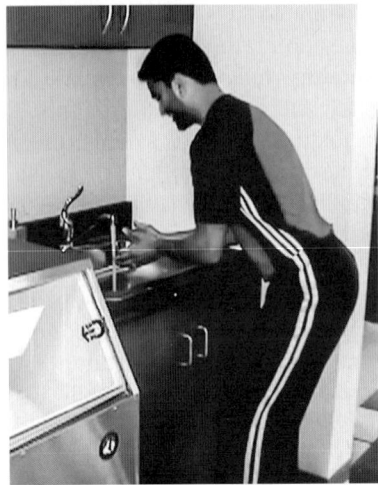

FIG. 5: Correct posture at sink

begin. Anti-inflammatory medications and modalities such as ice and electrical stimulation to reduce pain and swelling are indicated in this phase. Further information on the use of modalities can be read in text by Arnheim.[17]

Neutral Spine

Next, the patient must learn how to control the position of their lumbar and cervical lordosis to avoid reinjuring healing tissue during basic activities of daily living (ADL's). This is accomplished by teaching the patient the concepts of a "neutral spine". Neutral spine is a zone of spinal motion, not a single point, that minimize their pain (hopefully eliminate the pain), is usually between the extremes of spinal flexion and extension and allows the patient to gain cognitive awareness of the targeted muscles contracting to prevent painful movements. This neutral zone places the spinal segment in a mid-range to minimize compression or tension forces and keeps the loads below painful thresholds. Based on the history and objective examination, the patient's neutral spine is biased away from the painful motion e.g. flexion bias is used to move away from painful extension activities.

When teaching a patient how to define their lumbar neutral spine position they begin in hook laying and must master three basic principles. First the patient experiences and practices moving the pelvis between anterior and posterior pelvic tilts and notes how this changes their lumbar lordosis. Then the influence of the extremities, especially of the lower extremities, on the position of the pelvis is demonstrated by again moving the pelvis this time with legs extended and in hook laying. The patient notes the challenge this places on moving the pelvis. A posterior pelvic tilt will be more difficult to perform with the legs extended than in hook laying. Finally, patients, especially if they demonstrate fear avoidance, must understand the concept that "It is not what they do but how they do it." which causes their pain. A patient's proficiency for defining their neutral spine can be tested in multiple body positions such as sitting, standing and quadruped.

When teaching patients to control their cervical lordosis they are educated on the same principles to control their lumbar spine lordosis in addition to two others. The patient practices moving C0-C1 through a range of flexion to extension and feels how this changes their cervical lordosis. The patient next learns to "place their ears vertically over their shoulders" and correct for any head forward or head retracted postural faults. The head retracted postural fault is frequently associated with reduced thoracic kyphosis and scapular winging. The head forward postural fault is associated with increased thoracic kyphosis and scapular protraction. These postural faults all result in a flattening of the cervical curve.

Once the patient has mastered finding and maintaining their neutral spine, they work on the idea of "bracing" to set their trunk muscles to increase stiffness of the spinal segment without causing a Valsalva maneuver. Correct bracing results in narrowing of the waist with a firm abdominal muscle tone.

In the acute phase, the tendency to contract muscles forcefully should be discouraged to minimize compressive forces. The use of surface EMG can assist the patient to obtain sufficient muscle contraction. Patients learn to volitionally contract the transverse abdominus and lumbar multifidi per recommendation by Hides et al.[18] A corset or brace can also be helpful at this phase. To avoid muscle atrophy and dependence on the brace, the patients should be instructed to "narrow the waist" more than the corset's effect.

Applying tape to the lumbar spine in prone is a very an effective way to teach patients to avoid flexing their lumbar spine and change their movement patterns (Fig. 6). Further functionality is practiced by using hip hinging (Figs 7A and B) for spinal pain. Hip hinging involves having the patient move their spine from vertical to incline without flexing the spine but rather flexing at his or her hips. The patient initially practices using a dowel or stick, placed along the length of the spine from sacrum to occiput. Hip hinging is practiced in standing, sitting (Figs 7C and D) and squatting. Proficiency is tested by having the patient hip hinge without the dowel but being able to still maintain their neutral position.

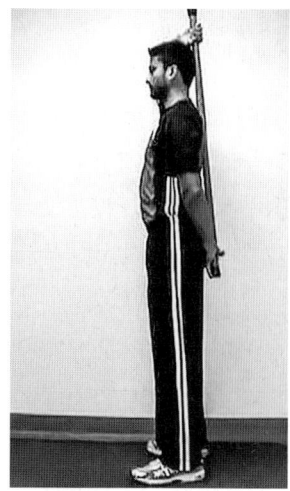

FIG. 7A: Hip hinge in standing starting position

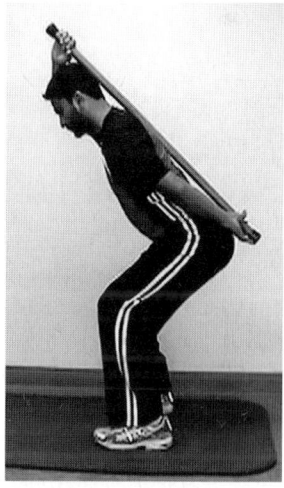

FIG. 7B: Hip hinge ending position with spine moving from vertical to inclined and the motion occurring at the patient's hips and knees

First Aide Positions

In the inflammatory phase of healing, the physical therapist works with the patient to learn positions and posture to help reduce their pain level and not impede their healing. These positions can be considered first aide positions and include resting in side laying, correct sitting posture and even maintaining

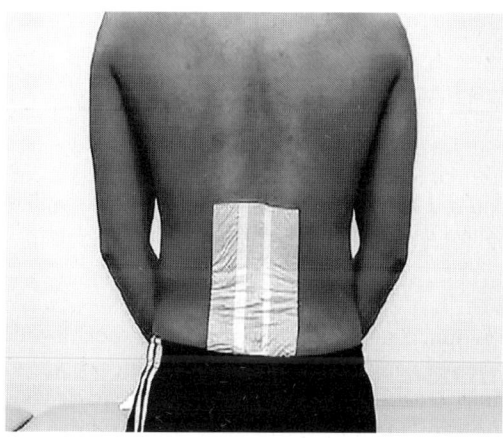

FIG. 6: Taping the lumbar spine helps patient become of maintaining their lumbar lordosis

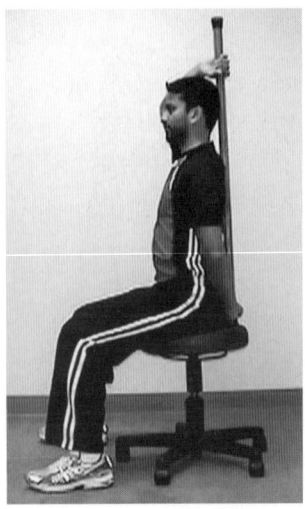

FIG. 7C: Hip hinge in sitting starting position

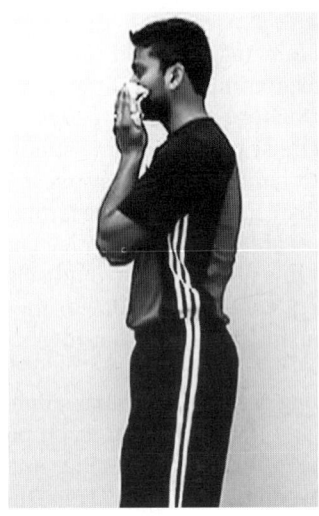

FIG. 8: Patients need to protect their spine in spontaneous motions such as sneezing

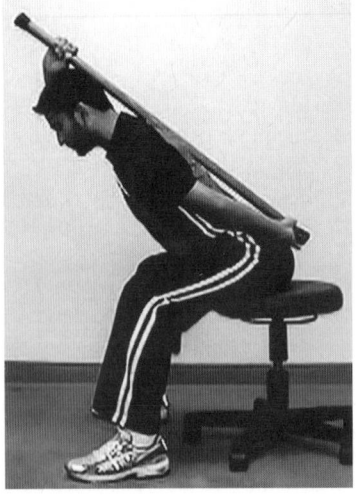

FIG. 7D: Hip hinge in sitting end position with spine moving from vertical to inclined and the motion occurring at the patient's hips

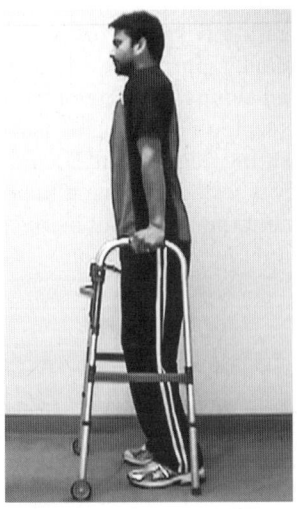

FIG. 9A: Patients may reduce their pain by "unloading" with a walker

the spine in neutral when sneezing (Fig. 8). To relieve compression forces the patient can try "unloading" their spine with the use of a walker (Fig. 9A) or by suspending themselves by way of their hands and a towel over the edge of an open door (Fig. 9B).

Once again the neutral spine position of the cervical and lumbar spine is incorporated into treatment but this time the patient is positioned and supported with pillows or bolsters so they can rest their muscles. They are not to brace their spine. Side laying in

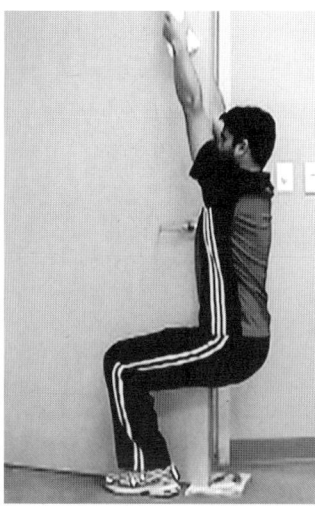

FIG. 9B: Patients may reduce their pain by "unloading" with a towel over an open door

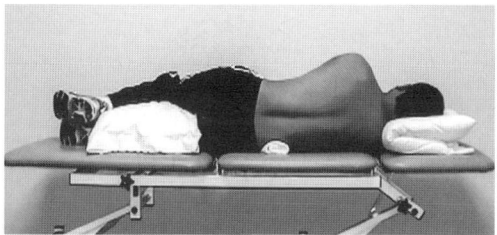

FIG. 10: Side lying with pillows positioned under the cervical spine and head, between the knee and a towel roll under the waist can maintain neutral spine position and allow the patient's muscle to rest

bed is a frequently pain-relieving position. Pillows positioned between the patient's knees, under the head and cervical spine and a towel roll under their waist can maintain the spine in its neutral position (Fig. 10). Flexing of the patient's hips and knees will help bias the lumbar spine toward flexion and open intervertebral foramina.

Sitting is a common aggravating activity for patients with spinal pain. Patients frequently need to sit in chairs for work or transportation but they may also need to sit on the floor. These positions place the spine in flexion. The flexion posture places tensile loads along the posterior aspect of the spine and compressive forces on the intervertebral disk and vertebral body. Few patients have the muscle endurance and body awareness to vigilantly correct this tendency for an extended duration. The physical therapist can work with the patient to use pillows to again position the spine toward neutral and reduce the need for muscle contraction. With sitting in a chair for driving or relaxing a pillow behind their back can help maintain the lumbar lordosis. (Fig. 11A). But when sitting at a desk or for meals a patient will lean forward to actively engage the task. This active sitting position will move away from a lumbar support. Pillow support under the pelvis will help hold the pelvis in an anterior pelvic tilt, which restores the lumbar and cervical lordosis (Figs 11B to D).

The patient in the inflammatory phase of healing often finds bending to reach the ground difficult and painful. This habitual movement patterns includes spinal flexion and rotation, which should be avoided to protect the healing of injured tissue such as the posterior annular fibers. Again, educating patients on new movement patterns can protect them. An alternative manner to reach the ground starts with the patient lowering themselves from standing to kneeling by

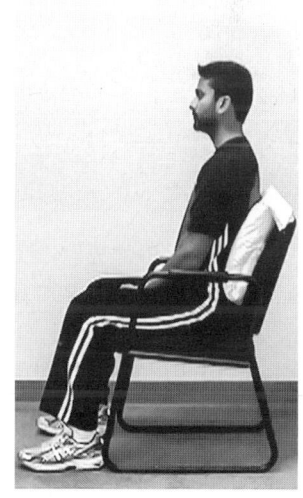

FIG. 11A: Sitting with lumbar support

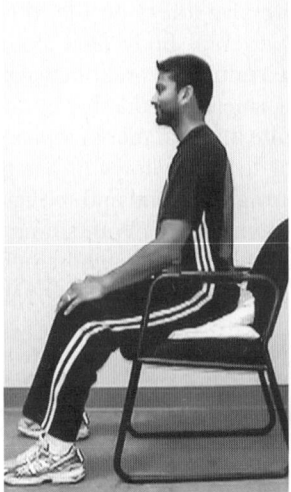

FIG. 11B: Sitting with pelvic support helps with patient in active sitting

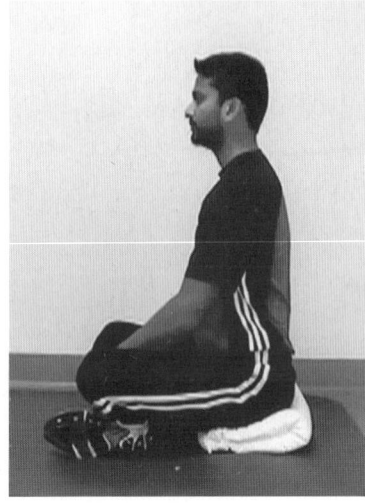

FIG. 11D: Sitting on the floor places with a pillow under the pelvis places the spine toward neutral and reduces the need for muscle contraction

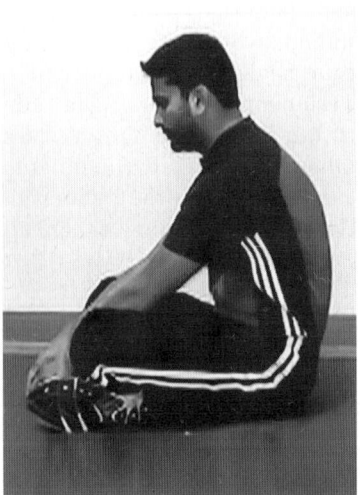

FIG. 11C: Sitting on the floor places the spine in flexion

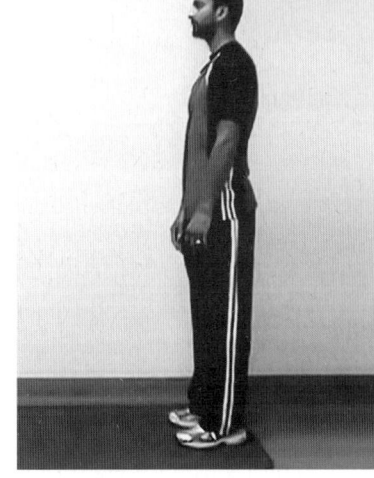

FIG. 12A: Transition standing to resting on the floor

genuflexion (Figs 12A to I). Once kneeling, the patient uses the hip hinge strategy to reach the ground. The patient walks their hands forward to support themselves as they move into quadruped. From quadruped most patients can lower themselves to the ground by a push-up manner. Once on the ground the patient rolls to their side and into hook laying while maintaining their shoulders and pelvis in the same plane and not twisting the spine. As the patient progress to other phases of healing during rehabilitation, they use this sequence to get to the ground to perform many of their strengthening exercises. To return to standing the patient reverses this sequence. For the physical therapist,

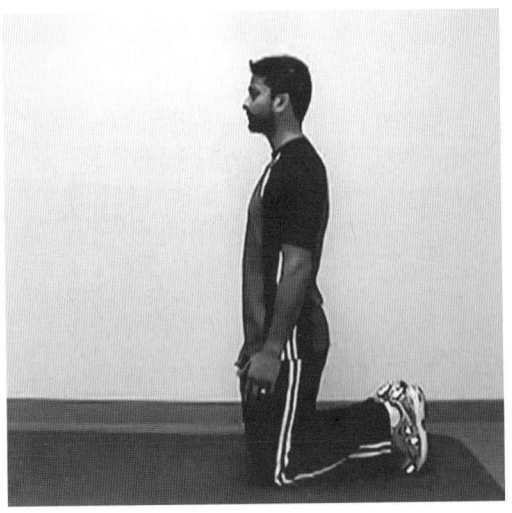

FIG. 12B: Genu flex to kneeling

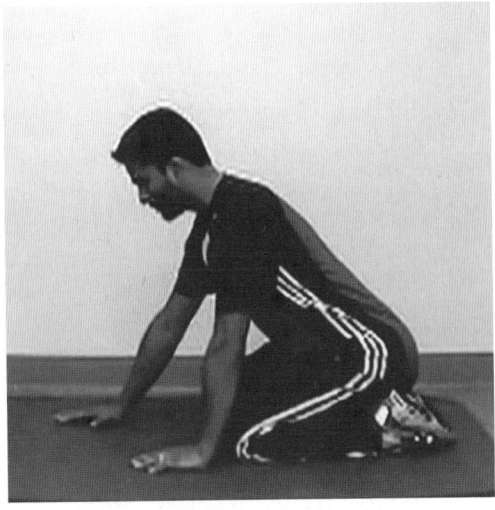

FIG. 12D: Patient reaches the ground and walks hands forward

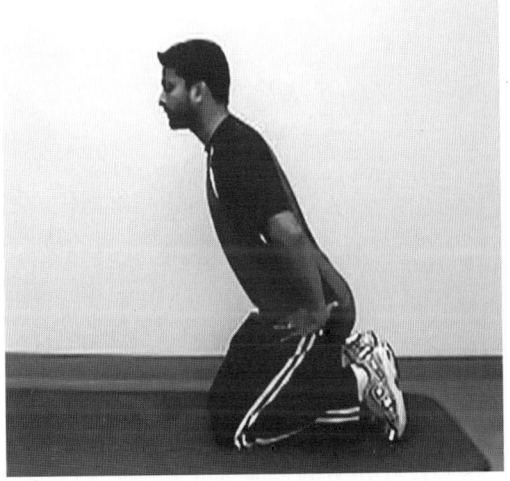

FIG. 12C: In kneeling hip hinge forward to reach the floor

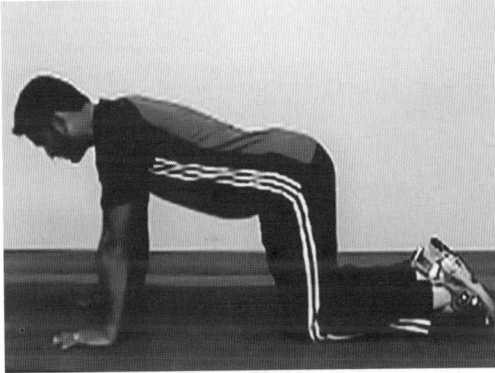

FIG. 12E: Patient moves to quadruped

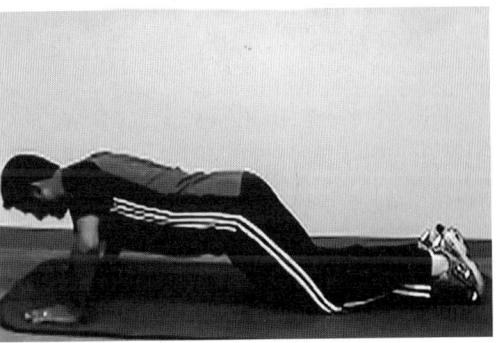

FIG. 12F: Patient lowers themselves to the ground

observing this sequence can identify the patient's areas of weakness or limited mobility which compromise their healing.

Once the patient has demonstrated proficiency with the identifying their spine's neutral zone, hip hinging, transferring from standing to the ground, they are instructed in pushing and pulling activities and alternative lifting movement patterns. To

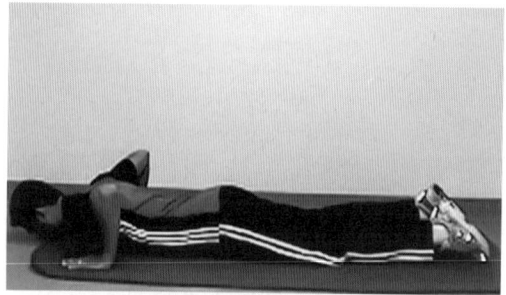

FIG. 12G: Patient in prone

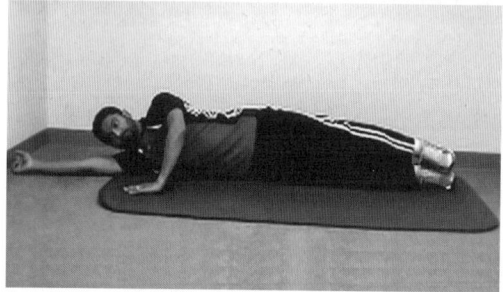

FIG. 12H: Patient rolls to side lying without twisting their spine

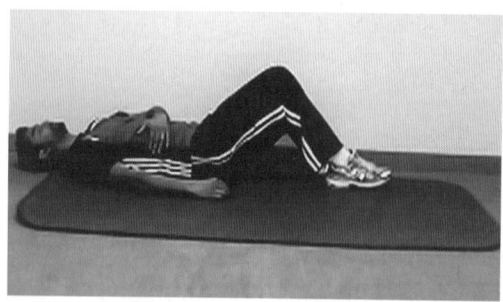

FIG. 12I: Patient in hook lying

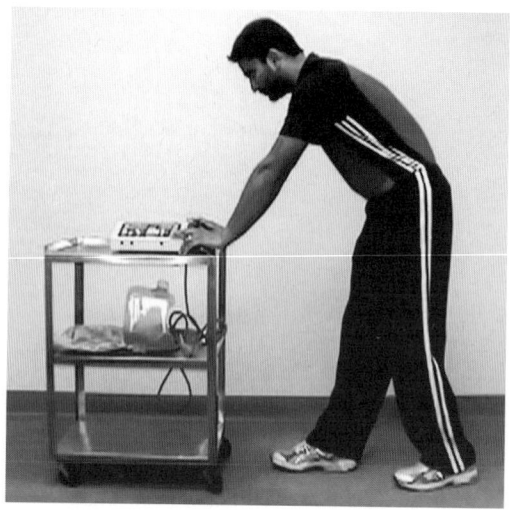

FIG. 13A: Incorrect body mechanics with pushing activities

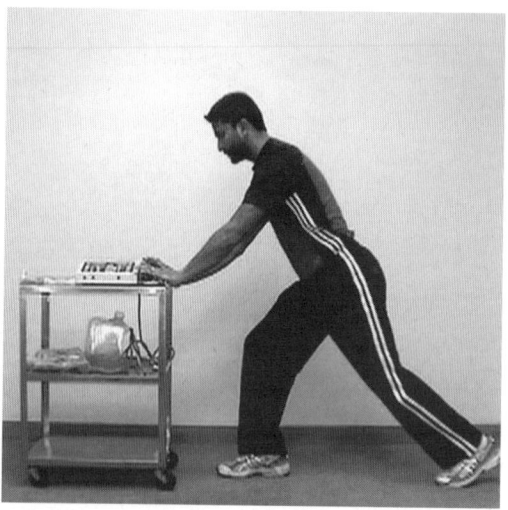

FIG. 13B: Correct body mechanics with pushing activities

be done correctly these activities need the patient to brace their spine with muscle effort in order to avoid injurious movements. Pushing incorrectly leads to excessive lumbar flexion or extension with forward translation forces while pulling incorrectly may lead to excessive lumbar flexion (Figs 13A to D).

Correct lifting has also been shown to reduce excessive loads on the spine and helps reduce the patient's pain. Lifting heavy objects should be completed with a "squat lift" to use the strong leg muscles (Fig. 14A) and allows for objects to be carried closer to the spine. "Lunge lifting" is effective to lift moderate weights from the ground and also allows the object to be kept close to the patient

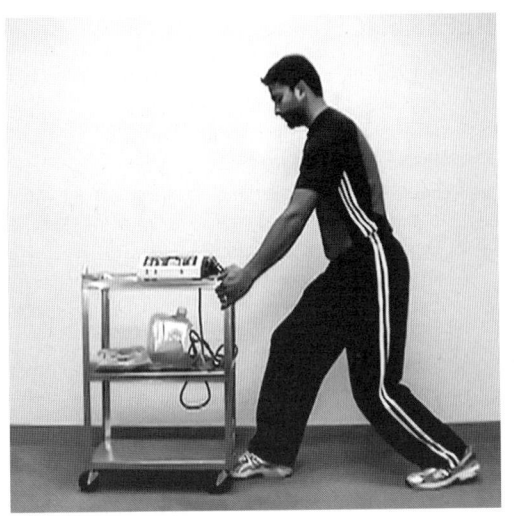

FIG. 13C: Incorrect body mechanics with pulling activities may result in excessive flexion motions of the lumbar and cervical spines

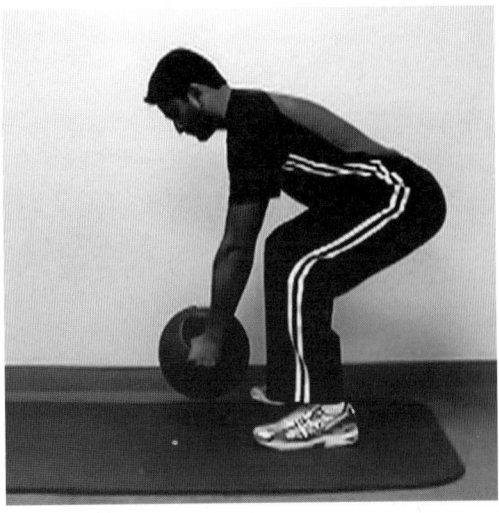

FIG. 14A: Squat lifting technique

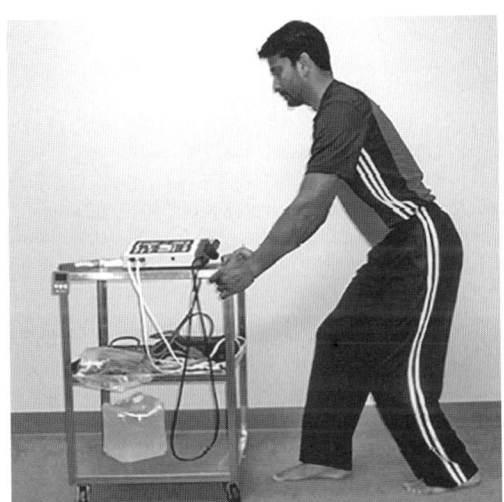

FIG. 13D: Correct body mechanics with pulling activities

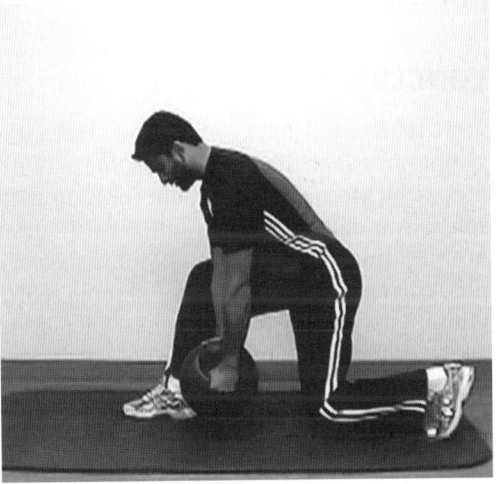

FIG. 14B: Lunge lifting technique

(Fig. 14B). This reduces to the leverage of the object. A "Golfer bow" technique of lifting, balancing on one leg and leaning forward, is optimal to reduce the energy expenditure of squats but only recommended for light objects (Fig. 14C).

Patients with acute onset of back or neck pain are looking for immediate assistance and can present significant challenges for clinicians. A treatment approach based on soft tissue healing provides an organized and predictable progression for clinicians. Physical therapists are uniquely qualified to provide treatment and especially education regarding movement re-education, postural training and the use of good body mechanics for the patient

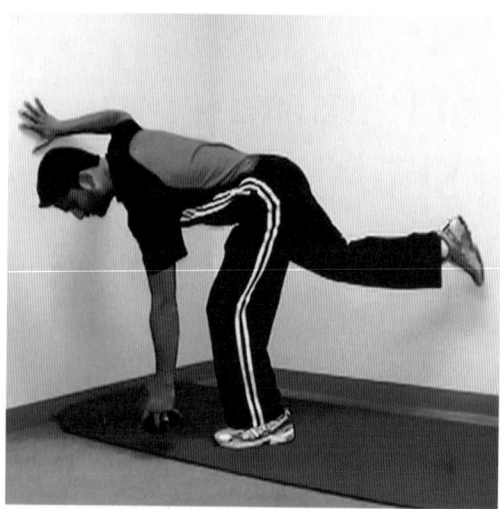

FIG. 14C: Golfer bow lifting technique

in the inflammatory phase of healing with back or neck pain.

CONCLUSION

Low back and neck pains are common symptoms which many patients suffer around the world. Most of these patients present with soft tissue damage, which follows a natural healing time line including inflammatory phase, reparative phase and remodeling phase. Knowing the patient's phase of healing allows a more specific and appropriate treatment tactic. The inflammatory phase is usually treated with oral and topical medication and therapeutic injections but the use of physical therapy during this phase is underutilized. Based on their evaluation, Physical Therapists can educate patients how to use a "neutral" spine postures and correct body mechanics and "unloading principles" to reduce their pain levels and protect the healing tissue to promote rapid return to daily activities.

REFERENCES

1. Manchikanti L. Epidemiology of low back pain. Pain Physician. 2000;3:167.
2. Hoy D, et al. The Epidemiology of Low Back Pain. Best Pract Res Clin Rheumatol. 2010;24:769.
3. Fejer R. The Prevalence of neck pain in the world population: a systematic critical review of the literature. Eur Spine Journal. 2006;15:834.
4. Torgerson WR Dotter WE, Comparative roentgenographic study of the asymptomatic and symptomatic lumbar spine. Bone Joint Surg Am.1976;58:850-3.
5. Saal J, et al. high levels of inflammatory phospholipase A2 activity in lumbar disc herniations. Spine. 1990. pp.674-8.
6. McCall I, et al. induced pain referral from posterior lumbar elements in normal subjects. Spine. 1974.pp.441-446.
7. Schwarzer A. C aprill CN, Bogduk N. The sacroiliac joint in chronic low back pain. Spine. 1995;20:31-7.
8. Aprill C. Dwyer A, Bogduk N. Ccervical zygapophyseal joint pain patterns part II. A clinical evaluation. Spine. 1990;15:458-61.
9. Woo S, Buckwalter J. Injury and repair of the Musculoskeletal soft tissues. American Academy of Orthopedic Surgeons; 1988.
10. Kirkaldy-Wills WH Managing low back pain. Churchill Livingstone. 1988.pp.3-14.
11. McGill S. Low Back Disorders Evidence-Based Prevention and Rehabilitation Human. Kinetics; 2002.pp.29-44.
12. Nachemson A. The effect of forward leaning on lumbar intradiscal pressure. Acta Orthop Scand. 1965;35: 314-28.
13. Sahrmann S. Diagnosis and treatment of movement impairment syndromes. Mosby; 2002:4.
14. Maitland GD. Vertebral Manipulation, 4th ed. Butterworths; 1977.pp.10-81.
15. Fairbanks J, et al. The oswestry low back pain disability questionnaire. Physiotherapy. 1980;66(8):271-3.
16. Butler D, Moseley L. Explain Pain. 2nd ed. Noigroup Publications, 2013.
17. Arnheim D. Modern. Principles of Athletic, 7th ed. Training Times Mirror Mosby College Publishing. 1989. pp.350-85.
18. Hides J, et al. Long-term effects of specific stabilizing exercises for first episode low back pain Spine. 2001;26(11): E243-8.

CHAPTER 47

Role of Physiotherapy in Treatment of Spinal Pain During Subacute/Reparative Phase

Neeraj D Baheti

INTRODUCTION

Acute episodes of spinal pain typically resolve by themselves. The reparative phase follows, once the acute, inflammatory and severely painful phase of spinal pain has passed. Depending on the tissue involved, it can take from 3 to 14 days for the reparative phase to start.[1] The start of this phase depends upon several factors, such as the patient's age, overall health, existing medical conditions and social habits, etc. The reparative phase can last from 7 to 12 weeks.[2] Pain lasting longer than that is considered as chronic pain. While the patient in the reparative phase, is no longer in acute pain, but still has to be cautious of acute exacerbation. The patient is not yet able to exercise independently, as they could easily re-injure themselves. The patient in the reparative phase often demonstrates fear-avoidance behavior. The reparative phase is characterized by the replacement of damaged cells with new-like cells.[1] If these new-like cells are damaged, and then the healing process may not be as good. Clinicians have to give close consideration to healing in order to enable the patient to move forward on the road to recovery. The patient in the subacute/reparative phase is an ideal candidate for physical therapy. If at any time during this phase, it is established that the patient is regressing, or is not recovering as fast as expected, then it is prudent to seek further medical advice and intervention.

GOALS OF PHYSICAL THERAPY TREATMENT

1. *Protection:* It is important to protect the spine from further damage. The patient should be encouraged to wean off the external cervical or lumbar support. In turn, proper spinal positioning, during activities of daily living, should be taught and verbal and tactile cues should be utilized as necessary. Review head and neck positioning, along with basic posture control in various body positions such as sitting, standing, squatting, etc. in order to protect the nerve and other healing tissues like nucleus pulposus and longitudinal ligaments.
2. *Body awareness:* Patient should be able to identify bad postures and self correct.
3. *Initiate basic trunk stabilization:* Re-educate the voluntary recruitment of abdominal and multifidus muscle. Biofeedback techniques can be utilized for this purpose if desired.
4. Initiate lower extremity strengthening and scapula-thoracic strengthening.

5. Start cardiovascular endurance exercises.
6. Improve patient confidence to address any underlying psychosocial issues that could be driving the patient's pain. If the psychological issues are not addressed, then the movement patterns may not normalize.[3]

SIGNS AND SYMPTOMS

Signs
1. Compared to the acute phase, the patient has improved scores on self-reported questionnaires such as Neck Disability Index[4] and the Oswestry questionnaire.[5]
2. Improved neurological exam, including sensations and deep tendon reflexes.
3. Improved cervical and lumbar active range of motion (AROM).
4. Patient is now able to perform spontaneous motions, without severe pain.
5. Lateral shift (if present during the acute phase) improves.
6. Antalgic posture and antalgic gait lessen.

Symptoms
1. Centralizing of arm and leg pain (if present during the acute phase) starts to occur.
2. Pain is controlled by posture better.
3. Symptoms lessen with increased activity and patient demonstrates improved confidence.

CLINICAL EXAMINATION

In the subacute phase, the physical therapy examination includes and extends beyond the areas covered in the acute phase. Additional clinical examination includes strength, gait, and balance testing. This examination should be performed in addition to any diagnostic investigations that may have been performed.
1. Postural examination should be performed in static and dynamic activities, with the goal of identifying the provocative and alleviating postures/motions.
2. Compression and perturbations should be performed in various body positions, to assess stability of postural curves.
3. *Cervical and lumbar AROM:* Identify patterns of limitation. Determine if the patient is having pain/symptoms in a certain direction of movement. This could be a sign of a facet joints involvement, a disk issue, etc.
4. Thorough neurological examination should be performed to assess for any residual neurological signs.
5. Muscular strength and endurance testing of the following muscle groups:
   a. *Cervical:* Scapular and shoulder muscles, deep neck flexors, cervical multifidi.
   b. *Lumbar:* Trunk, lower extremity strength.[6]
6. *Flexibility:* Lower extremity and upper extremity.
7. *Gait analysis:* Dynamic assessment of the lower body biomechanics looking for dysfunction of the kinetic chain.
8. *Balance testing:* Static and dynamic.

INVESTIGATIONS SUGGESTED

As mentioned earlier in this chapter, if it is established that the patient is regressing or is not improving as rapidly as expected, it might be a good idea to refer the patient to a specialist, who might request radiological investigations. In turn, if the patient is progressing well, it is a good idea to learn more about their other associated pathologies, e.g. cardiovascular status, osteoarthritis, etc. in order to advance them to the next phase of treatment.

PHYSICAL THERAPY TREATMENT

The treatment plan is guided by the goals as laid out for this reparative phase, and by the findings of the clinical examination.

Body Mechanics and Postural Education

It is essential that the patient understands the concept of the lumbopelvic clock, and is able to identify and demonstrate his/her lumbar neutral-spine in various body positions. Neutral spine has been defined as the region of minimal stiffness in all directions of the spinal movement.[7] Similarly, the patient should be able to assume a neutral head and neck position to minimize injury and promote further healing.

Muscle Re-education

Patients with current or recent spinal pain lose their involuntary ability to sequentially recruit the transverse abdominus and multifidi muscles in order to stabilize the lumbar spine.[8,9] Hence, it is essential to utilize techniques to re-educate these muscles and restore the natural sequencing. This can be done via various feedback mechanisms, such as surface EMG or blood pressure cuff.[10] Similarly, it is important for the patients to be able to recruit deep neck flexors and cervical extensor muscles voluntarily to stabilize the cervical spine.

Manual Therapy

Various manual therapy techniques are appropriate in this phase of rehabilitation. These include, but are not limited to cervical, thoracic, or lumbar joint mobilization,[11,12] manual cervical or lumbar traction,[13] soft tissue mobilization, and massage.

Therapeutic Exercises

The benefits of therapeutic exercise are well documented.[14,15] In the subacute/reparative phase; you want to avoid concentric contractions of the trunk and cervical muscles. The trunk and cervical muscles should be strengthened by engaging them isometrically. Below are some examples of such exercises. These exercises are the focus of this chapter. It should be noted that these exercises should initially be performed as in low repetitions and with sufficient rest in between. Also they should be performed with low load and low velocity to minimize re-injury.[16] You can also find videos and detailed explanations of some of these exercises at the following website: *http://www.ptoflosgatos.com*.

1. *Abdominal bracing in hooklying:* progression series. This exercise can start with alternate single leg marching (Fig. 1), and then be progressed in the following order. Alternate knee extension (Fig. 2); bilateral arm raise, with or without weight (Fig. 3); and simultaneous raising of opposite arm and leg (Fig. 4).

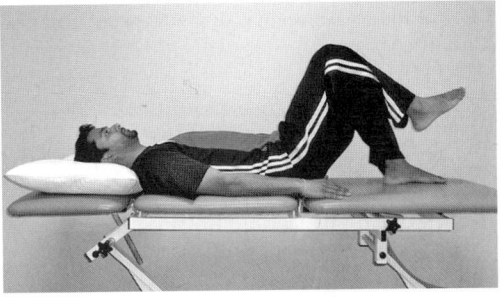

FIG. 1: Abdominal bracing with alternate leg marching

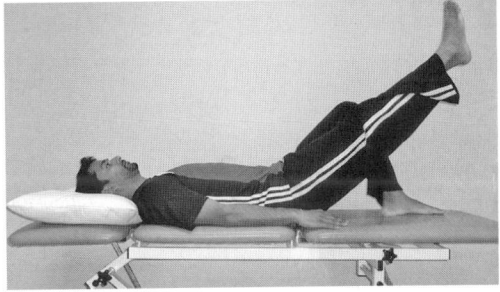

FIG. 2: Abdominal bracing with alternate knee extension

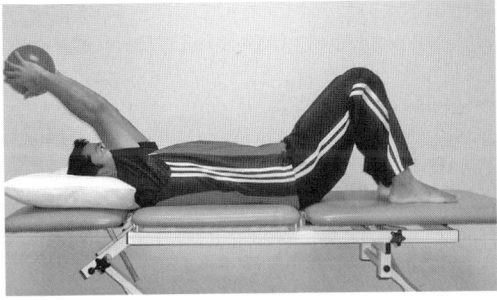

FIG. 3: Abdominal bracing with bilateral arm raise. Demonstrated here with 9 lb medicine ball

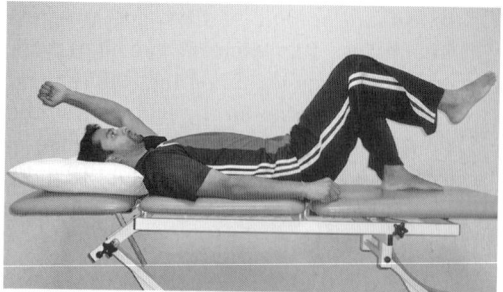

FIG. 4: Abdominal bracing with simultaneous opposite arm and leg raise

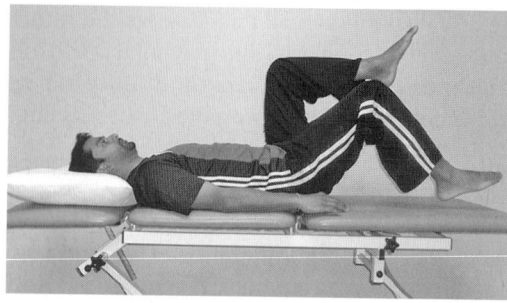

FIG. 7: 90-90 abdominal holds with alternate heel taps

2. *90-90 Abdominal holds progression series*: This exercise series involves holding 90° of hip flexion and 90° of knee flexion (Fig. 5). This can then be gradually progressed in the following order: alternate heel taps (Fig. 6), alternate knee extension (Fig. 7); bilateral arm raise, with or without weight (Fig. 8); and simultaneous extension of opposite arm and leg (Fig. 9).

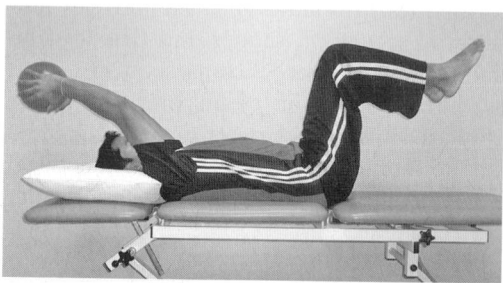

FIG. 8: 90-90 abdominal holds with bilateral arm raise. Demonstrated here with 9 lb medicine ball

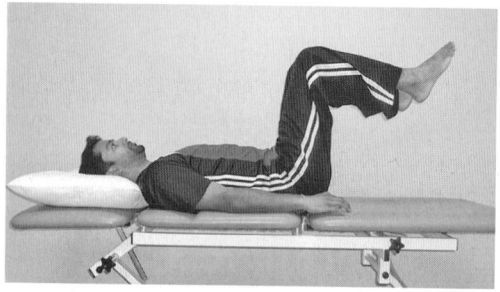

FIG. 5: 90-90 abdominal holds

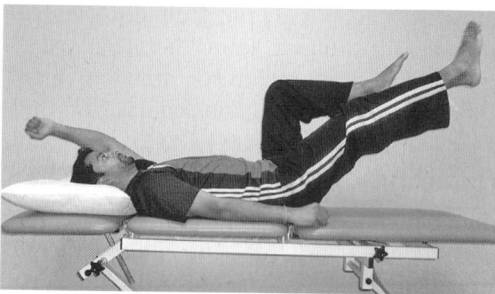

FIG. 9: 90-90 abdominal holds with opposite arm and leg raise

3. *Ball in lap with abdominal muscles working isometrically* progression series. This series comprises of a Swiss ball being placed in the lap of the patient, but not touching the abdominal muscles. The patient then squeezes the ball between their hands and thighs (Fig. 10). This exercise can then be progressed as follows: 90-90 abdominal holds with ball squeeze

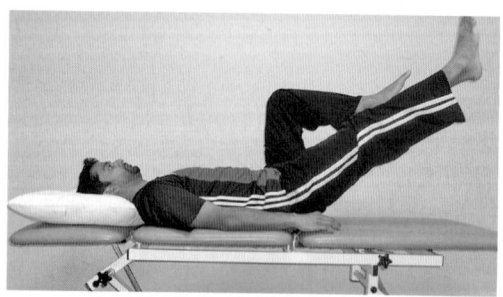

FIG. 6: 90-90 abdominal holds with knee extension

Chapter 47: Role of Physiotherapy in Treatment of Spinal Pain During Subacute/Reparative Phase

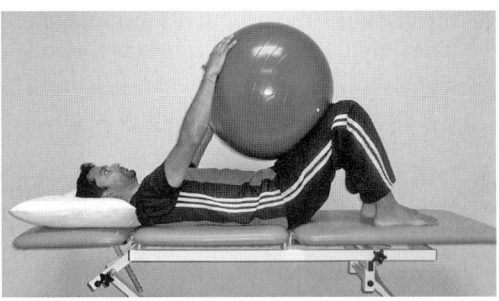

FIG. 10: Hook-lying with ball squeeze

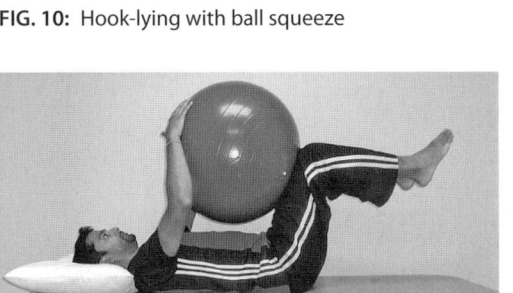

FIG. 11: 90-90 abdominal holds with ball squeeze

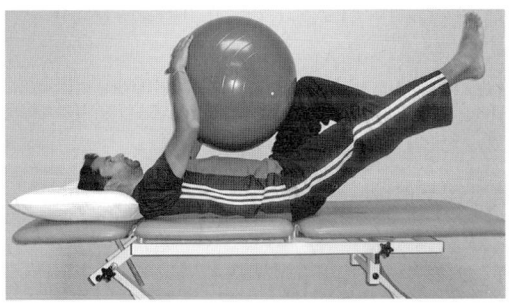

FIG. 12: 90-90 abdominal holds with single knee extension and ball squeeze

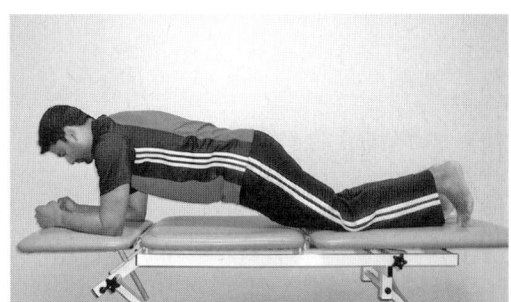

FIG. 13: Front plank on elbows and knees

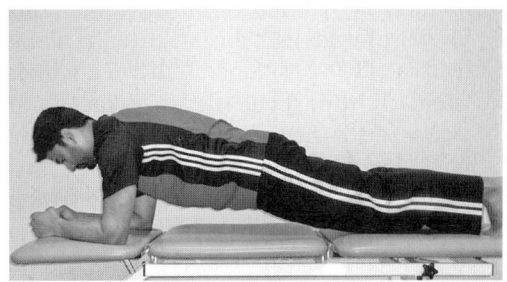

FIG. 14: Front plank on your elbows and feet

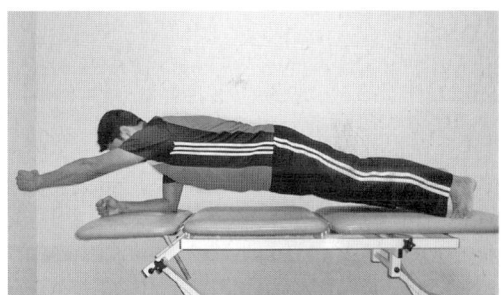

FIG. 15: Front plank with single arm raise

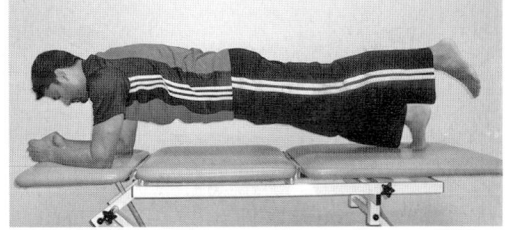

FIG. 16: Front plank with single leg raise

(Fig. 11); 90-90 abdominal holds position with ball squeeze and alternate knee extension (Fig. 12).

4. *Front plank progression:* The front plank can be performed by starting on elbows and knees (Fig. 13). The patient's ears, shoulders, hips, and knees should be in a straight line. This exercise can be advanced as follows: Front plank on elbows and feet (Fig. 14); Front plank with single arm raise (Fig. 15); Front plank with single leg raise (Fig. 16); and Front plank with opposite arm and leg raise (Fig. 17).

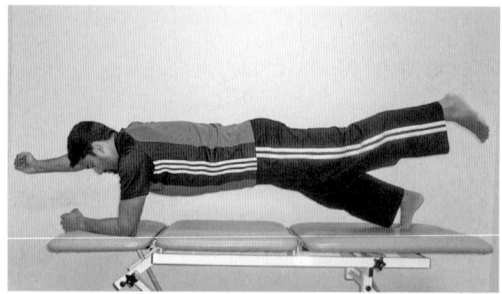

FIG. 17: Front plank with opposite arm and leg raise

this position, the patient needs much more kinesthetic awareness, in order to maintain a neutral spine. This exercise is advanced in the following order: alternating single arm raise (Fig. 20), alternating single leg raise (Fig. 21), and opposite arm and leg raise (Fig. 22).[17] There is an additional benefit to holding the Figure 22 position for a few seconds.[18]

5. *Multifidus training progression*: This exercise begins with the patient lying prone with a pillow positioned underneath their stomach. They should flex their knees and squeeze the heels together, while lifting their knees off the plinth (Fig. 18). This exercise can be progressed into being in a Quadruped position (Fig. 19). The quadruped position will be the first time that the patient's lumbar and cervical spine is not supported during exercise. In

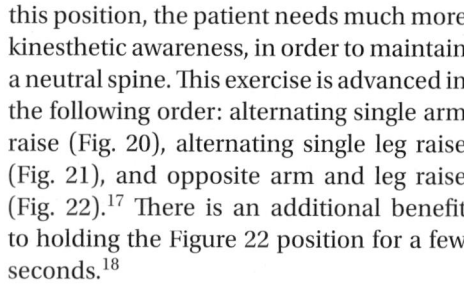

FIG. 20: Quadruped position with alternating single arm raise

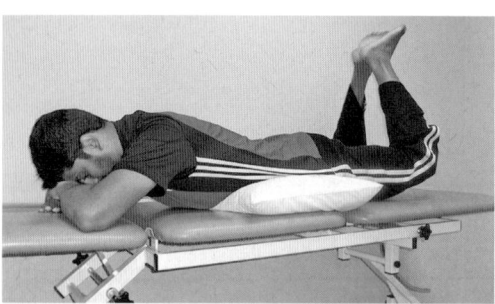

FIG. 18: Prone heel squeeze

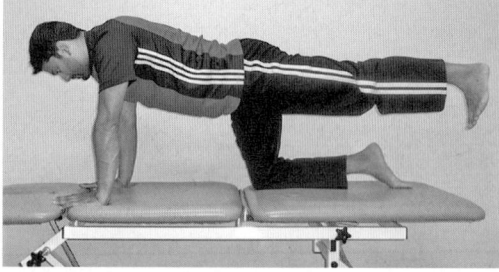

FIG. 21: Quadruped position with alternating single leg raise

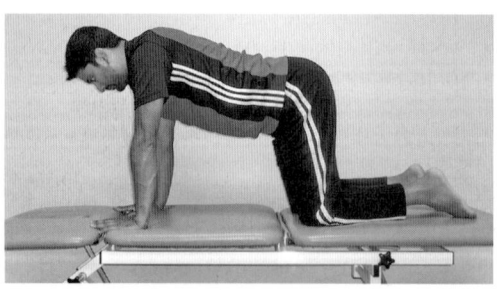

FIG. 19: Quadruped position

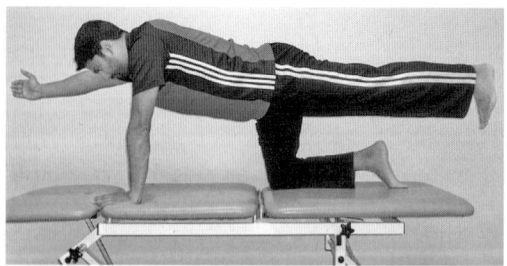

FIG. 22: Quadruped position with opposite arm and leg raise

Chapter 47: Role of Physiotherapy in Treatment of Spinal Pain During Subacute/Reparative Phase

6. *Side plank progression*: This exercise is performed to strengthen the external oblique abdominis muscles.[19] The side plank can be started by performing a modified side plank on the elbow and knees (Fig. 23). This can then be advanced by performing a dynamic arm raise with the opposite arm (Figs 24A and B). The exercise

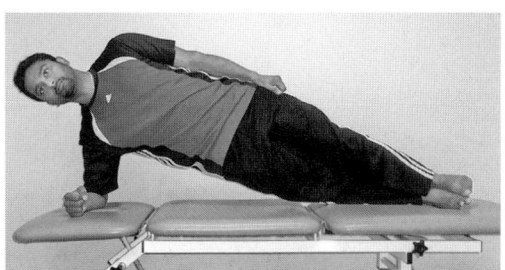

FIG. 25: Regular side plank on elbow and feet

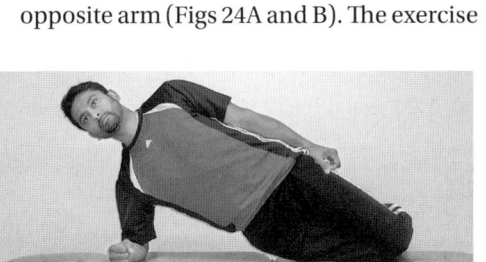

FIG. 23: Modified side plank on elbow and knees

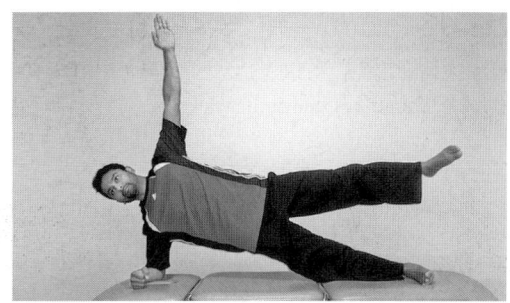

FIG. 26: Regular side plank with star pose

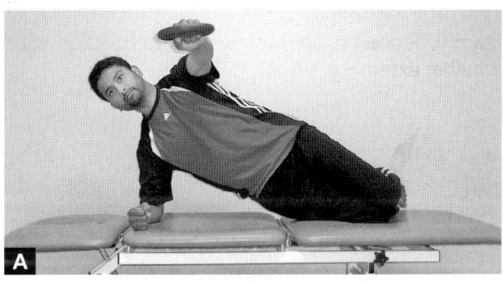

FIG. 24A: Modified side plank with opposite arm raise (position 1). Demonstrated here with 5-lb weight

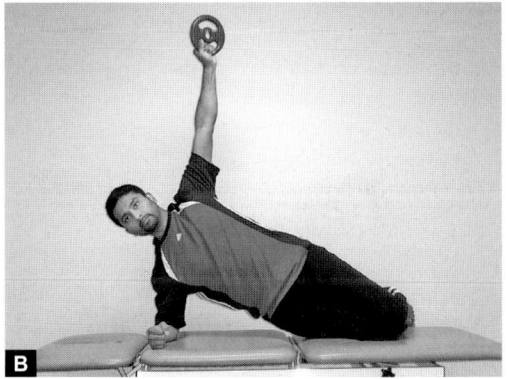

FIG. 24B: Modified side plank with opposite arm raise (position 2). Demonstrated here with 5-lb weight

can be further advanced by performing the regular side plank on the elbow and feet (Fig. 25). Further, you can perform the side plank with star pose (Fig. 26).

7. *Squatting progression*: This is a good starting exercise to initiate lower extremity strengthening. In this phase, it is prudent to perform squatting with external support for the lumbar spine as it provides some protection. Patient should be reminded to maintain their neutral spine and the natural lumbar lordosis while performing this exercise. The exercise can be performed with wall support, with or without a Swiss ball (Figs 27 and 28).

8. *Prone on ball with arm motion progression*: In this exercise, the patient continues to challenge their lumbar and cervical extensor muscles isometrically, by holding themselves in a straight line from their ears, shoulders, hips, knees, and feet. Patients can then perform various arm motions in increasing order

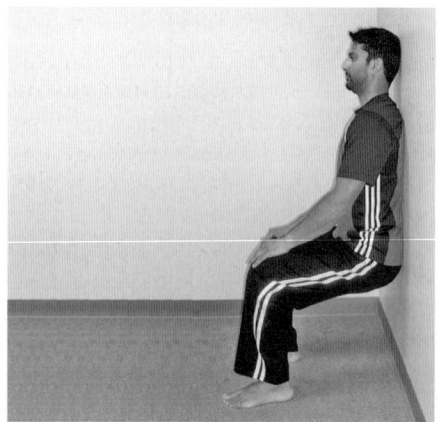

FIG. 27: Squatting against the wall

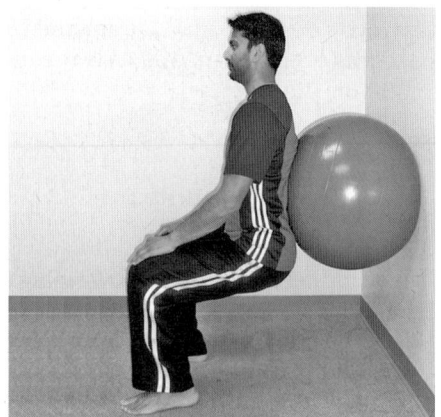

FIG. 28: Squatting against the wall using a Swiss ball

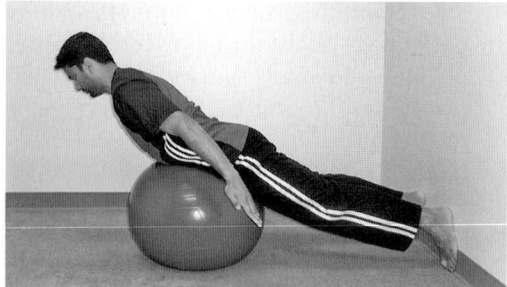

FIG. 29: Prone on ball with bilateral arm extension

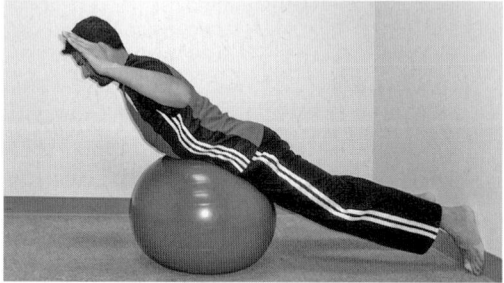

FIG. 30: Prone on ball with scapular retraction with shoulder external rotation

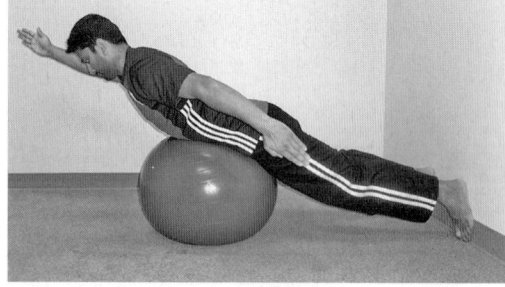

FIG. 31: Prone on ball with alternate arm raise and extension

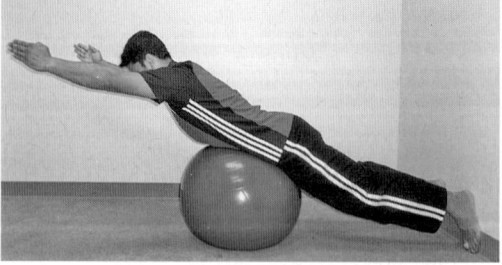

FIG. 32: Prone on ball with bilateral arm raise

of difficulty (Figs 29 to 32). The prone on ball series can be started with the patient's feet supported against the wall and then advanced to no foot support.

9. *Cervical exercises:* Most of the exercises discussed above, will also apply to cervical pain patients. Below are examples of some exercises, which are specific for training and strengthening of the cervical musculature. Cervical isometric exercises should be performed in front of a mirror, to correct for any rotation or side bending of the cervical spine. Figures 33 to 35 demonstrate cervical isometric exercises for muscles in the front, back, and sides of the neck respectively.

Cardiovascular Training

It is recommended to start performing cardiovascular exercise for spinal patients during this phase. This helps to improve overall mobility, boost patient confidence, and provides an overall sense of accomplishment. Standard techniques are utilized to calculate the patient's cardiovascular training zone, in terms of heart rate.[20] If there is a concern about the patient's ability to bear load on their spine, then the modified cycling techniques, as demonstrated in the figures below should be used. For example, stationary cycling in supine (Fig. 36). It is important to ensure that the patient is maintaining a neutral spine, while cycling. Alternatively, you can have the patient cycle on an upright bike and then have them occasionally use a walker for reducing the compression load on their spine (Fig. 37).

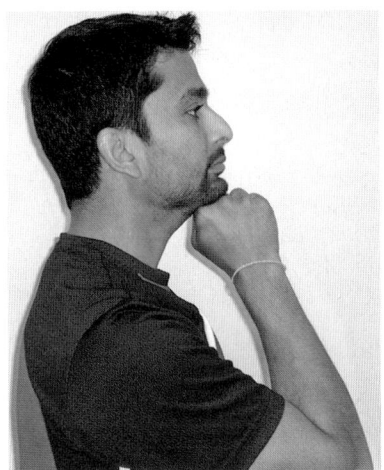

FIG. 33: Cervical isometrics for deep neck flexors

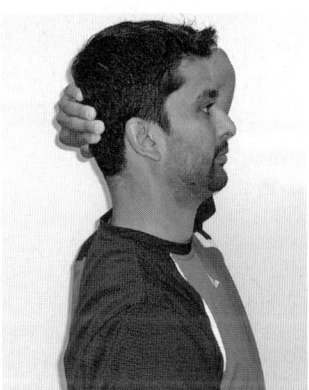

FIG. 34: Cervical isometrics for cervical extensor muscles

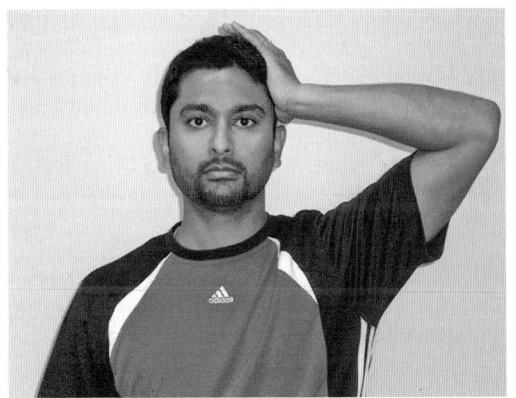

FIG. 35: Cervical isometrics for lateral cervical musculature

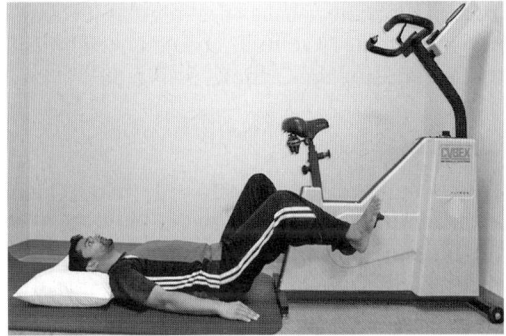

FIG. 36: Riding a stationary bike in supine

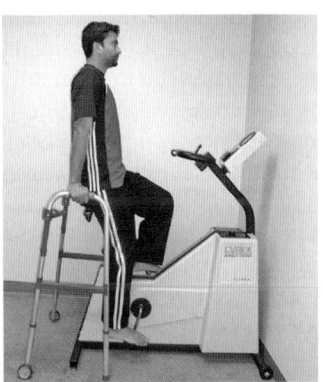

FIG. 37: Riding an upright bike with occasional use of a walker for unloading the spine

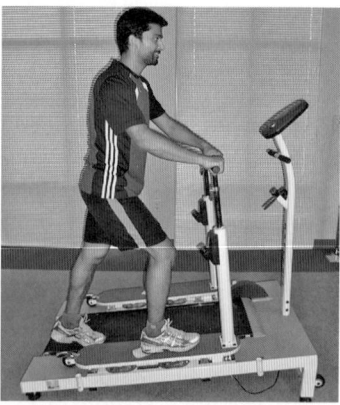

FIG. 38: Using the OrthoKick. Printed with inventor's permission

Other methods of performing cardiovascular exercise, which might be appropriate in the subacute phase, are regular cycling, walking on a Treadmill, using an Elliptical trainer, or using the OrthoKick (Fig. 38).

CONCLUSION

This chapter has discussed the goals and treatment options for patients in the subacute or reparative phase. If normal healing is occurring, the patient will transition into the maintenance or maturation phase. As discussed above; in the sub-acute phase, we recommended that the patient exercises their spinal muscles primarily in an isometric manner. Although in the maintenance phase it is considered safe to exercise the spinal muscles in a dynamic manner (e.g. abdominal crunches). It is critical to stress the healing tissue to an optimal level without damaging it during all phases. It is important to keep these concepts of healing in mind at all times, when preparing the treatment plan, as it will facilitate the patient's ability to reach their final goal, such as returning to working full-time or playing their favorite sport.

REFERENCES

1. Buckwalter J, et al. Injury and repair of the musculoskeletal soft tissue. American Academy of Orthopaedic Surgeons Symposium. 1998.
2. Dionne CE, Dunn KM, Croft PR, et al. A consensus approach toward the standardization of back pain definitions for use in prevalence studies. Spine. 2008; 33(1):95-103.
3. O'Sullivan P. Classification of lumbopelvic pain disorders--why is it essential for management? Man Ther. 2006; 11(3):169-70.
4. Macdermid, Joy C, et al. "Measurement properties of the neck disability index: a systematic review." Journal of Orthopaedic & Sports Physical Therapy. 2009;39(5): 400-17.
5. Fairbanks J, et al. The Oswestry Low Back Pain Disability Questionnaire. Physiotherapy. 1980; 66(8):271-3.
6. McGill S. Low Back Disorders. 3rd Edition With Web Resource: Evidence-Based Prevention and Rehabilitation. 3rd edition. Champaign, IL: Human Kinetics. 2015:247-90.
7. Smit TH, van Tunen MS, van der Veen AJ, Kingma I, van Dieën JH. Quantifying intervertebral disc mechanics: a new definition of the neutral zone. BMC Musculoskelet Disord. 2011;12:38.
8. Allison, et al. Feedforward responses of transverse abdominis are directionally specific and act asymmetrically: implications for core stability theories. Journal of Orthopaedic & Sports Physical Therapy. 2008;38:228-37.
9. Cleland J, et al. The Use of a Lumbar Spine Manipulation Technique by Physical Therapists in Patients Who Satisfy a Clinical Prediction Rule: A Case Series. Journal of Orthopaedic & Sports Physical Therapy. 2006;36(4):198-9.
10. P Hodges, et al. Therapeutic Exercise for Spinal Segmental Stabilization in Low Back Pain–Scientific Basis and Clinical Approach. Churchill Livingstone. 1998.
11. Childs, et al. A clinical prediction rule to identify patients with low back pain most likely to benefit from spinal manipulation: A validation study. Ann Intern Med. 2004; 141:920-28.
12. Gonzalez-Iglesias, et al. Thoracic spine manipulation for the management of patients with neck pain: A randomized Clinical Trial. Journal of Orthopaedic & Sports Physical Therapy. 2009;39(1):20-7.
13. Takasaki, et al. The influence of cervical traction, compression, and spurling test on cervical intervertebral foramen size. Spine. 2009;34:1658-62.

14. Costa, et al. Motor control exercise for chronic low back pain: A Randomized Placebo-Controlled Trial. Physical Therapy. 2009;89(12):1275-86.
15. Hides, et al. Long-term effects of specific stabilizing exercises for first-episode low back pain. Spine. 2001;26(11):E243-E248.
16. Solomonow M, Zhou BH, Lu Y, King KB. Acute repetitive lumbar syndrome: a multi-component insight into the disorder. J Bodyw Mov Ther. 2012;16(2):134-47.
17. Hides, et al. Effect of stabilization training on multifidus muscle cross-sectional area among young elite cricketers with low back pain. Journal of Orthopaedic & Sports Physical Therapy. 2008;38(3):101-08.
18. Danneels, et al. Effects of three different training modalities on the cross sectional area of the lumbar multifidus muscle in patients with chronic low back pain. British Journal of Sports Medicine. 2001;35:186-91.
19. Ekstrom, et al. Electromyographic Analysis of Core Trunk, Hip, and Thigh Muscles During 9 Rehabilitation Exercise. Journal of Orthopaedic & Sports Physical Therapy. 2007;37(12):754-62.
20. P Maffetone, Training for Endurance–Guide for Endurance Athletes of All Levels. 2000.

CHAPTER 48

Physiotherapy in Management of Chronic Pain

Saroj M Sanghavi, Dakshesh M Sanghavi

INTRODUCTION

Physiotherapy is that aspect of healthcare, which deals with restoration or maintenance of the human function and movement utilizing physical agents such as touch, heat, light, sound, etc. along with exercises and manual therapy techniques. It combines the knowledge of anatomy and physiology and applies that to the understanding of pathology and kinesiology to optimize human function. Physiotherapists view the patient as a "whole" rather than an isolated injury or impairment in a person.[1]

Pain is one of the most common sensations that prompt a person to seek the services of a physiotherapist. It is nature's indication that there is some damage to the tissues, be it musculoskeletal pain, sports injuries, post-operative pain, or labor pain. However, this broad explanation of pain does not always apply to chronic pain. It cannot be usually attributed to a specific system (e.g. neuromuscular or musculoskeletal) and is typically reported long after the damaged tissues have healed pathologically. This phenomenon, therefore, makes treating chronic pain difficult. The patient with chronic pain does not always get the treatment he/she deserves, as the healthcare professional tries to understand and treat the pain using the construct of a specific body system. Quite often, such patients are dismissed as being "problem patients" who do not have "real" pain.[2] Although the exact time frame that is used to determine the chronicity of pain is not specified in literature, most pain management specialists agree that pain that has lasted more than three to six months is considered to be chronic. It must be noted that when pain becomes chronic, it is no longer a symptom but a disease.[3] The cause of chronic pain is difficult to determine as it is rarely due to a single pathology.

CAUSES

The causes for chronic musculoskeletal pain may be many and are often overlooked if there are other existing pathologies and comorbidities. Patients with chronic pain typically end up seeking physiotherapy intervention after a long lapse of time since the onset of the pain. Whether this delay in intervention caused the acute pain to become chronic or was the pain slated to become chronic cannot be explained fully. However, physiotherapy does play a role in the management of chronic pain relief. Repetitive stress disorder may cause musculoskeletal pain due to overuse of certain muscles accompanied with poor positioning or posture, as typically encountered in people that use the computer or handheld devices for prolonged periods.

EVALUATION/ASSESSMENT

Prior to commencement of the treatment plan, a comprehensive evaluation is necessary. This includes, but is not limited to:
- Review of prior medical and surgical history (including premorbid conditions such as diabetes, pulmonary problems, cardiovascular conditions, etc.)
- Past functional status and present functional problems
- Onset and type of pain
- Location of pain (a body diagram may be very helpful)
- Specific time or activities that alleviate and/or relieve the pain
- Impact of pain on sleep
- Psychological and psychosocial aspects including cognition, arousal, and attention (fear of pain may lead to avoidance of physical activity and this may contribute further to anxiety and pain and functional impairments)
- Posture analysis and ergonomic considerations (workplace assessment may be indicated)
- Need for assistance or independence in activities of daily living (ADL)
- Impairments in range of motion and contractures and deformities
- Impairments in strength of specific muscles or muscle groups
- Neurological examination, including sensory deficits related to temperature, light touch, perception, reflexes, etc.

This assessment should be individualized and relevant to the patient and his/her functional status.[4] The information thus gathered should be correlated to other findings although it must be remembered that chronic pain will not always correspond to specific diagnoses, pathologies and syndromes.[5]

A Pain Clinic utilizes a multidisciplinary team to manage the multiple problems associated with chronic pain; a team that manages various issues is a preferred approach rather than isolated care. A comprehensive evaluation including laboratory and radiological findings complements the assessment by various disciplines such as a pain management physician, anesthesiologist, physiotherapist, orthopedic surgeon, neurologist and/or neurosurgeon, psychologist, nurse, dietician and vocational/recreational therapists. However, such specialty clinics are not a common feature of most hospitals or medical centers and access to them may be difficult.

GOALS OF TREATMENT

The following are goals that are usually involved in the treatment of chronic pain:
- Relief of pain and/or muscle spasm
- Prevention of contractures and deformity
- Improve and/or maintain the range of motion and strength
- Optimize functional abilities to premorbid levels.

The presence of pain will typically decrease a person's activity and therefore assessing the functional levels objectively is important. Several scales that measure ADL are available such as Barthel Index, Katz Index of ADL, human activity profile, sickness impact, which profile, etc. Such scales are invaluable in objectifying the impact, which pain has on the person's ability to function. Scales that are specific to the body part such as disability of arm shoulder and hand (DASH) or lower extremity functional scale (LEFS) or Oswestry low back pain scale provide a measure of the functional impairment in that limb or body part. They are standardized and validated, quick to use, patient-centered, able to be completed by the patient/caregiver and can be used to measure progress over the course of therapy. They can be easily incorporated in electronic records to provide an ongoing measure of objective progress, or lack thereof.

Pain scales such as visual analog scale (VAS), McGill pain questionnaire, etc. may be used to determine the intensity and monitor pain relief. For patients that may not be able to self-report pain, the use of Faces Pain Scale[6] (FPS) is recommended. This scale is often used in young children and cognitively impaired individuals, such as those in persistent vegetative state.

INTERVENTIONS FOR PAIN MANAGEMENT

The procedural interventions used by physiotherapists include:
- Therapeutic exercise-range of motion, active, active assistive or resistive/strengthening
- Functional training in self care and home management
- Functional training in community and work reintegration
- Manual therapy techniques
- Orthotic/adaptive device prescription and training
- Physical agents and modalities
- Electrotherapeutic modalities.

ELECTROTHERAPEUTIC MODALITIES

A full review of modalities and all the other interventions listed above is beyond the scope of this chapter and more information can be obtained from other sources. Most of the common electrotherapeutic modalities that are used in pain relief by physiotherapists are as follows:

Short-wave Diathermy

Short-wave diathermy (SWD) converts high-frequency electromagnetic waves to heat the body's tissues; the frequency used is 27.12 MHz. There are two forms. Pulsed or continuous and the use depends on the heating effect that is desired.

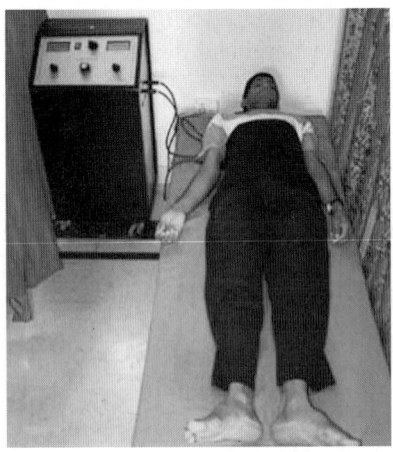

FIG. 1: Short-wave diathermy

- *Indications:* Musculoskeletal spasm, inflammation, arthritis, etc.
- *Physiological effects:* Increased vascularity and vasodilatation decreases inflammation, and reduces excitability of sensory nerves, helps in reducing muscle spasm.

Contraindications: Pacemakers, metal implants, active tuberculosis of joints, malignant tissues, venous thrombosis and hemorrhages[7] (Fig. 1).

Ultrasound

It converts sound waves at very high frequencies (0.8 MHz to 3 MHz), in pulsed or continuous modes, to deep heat; since it involves transmission of sound waves, it needs coupling agents like gel or water to create an interface between the sonicator and the skin. This form of therapy can also be used to introduce medication such as a steroidal or anti- inflammatory ointment to a specific area and this is referred to as phonophoresis.

- *Indications:* Soft tissue shortening (e.g. contractures, scarring, etc.), chronic inflammation, muscle spasm, trigger points. As it produces localized heat, ultrasound (US) is generally used for conditions that cause pain in a specific site, such as tendonitis, planterfascitis, tennis elbow, scar, etc.

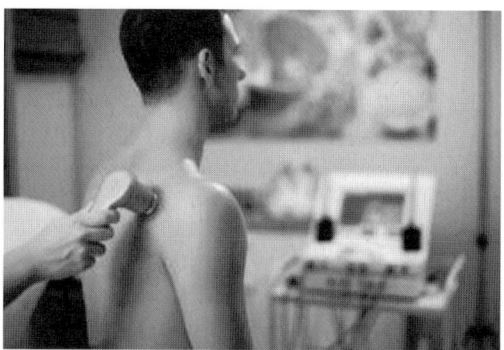

FIG. 2: Ultrasound therapy

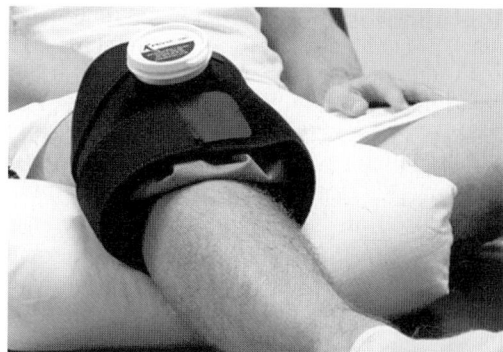

FIG. 4: Cryotherapy

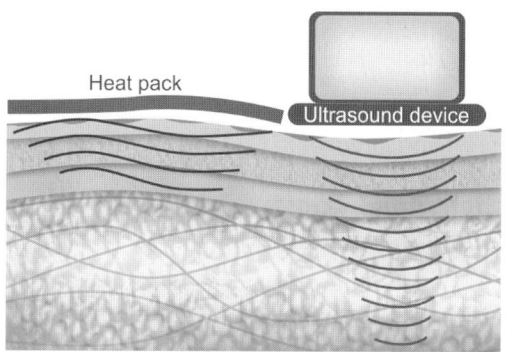

FIG. 3: Depth of penetration of ultrasound

- *Physiological effects:* The deep heat accelerates healing, increases extensibility of collagen; regenerates tissue and therefore used in wound repair.
- *Contraindications:* Acute sepsis, tumors, metal implants in the treated area and vascular conditions[8] (Figs 2 and 3).

Other forms of superficial heat therapy include moist heat packs, infra-red rays, microwave diathermy, paraffin wax bath, contrast bath, etc. These may be used to improve local circulation prior to exercising or manual therapy.

Cryotherapy

It is when the tissues are cooled to decrease metabolism and vasoactive agents to reduce inflammation and outward fluid filtration. It is most commonly used to decrease spasm, spasticity as it slows nerve conduction velocity. Ice massage or vapocoolant sprays are used over specific areas (e.g. trigger points) before deep massage or after cross friction massage to cool down the inflamed areas. Cold compression units are typically used after immediate trauma or postoperatively to minimize swelling and reduce pain[9] (Fig. 4).

Neuromuscular Electrical Stimulation

Neuromuscular electrical stimulation (NMES) utilizes electrical currents (alternating or direct) with various waveforms and different parameters of amplitude, frequency and pulse duration. Physiotherapists have the ability to choose from a variety of different forms of electrical outputs based on the desired outcome: pain relief, enhanced circulation, tissue healing or muscle retraining. Alternating currents (AC) or pulsed currents (PC) are most commonly used waveforms. These may be monophasic, biphasic—symmetric or asymmetric. Response to electrical stimulation is subsensory, sensory, motor or noxious.

- *Indications:* Chronic pain, muscle spasm, contractures
- *Physiological effect:* Increased vascularity and lymphatic drainage promoting venous return; stimulation of motor and sensory nerves promotes muscular contraction and relaxation of muscles which may re-educate muscles.

Iontophoresis

It is the introduction of medication to skin's underlying tissues using electrical current as a carrier. Medicated electrode patches are adhered to the skin at specific spots and direct current (DC) carries the medication. Common drugs used are dexamethasone (to decrease inflammation), lidocaine (for pain), acetic acid (for calcific tendonitis), salicylates (for joint pain), and etc.[10]

Transcutaneous Electrical Nerve Stimulation

Transcutaneous electrical nerve stimulation (TENS) uses high frequency, low-intensity electrical stimulation to control pain without motor stimulation. The intensity is 0-100 cycles/sec. and the frequency is adjusted as per the chronicity/acuity of pain. Since it is a portable unit, its use can be taught to the patient who can administer the treatment as necessary. There are several forms of TENS, which include conventional (frequency 10-100 Hz), Strong low-rate (frequency below 10 Hz), modulated (frequency and pulse durations are modulated from preset values). Typically, TENS is not used to produce muscle contraction but to regulate pain sensation.

Indications: Pain of neurogenic origin, e.g. neuralgias, postoperative pain, labor pain, primary dysmenorrheal, phantom pain to name a few.

Physiological effects: Gate Control mechanism was attributed to produce pain relief but more research indicates that it activates the descending pain suppression system which is mediated by endogenous opiates in the central nervous system.

Contraindications: Over carotid sinus and demand-type pacemaker.

Newer TENS units are wireless and the device is directly applied over the electrode on the skin. These are easier to use, and is of particular use to those who want pain relief while at work, or exercising or playing sports.[11]

Interferential Current

Interferential current (IFT) is produced by the interference of two different medium frequency electrical currents using vacuum or rubber electrodes.

Physiological effects: Stimulates autonomic nerves resulting in vasodilatation, release of endorphins, facilitates vascular and lymphatic drainage, reduces edema, and releases endogenous opiates.

Indications: Sports injuries, muscle spasm, chronic pain.

Contraindications: Pacemaker, thrombosis, fever and infection.[12]

Light Amplification by Simulation Emission of Radiation

It is a monochromatic, coherent and unidirectional form of electromagnetic radiation that has different uses in healthcare and other industries. Lasers used in physiotherapy are nondestructive. Different types of noninvasive light amplification by simulation emission of radiations (LASERs) that are used by physiotherapists are: Ruby, helium, neon, gallium arsenide (GaAs), diode with different wavelengths. The authors used GaAs with pulsed infrared (904 nm wave length that has 1.5-2 cm depth of penetration) with good results in various painful conditions.

Physiological Effects: Releases ACTH and Beta-endorphins; reduction of prostaglandin E and SOD activity, immunostimulant, balances intra-and extracellular activities and accelerates production of ATP and collagen synthesis.

Indications: Acute and chronic musculoskeletal pain, trigger points.

Contraindications: Over eyes, cancerous lesions, pregnancy, pacemakers, thrombosis and photochemical drugs[13] (Fig. 5).

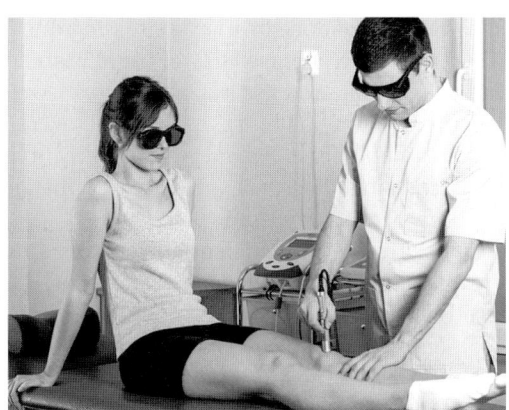

FIG. 5: Laser therapy

Electromyography Biofeedback

It provides a feedback of physiological function using audiovisual signals. It detects the tension in the muscle and enables the patient to be an active participant in relaxing the muscle. Different types like myoelectric feedback, electromyography (EMG) biofeedback, postural and stress-related devices are available and can be used for muscle relaxation causing pain relief.

Traction can be mechanical or manual. Newer traction units use computerized tables where the patient lies on and the force is directed to specific vertebral segments. The efficacy of mechanical traction is debated but is often used as an adjunct to other modalities to provide pain relief. Often home units are prescribed to allow patients to receive this treatment without traveling to the therapist.[14] However, a 2009 study developed a clinical prediction rule showing the most effective use of traction is in those individuals aged less than 30 years with non-manual labor jobs, low fear avoidance beliefs, and no neurologic deficits.[15]

The use of modalities in treatment of chronic pain must be judicious and the treatment plan altered as the pain reduces. Prolonged use of modalities is not the optimal treatment philosophy as this creates an artificial dependence on the modalities and does not allow the patient to progress to independence.

MANUAL THERAPY TECHNIQUES

Manual therapy techniques quite often complement physical modalities mentioned above. Physiotherapists that have sought specialized training in such techniques typically perform these procedures. Some of the techniques that can be used are:
- Soft tissue mobilization/Massage (cross-friction, kneading, etc.).
- Myofascial release (MFR) is an extremely gentle technique that involves application of a sustained, low pressure force to the myofascial structures to "free" restricted areas.
- Craniosacral therapy.
- Joint mobilization (spinal and peripheral joints) involves use of specifically targeted force on joints to mobilize the joint and improve flexibility.
- Muscle energy techniques.

Another form of supportive treatment is Kinesio taping. It is the application of a special tape in a very specific technique to promote appropriate muscle function and reduce pain. It is also reported to relax overused muscles and support muscles in movement during the entire day. The use of modalities and passive manual therapy techniques usually provide some pain relief but a proper exercise program is the cornerstone of an ideal chronic pain management program. Chronic pain may often lead to motor control problems due to kinesthetic impairments.[16]

Use of modalities must be cautious and not be the sole intervention during a physical therapy session. Modalities are often a supplement to exercise and manual therapy treatments. A systematic review by Yu, Cote et al on the use of passive modalities for shoulder pain included 1470 articles from which 11 met the criteria for inclusion—randomized control trials (RCT). Ultrasound and interferential current therapy were not found to be better than placebo treatments for non-specific shoulder pain. Low level laser therapy was found to be more beneficial than placebo or ultrasound in subacromial impingement syndrome.[17]

A well-developed exercise program is one that is customized to address the unique issues of that patient using specific exercises. A "one-size-fits-all" approach to exercise programs is most likely not going to produce the desired results and compliance to such a program will be limited.[18] Specific stretching and strengthening exercises should be taught to the patient to address his/her specific problems and these have to be carefully monitored and adjusted. Compliance to the exercise program and the instructions/precautions provided are necessary for a long-term successful rehabilitation process. Frequent follow-up with the healthcare provider may be recommended, especially for those patients that have more complex problems. Ergonomic considerations to modify worksite are invaluable, especially in repetitive stress disorders such as carpal tunnel syndrome, etc.

Exercises not only activate the muscle pump but also cause the improved vascularity and lymphatic flow that also disperses the chemically depolarizing/sensitizing agents, decreases edema, inhibits muscle spasm and reduces overall anxiety. It also improves range of motion, flexibility and strength of the muscles to optimize functional skills. The improved range of motion mobilizes the myofascium, which may be restricted and therefore inhibit optimal muscle contraction. Several studies have indicated that supervised exercise programs in elderly patients with osteoarthritis and rheumatoid arthritis showed improved pain control and fitness. Active and/or resistive exercises should be taught and an individualized home exercise program should be initiated from the early sessions of therapy. Yoga is an excellent adjunct to physiotherapy and may be considered when the patient is being weaned off modalities and led to independence in an exercise program.[19] The endorphin release that is usually noted after a regular exercise regimen, works well to improve the patient's mood and overall sense of fulfillment. This may particularly help in decreasing the sense of disability that is accompanied with chronic pain.

Assistive devices such as ambulatory aids (walkers, canes, quad canes, etc.) may be used to enhance functional activities without worsening the pain. The physiotherapist would determine the appropriate device and train the user to ensure optimal safety and efficacy of the device. Orthotic devices such as braces, shoe inserts, etc. should be judiciously prescribed and used to prevent dependency.

As technology advances, more modalities are emerging and scientists are studying their safety and efficacy. Two such modalities that may become common in the future are monochromatic infrared energy (MIRE) and extracorporeal shock wave therapy (ESWT). There is considerable evidence in the use of virtual reality (VR) in managing acute and chronic pain. Its efficacy has been demonstrated in acute burns, cancer pain, during medical procedures, and also in experimental studies in uninvolved humans. Its effectiveness is further validated with concurrent MRI studies that investigate brain activity during its use. This area of research is growing rapidly and commercial applications of VR for pain relief are expected to be available in the very near future.[20] However, the clinician is strongly encouraged to use an evidence-based practice approach to determine any modality or procedure's efficacy and applicability to clinical practice.[21]

CONCLUSION

Pain and function should not be viewed as distinct and separate entities but as integral elements, of the patient's report of the ability to perform their activities of daily living. An individualized exercise program and proper follow-up are invaluable components of a comprehensive pain management approach.

REFERENCES

1. Diullio R. Treating chronic pain in older patients. Rehab. Management: The interdisciplinary journal of Rehabilitation. 2010;23(9);18-23.
2. Goodman C, Snyder T. Differential Diagnosis for Physical Therapists. 4th ed. Saunders Elsevier; 2007;144-6.
3. O'Sullivan S, Schmitz T. Physical Rehabilitation. 5th ed. F. A Davis; 2007.pp.1124-27.
4. O'Sullivan S, Schmitz T. Physical Rehabilitation 5th ed. F A Davis; 2007.pp.115-8.
5. O'Sullivan S, Schmitz T. Physical Rehabilitation 5th ed. F A Davis; 2007.pp.1128-33.
6. Wong D.L, Wong's Essentials of Pediatric Nursing. 6th ed. Mosby; 2001.pp.1301.
7. Cameron M H, Physical Agents in Rehabilitation, 4th ed. Saunders; 2013.pp.202-12.
8. Cameron M. H, Physical Agents in Rehabilitation, 4th ed. Saunders; 2013.pp.173-88.
9. Cameron M. H, Physical Agents in Rehabilitation, 4th ed. Saunders; 2013.pp.129-37.
10. Cameron M. H, Physical Agents in Rehabilitation, 4th ed. Saunders; 2013.pp.272.
11. Cameron M. H, Physical Agents in Rehabilitation, 4th ed. Saunders; 2013.pp.257-9.
12. Hayes K. Manual for Physical Agents. 5th ed. Prentice Hall Health, 2001.
13. Cameron M. H, Physical Agents in Rehabilitation, 4th ed. Saunders; 2013.pp.292-8.
14. Cameron M H, Physical Agents in Rehabilitation, 4th ed. Saunders; 2013.pp.364-81.
15. Cai C, Pua YH, Lim KC. A clinical prediction rule for classifying patients with low back pain who demonstrate short-term improvement with mechanical lumbar traction. European Spine Journal. 2009;(184): 554-61.
16. Jull GA, Richardson CA. Motor Control Problems in Patients with Spinal Pain: A New Direction for Therapeutic Exercise. J of Manipulative Physiotherapy. 2000;23(2):115.
17. Yu H, Cote P, Shearer H, Wong J, Sutton D, Randhawa K, Varatharajan S, Southrest D, Mior S, Amis A, Stupar M, Nordin M, van der Velde G, Carroll L, Jacobs C, Taylor-Vaisey A, Abdulla S, Shergill Y. Effectiveness of passive physical modalities for shoulder pain: Systematic review by Ontario Protocol for traffic injury management collaboration. Physical Therapy. 2015;95(3):306-18.
18. Slade S, Molloy E, Keating J. People with non-specific chronic low back pain who have participated in exercise programs have preferences about exercise: a qualitative study. Australian Journal of Physiotherapy. 2009; 55(2):115-21.
19. Tekur P, Singphow C, Nagendra H, Raghuram N. Effect of short-term intensive yoga program on pain, functional disability and spinal flexibility in chronic low back pain: a randomized control study. Journal of Alternative Complementary Medicine. 2008;14(6): 637-44.
20. 16a Li A, Montano Z, Chen C, Gold J. Virtual reality and pain management: current trends and future directions. Pain management. 2011;1(2):147-57.
21. Michlovitz S L, Nolan T. Modalities for Therapeutic Intervention. 4th ed. F A Davis; 2005.pp.289-95.

SECTION 14

Psychotherapy

CHAPTER 49

Role of Psychiatric Medications in Chronic Pain Management

Harish K Shetty, Surbhi C Trivedi

INTRODUCTION

Pain has been defined by The International Association for the Study of Pain as "an unpleasant sensory and emotional experience which we primarily associate with tissue damage or describe in terms of such damage, or both".[1] Peripheral, spinal and supraspinal are the three levels at which pain pathway is controlled in the nervous system. With time there was a gradual progress in the way we understood the mechanism of pain—the initial concept was that painful stimulus generates a signal and this signal travels up along a specific pathway to the brain, where it is recognized as pain. After that came the Gate Control theory of pain which suggested that when there is a stimulus from the periphery, modulation of that stimulus occurs in the dorsal horn of spinal cord and it is the influences which are there at spinal level are the ones that play an important role in determination of pain. With the advent of functional imaging techniques for the brain it was established that not only the spinal level influences but also supraspinal influences play a role in determining the presence and severity of pain. The cortical regions sense pain in three different dimensions, which are—sensory, i.e. location and intensity of discomfort; affective, i.e. the emotional value of pain and cognitive, i.e. what one thinks about the pain.

CHRONIC PAIN

Acute pain (nociceptive pain) arises when there is activation of nociceptors which are the peripheral pain receptors. Acute pain is more of signals relayed by specific pain fibers in specific pain pathways in the nervous system and is usually protective and lasts for a short period of time unless the tissue injury is ongoing. Chronic pain (neuropathic pain) is pain that persists beyond the time of normal healing process after exposure to trauma or noxious stimulus. The duration of this pain is variable and can be from less than 1 month to more than 6 months.[1] It is the pain that lasts longer than might be reasonably expected to persist following the event that led to the onset of pain in the first place. Chronic pain is more a result of complex information processing network which is inefficient.

Acute pain if continues for a long time can go on to cause changes in the central nervous system pain mechanisms as a result of which the original pain is either enhanced or perpetuated or both leading to chronic pain, e.g. chronic low back pain. Modulation occurring at the level of other components of the pain pathway such as the peripheral neuron or the dorsal horn can also lead to neuropathic pain. Some other chronic pain conditions may never have a peripheral receptor involved in the pain and it may start at the center by itself, e.g. pain in depression, fibromyalgia. Such conditions may also have a number of other physical symptoms as well not explainable by any medical condition.

It can be said that for chronic pain there is a spectrum, where chronic pain can occur by itself without any other accompanying symptom, chronic pain can have certain additional physical, emotional or cognitive symptoms or it can be associated with syndromal psychiatric disorders. The relationship of chronic pain and psychological stress is probably bidirectional, i.e. each one can lead to and/or aggravate the other. However, both can also exist independent of each other. Though genetic studies do point to certain shared genetic and heritable components between chronic pain and disorders of mood,[2] neuroimaging studies have shown that in the brain the stress and pain processing circuits are independent of each other.[3] Studies on antidepressant drugs having analgesic effects have shown that as regards the analgesic effects they work well in patients with and without depression.[4] Hence, the treatment of chronic pain, which is a result of inefficient information processing in the pain pathway, will be the same irrespective of wherever it occurs in the spectrum.

WHY PSYCHIATRIC MEDICATIONS IN CHRONIC PAIN?

Out of the various pathways that are involved in regulating the pain circuit, two important descending inhibitory pathways which are implicated in chronic pain are those which use the neurotransmitters norepinephrine and serotonin. One is the descending norepinephrine pathway (originates in the locus coeruleus) where the descending noradrenergic neurons act on the α_2-adrenergic receptors and inhibit the release of neurotransmitters from afferent neurons at the level of dorsal horn.[5] The other one is the descending spinal serotonergic pathway (originates in the raphe magnus of rostroventromedial medulla), which acts via $5HT_{1B/1D}$ receptors to inhibit release of neurotransmitter from the afferent neurons at the level of dorsal horn.[5] The afferent neurons that these pathways inhibit are the ones that carry the sensation of pain from the peripheral receptors following the noxious stimulus. The descending norepinephrine and serotonin pathways are normally active in resting state and they help ignore the irrelevant input. If the inhibition by these pathways is not adequate, adequate masking may not happen and there may be perception of pain inspite of there being no noxious stimulus. However, at the same time it is to be noted that serotonin does have an excitatory effect as well via 5HT3 receptors in certain areas to facilitate the release of neurotransmitter from the afferent neurons.

Medications that will act on these monoamine systems of norepinephrine and serotonin and help enhance the inhibition of neurotransmitter release from the afferent neurons in pain pathway will hence help in conditions of chronic pain. This is the most popular theory on how the psychiatric medications help to treat chronic pain, though certain other mechanisms have also been implicated. A number of psychiatric medications (antidepressants) act on these monoaminergic systems and hence help in treatment of chronic pain disorders.

PSYCHIATRIC MEDICATIONS IN CHRONIC PAIN

Antidepressants

The various groups of antidepressants that have been found effective in treating chronic pain are:

Serotonin-norepinephrine Reuptake Inhibitors (SNRIs)

Serotonin-norepinephrine reuptake inhibitors (SNRIs) selectively inhibit the reuptake of serotonin and norepinephrine by acting on the serotonin reuptake transporter (SERT) and norepinephrine, transporter (NET). Another class of drugs, tricyclic antidepressants (TCAs), also inhibits the reuptake of serotonin and norepinephrine, but have their actions on numerous other receptors such as muscarinic, histaminergic and adrenergic receptors as well while SNRIs are more selective for serotonin and norepinephrine. Common side effects of this group are dry mouth, nausea, insomnia, dizziness, somnolence, sweating, sexual dysfunction, constipation, mydriasis and increase in blood pressure. Abrupt discontinuation can produce a withdrawal symptom. The various SNRIs are:

- *Venlafaxine:* It is a potent inhibitor of both serotonin and norepinephrine reuptake though the effect on norepinephrine reuptake is more pronounced at higher doses. Extended release formulation causes lesser side effects and is preferred over the immediate release preparation. Dose range is 75–375 mg/day and the maximum recommended dose for extended release formulation is 225 mg/day.[6,7]
- *Desvenlafaxine:* It is the active metabolite of venlafaxine. When compared to venlafaxine, desvenlafaxine has a relatively greater norepinephrine reuptake inhibition compared to serotonin reuptake inhibition. Dose range is 50–400 mg/day.[6,7]
- *Duloxetine:* It inhibits reuptake of serotonin slightly more than norepinephrine. Dose range is 20–120 mg/day.[6,7] With regards to side effects increase in blood pressure is probably lesser than that in venlafaxine.
- *Milnacipran:* It is the SNRI which has more potent effect on reuptake of norepinephrine compared to serotonin. Compared to other drugs of this group it cause more sweating and in some cases urinary hesitancy also. Dose range is 50–250 mg/day.[6,7]

Tricyclic and Tetracyclic Antidepressants (TCAs)

This class of drugs also blocks the reuptake of serotonin and norepinephrine. However, they also have their effects on muscarinic, adrenergic and histaminergic receptors. The doses of various TCAs are:[6,7]

- *Amitriptyline:* Dose range is 50–200 mg/day
- *Clomipramine:* Dose range is 10–250 mg/day
- *Imipramine:* Dose range is 50–200 mg/day
- *Nortriptyline:* Dose range is 30–150 mg/day
- *Doxepin:* Dose range is 30–300 mg/day.

Desipramine, trimipramine, protriptyline, are some of the other drugs of this group. Amoxapine, maprotiline are tetracyclic drugs.

The common side effects of this group of drugs are sedation, dry mouth, constipation, urinary retention, blurring of vision and arrhythmias.

Selective Serotonin ReuptakeInhibitors

The main mechanism of action is blocking serotonin transporter hence inhibiting the reuptake of serotonin from the synapses. They are found to be less effective in treating chronic pain compared to the SNRIs and TCAs as SSRIs act mainly on the serotonin levels and serotonin has both an inhibitory as well as a facilitatory action in the pain pathway. The dose ranges of various SSRIs are:[6,7]

- *Fluoxetine:* Dose range is 10–80 mg/day
- *Citalopram:* Dose range is 10–40 mg/day
- *Escitalopram:* Dose range is 10–20 mg/day
- *Fluvoxamine:* Dose range is 100–300 mg/day
- *Paroxetine:* Dose range is 10–60 mg/day
- *Sertraline:* Dose range is 25–200 mg/day.

The common side effects of this group of drugs are nausea, vomiting, diarrhea, sweating, anxiety, agitation, headache, hyponatremia and sexual dysfunction. On abrupt discontinuation, withdrawal symptoms may occur.

Monoamine Oxidase Inhibitors (MAOIs)

These act by inhibiting the monoamine oxidase (MAO) enzymes present on the outer mitochondrial membranes in the central and sympathetic nervous system and the gastrointestinal tract. MAO is the enzyme responsible for cytoplasmic and extraneuronal degradation of monoamine neurotransmitters. The various MAOIs are moclobemide, phenelzine, selegiline, tranylcypromine and isocarboxazid. Their side effects include insomnia, headaches, drowsiness, dizziness, postural hypotension, anticholinergic adverse effects, hepatotoxicity, leukopenia and hypertensive crisis. As a result of the higher incidence of side effects of MAOIs, they are not commonly used in practice.

PSYCHOTHERAPY

Psychotherapy helps not only in patients who have comorbid depression or anxiety along with chronic pain but also in those who do not have any psychiatric comorbidity. Cognitive behavior therapy (CBT) helps the patients learn how to cope effectively with the chronic pain.[8] Key components of CBT for chronic pain includes restructuring distorted cognitions by teaching the patients to understand and change the maladaptive thoughts; teaching relaxation techniques such progressive muscle relaxation, diaphragmatic breathing, guided imagery; giving homework assignments and teaching them how to be more active and to inculcate a healthy lifestyle. Group therapy and Family therapy are also useful in patients with chronic pain.

CONCLUSION

Chronic pain which is a result of inefficient complex information processing system requires multidisciplinary and multimodal approach for its management. Antidepressants and psychotherapy form important components of this multimodal treatment approach for patients with chronic pain irrespective of whether they have a comorbid psychiatric illness or not.

REFERENCES

1. Merskey H, Bogduk N. Classification of chronic pain: descriptions of chronic pain syndromes and definitions of pain terms, 2nd edition. Seattle (WA): International Association for the Study of Pain; 1994.
2. McIntosh AM, Hall LS, Zeng Y, Adams MJ, Gibson J, Wigmore E, et al. Genetic and environmental risk for chronic pain and the contribution of risk variants for major depressive disorder: a family-based mixed-model analysis. PLoS Med. 2016;13(8):1-6.
3. Giesecke T, Gracely RH, Williams DA, Geisser ME, Petzke FW, Clauw DJ. The relationship between depression, clinical pain, and experimental pain in a chronic pain cohort. Arthritis Rheum. 2005;52(5):1577-84.
4. Chan HN, Fam J, Yeong BN. Use of antidepressants in the treatment of chronic pain. Ann Acad Med Singapore. 2009;38:974-79.
5. Stamford JA. Descending control of pain. Br J Anaesth. 1995;75:217-27.
6. Taylor D, Paton C, Kapur S. The Maudsley—Prescribing guidelines in Psychiatry, 12th edition. West Sussex: Wiley Blackwell; 2015.
7. Sadock BJ, Saddock VA, Ruiz P. Kaplan and Saddock's Comprehensive Textbook of Psychiatry, 9th edition. Philadelphia: Lippincott Williams & Wilkins; 2009.
8. Ehde DM, Dillworth TM, Turner JA. Cognitive-behavioral therapy for individuals with chronic pain: efficacy, innovations, and directions for research. American Psychologist. 2014;69(2):153-66.

CHAPTER 50

Pain Psychology and Its Treatment Options

Anjali M Chhabria, Shrradha V Sidhwani, Juhi J Parmar

INTRODUCTION

Pain is defined as a physical, psychological and emotional discomfort. Once the physical element has been ruled out and treated by the practitioner, the psychosocial factors linger to intensify the pain. How can someone with chronic pain only suffer physically? Pain tires the body, causes fatigue, irritability and changes the behavior pattern of the individual. The ancient Greek believed that pain was associated with pleasure as the relief of pain was both pleasurable and emotional. Current theories on managing psychological aspects of pain suggest that pain is both a physical and psychological phenomenon.

Pain has been defined by the International Association for the Study of Pain (IASP) as 'an unpleasant sensory and emotional experience associated with actual or potential tissue damage, or described in terms of such damage.'[1] Pain is a complex experience that is influenced by effective, cognitive, and behavioral factors.[2] Physical pain fluctuates in intensity, severity and is sensitive to emotive, cognitive and situational factors. However, psychogenic pain remains fairly constant. Psychogenic pain generally begins abruptly and increases in severity for a few weeks or months. When pain persists in spite of medical treatment, as is the case in chronic pain syndrome, the issues become even more complex.

Chronic pain is both, individual and subjective. Pain that may be manageable for one person may be debilitating for another. Previously listed under Somatization Disorder and Undifferentiated Somatoform Disorder, the Diagnostic and Statistical Manual (DSM) of Mental Disorders—V categorizes pain disorder under Somatic Symptom Disorder (SSD). Somatic disorders refer to conditions wherein patients experience and communicate psychological and interpersonal problems in the form of physiological distress. Inability to function leads to a loss of role and self-esteem with the progressive intrusion of other problems such as financial hardship and strained relationships.[3] Pain leads to negative thoughts and negative evaluations of the world. It causes low frustration tolerance (LFT) which is poor ability to emotionally adapt in different situations. Memory and concentration are affected, and mood fluctuations are noticed.

Patients with pain disorder do not show any physical signs of pain even after repeated clinical evaluation and laboratory tests. However, they constantly complain of pain-related symptoms. The underlying causes of these disorders are heightened anxiety and fear, due to which the clients are unable to cope. Long-term effects of this negative anxiety lead to depression or even psychosis, termed 'Dysthymic Disorder' and 'Delusional Disorder'.[4]

CAUSES

Pain disorders without a significant physical symptomatology are generally caused by intrapsychic conflicts which are expressed through the body. According to the psycho-dynamic school of thought, defense mechanisms are unconscious thought patterns that protect the 'ego' from unpleasant emotions. Some of the defense mechanisms used by pain disorder patients are displacement (wherein an individual vents his aggression or frustration onto a person who is not the source of these emotions), substitution (wherein these 'inappropriate' feelings are expressed in a manner that is more socially acceptable) and repression (in which a person bottles up these emotions, without dealing with them, compartmentalizing them into a section of the subconscious so they do not have to confront these distressing events). In identification, another defense mechanism, the patient assumes the role of an ambivalent love object that also undergoes the same pain, e.g. parent. Suppressed aggression and repressed thoughts can be another factor causing unexplained psychological pain. Patients of pain disorders, who regard emotional pain as a sign of weakness and as non-justifiable, displace their feelings onto the body in order to fulfill dependency needs.

George Engel described the 'pain-prone personality' wherein pain symptoms are a result of long-standing feelings of guilt and worthlessness.[5] Some masochist personality types may feel that they are made to suffer and deserve the pain. Pain symptoms may intensify when they are rewarded by attentive behaviors of others or can be used as a manipulative strategy gaining advantage in interpersonal relationships. 'Secondary gain' is a concept that suggests that environmental factors are responsible for maintaining pain symptoms. Pain is, therefore, viewed as a way of communicating when people find it difficult to express their distress verbally.

SIGNS AND SYMPTOMS

Symptoms vary on the basis of the site of pain. Often patients find it difficult to describe the location, quality and depth of the pain. Constant discomfort despite taking medication is felt and symptoms are non-localized that encompass larger parts of the body. Irritability, passivity, insomnia and fatigue are some of the other identifiable symptoms. Pain may lead to inactivity and social isolation. Pain is viewed as an added burden to the normal demands of life and causes hindrance in the daily functionality. If not treated for a longer duration, symptoms cause major depression or dysthymia. Some patients even reach to the extremes of helplessness, hopelessness and suicide.[6]

PAIN AND DEPRESSION

Depression is a phase wherein, for more than 2 weeks, the patient feels sadness, irritability, lack of motivation, avolition, fatigue, sense of helplessness, and sleep and appetite disturbances. Pain symptoms such as fatigue, loss of mobility, do lead to depression. Major depressive disorder is present in about 20–25% of patients with pain disorder and dysthymic symptoms are reported in 60–100% of the patients (Kaplan). In a study of rheumatoid arthritis, depression was significantly high in patients and the level of depression increased with greater level of pain.[7] On the other hand, physical symptoms are also common in patients who suffer from major depression.[8] Approximately 60% patients with depression report pain symptoms at the time of diagnosis.[9]

PAIN AND ANXIETY

Patients suffering from pain disorder have a heightened sensation of their pain symptoms. Patients with a variety of chronic pain syndromes such as headache, neck pain and lower back pain have increased rates of both anxiety symptoms and anxiety disorders such as panic disorders and generalized anxiety disorders.[10] This behavior is reinforced by attention given from family members and practitioners. There is evidence that reinforcement of childhood illness behavior by anxious parents is associated with bodily preoccupation and anxiety in adulthood.[11] Fears, worries and preoccupation of having pain are secondary to actual experience of pain and these symptoms are resolved once the pain subsides.

Personality factors also enhance the above mentioned symptoms. Some complex personalities like to assume the "Sick Role" and feel intense sensation of pain. The patient here regards his condition as undesirable and he/she is not responsible for the symptoms, i.e. the condition cannot be reversed voluntarily.[12] Disturbed childhood, sexual or physical trauma and disturbed parenting styles can be some reasons why patients with pain symptoms are unable to fight the anxiety associated with it.

The fear-avoidance model highlights the relationship between pain symptoms and depression and anxiety state (Fig. 1). The model states that patients avoid physical movements or physical activities because of the fear that pain will make them worse.[13] Pain therapists also highlight the importance of anger management (suppression or expression of anger) while dealing with pain symptoms. Research shows high levels of pain symptoms were present in men with high hostility and suppression of anger. In women with chronic headaches, suppression of anger led to depression and expression of the negative state raised anxiety levels.[14]

DIAGNOSTIC CRITERIA

According to the DSM-V, what was previously known as pain disorder is now to be diagnosed as somatic symptom disorder with persistent pain, a marker for individuals whose somatic symptoms predominantly involve pain. This pain causes distress and interferes with the day-to-day functioning of the patient's life.

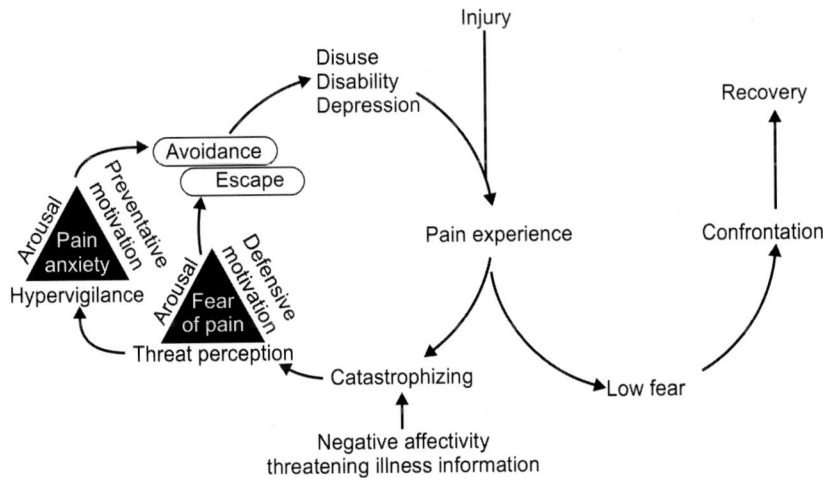

FIG. 1: The fear-avoidance model of chronic pain. Based on the fear-avoidance model of Vlaeyen and Linton (2000) and the fear-anxiety-avoidance model of Asmundson, et al. (2004)

Moreover, pain symptoms are not feigned or intentionally produced. There is the substantial evidence that psychological stressors play a significant role in causing the onset, severity or maintenance of the pain symptoms. Patients with pain disorder could have an intercurrent psychiatric disorder such as a mood disorder (depression, dysthymia), an anxiety disorder with generalized anxiety, panic disorder or phobic anxiety or an adjustment disorder related to their pain problem. Therefore, any other psychotic or mood disorders need to be excluded such as depression, delusional disorder. Pain is defined as acute if the duration is less than 6 months and is chronic if it persists for 6 months or more and is distinguished on the basis of etiology with psychological factors and with general medical condition (GMC). The International association for the study of pain classification defines pain on the basis of the region (head, face, mouth, abdomen, etc.), systems (musculoskeletal, nervous, gastrointestinal systems), temporal characteristics of pain (single episode, limited duration, non-fluctuating, etc.), patients evaluation of the intensity (mild, medium, severe), and etiology (degenerative, psychophysiological, psychological).[15] However, because of the extreme subjective nature of these criteria, the validity of the diagnosis is questionable and not used. The International Statistical Classification of Diseases and Related Health Problems (ICD) defines pain disorder or psychalgia on the basis of psychogenic pain or psychological pain, i.e. emotional pain that is caused by harm or threat to social connection, bereavement, embarrassment, shame and hurt feelings.

INVESTIGATIONS

The Minnesota Multiphasic Personality Inventory (MMPI) is the most widely used personality scale to measure somatic symptoms.[16] The hypochondriasis scale (Hs) measures a patient's level of concern over his/her bodily functions and malfunction. This scale also highlights the relation between pain symptoms and effective disorders such as depression. Also scale 3 Hysteria (Hy) is designed specifically to address concerns of somatic complaints that deny any emotional and interpersonal difficulty. 'Conversion V' with high scores on scales 1 and 4 in the MMPI is an indicator of these patients. The other test used is the Millon Clinical Multiaxial Inventory (MCMI) test. In the MCMI the items on the clinical somatoform disorder scale (scale H) is characterized by symptoms of fatigue, weakness, tension, aches, pains and physical discomfort. The above mentioned measures also reflect the patient's adjustment to chronic illness and can be found with patients who suffer from chronic health problems. Therefore, they may not be a good measure to reveal the identifiable organic etiology.[17]

Personality evaluations are helpful pointers that provide insight about an individual's disposition—their manner of reacting to situations, dealing with emotions; whether they express, or prefer to suppress feelings; whether they confront or avoid conflicts—all these sum up to indicate how a pain disorder may develop. Tests like the 16PF, the NEO-PI as also the MBTI, are other commonly used personality tests.

Additionally, projective tests such as the Thematic Apperception Test, Draw a Person, Sentence Completion Test, Picture Arrangement Test, to name a few, reveal underlying emotions that the individual himself may not be conscious of. The theory behind projective tests is that the seemingly ambiguous stimuli help us tap into the individual's subconscious, which reflects hidden conflicts and unresolved issues, which, in turn, help to pinpoint the problem areas and determine a course of action.

DIFFERENTIAL DIAGNOSIS

Persistent SSD is different from pain associated with sexual intercourse (Dyspareunia). In conversion disorder, symptoms of pain are more directed towards sensory and motor areas. Persistent SSD must not be confused with illness anxiety disorder, which is a constant preoccupation with having or acquiring a serious illness, i.e. somatic symptoms are not actually present, or present in a mild measure. It is the anticipation of contracting these symptoms that cause distress, as opposed to SSD, wherein a perpetual pain lingers.

TREATMENT

Numerous psychological factors can be evaluated while dealing with pain. Factors that lead to poor pain adjustment are pain catastrophizing, pain-related anxiety and fear of pain, and helplessness. Whereas factors leading to improve pain adjustment are self-efficacy pain-coping strategies, readiness to change, and acceptance of the individual.[18]

Psychoanalysis theorists believed that psychological pain was a result of early developmental conflicts with feelings of guilt and anger in the patient's life. Psychological pain is displaced and physical symptoms manifest as a result. Therefore, in therapy, one has to address the unconscious conflicts that contribute or maintain pain symptoms.

The initial form of psychological therapy for treating pain was behavior modification. Behavior therapists state that for a negative behavior to be extinguished, it must be punished and the positive behavior should be rewarded. In case of managing pain disorders, psychological pain symptoms are seen as a source of getting attention from desired sources, family, friends, and spouse. This concept is 'termed' as secondary gain'. Pain is used as a variable to manipulate people and the environment. However, therapist, also criticized that there are secondary losses that are part of pain disorders and the reducing pain disorder to a mere behavioral phenomenon was unjustified.

The most effective psychological therapy for pain has been cognitive behavioral therapy (CBT). This therapy emphasizes that the most fundamental factor causing pain is the patient's negative thinking and evaluations that he/she makes about himself. Moreover, CBT practitioners suggest that patients play an active role in maintaining these pain symptoms.[19] For example, the patient may develop negative beliefs that 'this will never end' or negative thoughts that 'I am worthless as I cannot work as effectively' or 'Why did this happen to me'. These negative beliefs and thoughts affect the patient's behavior and in turn his/her participation in pleasurable activities (he/she stops going to work or social gatherings). He/she is de-motivated and is likely to feel sad and is anxious to participate in activities of daily living. Some cognitive distortions highlighted in the CBT module are catastrophic thinking wherein the patient perceives the worst possible outcome "I will die of this pain". Other patients engage in arbitrary inference which is drawing conclusion on the basis of minimal evidence, e.g., "this pain is connected to the heart or is fatal".[20] Over-evaluating the pain symptoms and under-evaluating personal worth is generally seen in these patients. Patients tend to personalize the external circumstances and view pain as a source of punishment.

Awareness and Acceptance: This is the first step to recovery. The basics of acceptance and commitment therapy lies in teaching patients to accept negative thoughts and experiences as vital components of living a fulfill life rather than fighting or escaping from them. Acceptance of pain is an important factor in the patient's adjustment to pain symptoms. Acceptance involves psychologically training oneself to live each day as it comes, acknowledging limitations, accepting loss of self and believing that there is more to life than pain and relying (Risdon et al.).

Educating the patients on the pain and tension cycle is important. Once they have accepted the psychological basis of their pain symptoms, other procedures such cognitive restructuring can be introduced. Cognitive therapists believe that maladaptive thinking styles need to change for a patient to remove somatic pain symptoms. It is not only behavioral patterns that need to be changed but also the underlining schemas, e.g. "No matter what happens, I can manage", "I'm a survivor", "There's nothing much that can scare me". Therapists encourage patients to maintain a pain diary in which the daily patterns of pain are noted along with environmental stressors.

Techniques such as the 'Trains of Thought' are useful. Patients are encouraged to view their mind as a train station and their worrying thoughts as trains that they can either board or simply watch as it passes. Graded activity scheduling helps patients get back their functionality and confidence.[21] Therapists encourage patients to slowly increase activities in their daily life. Patients can be warned that this may increase their pain symptoms initially but eventually it will help achieve their goals of regaining themselves.

Systematic desensitization and imagery techniques are used when direct questioning does not reveal underlining cognitions.[22] In imagery, the patient is asked to visualize a scene that caused the distress and pain symptoms. Through relaxation, the therapist then helps the patient cope with the distressed situations without feeling the actual pain.

Rational Emotive Behavioral Therapist (REBT) suggests that pain results from disturbed emotions such as guilt, anger, low frustration tolerance, and anxiety. The REBT therapists believe that irrational beliefs are the fundamental causes of psychopathology. Some irrational beliefs are 'demanding and personalizing'. Patients tend to overuse terms such as 'shoulds, musts' and feel that they cannot handle situations. The client is over-expecting rather than accepting the reality and putting it into perspective. This self-defeating belief causes one to either perceive themselves or the world in extremes, i.e. good or bad terms "I should not feel this pain in my life", or "I am worthless because I have this pain". Patients succumb to irrational and inflexible thinking and distort reality.

In the therapy, a very effective strategy is to use pain as a tool to discuss emotional issues, e.g. "How does this pain make you feel? Does it get you down?" REBT helps patients give up these absolute beliefs and enables them to view life more rationally. Some techniques used by REBT practitioners are role playing where the patient is suggested to reverse his/her role with any other of the family and understand the irrational beliefs underlining pain symptoms. Shame attacking exercises help patients become bold and confront situations which they may otherwise find difficult. This helps in confidence building and self-acceptance. Using humor can bring about emotional benefits by pointing out absurdness in one's pattern of thinking and behaving.

Other techniques such as biofeedback, hypnosis, eye movement desensitization and reprocessing (EMDR) can be used. In biofeedback, electrical equipment is employed to measure the physiological functions of the body. In hypnotic therapy, the patient has to create a visual image of the pain and is encouraged to change or dissociate it from the rest of the body. The EMDR treatment assumes that physical pain is associated with stress. In cases where the pain is not associated with a traumatic event, a pain target is discussed and described in detail. Through the process of this therapy, the patients are taught to detach from their pain and get a better sense of control over their symptoms. A positive cognition is created pain-related memories are desensitized.[23] The application of which of the above mentioned techniques is most useful in pain management is still debatable.[24]

Hypnosis is a process through which the individual is guided into a state of consciousness wherein his focus and concentration are heightened, making it easier for him to recall incidents, and shut off distraction. When hypnosis is used for healing purposes, it is called hypnotherapy. During hypnotherapy, the therapist gets the client to revisit certain traumatic events, helping them to view these events objectively by stripping the memories of the attached emotions. By encouraging them to perceive these incidents as neither positive nor negative, but in neutral light, the therapist helps them to let go of the distressing emotions. Hypnoanalgesia is the process of making suggestions to the client, preferably when they are in the state of 'somnambulism' (the deepest state of sleep achieved through hypnosis), though it is effective in the earlier stages as well.[25] These suggestions play on the individual's subconscious, exuding control on their conscious mind as well, altering their distressed state.

It is important to note that since the pain disorder has been alleviated or relieved through hypnotherapy, it is not the proof of the fact that the pain was seated in their mind, and was thus imaginary. On the contrary 'while pain is felt at the site of injury, it is only experienced when the pain receptors in the brain have been alerted. Thus, even though the physical pain may have healed, the attached memories sometimes' need remedying too.

In October 2015, I took a course in Past Life Regression Therapy at the Weiss Institute, directed by Dr Brian Weiss. The basic essence of this therapy is the idea that physical pain may, sometimes, but not always, be rooted in the same physical area on the body—it may be transmitted onto the body through harbored distressing emotions, or even induced by stress. In past life regression therapy, the underlying belief is that unresolved issues from the past manifest as physical symptoms, as a result of which it becomes essential "to travel" to this period and confront the predicament. It is also helpful in terms of relaxation and its ability to put to rest emotional disturbances—often the root of pain disorders—at least temporarily.

At our clinic, "Mindtemple" we have tailor-made treatments to fit every individual. We work closely with pain psychologists, who often refer cases for emotional stress alleviation.

I always start with a personality profile work-up, which indicates the problem areas and sources of pain—a reserved individual, or an emotionally reactive one may be more prone to a pain disorder than their sociable or emotionally stable counterparts. Moreover, it also works as an indicator of which approach to use for a certain individual based on their behavioral history.

Therapy also focuses on relapse prevention. This means that one can foresee bad times will occur and plan how to cope with life's situations. Pain management involves integrating the physical psychological modalities of pain.

Important Tips for Medical Practitioners

- Build an effective therapeutic alliance with the patient.
- Do not underestimate or consider the pain as imaginary.
- Understand the sociocultural and background history of the patient.
- Assess the pain and its physical and psychological parameters.
- Engage the patient as a collaborator in the process of identifying the problems and thinking through the treatment process.
- Assess the possibility of relapse.

CONCLUSION

It is paramount to recognize the role of psychogenic factors which contribute to and precipitate pain disorders. At times, a physical pain site may not be present; however, this does not make the pain any less real. Anxiety and depression are the most commonly associated psychological maladies with pain disorders. If not addressed, this pain exacerbates one's mental health, which further aggravates the pain, turning into a vicious cycle leading to maladjustment and social withdrawal. Each case needs to be evaluated separately, and treatment options tailor-made—there is no blanket treatment for psychological disorders associated with pain. Various approaches are effective for different individuals—cognitive, behavioral, psychodynamic, pharmacotherapy, to name a few. A comprehensive treatment plan should be applied while treating pain symptoms to ensure that both pain and psychological trauma are dealt with effectively.

REFERENCES

1. Merskey, et al. Pain terms: a current list of definitions and notes on usage. Pain Supplement; 1986.pp.215-21.
2. Meldrum ML. A capsule history of pain management. Journal of American Medical Association. 2003;290: 2470-75.
3. Fordyce WE. Pain and suffering. American Psychologist. 1988;43:276-83.
4. Levenson. Textbook of Psychosomatic Medicine. Pain. The American Psychiatric Publishing; 2005. pp.827-66.
5. Engel GL. Psychogenic pain and the pain-prone patient. American Journal of Medicine. 1959;26:899-918.
6. James FR. The meaning of pain. In: Psychological investigations of the experience of chronic pain [Thesis], chapter IV. Auckland: University of Auckland; 1991. pp.60-72.
7. Dickens C, McGowan L, et al. Depression in rheumatoid arthritis: a systematic review of the literature with meta-analysis. Psychosomatic Medicine. 2002;64:52-60.
8. Lipowski Z. Somatization and Depression. Psychosomatics. 1990;31:13-21.
9. Magni G, Schnifano F, et al. Pain as a symptom in elderly depressed patients: relationships to diagnostic subgroups. European Archives of Psychiatry and Clinical Neuroscience. 1985;235(3):143-5.
10. Devlen J. Anxiety and depression in migraine. Journal of the Royal Society of Medicine.1994; 87:338-41.
11. Kirmayer L, Taillefer S. Somatoform disorders. In: S. M. Turner, et al. (Eds). Adult Psychopathology and Diagnosis, 3rd edition. New York, Wiley, 1997.
12. Parsons T. Social Structure and Personality. New York: Free Press, 1964.
13. Greenberg J, Burns JW. Pain anxiety among chronic patients: specific phobia or manifestation of anxiety sensitivity? Behavioral Research Therapy. 2003;41:223-40.
14. Veneable VL, Carlson CR, et al. The role of anger and depression in current headache. Headache. 2001;41: 21-30.
15. Merskey H, Bogduk N, International Association for the Study of Pain Classification of Chronic Pain. Seattle, WA, IASP Press, 2nd edition,1994.
16. Hatchway S, Mckinley JC. Minnesota Multiphasic Personality Inventory-2. Minneapolis, University of Minnesota, 1989.
17. Naliboff BD, et al. Does the MMPI differentiate between chronic illness and chronic pain? Pain.1982;12:333-41.
18. Francis K, Meredith R, et al. Psychological aspects of persistent pain: current state of science. The Journal of Pain. 2004;5(4):195-211.
19. Turk DC, Meichenbaum D, et al. Pain and behavioral medicine: A cognitive-behavioral perspective. New York: Guilford Press.1983.
20. Hales, Yudofsky, et al. Textbook of Psychiatry. Cognitive Therapy. The American Psychiatric Publishing, 5th edition, 2008;1211-48.
21. Sharpe M, et al. The psychological treatment of patients with functional somatic symptoms: A practical guide. Journal of Psychosomatic Research. 1992;36:515-29.
22. Tasman, Kay et al., Psychiatry. Cognitive and Behavioral Therapies. John Wiley & Sons, 2nd edition, 3;1753-77.
23. Marilyn L. Eye Movement Desensitization and Reprocessing (EMDR) Scripted Protocols. Springer publishing company, 2010.pp.517-99.
24. Hales R, Yudofsky S. The Textbook of Clinical Psychiatry. Pain Disorders. The American psychiatric publishing, 4th edition. 2003.pp.1023-43.
25. Montgomery H Guy, Duhamel N Katherine, and Redd H William. A meta-analysis of hypnotically induced analgesia: How effective is hypnosis? International Journal of Clinical and Experimental Hypnosis. 2008. pp.138-153.

SECTION 15

Allied Therapy

Role of Radiation in Cancer Pain

Krishna A Balkundi, Pallavi B Patil

INTRODUCTION

Cancer pain is caused by variety of factors—bony pain due to infiltration of bone by cancer, nerve pain due to pressure by the tumor mass, vascular pain due to tumor cell migration into vessels through blood stream, spine pain due to involvement of spine, etc. Such pain initially responds to analgesics, but eventually even cocktail of analgesics fail to suppress pain. In such situation, radiation is an option to alleviate pain.

TYPES OF RADIATION

These are three types of radiation—(1) alpha, (2) beta and (3) gamma radiations. All of them are used in killing cancer cells. However, for pain relief, gamma radiation is most commonly used. The radiation is also classified as external and internal radiation. The external radiation is given from an outside machine—linear accelerator, cobalt unit. The internal radiation is of two types: (1) sealed and (2) unsealed sources. The sealed sources are implanted in the organ and this form of radiation is called *brachytherapy*. The unsealed sources are isotopes, which are in liquid form and given either orally or intravenous route. They localize in cancer sites and deliver radiation selectively.

MECHANISM OF PAIN RELIEF BY RADIATION

The exact mechanism by which radiation alleviates the pain is not known. One of the mechanisms is that radiation reduces the tumor size by killing cancer cells and thus the pressure effect from the tumor mass is relieved, which results in pain palliation. Another mechanism is inhibition of chemical mediators of pain. In bone pain, osteolysis is reduced and thus pain is reduced. The rapid onset of pain relief—within days—is attributed to the decrease of various chemical pain mediators, whereas tumor shrinkage and recalcification of osteolytic bone lesions contribute to the long-lasting effect.[1]

METASTATIC BONE PAIN MANAGEMENT

In case of solitary bony lesion causing pain, external radiotherapy (RT) is given over 2 weeks, which results in pain relief in 60–70% of patients.[2]

Isotope Therapy for Metastatic Bone Pain

Isotopes play major role in alleviating pain in many cancer patients. The various isotopes used are phosphorus-32, strontium-89, samarium-153, rhenium-188, 177-lutetium, radioiodine (131-I) and radium-223.³

Mechanism of Action

These isotopes predominantly emit beta particles which have short distance of penetration (2–3 mm). These isotopes localize around the metastatic sites and selectively deliver radiation to all metastatic sites simultaneously. The isotopes deliver radiation for many days depending upon the half-life. There is no significant radiation to other organs since they have short track length. The advantages of isotope therapy over external RT are:
- Simultaneous radiation to multiple sites
- Sparing of adjoining structures.

The pain relief is seen in 60% of patients by 2–3 weeks and lasts for 6 months. It can be repeated if pain recurs. The hematological toxicity is in the form of bone marrow suppression needing blood transfusion in 10% of patients.

The ideal candidates for isotope therapy are those with life expectancy more than 3 months, enough medullary reserve, failed chemotherapy and whose analgesic requirement is multiple cocktail of drugs with poor response.

Targeted Isotope Therapy

This is a new approach to pain palliation wherein a receptor, antigen or antibody specific to a particular cancer is labeled with a therapeutic isotope and delivered through infusion. After localizing in the metastatic sites the isotope delivers intense radiation resulting in pain relief and in some cases reduction in disease activity due to killing of cells.

177-Lutetium-PSMA Therapy for Bone Metastases from Prostate Cancer

In this technique, the prostate-specific membrane antigen (PSMA) is labeled with 177-lutetium isotope and administered through infusion over 30 minutes. The isotope

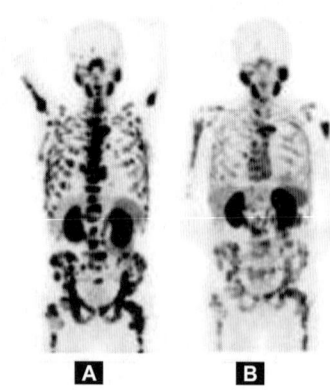

FIGS 1A and B: Ga-68 prostate-specific membrane antigen (PSMA) scan before (A) and after therapy; (B) Shows patient of prostate cancer with extensive bone metastases with significant reduction in disease on follow-up image and prostate-specific antigen (PSA) values after 177-Lu-PSMA therapy

delivers significant radiation to metastatic sites and pain relief occurs in 60–70% of patients by 2 weeks. It is also shown to kill tumor cells as seen by considerable fall in prostate-specific antigen (PSA) values (Figs 1A and B).There are no major side effects from this therapy. It is the current treatment of choice in all hormone refractory prostate cancer patients.⁴

223-Radium Alpha Radiation Therapy for Metastatic Prostate Cancer

Radium is an alpha particle emitter which deposits intense radiation at the site of its concentration. When given intravenously to a patient with skeletal metastases from prostate cancer, the alpha particles penetrate the tumor cells resulting in cell death and relief from bone pain.² It is given for 3 cycles at the interval of 6 weeks and the pain relief is seen in about 60–70% of patients. Unlike chemotherapy and 32-P isotope therapy, treatment with radium does not produce significant hematological toxicity. This form of therapy is currently the standard of care in European countries for unremitting pain due to bone metastases from prostate cancer.

Since it is very expensive and not available in India at present, the other indigenously produced isotopes, like 32-phosphorus and 153-samarium are currently used in India for alleviation of pain.[5]

177-Lutetium-DOTATATE Therapy for Neuroendocrine Tumor Patients

In metastatic neuroendocrine lesions in the bone and liver with unremitting pain, the isotope labeled therapy with 177-lutetium DOTATATE given intravenously not only alleviates pain in 70–80% of patients but also reduces disease burden resulting in progression free survival of 30–35 months (Figs 2A and B).[6]

Yttrium-90 (Y-90) Radioembolization Treatment for Liver Cancer

In liver cancer, the 'Yttrium-90 microspheres' are deposited directly into the tumor through the hepatic artery. The microspheres are unable to pass through the vasculature of the liver due to arteriolar capillary blockade and are trapped in the tumor. The isotope radiation produces significant reduction in tumor mass (Figs 3A and B) and thus pain is alleviated and life is prolonged.[7]

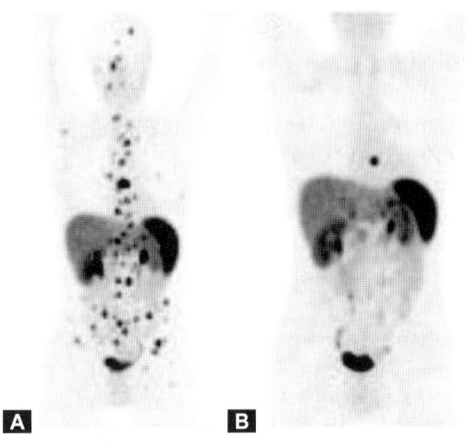

FIGS 2A and B: Ga-68-DOTANOC scan shows a patient with extensive bone metastases from carcinoid tumor pre- (A) and post-therapy; (B) Significant reduction in disease after therapy and almost completely pain free after 4 weeks

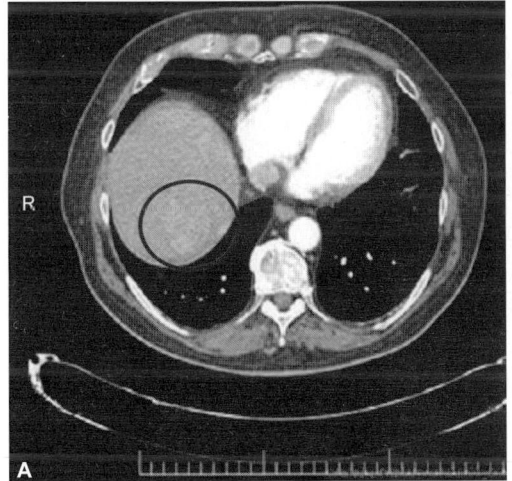
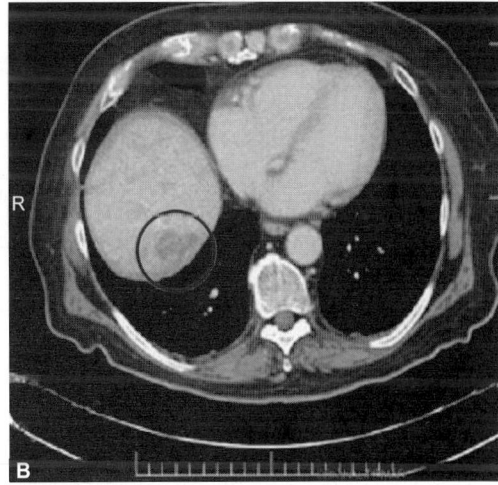

FIGS 3A and B: A computed tomography (CT) scan of a patient before and after Y-90 treatment. (A) In the pre-treatment CT on the left, the arterial phase shows a tumor with early arterial enhancement; (B) The post-treatment CT in the washout phase, on the right, shows exaggerated decreased contrast enhancement in the area of the tumor due to necrosis after Y-90 treatment

Radioiodine (131-I) Treatment in Thyroid Cancer

In thyroid cancer with bone metastasis with severe pain, the specific radiation treatment with 131-I alleviates the pain in 80% of patients. This treatment can be repeated as and when pain recurs. The advantage of this treatment is concomitant radiation to all metastatic sites apart from the painful site giving survival benefit (Figs 4A and B).[8]

131-I-MIBG Therapy for Metastatic Neuroblastoma

I-131 metaiodobenzylguanidine (MIBG) therapy has been used since the 80s as a palliative agent in relapsed patients. Figures 5A and B shows an example of a patient with metastatic neuroblastoma who was in remission after two cycles of I-131 MIBG.

ROLE OF EXTERNAL RADIATION THERAPY IN CHRONIC PAIN MANAGEMENT

External RT in Brain Tumors

The severe headache due to compressive effect of brain tumor is relieved by external RT by reducing the size of the tumor. This occurs in 80% of patients. Whole brain irradiation in multiple brain metastases relieves headaches and other symptoms in 60–80% of patients.

Pain due to Infiltration or Plexus or Peripheral Nerve

Tumor can grow and involve peripheral nerve producing severe pain and sensorimotor deficits. The most common sites are brachial and lumbosacral plexus involvement from breast and rectal cancers respectively. The

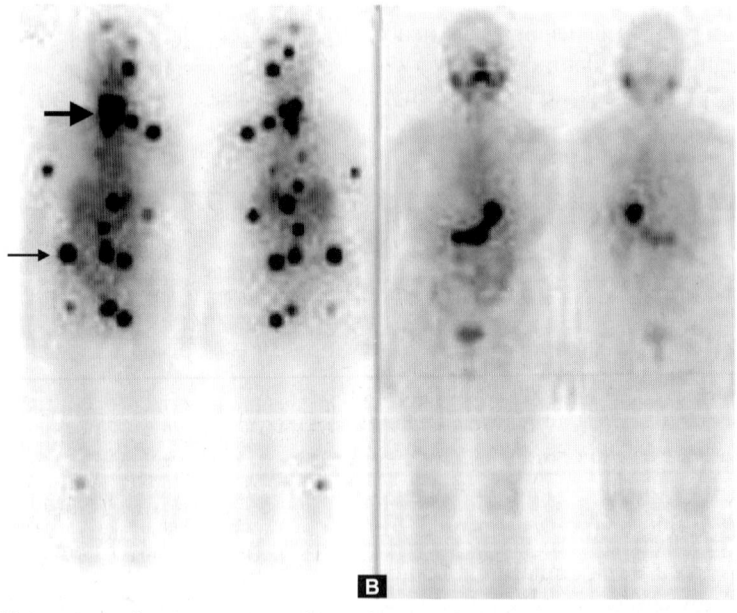

FIGS 4A and B: (A) Anterior and posterior views of post-therapy whole body scans (WBS) acquired 7 days after oral administration of 100 mCi 131-I, showing significant radiopharmaceutical accumulation in thyroid remnants (red arrow) and bone lesions (blue arrow); (B) Anterior and posterior views of diagnostic WBS acquired 48 hours after 131-I administration, 8 months after radioactive iodine (RAI) therapy, showing a complete disappearance of iodine uptake both in thyroid remnants and bone lesions

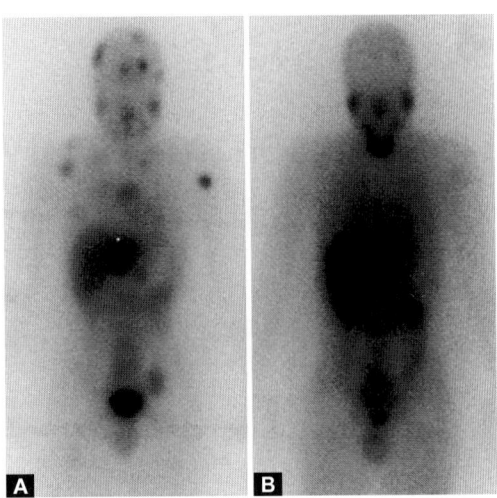

FIGS 5A and B: Treatment of metastatic neuroblastoma with I-131 meta-iodobenzylguanidine (MIBG). (A) I-131-MIBG scintigraphy before treatment: extensive bone metastases; (B) I-131-MIBG scintigraphy after two administrations of I-131-MIBG: no evidence of disease activity

neuropathic pain is severe with bad prognosis. Radiation in doses of 40–50 Gy in 4–5 weeks gives significant relief of symptoms in 80% of patients. However, the relief is of short duration.

Brachytherapy

These are sealed radiation sources (125 I) which are in pellet form. They are implanted in the tumor tissue and the beta rays kill tumor cells resulting in tumor shrinkage and alleviation of pain. This form of therapy is used in carcinoma cervix and bladder cancer.

CONCLUSION

The above resume of "radiation and pain" highlights the effective role of radiation in pain palliation in cancer patients. The radiation therapy includes isotope therapy, brachytherapy as it helps in reduction of chronic cancer pain. Since it has added tumoricidal effect, radiation is the first preferred method for pain palliation. The isotope labeled targeted radiation therapy is gaining momentum in view of selective radiation effect sparing normal organs with comparatively lesser complications than external RT.[4] The future will see more of targeted isotope therapy approaches. Since radiation therapy has attendant complication, it should be used judiciously to achieve maximum palliation with minimum complications.

REFERENCES

1. Mercadante S. Malignant bone pain: pathophysiology and treatment. Pain. 1997;69:1-18.
2. Yarnold JR. A prospective randomised trial comparing a single dose of 8 Gy and a multi-fraction radiotherapy schedule in the treatment of metastatic bone pain. Br J Cancer. 1998;78(Suppl.2):6.
3. Serafini AN. Current status of systemic intravenous radiopharmaceuticals for the treatment of painful metastatic bone disease. Int J Radiat Oncol Biol Phys. 1994;30(5):1187-94.
4. Baum RP, Kulkarni HR et al. 177Lu-Labeled Prostate-Specific Membrane Antigen Radioligand Therapy of Metastatic Castration-Resistant Prostate Cancer: Safety and Efficacy. J Nucl Med. 2016;57(7):1006-13.
5. C. Parker, S. Nilsson et al. Alpha Emitter Radium-223 and Survival in Metastatic Prostate Cancer. N Engl J Med. 2013;369:213-23.
6. Öberg K. Molecular Imaging Radiotherapy: Theranostics for Personalized Patient Management of Neuroendocrine Tumors (NETs). Theranostics. 2012;2(5):448 58.
7. Lewandowski RJ, Salem R. Yttrium-90 Radioembolization of Hepatocellular Carcinoma and Metastatic Disease to the Liver. Semin Intervent Radiol. 2006;23(1):64-72.
8. Schlumberger, Martin; Challeton, Cecile; De Vathaire, Florent; Jean-Paul Travagli; et al. Radioactive iodine treatment and external radiotherapy for lung and bone metastases from thyroid carcinoma The Journal of Nuclear Medicine; New York. 1996;37(4):598-605.

Role of Chemotherapy in Cancer Pain Management

Ashish V Bakshi, Nilesh M Lokeshwar, Vibhay Pareek

INTRODUCTION

Cancer pain afflicts approximately 17 million people worldwide every year. Inspite of several advances in the understanding of pathobiology and management of cancer pain, it remains a major international health problem. Cancer pain is prevalent at all stages of the disease and may often be the first symptom of cancer. However, it is more common in the advanced and terminal cases. The prevalence is dependent on the site of the disease, type of cancer, its extent and ongoing treatment. In a recently published systematic review on prevalence of pain, pain prevalence rates were 39.3% after curative treatment; 55.0% during anticancer treatment; and 66.4% in advanced, metastatic, or terminal disease.[1]

Although reports vary widely, the range of reported prevalence of pain is highest for the following tumors:[2]
- Head and neck (67–91%)
- Prostate (56–94%)
- Uterine (30–90%)
- Genitourinary (58–90%)
- Breast (40–89%)
- Pancreatic (72–85%).

TYPES OF CANCER PAIN

Cancer pain could be either nociceptive or neuropathic in origin. It is important to differentiate between nociceptive and neuropathic pain to take appropriate treatment decisions.

CAUSES OF CANCER PAIN

Cancer pain can be caused due to the cancer infiltrating into the surrounding tissues or nerves, inflammation, obstruction, distention of abdomen, raised intracranial pressure, or bone metastases.[3]

TREATMENT MODALITIES FOR CANCER PAIN

The management of cancer pain requires careful clinical assessment of pain, recognition of pattern and intensity, and its impact on the host. Appropriate and early palliative care has been linked to improved survival.[4]

A multidisciplinary team of specialists, including surgical oncologists, medical oncologists, radiation oncologists, pain specialists, palliative care physicians, anesthesiologists, psychiatrists and counselors is required for comprehensive cancer pain management. As the causes of pain and its modifiers vary from individual to individual, there is a need for a personalized approach to pain management. A detailed counseling of patient and family members should be done before starting therapy explaining them the expected benefits, toxicities, cost and long-term outcome.

A number of treatment approaches are available for the treatment of cancer pain. Pharmacotherapy (opioids, nonsteroidal anti-inflammatory drugs, antidepressants) remains the mainstay of cancer pain in patients throughout all stages of the disease. In addition, in certain cancer types, antineoplastic therapies such as surgery, radiation, chemotherapy, targeted therapies and bisphosphonates do play a significant role in alleviating the pain due to primary or metastatic disease.[5] Combining cancer treatments with pharmacological and nonpharmacological methods of pain control can result in optimum pain management.

In this chapter, we will discuss the role of cancer-directed systemic therapies in the management of cancer pain. These modalities can be broadly classified as:
- Cytotoxic chemotherapy
- Biologic and targeted therapy
- Hormone therapy
- Bone-targeted agents.

Cytotoxic Chemotherapy

Patients with advanced cancer are often treated with cytotoxic chemotherapy with the intention of relieving symptoms (often primarily pain), improve quality of life and prolong survival.

Effect of Chemotherapy on Cancer Pain

In most of the cancers, the pain occurs due to physical reasons, such as infiltration of surrounding soft tissues and bone neural infiltration or compression, tissue edema, capsular invasion or obstruction. Relatively few malignancies cause pain due to paraneoplastic attributes such as peripheral neuropathy in plasma cell dyscrasias. Therefore, use of chemotherapy can provide substantial pain relief by cytoreducing the primary and/or metastatic disease and thus directly relieving the pressure effect and infiltration of surrounding structures or indirectly controlling the paraneoplastic manifestations. However, to optimally utilize the potential of chemotherapy in cancer pain control, following factors need to be considered.

Relation of Pain to the Cancer

Careful clinical and radiological evaluation is required to establish the etiology and mechanism of pain before embarking on chemotherapy as a modality for offering pain relief. Cytotoxic chemotherapy is useful for pain relief only in conditions where the tumor is directly responsible for pain due to infiltration of surrounding tissue. For example, in a breast cancer patient, chemotherapy will decrease the symptoms of brachial plexopathy, only if it is due to the tumor infiltration and not the one due to prior radiation therapy.

Chemosensitivity of the Underlying Cancer Type

The extent and rapidity of pain control is highly dependent on the chemosensitivity of the underlying malignancies (Table 1). Backache due to retroperitoneal lymphadenopathy, caused by germ cell tumor or lymphoma shows dramatic and complete response to chemotherapy as compared to the one caused by renal cell carcinoma. Some tumors such as thyroid carcinoma are inherently resistant to cytotoxic chemotherapy, and a temptation, to offer chemotherapy for pain relief in such patients is discouraged.

The durability of pain control is dependent on the chemoresponsiveness of the given cancer subtype and its stage. For example, neoadjuvant chemotherapy and concurrent chemoradiation can permanently relieve the pain due to de novo oropharyngeal cancers. On the other hand, cancer pain

TABLE 1: Causes and prevalence of cancer pain

Potentially curable	Highly responsive (Response rates >50%)	Moderately responsive (Response rates >30%)	Less responsive (Response rates <30%)
• Acute myeloid leukemia • Acute lymphocytic leukemia (childhood) • Chronic myelogenous leukemia • Hodgkin's disease • Non-Hodgkin's lymphoma (some subsets) • Hairy cell leukemia • Germ cell tumors • Gastrointestinal stromal tumors	• Breast carcinoma • Ovarian carcinoma • Androgen-dependent prostate cancer (hormonal therapy) • Small cell lung carcinoma • Osteogenic sarcoma • Multiple myeloma	• Non-small cell lung cancer • Colorectal cancer • Transitional cell carcinoma of the urothelial tract (e.g. bladder cancer) • Sarcoma (some subsets) • Endometrial carcinoma (hormonal therapy)	• Gastric carcinoma Esophageal carcinoma • Head and neck carcinoma • Pancreatic carcinoma Hepatocellular carcinoma • Renal cell carcinoma • Malignant melanoma • Mesothelioma • Anaplastic thyroid cancer • Islet cell and carcinoid tumors

due to recurrent squamous carcinoma of head and neck cancer can be alleviated for only a few weeks to months with the use of palliative chemotherapy. Use of multiagent chemotherapy is preferred for patients with pain due to curable cancers in contrast to the use of single agent chemotherapy in palliative setting.

Prior Use of Chemotherapy and its Response

Benefits of chemotherapy in palliative setting are limited in patients who have been exposed to chemotherapy earlier and have had stable disease or no response to previous regimens. On the other hand, long-treatment free or progression-free interval and use of noncross-resistant drugs may predict better response rates.

Performance Status

It is considered as one of the powerful prognostic factors for several malignancies and an important predictive factor for response to therapy. In advanced carcinoma lung the survival advantage with palliative chemotherapy is limited to patients with good performance status only (Eastern cooperative oncology group performance status—0, 1). Therefore, use of chemotherapy to control pain in advanced cancers should be limited to patients with good performance status. Some patients have low performance status due the disabling pain, and such patients can benefit with chemotherapy and targeted therapies. However, patients with potentially curable and previously untreated malignancies like lymphomas and acute leukemia should receive chemotherapy irrespective of performance status.

Comorbidities

Older age more than 60 years, comorbidities such as uncontrolled diabetes mellitus, hypertension, coronary artery disease, cerebrovascular disease, cardiac dysfunction, renal or hepatic impairment may preclude the use of chemotherapy for pain control and unfavorably tilt the risk-benefit ratio. Thus, it is imperative to do a careful evaluation of patient before starting chemotherapy.

In general, use of chemotherapy in pain management can be guided by the site or region of pain and underlying malignancies. Temptation to start palliative chemotherapy in elderly, frail and poor performance patients should be resisted.

Due to its adverse impact on quality of life, pain control has become an important end-point in clinical trials for development of chemotherapy drugs for potentially incurable malignancies.[6,7]

Biological and Targeted Therapies in Management of Cancer Pain

Over the years, a better understanding of biology and pathogenesis of malignancies has led to development of various biological and targeted therapies (Table 2). Several of these new agents help in disease control and thus the tumor pain. These drugs have better efficacy and toxicity ratio thus improve the quality of life and provide better control over pain due to primary and metastatic disease.

TABLE 2: Approved targeted therapies for management of cancer

Brain tumor	Kidney cancer
Bevacizumab, Everolimus	Bevacizumab, Sunitinib, Pazopanib, Axitinib, Sorafenib, Everolimus, Temsirolimus, Cabozantinib, Lenvatinib, Nivolumab
Head and neck cancers	**Bladder cancer**
Cetuximab, Nimotuzumab, Pembrolizumab, Nivolumab	Atezolizumab
Thyroid cancer	**Prostate cancer**
Cabozantinib, Vandetanib, Sorafenib, Lenvatinib	Enzalutamide, Abiraterone, Sipuleucel T
Lung cancer	**Ovarian epithelial/fallopian tube/primary peritoneal cancers**
Bevacizumab, Gefitinib, Erlotinib, Afatinib, Osimertinib, Crizotinib, Ceritinib, Alectinib, Ramucirumab, Nivolumab, Pembrolizumab, Atezolizumab, Necitumumab	Bevacizumab, Olaparib
Breast cancer	**Cervical cancer**
Everolimus, Trastuzumab, Lapatinib, Pertuzumab, Trastuzumab emtansine, Palbociclib	Bevacizumab
Adenocarcinoma of the stomach or gastroesophageal junction	**Leukemia**
Trastuzumab, Ramucirumab	Imatinib, Dasatinib, Nilotinib, Bosutinib, Ponatinib, Rituximab, Alemtuzumab, Ofatumumab, Obinutuzumab, Ibrutinib, Idelalisib, Blinatumomab, Venetoclax, Tretinoin
Pancreatic cancer	**Lymphoma**
Erlotinib, Everolimus, Sunitinib	Rituximab, Obinutuzumab, Siltuximab, Bortezomib, Brentuximab, Denileukin Diftitox, Ibritumomab tiuxetan, Vorinostat, Belinostat, Romidepsin, Bexarotene, Pralatrexate, Ibrutinib, Idelalisib, Nivolumab
Liver cancer	**Multiple Myeloma**
Sorafenib	Bortezomib, Carfilzomib, ixazomib, Panobinostat, Daratumumab, Elotuzumab

Contd...

Contd...

Colorectal cancer	Myeloproliferative disorders
Cetuximab, Panitumumab, Bevacizumab, Aflibercept, Regorafenib, Ramucirumab	Imatinib, Ruxolitinib
Gastrointestinal stromal tumors	**Systemic mastocytosis**
Imatinib, Nilotinib, Sunitinib, Regorafenib	Imatinib
Neuroendocrine tumors	**Basal cell carcinoma**
Lanreotide acetate	Vismodegib, Sonidegib
Melanoma	**Giant cell tumor of the bone**
Ipilimumab, Vemurafenib, Trametinib, Dabrafenib, Cobimetinib, Pembrolizumab, Nivolumab	Denosumab
Soft tissue sarcoma	**Kaposi sarcoma**
Pazopanib, Olaratumab	Alitretinoin
Dermatofibrosarcoma drotuberans	**Neuroblastoma**
Imatinib	Dinutuximab

Hormone Therapy in the Management of Cancer Pain

Breast and prostate cancer are hormone-dependent cancers (estrogen and testosterone respectively) and certain subsets of these cancers respond to hormonal manipulation. Both breast and prostate cancers account for a large number of patients who present with metastatic disease and have cancer pain due to locoregional disease and bone metastases.

Breast cancer may respond to second- and third-line hormone treatment using antiestrogen drugs like tamoxifen or toremifene, aromatase inhibitors such as anastrozole and letrozole, progestogens, such as megestrol or medroxyprogesterone acetate, and occasionally, androgens.[8] These hormone maneuvers may be used sequentially, with useful responses for the patient with widespread disease and metastatic pain.

Antiandrogen therapy for prostate cancer results in dramatic pain relief for many patients, with response rates of over 90% on initial exposure but the median duration of response is between 18 months and 24 months.[9]

Steroids like dexamethasone and prednisolone are an important component of cancer pain management strategies. Certain tumors like lymphoma, leukemia, myeloma and prostate cancer are steroid responsive and these drugs can induce dramatic reduction of pain in these tumors. Painful vertebral and other bone lesions in patients with multiple myeloma show remarkable response to pulse dexamethasone.[10]

Steroids also reduce the tissue edema and thus the resultant pain perceived through nociceptors. Steroids play an important role in controlling pain due to cord compression and radiculopathy. Similarly, headache due to brain metastases from various cancers, and leptomeningeal involvement in leukemia and lymphomas can be substantially relieved with steroids.

Bone-directed Therapies in the Management of Cancer Pain

Bone metastases secondary to solid tumors increase the risk of skeletal-related events (SREs), like occurrence of pathological fracture, radiation to bone, surgery to bone, and spinal cord compression. The SREs are associated with increased pain and analgesic use in patients with bone metastases. Treatments that prevent SREs may decrease pain and the need for opioid analgesics and reduce the impact of pain on daily functioning. A variety of bone-modifying agents have been developed which reduce cancer pain and skeletal-related events in certain types of metastatic bone cancers. These drugs do not have a significant anticancer activity on the tumor per se but work on the bone microenvironment.

Bisphosphonates (clodronate, pamidronate, zoledronic acid and ibandronate) are structural analogs of pyrophosphates, a naturally occurring component of bone crystal deposition. Different side chain modifications of the basic pyrophosphate structure give rise to the different generations of bisphosphonates, with different levels of activity. The mode of action of bisphosphonates is multiple. Predominantly, through strong affinity to bone, bisphosphonates provide physicochemical protection by absorbing calcium phosphate, suppressing the normal functioning of mature osteoclasts, and prevent maturation of osteoclast precursors. Data from systematic review suggests that bisphosphonates provide modest pain relief for patients with painful bony metastases.[11] These drugs are integral to the management of painful bone metastases in patients with breast cancer, androgen independent prostate cancer and multiple myeloma.

Tumor-induced bone destruction is largely caused by activation of bone-resorbing osteoclasts. RANKL, the key activator of osteoclasts, is the main mediator of this bone resorption through tumor-secreted growth factors and cytokines. Denosumab is a monoclonal antibody against RANK ligand (RANKL) and has been shown to be non-inferior to Zoledronic acid in preventing skeletal-related events in patients with bone metastases due to solid tumors and multiple myeloma. Denosumab also significantly delayed time to development of moderate or severe pain [hazard ratios (HR), 0.81; 95% confidence interval (CI), 0.66–1.00], pain worsening (HR, 0.83; 95% CI, 0.71–0.97), and worsening pain interference in patients with no/mild baseline pain (HR, 0.77; 95% CI, 0.61–0.96) as compared to zoledronic acid.[12,13]

HOW TO INTEGRATE CANCER-DIRECTED SYSTEMIC THERAPIES IN MANAGEMENT OF CANCER PAIN?

Cancer-directed systemic therapies are often used with the intention of controlling pain and other symptoms in patients with cancer. As compared to opioid and nonopioid analgesics, these treatments often induce regression in tumor, improve quality of life and prolong survival. In responding patients, the need for pain medication is reduced or eliminated.

However, patients with metastatic cancer almost invariably recur and often pain is a manifesting symptom for recurrence. Therefore, it is recommended that a longitudinal assessment for pain should be continued during follow-up of cancer patients.[14]

A major drawback of using cancer-directed systemic therapies for management of cancer pain is the side effect profile of these drugs. These drugs often have multisystem side effects, which may impair the quality of life in cancer patients. Special attention and dose modifications may be required in patients in pediatric and geriatric age group. Cancer treatments can have potential interactions with the analgesics and other pain adjunctive therapies and appropriate dose modifications should be performed whenever needed.

Cancer-directed systemic therapies can themselves induce pain due to treatment (e.g. painful peripheral neuropathies, mucositis, palmoplantar erythrodysesthesia) which can be very prolonged and debilitating.[15] Hence a careful monitoring and prompt management of these side effects should be done. Certain drugs like intravenous vinorelbine can cause acute pain at tumor site during treatment administration, which can be avoided by using the oral route of the drug in patients experiencing such pain.[16]

Another limitation in using cancer-directed therapies is the high cost of these treatments, which are often palliative in nature. Therefore, patients should be counseled about the treatment benefits, toxicities and financial aspects of treatment before initiating these therapies.[17]

WHEN TO STOP CANCER-DIRECTED SYSTEMIC THERAPIES

Cancer patients are often treated with multiple lines of therapy to keep the disease under control and to prolong survival. At certain point of time, the tumors acquire mutations and start becoming resistant to therapies or the side effects of therapies override their benefits. Patients should be closely monitored for resistance or intractable side effects at which point of time, a decision should be taken to stop cancer-directed systemic therapies and a transition should be done to palliative care alone.

CONCLUSION

Cancer pain prevalence is on the rise in cancer patients. The chemotherapy does play a role both in relief of pain and cure. The newer and newer drugs are playing vital role.

REFERENCES

1. Van den Beuken-van Everdingen MH, Hochstenbach LM, Joosten EA, Tjan-Heijnen VC, Janssen DJ. Update on prevalence of pain in patients with cancer: systematic review and meta-analysis. J Pain Symptom Manage. 2016;51(6):1070-90.
2. http://www.iasp-pain.org/files/Content/ContentFolders/GlobalYearAgainstPain2/CancerPainFactSheets/Epidemiology_Final.pdf.
3. Falk S, Dickenson AH. Pain and Nociception: Mechanisms of Cancer-Induced Bone Pain. J Clin Oncol. 2014;32(16):1647-54.
4. Temel JS, Greer JA, Muzikansky A, Gallagher ER, Admane S, Jackson VA, et al. Early palliative care for patients with metastatic non-small-cell lung cancer. N Engl J Med. 2010;363:733-42.
5. Scheithauer W, Rosen H, Kornek GV, Sebesta C, Depisch D. Randomised comparison of combination chemotherapy plus supportive care with supportive care alone in patients with metastatic colorectal cancer. Br Med J. 1993;306:752-5.
6. Burris HA, Moore MJ, Andersen J, Green MR, Rothenberg ML, Modiano MR, et al. Improvements in survival and clinical benefit with gemcitabine as first-line therapy for patients with advanced pancreas cancer: a randomized trial. J Clin Oncol. 1997;15:2403-13.
7. Tannock IF, Osoba D, Stockler MR, Ernst DS, Neville AJ, Moore MJ, et al. Chemotherapy with mitoxantrone plus prednisone or prednisone alone for symptomatic hormone-resistant prostate cancer: A Canadian randomized trial with palliative end points. J Clin Oncol. 1996;14:1756-64.
8. Buzdar AU. Advances in endocrine treatments for postmenopausal women with metastatic and early breast cancer. Oncologist. 2003;8:335-41.
9. Logothetis CJ, Millikan R. Update: NCCN practice guidelines for the treatment of prostate cancer. Oncology. 1999;13:118-37.
10. Snowden JA, Ahmedzai SH, Ashcroft J, D'Sa S, Littlewood T, Low E, et al. Guidelines for supportive care in multiple myeloma. 2011;154:76-103.
11. Wong R, Wiffen PJ. Bisphosphonates for the relief of pain secondary to bone metastases. Cochrane Database Syst Rev. 2002:CD002068.
12. Henry D, Vadhan-Raj S, Hirsh V, von Moos R, Hungria V, Costa L, et al. Delaying skeletal-related events in a randomized phase 3 study of denosumab versus zoledronic acid in patients with advanced cancer: an analysis of data from patients with solid tumors. Support Care Cancer. 2014;22:679.
13. Von Moos R, Body JJ, Egerdie B, Stopeck A, Brown JE, Damyanov D, et al. Pain and health-related quality of life in patients with advanced solid tumours and bone metastases: integrated results from three randomized, double-blind studies of denosumab and zoledronic acid. Support Care Cancer. 2016;24:1327.
14. Fujii A, Yamada Y, Takayama K. Longitudinal assessment of pain management with the pain management index in cancer outpatients receiving chemotherapy. Support Care Cancer. 2016.
15. Ripamonti CI, Bossi P, Santini D, Fallon· M. Pain related to cancer treatments and diagnostic procedures: a no man's land? Ann Oncol. 2014;25(6):1097-106.
16. De Pas T, Sbanotto A, Catania C, Banfi MG, Curigliano G, Nolè F, et al. Oral administration of vinorelbine can overcome intractable endovenous-vinorelbine-associated acute tumor pain. Support Care Cancer. 2005:13:194.
17. Lal M, Raheja S, Kale S, Bhowmik KT. Palliative care tailored towards the needs of the poor in India. Indian J Surg Oncol. 2015;6:227.

CHAPTER 53

Oncosurgery and Cancer Associated Pain

Deepak Chabbra

INTRODUCTION

Cancer-related pain is a difficult problem, often with limited effective treatments. Local excision, radiation, brachytherapy, and nerve blocks are a part of the conventional interventional treatments of metastatic pain. Though each modality has advantages, it accompanies certain shortcomings as well. Primary or revision surgery is not only invasive but is often limited and morbid. Radiation offers a noninvasive means of treatment, but collateral damage to adjacent healthy tissue is inevitable, and maximum doses are often reached. Brachytherapy offers the advantage of treating tumors from the middle of the mass outward, but is technically difficult, expensive and similar to radiation it is susceptible to damaging normal adjacent tissue. Nerve blocks with local anesthetic can provide effective pain relief, but the effects are usually short-lived and 20–50% of patients do not benefit from the local anesthetics.[1] Local neurodestructive techniques are subject to unwanted sensorineural deficits. Pharmacologic management remains a common method of treating cancer pain[2] but sedation from opiates can often impair mental function.

DEFINITION AND UNDERSTANDING CONCEPTS IN SURGICAL PALLIATION FOR CANCER

Pain is commonly associated with cancer, occurring in about one quarter of patients with newly diagnosed cancer and in nearly three quarters of cancer patients with advanced disease.[3] A meta-analysis revealed that pain is reported in 59% of patients undergoing treatment, in 64% patients with advanced disease, and in 33% of patients after curative treatment.[4]

Etiology of cancer pain includes direct tumor involvement/infiltration of organs (85% cases), cancer therapies themselves (15%) as well as noncancer related problems (3–10%) that include psychological distress, cancer fatigue and breach in spirituality and existential dimensions.[5] In addition, various factors may influence prevalence of cancer pain, viz. primary tumor type (breast and prostate cancer are associated with greater incidence of cancer pain than lymphomas), tumor Stage (nonmetastatic cancer patients have significantly less cancer pain compared to advanced cancer cases; <15% vs 60–80%), tumors in close proximity to neural structure, and patient's variables including anxiety, depression and threshold levels.[6]

Surgical procedures performed for cancers frequently revolve around well-defined principles and a curative intent. Recurrent cancer is not uncommon despite an initial curative surgical attempt. Despite advances in diagnosis, many patients are detected with an unresectable disease at presentation.

Palliative interventions, (both operative and nonoperative) are used with noncurative intent to improve quality of life, pain control, symptom relief and possibly survival. The indications and goals for the appropriate use of these palliative interventions are less clearly defined. Inconsistent and inappropriate definitions of palliative care have also complicated the understanding of the role of surgery in managing patients with advanced malignancies.[7,8]

Surgical palliation of cancer may be defined best as *"a deliberate use of an operative procedure on behalf of a patient with incurable disease with the primary intention of improving quality of life by relieving symptoms and minimizing psychic distress caused by an advanced malignancy, the effectiveness of which should be judged by the presence and durability of patient-acknowledged symptom resolution."*[9,10]

INDICATIONS FOR SURGICAL PALLIATION

Surgical palliative procedures fall generally into three areas of concern, viz. bleeding, obstruction and perforation, and decisions to advocate operative procedures for cancer related pain are often based on individual expectations and anecdotal experience.

The two primary indications for surgical intervention for pain relief in advanced malignant lesions are:
- When other less invasive means have failed or
- When selected therapy results in intolerable side effects.

The surgery may not necessarily aim to eradicate cancer tissue in the patient. In fact, palliative surgery is often deemed as worthwhile and feasible by cancer specialists when the disease is not responsive to any type of curative treatment (Fig. 1). Palliative surgery which removes cancer tissue is recorded as cancer-directed surgery (Figs 2A to C). Palliative procedures such as a nerve block procedure to interrupt pain signals in the nervous system, or a stent placement to alleviate obstruction, etc., which does not remove cancer tissue are recorded as noncancer directed surgery.[11]

PATIENT SELECTION FOR PALLIATIVE SURGERY

The selection of patients for palliative cancer directed surgery should include:
- A careful assessment of symptom severity, whether the pain is refractory to less invasive pain management modalities
- Likelihood that surgery will alleviate the pain
- Suitability of the patient to tolerate surgery
- Possible morbidity of the proposed operation
- Anticipated life expectancy and expected disease course
- Tumor biology.

A surgeon's willingness to contribute to effective pain management needs to be balanced against

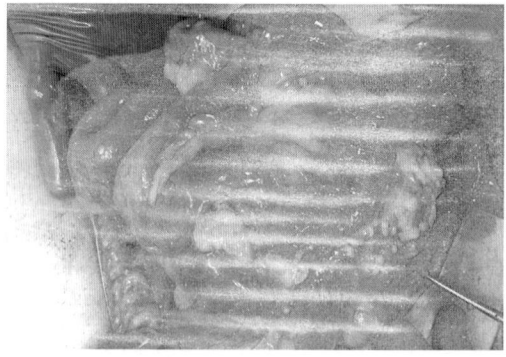

FIG. 1: Intraoperative photograph of a patient with advanced peritoneal carcinomatosis. Palliative major bowel resection was done for large mesenteric tumor deposits involving multiple small bowel loops causing obstruction *(For color version, see Plate 15)*

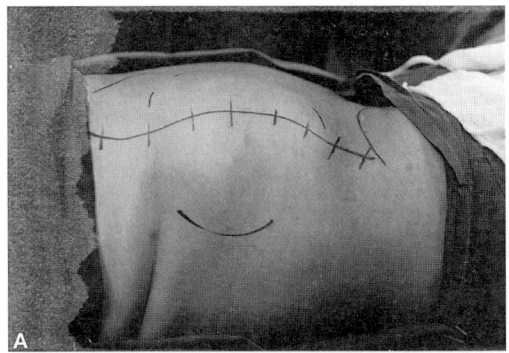
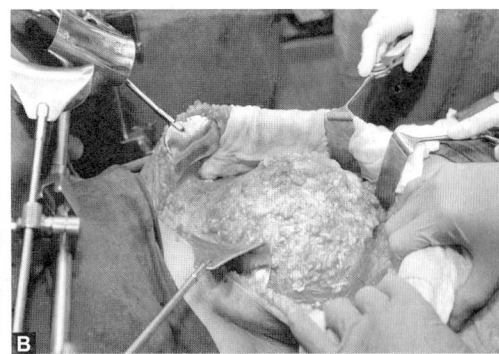
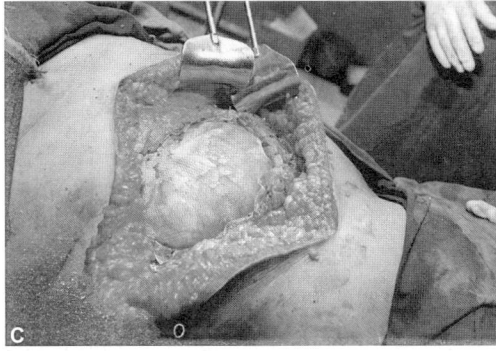

FIGS 2A to C: (A) Patient with a recurrent and metastatic hepatocellular carcinoma planned for palliative surgery; (B) Palliative resection of extra-abdominal tumor done for compression symptoms; (C) Abdominal wall reconstruction after tumor excision *(For color version, see Plate 15)*

the likelihood of an often frail, nutritionally compromised patient recovering uneventfully from possibly major surgery.[12]

The biological aggressiveness of underlying cancer could be an important determinant for a judicious decision making for palliative surgery, e.g. a cautious therapeutic approach is warranted for a metastatic pancreatic adenocarcinoma while a metastatic pancreatic neuroendocrine tumor may remain indolent for years and may be well suited to the aggressive management of disease symptoms because of their long life expectancy and their excellent performance status.

Two very important key questions that need to be addressed while offering a palliative surgery for pain are: (1) is there any evidence to support the use of palliative surgery for pain treatment? and (2) are the outcomes with palliative surgery for cancer favorable?

THE EVIDENCE AND THE OUTCOMES

The current medical literature lacks information on the range of data required to guide sound decisions for the use of palliative surgery for end-stage cancer patients;[13] however, symptom resolution form a palliative surgical intervention has also been reported to be as high as 80–90%.[14] In a landmark study, by Miner et al., that involved prospective, symptom related outcomes analysis of 1,022 palliative procedures for advanced cancer, median symptom free survival and the median survival after palliative surgery was 135 days and 194 days, respectively[15] suggesting that palliative surgical approaches can offer improvement in the quality of life for patients in the final stages of their existence. This has been especially true in the setting of sarcomas and melanomas involving the limbs. A study of 15 patients with palliative major amputations of fungating painful melanomas though reported a short median survival of 5 months, 14 of the 15 patients (93%) were able to survive to leave the hospital.[16] Similarly, Malawer et al.[17] reported a dramatic pain relief and survival beyond 1 year in 11 patients who underwent major palliative amputations for the management of advanced melanoma, sarcoma, and carcinoma. In this series, previous treatment modalities directed at pain relief that had failed in all patients.

In a large survey by the Society of Surgical Oncology in the United States that involved more than 400 surgeons with largely cancer-focused practices, it was estimated that palliative surgery made up more than 20% of all cancer operations.[18] The survey identified goals of greatest importance in palliative surgery as achieving patients' pain relief, other symptom relief, and maintaining patients' independence and function. Improving patient survival was identified as the least important goal of palliative surgery.

Postoperative morbidity remains a major concern in end-stage cancer patients who have many surgical risk factors such as malnutrition, anemia and other systemic side effects from possible palliative chemotherapy. While postoperative morbidity rates have been reported between 20% and 40%.[19,20] One prospective study examining palliative surgery demonstrated that patients were most likely to opt for palliative surgery as a means to resolve symptoms leading to improvement in quality of life and very few patients expressed concerns about perioperative morbidity.[21]

It is thus imperative to have a robust evidence to support the concept of palliative surgery in cancer related pain. Unfortunately, few high-quality studies have been done that carefully evaluate symptom relief in patients undergoing palliative surgery. Miner et al. reviewed literature from 1990 to 1996 and noted that studies rarely reported quality of life (17%) or pain relief (10%) as end-points of measurement[13] and only 9% of the literature in this time frame was prospective.

Surgical oncology literature in general has always focused on surgeries performed with the intent to cure. Data on outcomes other than survival are lacking.[22] Among literature focused on palliation alone, reports of outcomes have been physicians' impressions rather than patient-reported data. Physician-reported outcomes cannot reflect actual patient impressions when compared with patient-reported data.[23]

A prospective evaluation of patients undergoing surgery for the palliation of an advanced malignancy enrolled 26 patients between 1997 and 1999.[24] This was the only study that highlighted the importance of a critical palliative triangle (in palliative surgical decision-making) between the patient, family member, and surgeon that clarified and defined the goals of each patient's individual treatment (Fig. 3). Through the dynamics of the triangle, the patient's complaints, values, and social and emotional support were considered against the medical and surgical alternatives. Before surgery, the patient, a significant family member, and the attending surgeon all expressed a primary goal, which they hoped, would be achieved by the operation. All of the patients expressed a desire for resolution of their chief complaint. Despite acknowledging the palliative intent of the proposed operation, 46% (12 of 26) of the patients also expressed

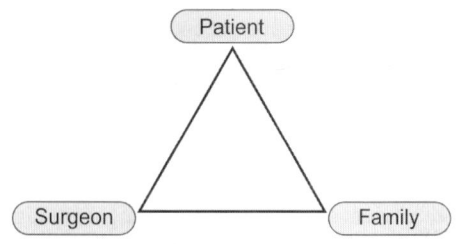

FIG. 3: An ideal palliative triangle. Equal interactions between the patient, the family member, and the surgeon guide individual decisions regarding palliative care. The dynamic of this interaction is influenced by unique factors provided by each participant

a hope that no evidence of disease would be found at the time of surgery. Although 38% (10 of 26) stated that they additionally sought a prolongation of life, 27% (7 of 26) of the patients reported that they did not expect to survive the proposed operation. After a palliative operation, only 46% (12 of 26) showed clinical improvement. Clinical gains were noted at 30 days after the palliative procedure in all patients who experienced a benefit. Improved quality of life or pain perception was maintained in these patients for a median of 108 days but 75% (9 of 12) patients experiencing a clinical benefit died before the termination of the study. 35% (9 of 26) of the patients had a significant postoperative complication, and 89% (8 of 9) of these patients were never discharged from the hospital after their surgery and died as a result of either complications or progression of disease.

Despite the effective interactions between members of the palliative triangle, the majority (54%) of patients in this study did not obtain a significant benefit after undergoing a palliative operation. These patients did not experience an improvement in quality of life or pain perception or subjective improvement after surgery. Patients had relatively long hospitalizations, and many died in the hospital as a result of complications of the surgery, progression of disease, or both. There were no significant differences among patients who survived in the perioperative period and those who did not. The high mortality associated with palliative surgery in this series is very discouraging and only puts a question mark on the benefits of offering a surgical procedure for palliation in general.

CONCLUSION

Most patients with incurable disease will not need major surgical intervention; however, as part of a multidisciplinary team, surgeons must be aware of the proper patient and proper time to intervene with palliative surgical intent. A surgeon is frequently confronted with a range of multidisciplinary treatment options and technical considerations that could potentially relieve some of the symptoms of an advanced malignancy but current medical literature lacks information and is unable to guide sound decisions for palliative surgeries that are often being offered on basis of the individual experiences. In all fairness, the patient should be fully informed that complications arising out of a palliative surgery could lead to worsening, unresolved, or new symptoms and perhaps even hasten their demise. While all possible complications cannot be accurately predicted, open and advance communication about these possibilities usually facilitates a deep sense of personal trust between surgeons, their patients and patient family members. With the incorporation of pain management teams as a part of multidisciplinary cancer care and improved pharmacotherapeutics with longer acting opioids such as slow release oxycodone or morphine and transcutaneous fentanyl patches, surgery is nowadays sparingly used for the treatment of cancer pain and minimally invasive techniques, such as nerve blocks, radiofrequency ablations or neurolytic destructions, etc. are increasingly being promoted in the wide cancer pain management arsenal.

ACKNOWLEDGMENTS

I am thankful to Dr Sarika Lamba (Associate Consultant in Surgical Oncology at Narayana Multispeciality Hospital, Jaipur) for helping me in preparing this manuscript.

REFERENCES

1. Jacox A, Carr DB, Payne R. New clinical-practice guidelines for the management of pain in patients with cancer. N Engl J Med. 1994;330:651-5.
2. Zekry HA, Reddy SK. Opioid and nonopioid therapy in cancer pain: the traditional and the new. Curr Rev Pain. 1999;3:237-47.
3. Cleeland CS, Gonin R, Hatfield AK, Edmonson JH, Blum RH, Stewart JA, et al. Pain and its treatment in outpatients with metastatic cancer. N Engl J Med. 1994;330:592-6.

4. van den Beuken-van Everdingen MH, de Rijke JM, Kessels AG, Schouten HC, van Kleef M, Patijn J. Prevalence of pain in patients with cancer: a systematic review of the past 40 years. Ann Oncol. 2007;18(9):1437-49.
5. Benedtti C, Brock C, Cleenland C. NCCN Practice Guideline for cancer pain. Oncology. 2000;(11A):135.
6. Chochinov H, Breithart W. Handbook of psychiatry in palliative medicine. New York: Oxford University Press; 1999.
7. Miner TJ, Jaques DP, Karpeh MS, Brennan MF. Defining non-curative gastric resections by palliative intent. J Am Coll Surg. 2004;198:1013-21.
8. McCahill LE, Krouse RS, Chu DZ, Juarez G, Uman GC, Ferrell BR, et al. Decision making in palliative surgery. J Am Coll Surg. 2002;195:411-22.
9. Miner TJ. Palliative surgery for advanced cancer, lessons learnt in patient selection and outcome assessment. Am J Clin Oncol. 2005;28:411-4.
10. Miner TJ. Communication as a core skill of palliative surgical care. Anesthesiol Clin. 2012;30:47-58.
11. Palliative and Reconstructive surgeries: National Cancer Institute (NIH). NCI SEER training module.
12. McCahill LE, Ferrell B. Palliative surgery for cancer pain. West J Med. 2002;176(2):107-10.
13. Miner TJ, Jaques DP, Tavaf-Motamen H, Shriver CD. Decision making on surgical palliation based on patient outcome data. Am J Surg. 1999;177:150-4.
14. Miner TJ, Cohen J, Charpentier K, McPhillips J, Marvell L, Cioffi WG. The palliative triangle: improved patient selection and outcomes associated with palliative operations. Arch Surg. 2011;146:517-22.
15. Miner TJ, Brennan MF, Jaques DP. A prospective, symptom related, outcomes analysis of 1022 palliative procedures for advanced cancer. Ann Surg. 2004;240:719-26.
16. Jaques DP, Coit DG, Brennan MF. Major amputation for advanced malignant melanoma. Surg Gynecol Obstet. 1989;169:1-6.
17. Malawer MM, Buch RG, Thompson WE, Sugarbaker PH. Major amputations done with palliative intent in the treatment of local bony complications associated with advanced cancer. J Surg Oncol. 1991;47:121-30.
18. McCahill LE, Krouse R, Chu D, Juarez G, Uman GC, Ferrell B, et al. Indications and use of palliative surgery: results of Society of Surgical Oncology survey. Ann Surg Oncol 2002;9:104-12.
19. Badgwell BD, Smith K, Liu P, Bruera E, Curley SA, Cormier JN. Indicators of surgery and survival in oncology inpatients requiring surgical evaluation for palliation. Support Care Cancer. 2009;17:727-34.
20. Howard JH, Pollock RE. Palliative Surgery for Sarcoma. ESUN. 2014:11(6).
21. Collins LK, Goodwin JA, Spencer HJ, Guevara C, Ferrell B, McSweeney J, et al. Patient reasoning in palliative surgical oncology. J Surg Oncol. 2013;107:372-5.
22. Porter GA, Skibber JM. Outcomes research in surgical oncology. Ann Surg Oncol. 2000;7:367-75.
23. Blazeby JM, Williams MH, Alderson D, Farndon JR. Observer variation in assessment of quality of life in patients with oesophageal cancer. Br J Surg. 1995;82:1200-3.
24. Miner TJ, Jaques DP, Shriver CD. A Prospective evaluation of patients undergoing surgery for the palliation of an advanced malignancy. Ann Surg Oncol. 2002;9(7):696-703.

CHAPTER 54

Management of Ophthalmic Pain

Salil A Mehta

INTRODUCTION

Physiology of ophthalmic pain: Specialized nerve endings (nociceptors) exist within ocular tissue. These may be activated by a wide variety of stimuli including chemical and mechanical.

There is a complex biochemical process that involves prostaglandins (PGE2) and leukotrienes that sensitize the pain receptors to bradykinin and histamine. Substance P then stimulates the nerve endings. Substance P also causes a cascade release of more histamine, prostaglandins and bradykinins, causing further pain. Afferent fibers that transmit the pain signal, synapse in the dorsal root ganglion and travel to the spinothalamic tract to further synapse in the thalamus. In the thalamus, there is a final synapse with the primary sensory cortex fibers that occurs in the thalamus. Ophthalmic pain is primarily transmitted via the trigeminal (V) nerve. This has three main branches—maxillary, mandibular, and ophthalmic. The ophthalmic branch is responsible for the transmission of pain stimuli in most cases. The corneal nerves as well as the nerves that innervate the iris all use the ophthalmic branch to transmit pain thus accounting for the pain that is felt in these two common conditions. The facial nerve (VII) transmits impulses of pain from the eyelid and the optic nerve (II) transmits pain impulses due to neuritis or compression.

Ophthalmic pain may be acute or chronic. *The common causes of acute pain include*:

Conjunctivitis is a common cause. The etiology may be an allergy or infective (viral or bacterial). The conjunctiva is congested, inflamed and usually associated with mild pain. Treatment is with local applications of antibiotic or antiviral drops or ointments.

Corneal injuries (abrasions and ulcerations) may caused by foreign bodies, contact lens related pathology or may be due to infections. Corneal lesions tend to be profoundly painful and are marked by epithelial loss, infiltrates or stromal edema. Treatment focuses on the restoration of epithelial cover and the elimination of any infection.

CHEMICAL INJURIES

Burns may result from exposure to acid or alkalis, both within the household or industrial. Arc welding may produce ultraviolet related corneal injuries. Treatment includes removal of the offending agent, irrigation and use of local steroid drops to ameliorate inflammation.

Local infections such as styes or chalazia are common causes. They are marked by red, painful, tender swellings that may arise on either eye lid. Treatment is via local and systemic antibiotic treatment.

Acute Glaucoma

Glaucoma is defined as an increase in the intraocular pressure from the normal upper limit of 21 mmHg. The causes are diverse and may be primary or secondary to other ocular diseases. Primary glaucoma may be due to an obstruction of the outflow channels by a narrow anterior chamber which is termed as narrow angle glaucoma. The more common variant is open angle glaucoma which is defined by open angles and raised intraocular pressure. While mild increases of intraocular pressure are painless, significant increases beyond 30 mmHg are usually symptomatic. The treatment focuses on decreasing the intraocular pressure with the use of antiglaucoma medications. These may be delivered via local drops (beta blockers or prostaglandin analogues) or orally (acetazolamide).

UVEITIS

Uveitis is defined as the inflammation of the uvea. Uveitis may be classified according to its location (anterior, intermediate or posterior uveitis) or etiology (autoimmune, infective or idiopathic). Uveitis produces pain ranging from mild to severe depending on the extent and severity of inflammation. Investigations are mandatory and are usually focused on ruling out an infective etiology. The mainstay of treatment is immunosuppression usually with the use of steroids (orally or topically). More recalcitrant cases need the use of stronger immunosuppressives such as methotrexate, cyclosporine or azathioprine.

Optic neuritis is a demyelination of the optic nerve usually due to autoimmune disease. The pain is typically mild, dull and exacerbated on lateral movements of the eyeball. It is classically diagnosed by the typical scotomas on perimetry and reduced amplitudes and latencies on visual evoked potential assessment. Systemic steroids such as injectable methyl prednisolone are the mainstay of treatment.

Commonly Encountered Causes of Chronic Pain Include

Ischemic Etiologies

Neovascular glaucoma with total closure of the angle (NVG) (Fig. 1).

Several ocular and systemic diseases produce retinal ischemia/hypoxia and the consequent release of an angiogenesis factor. This causes the formation of new blood vessels from preexisting vessels. This causes glaucoma either through open-angle or closed-angle mechanisms. Angle closure occurs due to the growth of a fibrovascular membrane over the trabecular meshwork in the angle, resulting in its obstruction, often associated with peripheral anterior synechiae (Fig. 1).

Retinal ischemia is the most common mechanism in practically all cases of NVG. This ischemia leads to the production of a angiogenesis factor that has recently been suggested to be vascular endothelial growth factor (VEGF). This factor diffuses into the anterior segment and causes neovascularization at the pupillary border and iris surface [neovascularization of the iris (NVI)] (Fig. 2) and over the iris angle [neovascularization of the angle (NVA)] (Fig. 3).

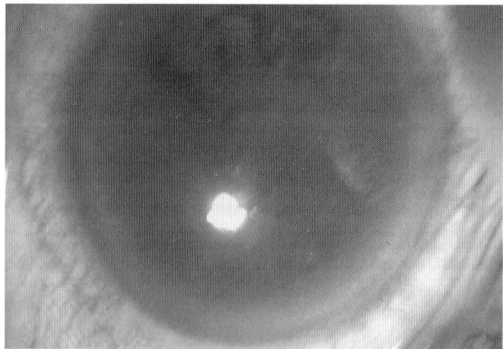

FIG. 1: Color photograph showing a congested painful eye with advanced neovascular glaucoma. extensive neovascularizaration of the iris is seen *(For color version, see Plate 16)*

The neovascularization is accompanied by a fibrovascular membrane that can occlude the angle and cause closed angle glaucoma. Further maturation of these membranes causes the formation of peripheral anterior synechiae and progressive angle closure and an elevated IOP.

The clinical presentation of NVG can be divided into the early stage and the advanced stage.

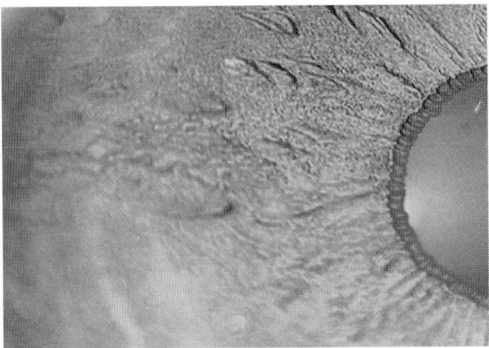

FIG. 2: Color photograph showing new vessels on the iris *(For color version, see Plate 16)*

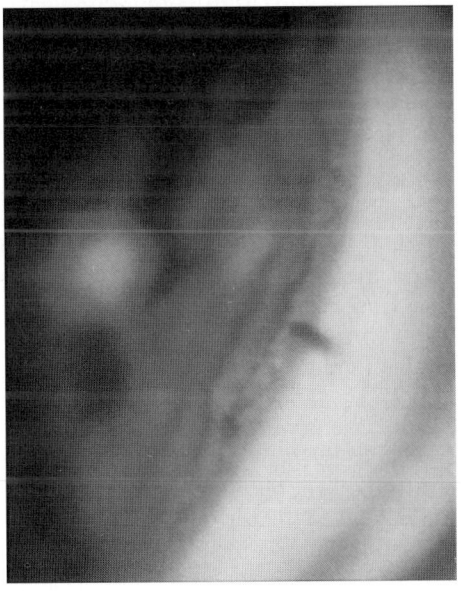

FIG. 3: Photograph of the angle showing new vessels of the angle *(For color version, see Plate 16)*

- *Early stage (rubeosis iridis):* This is marked by a normal intraocular pressure in the presence of visible neovascularization in the anterior segment (at the pupillary margin, iris or the angle).
- *Advanced stage:* There is additionally elevated intraocular pressure (often above 60 mmHg), reduced visual acuity and acute distress in the form of acute severe pain, headache. Hyphema may be present along with peripheral anterior synechiae, severe rubeosis and optic nerve cupping may be seen in the late stages.

Common Causes of NVG Include

- Central retinal vein occlusion (CRVO)
- Proliferative diabetic retinopathy
- Carotid artery occlusive disease (CAOD).

General Principles Include

- *Identifying the underlying causative agent:* This includes searching for evidence of central retinal vein occlusion or diabetic retinopathy commonly.
- *Prophylactic treatment:* This focuses on ablating the ischemic retina to reduce the production of angiogenetic factors. Ablation of nonviable retina is known to inhibit and may even reverse neovascularization of the anterior segment. Retinal ablation is commonly achieved via panretinal photocoagulation (PRP) or cryotherapy if media opacities preclude PRP. PRP can be delivered in the following three ways: slit lamp delivery system, indirect laser, or endolaser at time of vitrectomy. Current guidelines suggest 1500–2000 burns, with a spot size of 500–800 μm in the periphery as adequate to achieve sufficient retinal ablation. Cryotherapy uses a retinal cryoprobe is used to create burns. Prophylactic PRP is recommended in cases with extensive capillary nonperfusion. For patients with diabetic retinopathy, good glycemic control is mandatory. If

proliferative diabetic retinopathy exists, then complete PRP is necessary.

- *Early-stage treatment*: Treatment is the same as for the prophylactic stage PRP (filler PRP if needed), panretinal cryotherapy, and medical therapy. Medical therapy at this stage includes topical atropine 1% to reduce ocular congestion and topical steroids (e.g. prednisolone to reduce the inflammation. Antiglaucoma medications to treat the open-angle glaucoma include topical beta-blockers (e.g. levobunolol, timolol, topical brimonidine, topical carbonic anhydrase inhibitor (e.g. dorzolamide), and oral carbonic anhydrase inhibitor (e.g. acetazolamide).
- *Advanced-stage treatment*: This stage is characterized by synechial closure of the angle and subsequent angle-closure glaucoma. PRP is still the firstline treatment. It reduces further neovascularization and helps achieve optimal surgical outcomes. Medical therapy is as above with topical atropine and steroids being the most used. Antiglaucoma medications, topical beta-blockers, and carbonic anhydrase inhibitors may also be used.
- *Anti-VEGF therapy*: The use of anti-VEGF therapy is now increasingly being accepted.[1,2] Anti-VEGFs such as bevacizumab (Avastin), aflibercept (Eylea) and ranibizumab (Lucentis) reduce neovascularization by blocking VEGF receptors within the ocular tissues. These (VEGF) are angiogenic factors that promote the formation of new vessels. Aqueous growth factors have been shown to significantly decrease after intravitreal anti-VEGF.[3] Several studies suggest the use of anti-VEGF agents along with panretinal photocoagulation (PRP), with or without vitrectomy.[4]

Intravitreal bevacizumab is the most used anti-VEGF due to its lower costs. A systematic review of the efficacy and safety of intravitreal bevacizumab (IVB) suggests that bevacizumab is well tolerated, effectively stabilizes INV activity, and controls IOP in patients with INV when used alone and at an early-stage of NVG.[5]

END-STAGE TREATMENT

There is complete angle closure with no useful vision. The primary goal is pain relief. Medical therapy includes topical atropine 1% and steroids. In cases of corneal decompensation occurs, a bandage contact lens can be used. Cyclodestructive procedures may be used if medical therapy fails to provide pain relief. Cyclocryotherapy achieves IOP lowering by destroying the ciliary epithelium that secretes aqueous and by reducing blood flow to the ciliary body.

Retrobulbar alcohol injection is used after all other options have been tried and the patient does not permit eye removal. Enucleation is indicated only if intractable pain is present and is not relievable by any other modality.

Surgical care is necessary in patients with remaining useful vision. Surgical modalities include trabeculectomy with or without an antifibrotic agent and valve implant surgery.

Trabeculectomy with the antifibrotic agents mitomycin-C and 5-fluorouracil (5-FU) is one surgical option. Standard trabeculectomy in NVG has a high failure rate due to fibrosis of the bleb but injections of 5-FU subconjunctivally in the postoperative period have enhanced the surgical success.

A retrospective cohort study of 101 eyes suggested that factors responsible for the failure of trabeculectomy with MMC for NVG were younger age and a previous vitrectomy in patients with NVG.[6]

Valve implant surgery is another surgical option and may be used when trabeculectomy fails or extensive conjunctival fibrosis or scarring is present precluding a routine filtering procedure. Molteno, Krupin, and Ahmed valve implants commonly are used.

Complications include postoperative hypotony with associated complications, blockage of the internal opening and fibrosis of the filtering bleb.

Infective and Neuropathic Causes

Varicella-zoster virus (VZV) and postherpetic neuralgia: VZV usually causes a febrile illness (chicken pox) but any subsequent immunosuppression or stress permits the reactivation of the latent infection and results in a localized skin rash in a single dermatome. This is termed herpes zoster (HZ).

When the HZ involves the first division of the trigeminal nerve it is termed herpes zoster ophthalmicus. HZO accounts for as many as 10–25% of HZ and is a common cause of debilitating ocular pain as also chronic inflammation and visual disability.

Pathophysiology

After a initial infection the virus enters the dorsal root ganglia where it remains latent. In response to stress, the virus is released from the trigeminal ganglion, and moves down the ophthalmic nerve to the nasociliary nerve. The nasociliary nerve is responsible for innervation of the ocular surface and skin of the nose (especially the tip).

Clinical Presentation

The prodrome typically includes a mild flu like illness with fatigue and a low-grade fever that presents for 5–7 days prior to the appearance of the unilateral rash over the forehead, upper eyelid, and nose. Often there is some localized pain. The initial clinical sign is an erythematous macular rash that forms clusters of papules and vesicles. Pustule formation is common along with crusting and the lesions soon heal completely. There is usually some scarring and hypopigmentation or hyperpigmentation.

Ocular Complications Include

- Periorbital and conjunctival edema
- Secondary bacterial infections leading to scarring
- Corneal lesions including punctate epithelial keratitis, dendritic keratitis and stromal keratitis
- Neurotrophic keratopathy
- Uveitis with secondary glaucoma and cataract.

The most common complication of HZO is postherpetic neuralgia. This is a neuropathic pain that can persist weeks or even years.

Treatment of HZO

Emergency care includes local care, adequate pain control and early antiviral and antibiotic treatment.

Antiviral Treatment

Oral acyclovir (5 times/d) reduces the duration and severity of symptoms. However, it has no effect on reduction of the severity of postherpetic neuralgia. Famciclovir (500 mg tid) and valacyclovir (1 g tid) have been shown to be effective as acyclovir. Shafran has found that a once-daily regimen of famciclovir 750 mg caused a reduction of cutaneous symptoms and pain as much as current standards of care. All regimens need to be used for at least 7–10 days.[7]

Corticosteroid Therapy

Their use reduces the duration of pain and increases the rate of cutaneous healing. The should be used only in conjunction with antiviral agents.

Treatment of Ophthalmic Complications

- Blepharitis/conjunctivitis—topical lubrication and antibiotics
- Stromal keratitis—Topical steroids
- Neurotrophic keratitis—Topical lubrication and topical antibiotics, bandage contact lenses
- Uveitis—local steroids; systemic steroids; systemic acyclovir; cycloplegics
- Scleritis/episcleritis—local NSAIDS, steroids
- Acute retinal necrosis/progressive outer retinal necrosis—Intravenous acyclovir (1500 mg/m^2/day divided into 3 doses) for 7–10 days, followed by oral acyclovir

(800 mg orally 5 times daily) for 14 weeks followed by barrage laser if required.
- Surgical treatment—some patients may need a lateral tarsorrhaphy or lid traction sutures.

Treatment of Postherpetic Neuralgia

The appearance of severe pain at any point of time when the vesicles appear or after should raise the possibility of postherpetic neuralgia. Pavan-Langston[8] has suggested that the following protocol may be used.
- Tricyclic antidepressants—amitriptyline, or desipramine 25 mg with dosage increases up to 75 mg (at bedtime)
- Topical treatment with capsaicin ointment daily up to 4 times/day (qid) or lidocaine patches
- Gabapentin (30–600 mg tid).

In a study by Kanai et al.[9] the use of lidocaine 4% eye drops caused significant reduction in eye and forehead pain. Analgesia was noticed within 15 minutes after instillation and persisted for up to 36 hours.

Several anesthesia-based interventions have been described. These include.
- *Local anesthetic blocking of sympathetic nerves or stellate ganglion blockade*: The stellate ganglion is part of the sympathetic network and is formed by the inferior cervical and first thoracic ganglia. It is found just anterior to the head of the first rib and receives input from the paravertebral sympathetic chain and provides sympathetic efferents to the upper extremities, head, neck, and heart. The traditional blocks have involved infiltrating local anesthetic by palpating the transverse process of C6. If enough anesthetic reaches the ganglion, the block is effective.

Image-guided stellate ganglion blocks have several advantages of which the increased safety and accuracy care are primary.

FLUOROSCOPIC TECHNIQUE

The C7 vertebral body is identified and a a 25-gauge spinal needle is used to inject 10 mL of 0.25% bupivacaine at the junction of the body and the transverse process of C6.

CT-GUIDED TECHNIQUE

Under CT guidance: A 25-gauge spinal needle is maneuvered onto the head of the first rib. This should be as close as possible to the vertebral body. Bupivacaine (up to 1–2 mL) is slowly injected.
- Transcutaneous electric nerve stimulation and, if necessary, neurosurgery (e.g. thermocoagulation of substantia gelatinosa Rolandi) has been found to be effective in some cases.

Inflammatory Causes: These Include

- Nonspecific orbital inflammation (NSOI) (orbital pseudotumor) is the most common cause of painful orbital mass in adults. NSOI may present in one of two forms—localized or diffuse. The localized or discrete version can affect any orbital tissue including the extraocular muscles (myositis), sclera (scleritis), lacrimal gland (dacryoadenitis) or the superior orbital fissure and cavernous sinus (Tolosa-Hunt syndrome). Alternatively, the diffuse form may involve the intraorbital fatty tissues. Infectious and immune-mediate etiologies may be responsible for this disease. Orbital pseudotumor usually presents with acute onset of pain, proptosis, swelling and erythema. Unilateral presentation is more classic. Pain is the most common symptom in adult patients and occurs about 60% of the time. Diplopia is less common (30%). Periorbital edema, proptosis, chemosis, reduced and ptosis are the most common signs. Laboratory work-up includes complete blood count, thyroid function studies, erythrocyte sedimentation rate, antineutrophil cytoplasmic antibodies, angiotensin-converting enzyme level, rapid plasma reagin test, antinuclear antibodies, and rheumatoid factor. Radiological investigations include high-resolution computed tomography (CT) or contrast-enhanced magnetic resonance imaging (MRI). Treatment options are varied and can include surgery, steroids, chemotherapeutic agents and irradiation.

Specific Orbital Tumors: Common Types Include

Lymphoma: These are usually the non-hodgkins, B-cell type. These patients are usually 50 + years old, no specific sex predilection, and present with diplopia, epiphora, and painless proptosis. Signs, include eyelid swelling and ptosis. Radiological investigations may reveal an orbital or subconjunctival mass. Therapy includes external beam radiation therapy or a combination of chemotherapy and radiation therapy

Meningioma: Meningiomas are neurogenic tumors originating from the optic nerve sheath or sphenoid ridge. They are slow-growing and cause pressure relayed symptoms. Visual loss is common and is seen in more posterior tumors. The management of optic nerve sheath meningiomas involves vision preserving radiation therapy.

Cavernous hemangioma: It is the most common benign orbital tumor in adults and is common in middle-age women. It is usually unilateral, and a slowly progressive orbital tumor. The treatment is usually excision.

Carotid–cavernous fistula: These are acquired arteriovenous shunts and are usually caused by trauma. These traumatic shunts which are usually high-flow lesions, produce orbital swelling, chemosis, increased episcleral venous pressure and pulsatile proptosis. Treatment is primarily surgical. Other entities include:

- Lacrimal gland epithelial tumors
- Pleomorphic adenomas
- Adenoid cystic carcinoma.

CONCLUSION

Ocular pain remains a commonly encountered problem and one which may be significantly distressing to the patient. It may present in both its acute and chronic forms and may need a variety of surgical and medical regimens for its treatment.

REFERENCES

1. Hasanreisoglu M, Weinberger D, Mimouni K, Luski M, Bourla D, Kramer M, et al. Intravitreal bevacizumab as an adjunct treatment for neovascular glaucoma. Eur J Ophthalmol. 2009;19(4):607-12.
2. Andreoli CM, Miller JW. Anti-vascular endothelial growth factor therapy for ocular neovascular disease. Curr Opin Ophthalmol. 2007;18(6):502-8.
3. Tripathi RC, Li J, Tripathi BJ. Increased level of vascular endothelial growth factor in aqueous humor of patients with neovascular glaucoma. Ophthalmology. 1998;105(2):232-7.
4. Simha A, Braganza A, Abraham L, Samuel P, Lindsley K. Anti-vascular endothelial growth factor for neovascular glaucoma. Cochrane Database Syst Rev. 2009;3.
5. Ehlers JP, Spirn MJ, Lam A, Sivalingam A, Samuel MA, Tasman W. Combination intravitreal bevacizumab/panretinal photocoagulation versus panretinal photocoagulation alone in the treatment of neovascular glaucoma. Retina. 2008;28(5):696-702.
6. Takihara Y, Inatani M, Fukushima M, Iwao K, Iwao M, Tanihara H. Trabeculectomy with mitomycin C for neovascular glaucoma: prognostic factors for surgical failure. Am J Ophthalmol. 2009;147(5):912-8.
7. Shafran SD, Tyring SK, Ashton R, Decroix J, Forszpaniak C, Wade A, et al. Once, twice, or three times daily famciclovir compared with aciclovir for the oral treatment of herpes zoster in immunocompetent adults: a randomized, multicenter, double-blind clinical trial. J Clin Virol. 2004;29(4):248-53.
8. Pavan-Langston D. Herpes zoster antivirals and pain management. Ophthalmology. 2008;115(2 Suppl):S13-20.
9. Kanai A, Okamoto T, Suzuki K, Niki Y, Okamoto H. Lidocaine eye drops attenuate pain associated with ophthalmic postherpetic neuralgia. Anesth Analg. 2010;110(5):1457-60.

INDEX

Page numbers followed by *f* refer to figure and *t* refer to table.

A

Abdomen 265
Abdominal pain
  chronic 96
  upper 264
Abdominal ultrasound 236, 266
Abdominal wall myofacial pain 218
Abduction 55, 199f
Abiraterone 481
Abortive therapy 129
Abuse
  alcohol 46, 169
  drug 53, 498
Acetaminophen 38, 192, 389
Acetylsalicylic acid 37, 38
Achilles reflexes 54
Achilles tendon 414f
Acid-base status 38
Acyclovir 379
Adenocarcinoma 274
Adenomyosis 98, 218, 272
Adenosine
  diphosphate 409
  triphosphate 409
Adhesions 218, 234
Adnexal cysts 218
Adventitial cystic disease 309
Afatinib 481
Aflibercept 482
Alectinib 481
Alemtuzumab 481
Alien face 69, 70f
Alitretinoin 482
Allergic dermatitis 224
Allodynia 20
Alteplase 314
Aluminum toxicity 403
Amitriptyline 461
Amputation 368
Anal fissures 218
Analgesia, patient-controlled 245, 259
Analgesics 266
Anaplastic thyroid cancer 480
Anderson's lesion 89
Androgen-dependent prostate cancer 480
Abdominal
  angina 234t
  aortic aneurysm 167b
Ankle-brachial index 312, 316
Ankylosed spine, fracture of 89
Ankylosing spondylitis 67f, 167, 170, 202
Ankylosis 89
Anorectal pain 218
Anorectal pain syndromes 225
Anorexia 29
Anticoagulation therapy 405
Anticonvulsants 167, 228, 336
Antidepressant 328, 460, 479
  drugs 389
Antiepileptic
  agents 30
  drug 32t, 389
Antinuclear antibody profile 200
Antispasmodics 266
Anti-VEGF therapy 494
Antiviral treatments 378, 495
Anxiety 127, 234, 265, 465
Anxiolytics 335
Aortic coarctation 309
Arm extension, bilateral 444f
Arnold nerve infiltration 71
Arterial
  dissection 309
  embolism 309
  fibrodysplasia 309
  occlusive disease peripheral 309
  thrombosis 309
  tumors 309
Arthritis 64f, 199, 387
  of apophyseal 89
  reactive 167
Articular process
  inferior 65f
  superior 65f
Atezolizumab 481
Atlantoaxial joint 62f, 158
Atlanto-occipital joints 158
Auscultation 266
Axitinib 481
Anterior cervical diskectomy and fusion 160
Anterior labial nerve 343

B

Babinski's reflex 54
Bacillus calmette guerin 274
Back pain
  chronic low 172
  low 52, 53, 85, 164, 187, 218, 234, 324
Bacterial prostatitis
  acute 220
  chronic 220
Balanitis 218
Balloon compression 138, 143
Balloon microcompression 136-138, 140
Basal cell carcinoma 482
Behçet's disease 224
Belinostat 481
Bevacizumab 481, 482
Bexarotene 481
Biocellular chemistry 408
Bipolar personality disorder 218
Bisphosphonates 111, 404
Bladder
  cancer 480, 481
  dysfunction 192
  neoplasm 218
Bladder pain syndrome 222, 223f
Blinatumomab 481
Blood
  investigation 397
  tests 148, 266
Bone
  disease 167

marrow
  density 167
  pathologies 94
mass 113
mineral density 109, 110
  normal 113f
morphology 66
scan 83, 387
scintigraphy 362
tumors, primary 167
Bony tumors of pelvis 274
Bortezomib 481
Bosutinib 481
Botulinum toxin 136, 250, 328
Brachial
  plexopathy 255
  plexus
    infiltration 259f
    neuralgia 149
Brachytherapy 473, 477
Brain tumor 481
Breakthrough pain 245, 250
Breast 478
  cancer 248, 481
  carcinoma 67f, 480
  surgery 10
Brentuximab 481
Buprenorphine 35
Bupropion 32, 33
Burger's disease 309
Butorphanol 35

C

Cabozantinib 481
Caffeine 250
Calciphylactic lesions 402f
Calciphylaxis 400
  causes and association 403t
  clinical features 401
  diagnosis 401
  epidemiology 401
  pathogenesis of 401
  treatment 403
Calcitonin 109, 111, 250
Calculi 234
Cancer 22, 168
  directed systemic
    therapies 484
  pain 239, 473, 478
    causes of 478, 480t
    etiology of 485

management of 478, 481-483
management 478
prevalence 480t
treatment for 478
types of 478
related pain 241, 485
surgical palliation for 485
Carbamazepine 31, 32, 397, 398
Carcinoma in situ 270
Cardiovascular
  disease 316
  exercise 445
Carfilzomib 481
Caroticocavernous fistula 144
Carotid artery puncture 144
Carotid-cavernous fistula 497
Catechol-O-methyltransferase 11
Caudal epidural
  injection 391
Cavernous hemangioma 497
Celiac
  ganglia 71
  neurolysis 80f
  plexus 267f
    needle position 267f
Cell carcinoma, transitional 480
Cell lung cancer 480
Central canal stenosis 180
Central nervous system 359
Central nucleus, degeneration
  of 83
Cerebrospinal fluid 73, 333, 347, 380
  examination 127
Ceritinib 481
Cervical
  cancer 481
  diskogenic pain 157
  diskography 159, 159f, 160
  epidural steroid injection 150
  exercises 444
  extensor muscles 445f
  facet joint 158
  pain 152
  lordosis 44f
  malignancies 98
  myelopathy 46
  nerve root 49f
  nucleoplasty wand 150f
  pain 121
  polyps 218

radiculopathy 146, 146f
pain 146
root injections 72, 73f
selective sensory
  neurolysis 259f
spine 43, 45f, 61, 62f, 70f, 71, 88, 431f, 435f
  lateral projection 62f
  normal X-ray 61f
  neuromusculoskeletal
    examination of 47
stenosis 218
traction 150
vascular disorder 125
Cetuximab 481, 482
Chemical neuromodulatory
  therapies 379
Chemotherapy 243, 245, 249
  on cancer pain, effect of 479
Chlamydial endometritis 218
Cholecystectomy 10
Chondrosarcoma 274
Chordoma 167
Chronic pain 13, 19, 20, 22, 459, 460
  causes of 492
  management of 27, 448, 459, 476
  medications 30
  syndromes 365
Citalopram 33, 461
Claudication 314, 315
Clitorial pain 218
Clomipramine 461
Clonazepam 397, 398
Cluster headache 76, 129
Cobimetinib 482
Coccydynia 275
Coccygeal nerve block 206
Coccygeoplasty 206
Coccygodynia 204, 207, 218, 227
Coccyx 204
Codeine 34
Coeliac ganglia neurolysis 78
Cognitive behavioral therapy 335, 467
Colitis 218
Colon, carcinoma of 218
Colorectal cancer 480, 482
Complete blood count 127
Complex regional pain
  syndrome 22, 359

Compression
  acute 92f, 104
  chronic 92f, 104, 234
Condyloma 273
Congenital seminal vesicle
  obstruction 218
Constipation 218, 265
Corneal ulceration 144
Cortical bone 109
Corticosteroid 129, 415
  therapy 495
Costovertebral joint 71, 89
Crane neck, posture correction
  of 327f
Cranial neuralgias 125
C-reactive protein 200, 236
Cremasteric muscle 342
Critical limb ischemia 315
Crizotinib 481
Crohn's disease 224
Cryotherapy 451, 451f
Cutaneous nerve entrapment,
  abdominal 218
Cystitis
  acute 218
  radiation 218
Cystoscopy 222
Cytotoxic chemotherapy 479
Chronic obstructive pulmonary
  disease 316

D

Dabrafenib 482
Daratumumab 481
Dasatinib 481
Degenerative disk disease 187
Delusional disorder 464, 466
Denileukin diftitox 481
Denosumab 482
Depression 218, 234, 265, 464,
  466
Dermatofibrosarcoma
  drotuberans 482
Dermatomes, abdominal 329f
Desvenlafaxine 461
Detrusor-sphincter
  dyssynergia 218
Dextrose prolotherapy 206
Diabetes 46, 312, 316
  mellitus 396, 400
Diabetic neuropathy 22

Diaphragmatic pain 255
Diarrhea, transient 268
Diathermy, short-wave 450, 450f
Dihydroergotmine 129
Dinutuximab 482
Diplopia 32
Diskogenic pain 164,165, 166, 201
Disk 218
  height 68
  herniation 88f
  location of 86f
Diskitis 89, 167
Diverticular disease 218
Diverticulitis 234
Dizziness 32
Dopamine 397
Doxepin 461
Ductal obstruction 98f
Duloxetine 32, 461
Duodenal tumor 264f
Dysmenorrhea, atypical 218
Dyspareunia 466
Dysthymia 466
Dysthymic disorder 464
Degenerative spinal disease 83

E

Eating disorders 234
Ectopic pregnancy, chronic 218
Elbow
  extension 147
  flexion 147
  joints 50
Electromyography 106, 148
Electroneuromyography 100, 105
  limitations of 105
  tests 101
Elotuzumab 481
Embryonic stem cells 409
Endometrial
  carcinoma 480
  malignancies 98
  polyps 218
Endometriosis 98, 218, 234, 272
Endometritis, chronic 218
Endometrium 98f
  cancer 273
Endosalpingiosis 218
Endothelial nitric oxide 367
Enteropathic arthritis 167
Enzalutamide 481

Enzyme-linked immunosorbent
  assay 412
Epicondylitis, lateral 324
Epidermal growth factor 409
Epididymitis 218
Epidural
  abscess 167
  drug delivery system 276
  nerve block 276
  neurolysis 278
  neurolytic block 278
  neuroplasty 391
Epiduroscopy 391
Epinephrine inhibitor 32
Episcleritis 378f
Epithelial growth factor 195
Ergot toxicity 310
Erlotinib 481
Erogtamine tartrate 129
Erythrocyte sedimentation
  rate 127, 200, 236
Escitalopram 461
Esophageal carcinoma 480
Estrogen 109, 111
Everolimus 481
Ewing's sarcoma 274
Extra-pyramidal syndrome 397

F

Faber's test 54, 55, 55f, 199, 199f
Facet
  blocks 390
  cyst, puncture of 75f
  injection 73f
  joint 68, 71, 85, 164f, 173
    arthritis 68f
    normal 86f
    pain 45f, 164-166, 383
    subluxation of 87f
    synovial cyst 87f
  mediated pain 173
Facial nerve palsy 144
Facial pain 125
  central causes of 125
  primary 125
Fallopian tube 481
Famcyclovir 379
Familial mediterranean fever 218
Fascia 158, 342
Fear-avoidance model of chronic
  pain 465f

Female genitilia 218
Femoropopliteal artery stenosis 316
Fibroblast growth factor 409
Fibroid 234
 of uterus 167
Fibromyalgia 22, 332, 334, 335
 cause of 333
 syndrome 11
Fibromyositis 218
Fibrosis 208
 radiation 310
Fibrous joint 65
Finger
 extension 147
 flexion 147
 test 199
Flexion 55, 199f, 209, 209f
 coccygodynia 205f
Fluid cleft 92f
Fluoroscopic technique 496
Fluoroscopy 267f
 guided piriformis injection technique 210
Fluorosis 167
Fluoxetine 33, 461
Fluvoxamine 33, 461
Focal
 back pain 163, 166, 168-170
 bone lesion 68f
 low back pain 163, 170
Foramen ovale 76f, 138f, 139f
Foraminal compression test 147
Foraminal stenosis 383
Fortin finger test 385f
Fracture 167
 line 90
Full blood
 count 236
 picture 200
F-waves 104

G

Gabapentin 30, 32, 363, 397, 398
Gabapentinoids 16
Gaenslen's test 54, 55, 199, 200f
Gallbladder disease 167
Gamma-aminobutyric acid 32
Gasserian ganglion 137, 140, 144
 radiofrequency thermo-coagulation of 136, 138
Gastric carcinoma 480
Gastrointestinal stromal tumors 480, 482
Gastrointestinal systems 466
Gate control theory 4
Gefitinib 481
Genital prolapse 218
Genitofemoral nerve 218, 342
 blocks 229
Genitourinary 478
Giant cell tumor of bone 482
Gingival hyperplasia 32
Glaucoma, acute 492
Glycerol injection 136, 138, 143
Golfer bow lifting technique 436f
Graft-versus-host disease 407
Growth factor, transforming 409
Gynecological diseases 98
Greater occipital nerve 71

H

Hairy cell leukemia 480
Head and neck 478
 cancer 241, 242, 481
  pain management 241
 carcinoma 480
Headache 11, 22, 123, 125
 disorders, primary 124
 primary 125, 128
 types of 125
Heel ulcer 107f
Hemangioma 66, 167
Hematoma 210
Hemopoietic stem cells 408
Heparin 167, 314
Hepatocellular carcinoma 97f
Hepatocyte growth factor 409
Hernias 218
Herniation 56
Herniorrhaphy 13
Herpes simplex 144, 273
Herpes zoster 149
Hip 10, 111
 hinge 429f, 430f
 mediated pain 56
Hodgkin's disease 480
Hoffman signs 148
Homeostasis, disorder of 125
Hormonal therapy 480, 482
Hormone replacement therapy 224
Horner's syndrome 77
Human leukocyte antigen 200, 408
Human papillomavirus 273
Hydrated nucleus
 pulposus 84f
Hydrocodone 34
Hyperalgesia 20
Hyperbaric oxygen therapy 367, 404
Hypercalcemia 403
Hyperlordosis 208
Hyperparathyroidism 167, 403
Hyperphosphatemia 403
Hyperreflexia 148
Hypertonia 148
Hypertrophy 208
Hypnosis 468
Hypogastric plexus block 277f
 superior 229, 237, 275, 276

I

Ibritumomab tiuxetan 481
Ibrutinib 481
Ibuprofen 38
Idelalisib 481
Idiopathic intracranial hypertension 130
Iliohypo-gastric nerve, neuroanatomy of 343
Ilioinguinal nerve, neuroanatomy of 342
Iliopsoas
 bursa 212f
 injection 212f
  procedure 211
 bursitis 211
 injection technique 211
 muscle 212f
Iliopsoas pain syndromes 208
Iliopsoas syndrome 211
Iliopsoas tendon injection procedure 212
Imatinib 481, 482
Imipramine 461
Implantable pulse generator 392
Infection 210
Inflammatory arthritis 202

Inflammatory bowel disease 218, 234
Inflammatory spondyloarthritis 89
Inflammatory spondyloarthropathy 67f
Inguinal
  canal 342
  nerves 344f
  pain
    chronic
      postoperative 341
      postsurgical 345
Inguinodynia, syndrome of 345
Insomnia 29, 265
Intermittent bowel obstruction, chronic 218
International Classification of Headache Disorders 124t, 133
Interstitial cystitis 218, 222, 223f, 224, 234
Interventional pain
  management 246
  treatment procedures 71
Intra-articular gas 68
Intracranial
  hemorrhage 130, 144
  pressure 130
Intradiskal
  electrothermal therapy 166, 194
  biacuplasty 194
  platelet-rich plasma 415f
Intrathecal
  drug delivery system 393, 393f
  pumps 360
Intrauterine
  contraceptive device 218
  devise 234
Iontophoresis 452
Iron
  dextran infusion 403
  sulfate 397, 398
Irritable bladder 11
Irritable bowel 234
  syndrome 11, 218
Ischemic pain 307
Ischial spine 218
Ivory vertebra 67f
Ixazomib 481

J

Joint
  disease, degenerative 218
  peripheral 50
  space 64f

K

Kaposi sarcoma 482
Keratitis 379f
Ketamine 16, 228, 328, 369
Kidney
  cancer 481
  disease, chronic 401
  failure 396
  function test 266
  tumor 265f
Knee 148
  joint, X-ray of 110f

L

Lanreotide acetate 482
Laparoscopic hernia repair 10
Lapatinib 481
Laser therapy 453f
Leg pain 311
Leg syndrome, causes of restless 396t
Leiomyomata 218
Lenvatinib 481
Leukemia 481
Levator ani syndrome 218, 225
Ligament
  defect, broad 234
  posterior longitudinal 89f
Ligamentum flavum, hypertrophy of 88f
Lignocaine infusion 336
Limb
  amputation 10
  ischemia
    acute 310, 311, 313
    chronic severe 315
  revascularization 405
  types of missing 373f
Lithium carbonate 129
Liver
  cancer 475, 481
  capsular pain 255
  mass 265f
  posterior segment of 97f

Lorazepam 369
Low back pain, nonmechanical causes of 167
Lower extremity functional scale 449
Lpilimumab 482
Lucilia sericata 405
Lumbar disk pain 187
  diskogenic back pain 187
  epidural injection 72, 73f
  facet joint 172
    injections 73
    nerve 176
    pain syndrome 172
  nerves, radiofrequency ablation of 177
  lordosis 429f
  pain 52
  periradicular injection 73
  plexus 71
    needle position 367f
    neurolysis 79
    spread of dye 366f
  spinal stenosis 180, 181
  spine 52, 63, 71, 83, 165
    lateral projection 66f
    normal X-ray 65f
    severe degeneration of 68f
  spondylolysis test infiltration 73
  sympathectomy 317
  sympathetic block 275
    bilateral 229
  synovial cyst infiltration 74
  vertebrae, compression of 218
Lumbosacral spine 110f
Lung
  cancer 481
  carcinoma 252
  parenchyma 255
  primary cancer of 252
Lutetium-Dotatate therapy 475
Lymphocytic leukemia, acute 480
Lymphoma 167, 481, 497

M

Magnetic resonance cholangio-pancreatography 97
Male genitilia 218
Mastectomy 13

Meckel's cave 142
Median branch blocks 165
Median motor conduction technique 102f
Medication overuse headache 130
Melanoma 482
  malignant 480
Meningioma 497
Meningitis 130, 144
Mesenchymal stem cells 415f
Mesenteric tumor 486f
Meshoma 342
Mesothelioma 255, 480
Metabolic diseases 199
Metastasis, typical appearance of 70f
Metastatic
  bone pain 473
    management 473
  tumors 167
    neuroblastoma 476
      treatment of 477f
    prostate cancer 474
Methadone 35
Methysergide 129
Microvascular decompression 132, 136
Migraine 11, 124, 128, 128t, 324
  abdominal 218
  pharmacotherapy of 129t
  triggers 127t
Mirror box manipulation 374
Monoamine oxidase inhibitors 462
Morphine 34
Motion palpation tests 199
Motor nerve conduction 102
Motor unit action potential 102, 103
Mucopurulent conjunctivitis 378f
Multiple myeloma 94f, 164, 167, 480, 481
Muscle 158
  abdominal 440
  anomalies 208
  atrophy 311
  contraction 432f
  re-education 439
  relaxants 327, 336, 389
  structure 324f
  weakness 147
Muscular
  sprains 218
  strains 218
Musculoskeletal pain, chronic 448
Myasthenia gravis 30
Myelogenous leukemia, chronic 480
Myeloid leukemia, acute 480
Myeloproliferative disorders 482
Myofascial pain 234, 321, 323, 325
  management of 323
  syndrome 201, 324, 354
  treatment of 327
Myofascial trigger point 324, 235
Myositis ossificans 208
Myotomes 50

N

Naltrexone, low dose 363, 370
Naproxen 38
Narcotic medications 379
Nausea 32, 265
Necitumumab 481
Neck
  disability index 425
  distraction test 148
  flexors, deep 445f
  pain 44, 104, 121, 436
    chronic 152
Needle electromyography 103f
Nerve
  block, peripheral 276
  conduction studies 101, 105, 182
  injury 12
  lesions 342
  peripheral 476
  root 147, 183f
    block 149
    compression, acute 104
    compression, chronic 104
    inflammation 384f
    pain 153
    stimulation, dorsal 347
Nerve entrapment syndrome 354
Neural elements 45f
Neuroblastoma 482
Neurocentral joint 63f
Neuroendocrine tumors 482
Neurologic dysfunction 218
Neurolysis 71, 81f
Neuroma formation 354
Neuromuscular electrical stimulation 451
Neuropathic causes, infective and 495
Neuropathic pain 311, 342, 355, 383, 459
Neuropathy, peripheral 396
Neutral spine 428
Nilotinib 481, 482
Nimotuzumab 481
Nitrazepam 397, 398
Nivolumab 481, 482
N-methyl-d-aspartate 4
  antagonists 228
Nociceptive pain 20, 459
  acute 19
Nonhealing necrotic ulcer over leg 402f
Nonhealing wound 311
Non-Hodgkin's lymphoma 480
Nonmetastatic cancer 485
Nonsteroidal anti-inflammatory drugs 5, 15, 37, 75, 129, 168, 184, 192, 209, 327, 415, 479
Nonvascular intracranial disorder 125
Nonviable limb 314
Noradrenaline reuptake inhibitors 335
Nortriptyline 461
Nucleoplasty 71, 79, 150
Nummular headache 125

O

Obinutuzumab 481
Occipital neuralgia 71
Ocular complications 495
Ofatumumab 481
Olaparib 481
Olaratumab 482
Opacification 81f
Ophthalmic complications, treatment of 495
Ophthalmic nerve 135
Ophthalmic pain, management of 491
Opiates 5
Opioid 5, 33, 228, 479

agonist 34
system 396
Oral
  mucositis 245
  transmucosal fentanyl
    citrate 250
Orchialgia 218, 221
Orthostatic hypotension 268
Osimertinib 481
Osteoarthritis
  hip joint pain 201
  of apophyseal joint 85
Osteoblastoma 167
Osteoblasts 109
Osteoclasts 109
Osteocytes 109
Osteogenic sarcoma 480
Osteoma 167
Osteomalacia 167
Osteopenia 114f, 115f
Osteophytic disease 63f
Osteophytosis 68
Osteoporosis 64f, 110f, 116f-118f, 166, 167
  monitoring of 111
Osteoporotic compression, benign 92f
Ovarian
  carcinoma 480
  dystrophy 218
  pathologies 98
Ovarian remnant syndrome 218, 234
Ovulatory pain 218
Oxycodone 34, 335, 397, 398
Oxymorphone 35

P

Paget's disease 66, 67f, 167
Pain 3, 45, 164, 242, 243, 249, 275, 464, 465, 476
  acuity of 36
  acute 6, 8, 459
  distribution of 45
  intensity 36
  interventions 390
  management 3, 405
    strategies 249
  pharmacological management of 245
  prevalence of 242
  psychology 463
  quality of 385
  radicular 153
  radiotherapy induced 245
  relief 317
    mechanism of 473
  symptoms 43
  syndrome, postsurgical 10t
  to cancer, relation of 479
  Z-joint 201
Painful ischemic necrosis 401
Palbociclib 481
Palliative surgery, selection for 486
Pancoast's tumor 149, 253, 255
Pancreatic cancer 481
Pancreatic carcinoma 480t
Pancreatic tumor 264f
Pancreatitis 167
  chronic 98f
Panitumumab 482
Panobinostat 481
Paraspinal muscle
  electromyography 102
Paraspinal soft tissue mass, large 69f
Parathyroid hormone 109, 111
Paroxetine 33, 461
Pars interarticularis 65f
Patellar tendon, pathological 416f
Patrick's test 199, 199f
Pazopanib 481, 482
Pelvic
  congestion 234
  syndrome 218
  inflammatory disease 167, 234
  pain 215, 270
    chronic 219f, 233, 234, 234t
    chronic nonmalignant 233
    malignant 270
    management of 275, 276t
    relief of 275
    syndrome, chronic 217, 220
  tumors 167
Pembrolizumab 481
Percutaneous cervical
  cordotomy 260f
Percutaneous laser disk
  decompression 81f
Percutaneous transluminal
  angioplasty 315
Performance status 480
Perineal numbness 192
Peripheral neuropathy,
  chemotherapy-induced 252
Periradicular infiltration 71
Peritoneal cancers, primary 481
Peritoneal cysts,
  postoperative 218
Pertuzumab 481
Pethidine 34
Phantom limb pain 372-374
  causes 373
  signs 372
  symptoms 372
  treatment 374
Phenytoin 31, 32
Physical therapy 437
Physiotherapy 421, 448
Piriformis 208
  muscle 210f
  syndrome 208, 218
Piriformis pain syndrome 201
Plasma protein
  electrophoresis 200
Plasmacytoma 94f
Platelet-derived growth
  factor 195
Platelet-rich plasma
  injection 195
Pleural mesothelioma 254f, 260f
Plexus nerve block 276
Ponatinib 481
Popliteal
  artery entrapment 310
  emboli 316
Porphyria 218
Positron emission
  tomography 254
Posthernioplasty pain 344f
Post-herniorrhaphy pain 341
Postherpetic neuralgia 377
  signs 377
  symptoms 377
  treatment of 496
  options 378
Post-irradiation pain 252
Post-laminectomy pain 383
  etiology 383
  examination 385
  investigations 386
  management 388
Post-pleurodesis pain 255

Postsurgical pain, chronic 10, 11, 13, 344
Post-thoracotomy pain 252, 254, 257f, 353
  syndrome 353
    treatment of 355
Pralatrexate 481
Pregabalin 397, 398
Pregnancy 111
Proctalgia fugax 218, 225
Proinflammatory proteins 360
Prone heel squeeze 442f
Propoxyphene 35, 397, 398
Prostadynia 218, 220, 234
Prostate 478
  cancer 274, 474, 474f, 481
  pain, chronic 220, 221f
  specific antigen 200, 274, 474f
  specific membrane scan 474f
  transurethral needle ablation of 221
Prostatitis 218, 220
  chronic 220
Proton pump inhibitor 255
Pseudo Arnold's neuralgia 72
Pseudoarthrosis 383
Pseudotumor cerebri 130
Psoas muscle 211, 344f
Psoriatic arthritis 167, 202
Psychiatric disorder 125
Psychotherapy 365, 457, 462
Pterygoid plate 77f
Pterygopalatine ganglion 76
Pudendal nerve
  block 229, 276
  entrapment 218, 226
Pudendal neuralgia 226

R

Radiation therapy 249
Radical cystectomy 274
Radiofrequency ablation 391, 415
Radium alpha radiation therapy 474
Ramucirumab 481, 482
Raphe nucleus magnus 23
Raynaud's syndrome 11
Red flag symptoms 45, 53, 147
Reflexive contraction, abdominal 426f

Regenerative injection 416f
Regional anesthesia 16
Regorafenib 482
Reiter's syndrome 202
Relaxation techniques 334
Renal
  cell carcinoma 480
  disease 167, 310
    end-stage 400
  failure, chronic 403
  insufficiency 192
Restless leg syndrome 395-397
  causes 395
  signs 396
  symptoms 396
  treatment protocol 397
Retrobulbar hemorrhage 144
Retroperitoneal fibrosis 310
Rheumatoid
  arthritis 62f, 167, 211, 396
  factor 200
Rhizotomy 177
Rib 255
  fractures 254
  metastasis 254
Rituximab 481
Romanus lesions 89
Romberg's maneuver 182
Romidepsin 481
Root lesions, multiple 105
Rotator cuff, disorders of 149
Royal College of Radiologists Guidelines 61
Rutherford categories 310
Ruxolitinib 482

S

Sacral
  foramen 201f
  foraminal nerve block 276
  nerve 218
    root block 277
    neuromodulation 229
    tumor 271f
Sacroiliac joint 65, 66f, 71, 75f, 198
  anatomy of 198f
  dysfunction 56
  injection 74, 391, 391f
  mediated pain 385f
  pain 164-166, 218

  syndrome 198
  syndrome, causes of 199
  acute 74
  chronic 74
Sacroiliac syndrome 209
Sacroilitis 167
Saddle block 278
Salicylate 37, 38
Salpingitis 218
Sarcoma 480
Scapula 255
Schmorl's node 90
Sciatic nerve palsy 210
Sclerosis, multiple 22, 134f, 144
Scottish terrier' dog appearance of vertebral body 65f
Scrotal nerve, anterior 343
Scrotal pain 222f
Secondary headache 130
  disorders 125
Sensory nerve
  action potential 101
  pain 415
Serotonin noradrenaline reuptake inhibitors 33
Serotonin receptor antagonists 336
Serotonin reuptake
  inhibitor 29, 33, 335, 336, 461
  transporter 461
Serotonin-norepinephrine reuptake inhibitors 460
Sertraline 461
Shocks 106
Shoulder
  abduction 147
  abduction test 148
  external rotation 444f
  joints 50
Sickle cell disease 167
Siltuximab 481
Sinusitis-associated headache 130
Sjögren's syndrome 224
Sleep
  disturbances 218
  studies 397
Small cell lung carcinoma 480
Sodium
  channel blockade 228
  thiosulfate 404

valproate 29
Soft tissue 69
  injury 167
  mass 91f
  sarcoma 482
Solitary sclerotic vertebra 67f
Somatic
  nerve block 276
  symptom disorder 463
Sorafenib 481
Soy isoflavones 251
Specific orbital tumors 497
Sphenopalatine ganglia 71, 76
Sphinx test 55, 55f
Spinal
  abscess, postoperative 96f
  canal stenosis 65f
  cord 13, 183f
    injury 22
    neoplasia of 218
    stimulation 206, 318, 319, 368, 392, 393
  dorsal root ganglion 73
  fixators 255f, 259f
  infection 93f, 94, 95f
  limitations 426t
  pain 423, 437
    causes of 424
    postoperative 95
  tumors 89
Spine
  functional motion of 427f
  infection of 169
  palpation of 48
  radiological anatomy of 61
Spinocerebellar ataxia 396
Spinothalamic tract 23
Splanchnic
  nerve 71
  neurolysis 77
  plexus 267f
Spondyloarthropathies 199
Spondylolisthesis 56, 66f
Spondylolysis 65f, 71
Spondylolytic defect 74f
Spondylosis 218
Spurling test 147
Squamous cell carcinoma 274
Squat lifting technique 435f
Stellate ganglion
  block 366f

neurolysis 77
Stem cells 409, 412
Sterile arachnoiditis, chronic 96
Sterile maggot therapy 405
Sternum 255
Steroids 167, 389, 404
Stevens-Johnson syndrome 30, 32
Stone 218
Stress 127
Stump neuromas 375
Subacute salpingo-oophoritis 218
Subarachnoid block 276
Subchondral sclerosis 68
  of sacroiliac joints 66
Subcostal nerve 342
Subcutaneous implantable pulse generator 392f
Subluxation 207
Sunitinib 481, 482
Sural sensory
  conduction technique 101f
  nerve action potential 102f
Surgery 150, 221, 249
  role of 244
Surgical palliation, indications for 486
Sympathetic
  nerve block 365, 375
  pain 149
Symphysis pubis
  dysfunction 218
Syndesmophytes 89, 170
Synovial facet cyst 74
Systemic lupus
  erythematosus 224
Systemic mastocytosis 482

T

Takayasu arteritis 309
Temporal arteritis 309
Temporary paraplegia 268
Temporomandibular joints 50
Temsirolimus 481
Tendonitis 211
Tension-type headache 124, 126, 129, 324
Testicular
  pain 221, 234
  tumors 274
Tetrahydrocannabinol 250

Tetrodotoxin 250
Therapeutic drug monitoring 27
Thoracic dermatome 377f
Thoracic outlet
  obstruction 309
  syndrome 149
Thoracic spine 63, 71
  lower 67f
Thoracolumbar region 63
Thoracolumbar spine lateral spine 64f
Thoracotomy 10, 13
Thumb nail blanches 333
Thyroid cancer 476, 481
Tiagabine 32
Tolerance 463
Total knee arthroplasty 16
Tramadol 327, 389, 397, 398
Trametinib 482
Transcutaneous electrical nerve stimulation 375, 452
Transforaminal epidural
  injection 390, 390f
  steroid 150
Trastuzumab 481
  emtansine 481
Trauma 309
Tretinoin 481
Triazolam 397, 398
Tricyclic antidepressants 32, 192, 228, 461
Trigeminal autonomic
  cephalalgias 124
Trigeminal ganglia
  neurolysis 75
Trigeminal glycerol injection 137, 142, 143f
Trigeminal nerve 71, 76f
Trigeminal neuralgia 132, 133, 136, 144
  classification of 133
Trigeminoautonomic
  cephalgias 129
Tubercular
  infection 93f
  spondylitis 91f
Tuberculous salpingitis 218
Tumor 249
  abdominal 167
  marker 168
  necrosis factor 14, 243

U

Ultrasound therapy 451f
Uncovertebral joint 63f
Urethral diverticulum 218
Urethral pain syndrome 224, 225f
Urethral syndrome 218, 224, 234
Urethritis, acute 218
Urinary tract infection,
    chronic 218, 234
Urine tests 266
Urogenital pain 218, 227, 229t
    chronic 217
    management,
        nonmalignant 217
Urokinase 314
Urolithiasis 218
Urothelial tract 480
Uterine 478
    leiomyoma 272
Uveitis 492

V

Valacyclovir 379
Vandetanib 481
Vascular
    calcification 403
    endothelial growth factor 409, 492
    malformations 167
Vasculitis 167
Vasospasm 309
Vemurafenib 482
Venetoclax 481
Venlafaxine 32, 33, 461
Verapamil 129
Vertebral body
    collapse 89
        causes of 90t
    end-plate of 68
    fracture 165, 166
    metastasis 258f
    multiple 94f
    posterior part of 92f
Vertebral
    fracture 111, 164
    osteomyelitis 167
    tumor, large 94f
Vertebral end-plate sclerosis 68f
Vertebroplasty 71, 81, 82f
Vigabatrin 32
Vincristine legs 271f
Vismodegib, sonidegib 482
Visual analog scale 414, 450
Vitamin D 109
Vorinostat 481
Vulvar condyloma 273
Vulvar pain syndrome 224
Vulvar vestibulitis syndrome 218
Vulvodynia 218, 224

W

Waddell signs 386
Winking eye 70, 70f
Wrist
    extension 147
    flexion 147

Z

Zoledronic acid 483
Zostavax 381